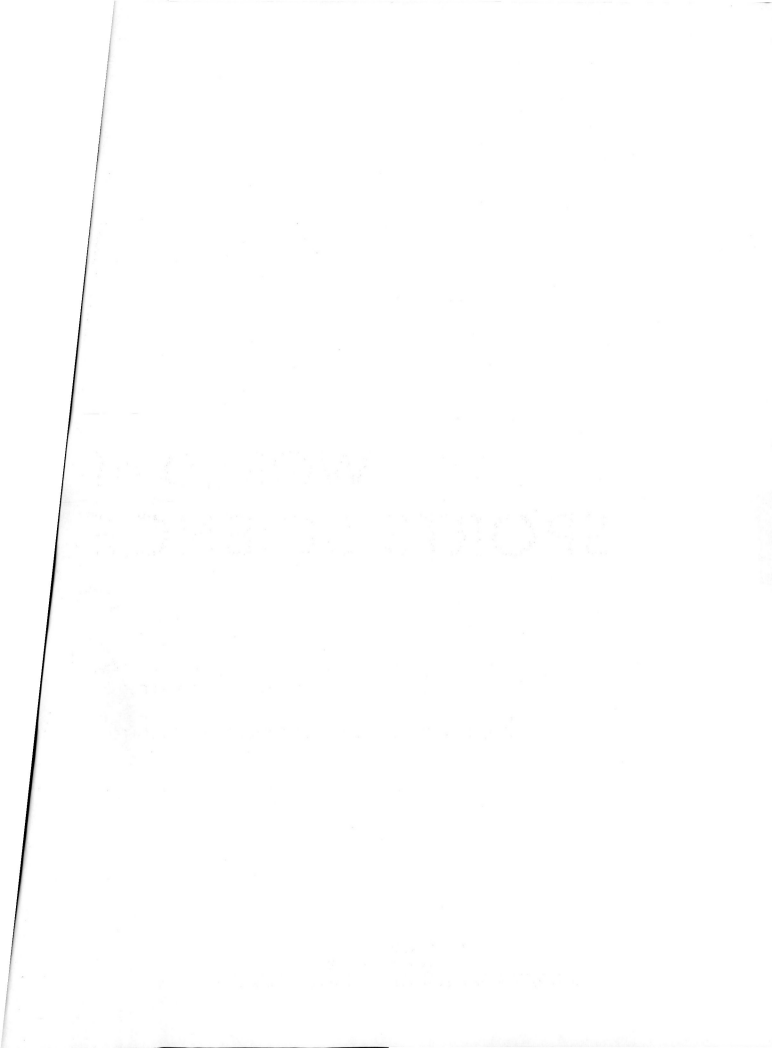

WORLD
SPORTS SCIENCE

# WORLD of
# SPORTS SCIENCE

VOLUME **2**
## M-Z

### GENERAL INDEX

K. Lee Lerner and Brenda Wilmoth Lerner, EDITORS

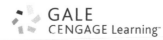

GALE
CENGAGE Learning

Detroit • New York • San Francisco • New Haven, Conn • Waterville, Maine • London

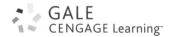

# World of Sports Science

K. Lee Lerner and Brenda Wilmoth Lerner, Editors

**Project Editor**
Kimberley A. McGrath

**Editorial**
Madeline Harris, Kristine Krapp, Paul Lewon,
Elizabeth Manar

**Editorial Support Services**
Andrea Lopeman

**Indexing**
Factiva, a Dow Jones & Reuters Company

**Rights and Acquisitions**
Margaret Abendroth, Kim Smilay

**Imaging and Multimedia**
Lezlie Light, Kelly Quin

**Product Design**
Tracey Rowens

**Composition**
Evi Seoud, Mary Beth Trimper

**Manufacturing**
Wendy Blurton, Dorothy Maki

LIBRARY OF CONGRESS CATALOGING-IN-PUBLICATION DATA

World of sports science / K. Lee Lerner and Brenda Wilmoth Lerner, editors.
    p. cm.
    Includes bibliographical references and index.
    ISBN-13: 978-1-4144-0614-5 (set hardcover : alk. paper)
    ISBN-10: 1-4144-0614-2 (set hardcover : alk. paper)
    ISBN-13: 978-1-4144-0615-2 (vol. 1 : alk. paper)
    ISBN-10: 1-4144-0615-0 (vol. 1 : alk. paper)
    [etc.]
    1. Sports medicine–Encyclopedias - 2.  Sports sciences–Encyclopedias. - I.  Lerner,
K. Lee. - II.  Lerner, Brenda Wilmoth.

    RC1206.W672007
    617.1′02703–dc22                                                        2006013088

| ISBN-13: | ISBN-10: |
|---|---|
| 978-1-4144-0614-5 (set) | 1-4144-0614-2 (set) |
| 978-1-4144-0615-2 (v1) | 1-4144-0615-0 (vol. 1) |
| 978-1-4144-0616-9 (v2) | 1-4144-0616-9 (vol. 2) |

This title is also available as an e-book,
ISBN-13: 978-1-4144-0613-8, ISBN-10: 1-4144-0613-4
Contact your Gale sales representative for ordering information.

Printed in the United States of America
4 5 6 7 8 9 14 13 12 11 10 09

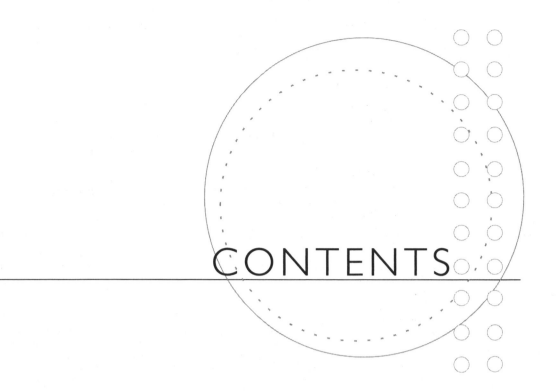

# CONTENTS

# ACKNOWLEDGMENTS

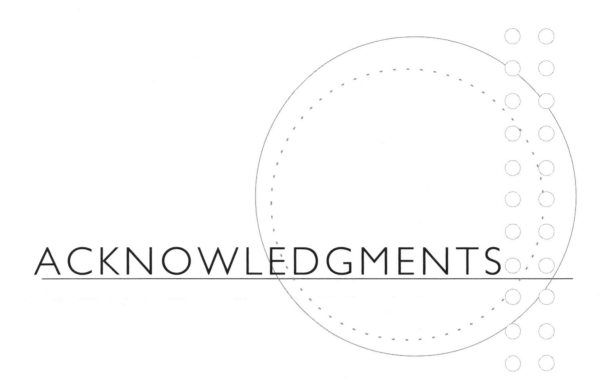

In compiling this edition, we have been fortunate in being able to rely upon the expertise and contributions of the following scholars who served as academic and contributing advisors for *World of Sports Science*, and to them we would like to express our sincere appreciation for their efforts to ensure that *World of Sports Science* contains the most accurate and timely information possible.

## Contributing Advisors

William Atkins, MS
Normal, Illinois

Bryan Davies, LLB
*Journalist (Sports Columnist) and Coach (Basketball)*
Whitby, Ontario, Canada

Antonio Farina, MD, PhD
University of Bologna
Bologna, Italy

Larry Gilman, PhD
Sharon, Vermont

Brian D. Hoyle, PhD
Nova Scotia, Canada

Peter Lonergan, MEd
*Director of Athletics and Head Coach, Women's Basketball*
Medaille College
Buffalo, New York

Bill Pangos, MPhysEd
*Sports Administrator and Head Coach, Women's Basketball*
York University
Toronto, Ontario, Canada

Alexandr Ioffe, PhD
Russian Academy of Sciences
Moscow, Russia

## Acknowledgments

The editors would like to extend thanks to Connie Clyde for her assistance in copyediting. The editors also wish to specially acknowledge Adrienne Wilmoth Lerner and Alica Marie Caferty for their diligent and extensive research on selected entries.

The editors gratefully acknowledge the assistance of many at Thompson Gale for their help in preparing *World of Sports Science*. The editors wish to specifically thank Carol Nagel and Debra Kirby for their help and advice in launching this project. Special thanks are also offered to Gale Senior Editor Kim McGrath for her timely, skilled, and gentle guidance through various project complexities.

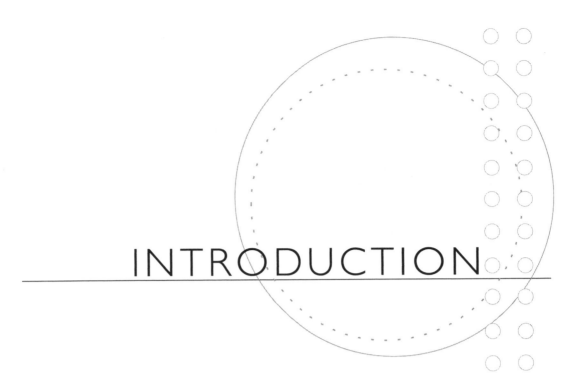

# INTRODUCTION

Sports offer both competition and a path to fitness. Accordingly, sports science has grown beyond the exclusive application of science toward improving competitive performance to applications that improve the quality of life and health. Sports and the advances in sports science have, however, increasing impact on broad segments of society—from advanced competitors wishing to enhance Olympic-caliber performance to those wishing modest improvement in the quality of their health and life through the practice of yoga or Pilates. Intended for high school-aged students and readers at the start of their studies of sports science, *World of Sports Science* is designed to be an interesting and useable introduction to the field.

Sports often captivate younger audiences, and *World of Sports Science* is specifically designed to allow younger students to relate fundamental terms and concepts taught in the science classroom to their often passionate pursuit of sports. In so doing the science becomes more relevant to their daily lives and, in turn, participation and capabilities in sport are enhanced by a greater understanding of issues related to exercise physiology, biomechanics, drug use, etc. The editors have not shied from the controversies in sport related to the use of performance-enhancing drugs and have taken special care to identify the dangers and ethical concerns related to such use. The controversy in the wake of the 2006 Tour de France, in which the winner Floyd Landis was reported to have tested positive for the use of a banned substance (testosterone, an anabolic steroid) took place after *World of*

*Sports Science* went to press. At the time of this writing, Landis proclaims his innocence and official action remains pending against Landis, who faces being stripped of his Tour title and a ban from professional cycling for two years. Such incidents are becoming increasingly common across the world of sport and although the editors can not forecast the news, *World of Sports Science* is designed to provide students and readers with resources and readings that enable them to more fully understand the complexities of such evolving news stories. For example, entries on the World Anti-Doping Agency, WADA director Richard Pound, the U.S. Anti-Doping Agency, and Court of Arbitration for Sport provide insight in to the agencies and processes used to investigate and enforce provisions against banned substances while entries on anabolic steroids, testosterone, cycling, and a specialized article on the Tour de France (Cycling: Tour de France) provide examples of entries offering essential background reading that empower critical thinking about events in the news.

*World of Sports Science* is a collection of nearly 600 entries that evidence the wide application of science to sport and that place special emphasis on the basic science related to introductory concepts related to muscular strength and endurance, cardiovascular efficiency, oxygen use, and the importance of flexibility—all critical elements of fitness and athletic performance. The science in this book is simplified so that the it offers straightforward but accurate descriptions of measurements of both general and specialized topics—ranging from entries related to anatomy, physiology, and kinesiology to more specialized treatments of injury prevention, nutrition, and the calculation of muscle to fat ratios.

In addition to students and a general readership, *World of Sports Science* is designed to be a valuable general reference for a range of specialized interests—from physical education teachers wishing to provide content-related readings that support their curriculum objectives to personal trainers wishing to give their clients fundamental reading material related to the changes in the body induced by exercise.

In an effort the enhance readability and interest, the editors include biographies of athletes and others involved in sport science, technology, and history who are more readily known to students and a general readership. This is not intended as insult to the thousands of men and women who skillfully labor to advance sports science, and who are due recognition in future volumes, but rather as a calculated attempt to capture student interest by, as exemplified in the entry on champion cyclist Lance Armstrong, relating athletic achievement to some aspect of sports science or technology.

The editors hope that *World Sports Science* serves to inspire students and readers to examine the linkage of science to sport, and encourages them toward further study.

K. Lee Lerner & Brenda Wilmoth Lerner
*Editors*
London, U.K.
July 2006

**How to Use the Book**

The articles in the book are meant to be understandable by anyone with a curiosity about the relation of science to sport. *World of Sports Science* carries specifically selected fundamental topics in genetics, anatomy, physiology, physics, etc., that provide a basis for understanding the application of science to sport.

This first edition of *World of Sports Science* has been designed with ready reference in mind:

- **Entries are arranged alphabetically**, rather than by chronology or scientific field.
- **"See also" references** at the end of entries alert the reader to related entries not specifically mentioned in the body of the text.
- The **Historical Chronology** includes many of the significant events in the advancement of sports science.
- A **Sources Consulted** section lists the most worthwhile print material and web sites we encountered in the compilation of this volume. It is there for the inspired reader who wants more information on the people and discoveries covered in this volume.
- A **comprehensive General Index** guides the reader to topics and persons mentioned in the book. Bolded page references refer the reader to the term's full entry.

A detailed understanding of biochemistry is neither assumed nor required for *World of Sports Science*. Accordingly, students and other readers should not be intimidated or deterred by the complex names of chemical molecules. Where necessary, sufficient information regarding chemical structure is provided. If desired, more information can easily be obtained from any basic chemistry or biochemistry reference.

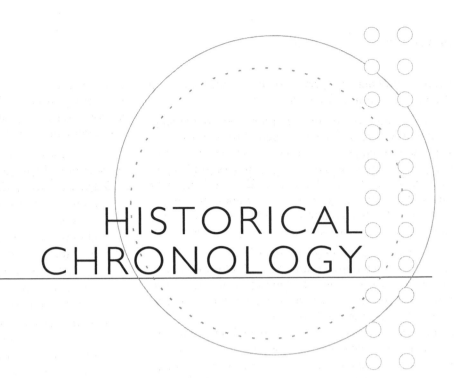

# HISTORICAL CHRONOLOGY

c. 5000    The first water craft are developed in various indigenous cultures throughout the world (canoes, kayaks, and wind-powered vessels).

c. 3500 BC    The traditional Indian holistic medicine practices known as Ayurveda are traced to this period, as is the practice of yoga.

c. 3000 BC    The oldest written references to traditional chinese medicine (TCM), including various herbal medicine techniques and acupuncture, are dated to this period.

c. 1000 BC    Baggataway, the forerunner to lacrosse, is first played by the indigenous peoples of North America during this period.

c. 1000 BC    The ancient Scottish highland sports, including the caber toss and putting the stone, originated with the clan gatherings of this period.

c. 800 BC    The Mayan peoples of southern Mexico participate in organized high diving from cliffs into the Pacific Ocean.

c. 776 BC    The first Olympic Games is held at Athens. The competitions are restricted to men only; the credo of the ancient Games, "Higher, Faster, Stronger," remains the inspiration of the modern Olympics.

c. 700 BC    The use of anatomical models is established in India.

490 BC    Phillipides, a messenger with the Greek army, dies after running from the site of the Battle of Marathon to the city of Athens to proclaim the victory over the Persian army. The modern marathon is named for his feat.

c. 275 BC    Herophilus's younger colleague, Eristratus (c. 310–c. 250 BC), asserts that veins and arteries are connected.

36 BC    The first swimming races are held in Japan, as a part of the training of the Samurai warrior class.

c. 100    The sport of sumo, a competition that first evolved within the Shinto religion of Japan as a means of appeasing the gods, was developed in this period.

c. 393    The Olympics are abolished by Roman emperor Theodosius I, on the grounds that the Games were pagan.

c. 850    Arab scholar Yaqub ibn-Ishaq al-Kindi (c. 800–870) advances an anatomical and physiological explanation of vision.

c. 1200    Versions of football (soccer) are being played in various regions of Europe.

c. 1275    William of Saliceto creates the first established record of a human dissection.

c. 1300    Cricket is being played in a variety of forms across the south of England.

1490    Leonardo da Vinci (1452–1519) designs the world's first bicycle.

1505    Leonardo da Vinci adds to a series of anatomical studies by creating the first wax cast of oxen brain ventricles.

1540 Servetus offers the first description of the pulmonary circulation of blood.

c. 1550 Early forms of tennis are being played in various regions of Europe.

1658 Dutch naturalist Jan Swammerdam publishes records of observations of red blood cells.

1660 Marcello Malpighi makes publishes works describing vascular capillary beds and individual capillaries.

1664 The idea of reflex action, formulated by René Descartes (1596–1650), French philosopher and mathematician, is made public. The assertion is included in a French edition of his posthumously published work on animal physiology. In his analysis Descartes applied his mechanistic philosophy to the analysis of animal behavior and first used the concept of reflex to denote any involuntary response the body makes when exposed to a stimulus.

1665 Robert Hooke publishes *Micrographia*, an account of observations made with the new instrument known as the microscope. Hooke presents his drawings of the tiny box-like structures found in cork and calls these tiny structures "cells." Although the cells he observes are not living, the name is retained. He also describes the streaming juices of live plant cells.

1680 Posthumous publication of *On Motion in Animals* by Giovanni Alfonso Borelli (1608–1679), Italian mathematician and physicist. Borelli studied the human body from the standpoint of Descartes's mechanistic philosophy, describing physiology as a branch of physics and offering a mechanical analysis of the skeletomuscular system.

1746 Pierre-Louis Moreau de Maupertuis publishes *Venus Physique*. Maupertuis criticizes preformationist theories because offspring inherit characteristics of both parents. He proposes an adaptationist account of organic design. His theories suggests the existence of a mechanism for transmitting adaptations.

c. 1750 Cricket increases in popularity throughout England. The rules are codified and formal cricket clubs are established in London.

1757 Albrecht von Haller 1757–1766), publishes the first volume of his eight-volume *Elements of Physiology of the Human Body*, subsequently to become a landmark in the history of modern physiology.

1770 Captain James Cook, English explorer, observes the sport of surfing practiced by native people in the Hawaiian Islands.

1771 Luigi Galvani (1737–1798), Italian anatomist, discovers the electric nature of nervous impulses.

1772 Joseph Priestley (1733–1804), English theologian and chemist, discovers that plants give off oxygen.

1774 Antoine-Laurent Lavoisier (1743–1794), French chemist, discovers that oxygen is consumed during respiration.

1796 Erasmus Darwin, grandfather of Charles Darwin, and Francis Galton, publishes his *Zoonomia*. In this work, Darwin argues that evolutionary changes are brought about by the mechanism primarily associated with Jean-Baptiste Lamarck, that is, the direct influence of the environment on the organism.

1820 First United States *Pharmacopoeia* is published.

1823 The invention of rugby is credited to William Webb Ellis at Rugby School, England. The rules of rugby are formalized in England in 1845, the first stage in a rise in rugby's popularity as a world game.

1829 The first Oxford-Cambridge rowing race is held on the Thames River, London.

1839 Theodore Schwann extends the theory of cells to include animals and helps establish the basic unity of the two great kingdoms of life. In *Microscopical Researches into the Accordance in the Structure and Growth of Animals and Plants*, Schwann asserts that all living things are made up of cells, each of which contains certain essential components. He also coins the term "metabolism" to describe the overall chemical changes that take place in living tissues.

1846 The first recorded game of organized baseball is played at Elysian Fields, New Jersey. Alexander Cartwright (1820–1892) had written the first comprehensive set of rules for baseball in 1845.

1848 The Cambridge Rules, the first codification of the rules of soccer, are created at Cambridge University, England.

1851 The first race of what would become the America's Cup yacht racing series was contested.

1854 Gregor Mendel begins his study of 34 different strains of peas. Eventually, Mendel selects 22 kinds for further experiments. From 1856 to 1863, Mendel will grow and test over 28,000 plants and analyze seven specific pairs of traits.

1855 Barolomeo Panizza (1785–1867), Italian anatomist, first proves that parts of the cerebral cortex are essential for vision.

1858 Rudolf Ludwig Carl Virchow publishes his landmark paper "Cellular Pathology" and establishes the field of cellular pathology. Virchow asserts that all cells arise from preexisting cells (*Omnis cellula e cellula*). He argues that the cell is the ultimate locus of all disease.

1859 Charles Robert Darwin publishes his landmark book *On the Origin of Species by Means of Natural Selection.*

1863 The Football Association, the world's oldest soccer league, is founded in London, England.

1870 Gustav Theodor Fritsch (1838–1927), German anatomist and anthropologist, and Eduard Hitzig (1838–1907), German physiologist and neurologist, discover that electric shocks to one cerebral hemisphere of a dog's brain produces movement on the other side of the animal's body. This is the first clear demonstration of the existence of cerebral hemispheric lateralization.

1870 Lambert Adolphe Jacques Quetelet shows the importance of statistical analysis for biologists and provides the foundations of biometry.

1873 Franz Anton Schneider describes cell division in detail. His drawings included both the nucleus and chromosomal strands.

1873 John Trudgen introduces a swimming stroke to swimmers in England that is a precursor to the modern front crawl. The Trudgen technique dramatically increases the speed and the efficiency of swimmers; the Trudgen stroke remains the staple in swim races for 30 years.

1873 Walther Flemming discovers chromosomes, observes mitosis, and suggests the modern interpretation of nuclear division.

1874 The first American football game, a variation of rugby, is played between McGill University (Montreal, ON, Canada) and Harvard. Harvard will play Yale in the first ever American intercollegiate game in 1875.

1875 The first organized ice hockey game is played in Montreal, ON, Canada.

1876 North American baseball's National League is founded.

1878 A.G. Spalding establishes the sporting goods company that bears his name in Chicago. Spalding products form the backbone of the first ever sporting goods empire.

1878 Charles-Emanuel Sedillot introduces the term "microbe." The term becomes widely used as a term for a pathogenic bacterium.

1881 FIG, the international governing body of gymnastics, is founded in Paris.

1882 Robert Koch (1843–1910), German bacteriologist, discovers the tubercle bacillus and enunciates "Koch's postulates," which define the classic method of preserving, documenting, and studying bacteria.

1882 Shihan Kano of Japan develops the sport of judo.

1882 Walther Flemming publishes *Cell Substance, Nucleus, and Cell Division,* in which he describes his observations of the longitudinal division of chromosomes in animal cells. Flemming observes chromosome threads in the dividing cells of salamander larvae.

1884 Elie Metchnikoff discovers the antibacterial activity of white blood cells, which he calls "phagocytes," and formulates the theory of phagocytosis.

1884 Louis Pasteur and coworkers publishes a paper entitled "A New Communication on Rabies." Pasteur proves that the causal agent of rabies could be attenuated and the weakened virus could be used as a vaccine to prevent the disease. This work serves as the basis of future work on virus attenuation, vaccine development, and the concept that variation is an inherent characteristic of viruses.

1887 The game of softball is invented by George Hancock in Chicago, Illinois.

1888 Heinrich Wilhelm Gottfried Waldeyer coins the term "chromosome." Waldeyer introduces the use of hematoxylin as a histological stain.

1891 Charles-Edouard Brown-Sequard suggests the concept of internal secretions (hormones).

1891 Hermann Henking distinguishes between the sex chromosomes and the autosomes.

1891 James Naismith, a physical education instructor with the YMCA, invents the sport of basketball in Springfield, Massachussets.

1893 Senda Berenson Abbott, a physical education instructor at Smith College, Massachussets, revises the Naismith rules of basketball to create a version of basketball for women.

1895 Physical education instructor William Morgan, a friend of James Naismith, invents volleyball in Springfield, Massachussets.

1896 The Olympic Games are revived by Baron Pierre de Coubertin (1863-1937), and are held in Paris. The International Olympic Committee is established to organize all successive Olympic Games.

1897 The inaugural Boston Marathon (26.2 mi [42.2 km]) is run on a course from Hopkington, Massachussets, to Boston; 15 runners take part. The Boston Marathon becomes the most famous road race in the world.

1897 The world's first bobsled run is constructed at St. Moritz, Switzerland.

1899 Scientist Felix Hoffman invents aspirin (acetysalicylic acid) in Germany. Aspirin, originally designed as an analgesic is the most consumed medication in history.

1900 Karl Landsteiner discovers the blood-agglutination phenomenon and the four major blood types in humans.

1901 Jokichi Takamine (1854–1922), Japanese-American chemist, and T.B. Aldrich first isolate epinephrine from the adrenal gland. Later known by the trade name Adrenalin, it is eventually identified as a neurotransmitter. This is also the first time a pure hormone has been isolated.

1902 Walter Sutton presents evidence that chromosomes have individuality, that chromosomes occur in pairs (with one member of each pair contributed by each parent), and that the paired chromosomes separate from each other during meiosis. Sutton concludes that the concept of the individuality of the chromosomes provides the link between cytology and Mendelian heredity.

1903 The first Tour de France is organized, a 1,500-mi (2,500 km) race. Over one hundred years later, the Tour de France is the most famous cycling race in the world.

1905 Nettie Maria Stevens, American geneticist, discovers the connection between chromosomes and sex determination. She determines that there are two basic types of sex chromosomes, which are now called X and Y. Stevens proves that females are XX and males are XY. Stevens and Edmund B. Wilson independently describe the relationship between the so-called accessory or X chromosomes and sex determination in insects.

1905 The Isle of Mann motorcycle races are organized for the first time. The Isle of Mann competition remains one of the most famous motorcycle challenges in the world.

1907 Ivan Petrovich Pavlov (1849–1910) investigates the conditioned reflex (1904–1907). A great stimulus for behaviorist psychology, his work establishes physiologically-oriented psychology.

1909 Jean de Mayer, French physiologist, first suggests the name "insulin" for the hormone of the islet cells.

1909 The Indianapolis Speedway is constructed; this race track becomes the permanent home of the annual Indianapolis 500 auto race.

1920 The National Football League (NFL) commenced play.

1923 German-born Joseph Pilates, developer of the exercise training program of the same name, opens his first studio in New York.

1928 Alexander Fleming (1881–1955), Scottish bacteriologist, discovers penicillin. He observes that the mold *Penicillium notatum* inhibits the growth of some bacteria. This is the first antibacterial, and it opens a new era of "wonder drugs" to combat infection and disease.

1928 The Summer Olympics held at Amsterdam are the first to provide a significant number of women's events.

c. 1930 Anabolic steroids are discovered by German scientists. The chemicals are not used in sport applications until the 1950s.

1930 The first World Cup of soccer is held in Uruguay; the host nation beat Argentina in the championship final. The World Cup is today second only to the Olympics in global sporting popularity.

1932 Charles "Chuck" Taylor puts his signature on the logo of the Converse All Star basketball shoe; Converse are the most popular basketball shoe in the world for almost 40 years.

1934 George Nissen of Iowa builds the first trampoline intended for the commercial market.

1935 Effa Manley becomes the first woman to both own and administer the day to day operations of a professional baseball club when she assumes control of the Newark Eagles of the Negro League.

1946 Bloch and Purcell develop nuclear magnetic resonance (NMR) as viable tool for observation and analysis.

1947 Jackie Robinson becomes the first black man to play major league baseball when he is signed to a contract by the Brooklyn Dodgers.

1948 The Stoke Mandeville Games for disabled persons, the forerunner to the modern Paralympics, are held at Stoke-on-Trent, England.

1949 Joseph Sobek of Conneticut creates a new game that he calls "paddleball" the game is ultimately named racquetball and it would be come a very popular sport by the 1970s throughout North America.

1950 The first Maccabiah Games to be hosted by the state of Israel are held in Tel Aviv. Styled in the manner of the Olympic Games for Jewish athletes from around the world, the Maccabiah Games become a quadrennial event in 1957.

1951 Rosalind Franklin obtains sharp x-ray diffraction photographs of DNA.

1954 Danny Biasone of the National Basketball Association (NBA) devises the 24-second shot to clock to speed the game. His innovation will become an integral part of the game both in the United States and in all international championships.

1954 Roger Bannister of England, a medical student, becomes the first person to run one mile in under four minutes. Bannister's rivalry with Australian John Landy and American Wes Santee to be the first sub-four-minute runner is one of the most compelling in the history of sport.

1956 Mary F. Lyon proposes that one of the X chromosomes of normal females is inactivated. This concept became known as the Lyon hypothesis and helped explain some confusing aspects of sex-linked diseases. Females are usually "carriers" of genetic diseases on the X chromosome because the normal gene on the other chromosome protects them, but some X-linked disorders are partially expressed in female carriers. Based on studies of mouse coat color genes, Lyon proposes that one X chromosome is randomly inactivated in the cells of female embryos.

1957 Francis Crick proposes that during protein formation each amino acid is carried to the template by an adapter molecule containing nucleotides, and that the adapter is the part that actually fits on the RNA template. Later research demonstrates the existence of transfer RNA.

1959 The Daytona 500 auto race, the most prestigious of the American NASCAR events, is first run at the Daytona speedway this year.

1961 "Wide World of Sports," the groundbreaking American weekly sports program, airs for the first time. "Wide World of Sports," featuring host Jim McKay, runs until 1998.

1962 James D. Watson, Francis Crick, and Maurice Wilkins are awarded the Nobel Prize in Medicine or Physiology for their work in elucidating the structure of DNA.

1965 A primitive form of the modern snowboard, the "Snow Surfer" is developed in the United States.

1965 Dr. Robert Cade of the University of Florida and a team of researchers create the sports drink Gatorade, a product that became the largest selling sports drink in the world.

1965 François Jacob, André Lwoff, and Jacques Monod are awarded the Nobel Prize in Medicine or Physiology for their discoveries concerning genetic control of enzymes and virus synthesis.

1966 Marshall Nirenberg and Har Gobind Khorana lead teams that decipher the genetic code. All of the 64 possible triplet combinations of the four bases (the codons) and their associated amino acids are determined and described.

1966 Sex testing (gender verification testing) is introduced at the European track and field championships.

1967 Kathryn Switzer becomes the first woman to enter and to complete the Boston Marathon.

1967 The sport of windsurfing claims a number of different inventors; it begins to receive popular attention this year.

1968 American long jumper Bob Beamon shatters the world record by over 21 inches (53 cm) at the 1968 Summer Olympics at Mexico City.

1968 Dick Fosbury, American high jumper, introduces a revolutionary style of jumping, nicknamed the "Fosbury Flop." Fosbury wins the Olympic gold medal in the event.

1972 Eleven Israeli Olympic team members are taken hostage and ultimately murdered by an Arab terrorist cell, "Black September" at the Summer Olympics at Munich.

1972 The shoe soon to be popularized as the Nike "waffle" sole is designed by U.S. track coach Bill Bowerman.

1972 The United States government passes Title IX of the Civil Rights Act into law; Title IX establishes a framework within which female athletes are entitled to equality of opportunity in all aspects of American amateur sport. Title IX was the impetus for the creation of female athletic scholarships and female sports organizations across the United States.

1973 Dr. Frank Jobe of Callifornia performs revolutionary elbow ligament surgery on American baseball pitcher Tommy John. This procedure will prolong the careers of thousands of athletes.

1973 The Iditarod sled dog race is run from Anchorage to Nome, Alaska. The Idiatord established a reputation as one of the toughest sporting challenges in the world.

1976 Romanian gymnast Nadia Comaneci, coached by Bela Karolyi, is awarded the first ever perfect score in the history of gymnastics at the Summer Olympics in Montreal.

1976 The International Olympic Committee institutes testing for anabolic steroids and other prohibited substances at the Summer Olympics in Montreal.

1978 The Hawaii Ironman is started as a 2.4-mi (4 km) swim, a 112-mi (191 km) cycle, and a 26.2-mi (42 km) run. Twelve athletes finish in the 15-person starting field. Ironman events are now held throughout the world.

1980 The United States men's hockey team defeats the favored Soviet Union to win the Olympic gold medal at Lake Placid.

1982 The United States Food and Drug Administration (FDA) approves the first genetically engineered drug, a form of human insulin produced by bacteria.

c. 1983 Dr. James Andrews continues to develop arthroscopic surgery techniques that both repair athletic injuries and reduce the time require for rehabilitation.

1984 Michael Jordan is selected in the National Basketball Association draft by the Chicago Bulls. Jordan wins six league championships with the Bulls and acclaim as the greatest player in NBA history.

1986 Former world-class marathoner Brian Maxwell invents the PowerBar, a popular energy bar used by endurance athletes.

1986 Greg Lemond of the United States becomes the first American to win the Tour de France.

1986 The United States Department of Energy officially initiates the Human Genome Initiative.

1988 Canadian Ben Johnson is disqualified as the Olympic men's 100-m champion and world record holder when he tested positive for steroids at the 1988 Summer Olympics. Johnson is the highest profile drug cheat in the history of sport.

1988 The Human Genome Project officially adopts the goal of determining the entire sequence of DNA comprising the human chromosomes.

1992 Jackie Joyner Kersee, American heptathlete, wins the Olympic gold medal at Barcelona, Spain, to become one of the most decorated female athletes in Olympic history.

1994 The United States passes the Dietary Supplements Health Promotion Act, a law intended to regulate aspects of the growing supplements market in America.

1998 Several cyclists in the Tour de France are found to have taken the hormone erythropoetin, EPO, a practice known as "blood doping." Allegations of EPO use will plague the Tour and leading riders such a seven-time champion Lance Armstrong through 2006.

1999 Scientists announce the complete sequencing of the DNA making up human chromosome 22. The first complete human chromosome sequence is published in December 1999.

1999 The World Anti-Doping Agency, WADA, is created after several years of international organizational efforts in the sports community. WADA will become one of the most influential sports organizations in the world.

2001 Tiger Woods becomes the only golfer in history to hold all four major championships simultaneously.

2003 Paul Lauterbur is awarded the Nobel Prize for Chemistry in recognition of his contributions to the invention of the magnetic resonance imaging technology, MRI; the technology is a extremely important diagnostic tool in assessing athletic injuries.

2003 The BALCO (Bay Area Laboratory Cooperative) scandal surfaces in the United States; BALCO principals are involved in the distribution of nandrolone, an anabolic steroid, and other prohibited substances, to high profile American athletes, including world record sprinter Tim Montgomery and baseball home run hitter Barry Bonds.

2003 Following initial publication in 2001, The Human Genome Project for the National Institutes of Health culminates in the completion of a more complete human genome sequence, published in the journal *Nature*.

2005 Lance Armstrong wins his record seventh Tour de France and retires from competition.

2005 Major League Baseball (MLB) players are subpoenaed to testify before Congress concerning the use of steroids in the sport.

2006 Several leading riders are banned from competition on the eve of the start of the 2006 Tour de France under suspicion of links to use of performance enhancing drugs raised by a Spanish sport and police inquiry.

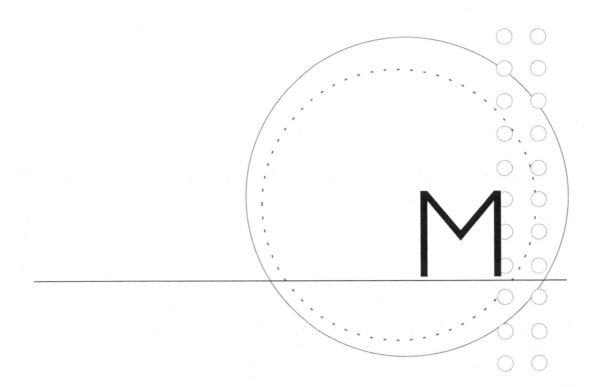

# Maccabiah Games

The Maccabiah Games are a quadrennial athletic festival held at the permanent host country, Israel, and open to Jewish athletes from around the world. Known as the Jewish Olympics, the Games are second only to the Olympics in both the number of participating countries and of competing athletes.

Judah Maccabee was a legendary Jewish warrior who battled the ancient Greeks in what was then Palestine in 160 BC. In 1927, the Jewish movement that had been founded to promote better physical fitness among the Jews living in the ghettos of European cities adopted the name of this warrior as their symbol. The Maccabi World Union was later founded to promote physical education within the broader Jewish heritage. In the face of rising social pressures on European Jews, particularly in Germany and in the Soviet Union, the Maccabi World Union soon became a symbol of the worldwide Zionist movement and the drive to create a Jewish homeland in Palestine. Today, it is under the auspices of the Maccabi World Union that the Games are staged.

The first Maccabiah Games was held in Tel Aviv (in the former Palestine) in 1932. The Games resumed in 1950, following the disruptions caused by World War II and the subsequent founding of the state of Israel in 1948. As of 1957, the Games have been held in Israel every four years, the seventeenth edition taking place in 2005, with 50 nations and over 6,000 athletes participating. The Maccabiah delegation from the United States, a country with a large Jewish community, included more than 900 athletes. The Games have a format similar to that of the Summer Olympics, with track and field events, swimming, boxing, soccer, basketball, and volleyball competitions.

The Maccabiah Games are a member of the Olympic movement headed by the International Olympic Committee (IOC). As with national Olympic organizing committees, the member countries of the Maccabiah Games have national Maccabiah organizations that direct the qualifying competitions for each Maccabiah Games in their respective countries.

Israel, the permanent home to the Maccabiah Games, is a country that has been in a state of war with a number of its Arab neighbors since its creation in 1948. The Games have been affected at various times by these regional tensions, but to a large degree, through a combination of comprehensive Israeli security measures and the fact that the Games are a demonstrably peaceful event, disruptive incidents have been few.

**SEE ALSO** International federations; International Olympic Committee (IOC); National governing bodies.

# Magnesium

Magnesium is the eighth most abundant element found within the human body; a 190-lb (86 kg) person possesses approximately 1 oz (23 gr) of magnesium in various places. Approximately 50% of the mineral is stored in the bone structures, and approximately 50% is located within various cells, and organ and tissue structures. One percent of all of the body's magnesium is contained within the cardiovascular system. Magnesium plays a role in more than 300 of the biochemical reactions that are essential to human performance, ranging from the maintenance of the skeletal structure and organ health to the function of the cardiovascular and central nervous systems.

While pure magnesium is an element found on the periodic table, it is not obtained in its natural state from the Earth due to its chemical composition, which makes magnesium react with a number of other elements to form compounds, particularly those involving oxygen, sulphur, and hydrogen. The active ingredient in the bitter water first discovered in an English well in the early 1600s, which later became known as the tonic, Epsom salts, is magnesium sulphate, or $MgSO_4$. The popular digestive aid, Milk of Magnesia, also uses magnesium in its composition.

Magnesium is an important component of chlorophyll, the chemical that makes living plants green. For this reason, many of the excellent dietary sources of magnesium are plant products such as green vegetables, most whole grains, beans, and nuts. Well water that is drawn from ground that has a significant mineral composition, sometimes referred to as hard water, will usually contain significant amounts of magnesium. Magnesium is typically contained in foods that also have significant amounts of potassium and dietary fiber.

As foods are digested, any magnesium is absorbed into the body through the small intestine. The magnesium not processed into the body is excreted through the kidneys in urine. It would be difficult to consume magnesium in quantities sufficient to induce a toxic reaction; magnesium deficiency is a far more important dietary issue. The recommended daily allowance (RDA) of magnesium is 420 mg per day for a male over 30 years of age; the RDA for a 30-year-old female is 320 mg per day.

While calcium, in combination with vitamin D, is the most significant mineral presence in the construction and the maintenance of the human bones, magnesium plays a significant role in the transport of calcium to the required areas of bone development.

The combined operation of trace minerals, including magnesium, is a preventative in the onset of osteoporosis, a common bone density disease, especially among post-menopausal women.

Magnesium is also a factor in the manner in which the skeletal muscles respond to the directions transmitted by the central nervous system. Although less crucial in this respect than sodium or potassium, magnesium is necessary in the manner in which signals are sent to working muscles during exercise.

Magnesium plays an important role in the determination of blood sugar (glucose) levels, as well as the manner in which proteins ingested through food are synthesized by the body. In a related fashion, magnesium also acts in the regulation of heartbeat and the functions of the immune system. As with the many influences of magnesium on the metabolisms of the human body, magnesium is not usually the lead actor, but works in a supporting capacity.

Magnesium levels within the body can be influenced by a number of factors, in addition to the obvious failure to consume sufficient magnesium-rich foods. Medications that possess a diuretic quality have been established as contributing to a negative impact on the body's ability to retain magnesium. The medications that are particularly reactive to magnesium in this fashion are those used in the treatment of disorders such as Crohn's disease, a serious illness of the intestinal system. In a similar fashion, the excess consumption of caffeine has the effect of reducing magnesium stores within the body.

A magnesium deficiency will not be manifested in a sudden or dramatic physical fashion. The early symptoms of a magnesium deficiency may include a loss of appetite, generalized weakness, and fatigue. If the condition worsens, the person will experience difficulties in concentration (similar to other electrolytic disruptions in the body), and ultimately, low levels of both calcium and potassium will occur. The most effective way to restore low levels of magnesium is by way of improved diet, especially through green vegetables and whole grains. In some circumstances, the levels may be increased through the use of magnesium supplements. Given the nature of the element, magnesium can be restored to its appropriate concentration in the body within a number of days. Magnesium is a component of a number of dietary and training supplements, in a variety of compounds.

**SEE ALSO** Calcium; Minerals; Sodium and sodium deficits.

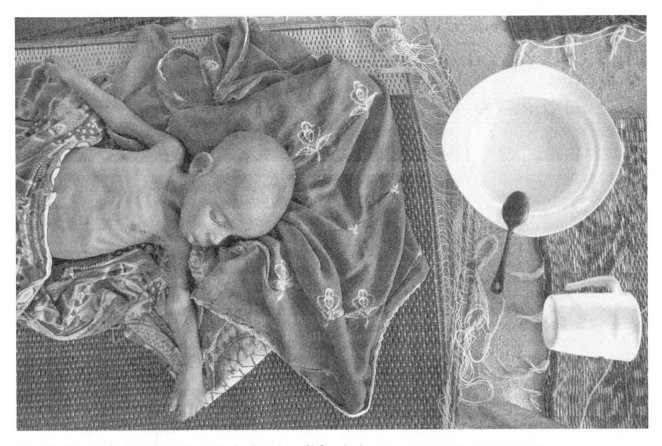

In less-developed countries, malnutrition is the leading cause of infant death. © FINBARR O'REILLY/REUTERS/CORBIS

## Male athletes SEE Gender in sports: Male athletes

## Malnutrition

Malnutrition is an imbalance in diet that occurs in one of two ways. In its first manifestation, malnutrition is caused by a diet that includes too little food, resulting in a caloric shortfall in the body. When the body cannot process sufficient food to generate the energy that it requires for its purposes, the person is stated to be malnourished.

Malnutrition is also the result of insufficient nutrients being consumed and available to the body through diet. In this form of malnutrition, it is possible for the body to be adequately nourished in terms of calorie consumption, but subject to deficiencies of both macronutrients such as protein, the building blocks used by the body for muscle and tissue construction and maintenance, and micronutrients, those trace amounts of vitamins and minerals that are essential to the function of a multitude of bodily processes.

A significant contributor to the two forms of malnutrition is the failure to provide adequate amounts of fiber in diet. Fiber is essential to the optimal digestion of all foods. Fiber is itself not a food group, it is not an energy source, and it is not digestible. However, fiber is often linked to foods that possess substantial quantities of various micronutrients; when fiber is below optimal levels, the body will not properly digest and process those foods.

Malnutrition is a matter of degree. In children, particularly those in less-developed nations, malnutrition is a leading cause of death. This worst-case aspect of malnutrition is the starvation of the child. In less pronounced but serious circumstances, children who are malnourished will not develop to their fullest physical or mental capabilities. A deficiency in the amount of calories consumed results in children who are undersized, as their bone and muscle development is stunted. The combination of an inadequate caloric intake and essential vitamins and minerals will often limit the intellectual development and mental capacity of the child.

An aspect of inadequate food intake is a condition known as protein energy malnutrition. The generation of energy by the body ultimately results in the generation of a substance known as adenosine triphosphate

(ATP), a process that occurs within the individual cells. Where the body has too few carbohydrates available to produce the energy source glucose, the body will break down its proteins to resolve the shortfall.

The deficiencies in various vitamins and minerals that result in malnutrition are reflected in a variety of conditions, some of which are capable of remedy, others of which are permanent in their physical consequences. Among the most prominent of these deficiencies is that involving the mineral calcium, a condition that often occurs in conjunction with a shortage of vitamin D. Calcium is the key mineral in the formation and maintenance of the skeletal bone structure; calcium is the most prominent mineral in the body. Vitamin D is essential to the processing of calcium in bone formation, maintenance, and repair. A shortage of either substance will result in structural problems in bone formation. A prolonged deficiency in either of these micronutrients will create permanent skeletal weaknesses.

A number of other conditions flow from vitamin and mineral deficiency. For the athlete whose body is subjected to the stresses of muscular activity and the competitive environment, even a small deficiency in one of the micronutrients can have a negative impact on athletic performance. For example, while a vitamin A deficiency impacts function of the immune system, a deficiency of the B complex has a broad range of negative impacts. The various components of the B vitamin complex are crucial to the breakdown of carbohydrates into useful energy sources, the maintenance of healthy skin and other organs. Vitamin C is essential to the maintenance of the health of the body's connective tissues, the central nervous system, and the function of the adrenal glands.

The deficiencies in other minerals, particularly sodium, potassium, iron, and magnesium impact on a number of essential human systems. As an example, when the presence of the electrolytic minerals such as sodium and capacity is reduced, as often occurs if the body is dehydrated, the fluid-leveling ability of the body is significantly impaired. Iron is crucial to the function of the ability of the cardiovascular system, through the red blood cell component hemoglobin, to transport oxygen in the creation of energy.

Nutritionists recommend that, whenever possible, both macronutrients and micronutrients should be obtained from food sources. Information concerning the best sources is widely available. Dietary supplements, including vitamin and mineral formulations, are commonly used by athletes to ensure that they have no hidden or undetermined deficiency that has arisen through the stresses of training.

**SEE ALSO** Carbohydrates; Minerals; Protein supplements; Vitamin C.

# Effa Manley

3/27/1900–4/16/1981
AMERICAN
NEGRO LEAGUES BASEBALL TEAM OWNER

In the 1930s and 1940s, Effa Manley was known as the Queen of the Negro Leagues. Manley first rose to prominence in the sport of baseball as the co-owner of the Brooklyn Eagles in 1935, a club she operated with her husband, Abe Manley. In 1935, major league baseball was an entirely segregated sport, and the Negro Leagues served to provide a professional baseball outlet for black players and their predominately black fan base in the cities of the northeastern United States.

During World War II, the Negro Leagues prospered and its teams developed many outstanding players. Many of these players ultimately moved to the major leagues after the Brooklyn Dodgers obtained the services of Negro League star Jackie Robinson in 1947, breaking baseball's color barrier.

Manley was a social activist during the 1930s, when she was instrumental in organizing a store boycott in Harlem to pressure white business owners to hire more black sales clerks. Manley was also a well regarded member of the National Association for the Advancement of Colored People (NAACP).

Manley achieved her greatest prominence in the Negro Leagues after 1936, when she and Abe Manley moved the Brooklyn Eagles to Newark, New Jersey. Manley was the driving force in the operation of the Newark franchise, where she was responsible for all financial and business decisions regarding the team. Manley was admired as an owner who cared abut the players welfare in all respects; she and her husband sponsored a team in the Puerto Rican winter leagues at that time to ensure that the Newark players had employment in the off-season.

After Jackie Robinson left the Negro Leagues in 1947, major league baseball began to sign other Negro League stars, including Newark's Larry Doby and Don Newcombe, both of whom would ultimately be enshrined in the Baseball Hall of Fame. The Negro League was no longer viable, and the league folded in 1948. Manley lobbied unsuccessfully for compensation from major league baseball for the loss of the players developed in the Negro Leagues.

Effa Manley was the only female owner in the history of the Negro League. In 2006, she became the first woman to be inducted into the Baseball Hall of Fame.

SEE ALSO Baseball.

# Marathon SEE Running: Marathon

# Mass, muscle SEE Muscle mass and strength

# Massage therapy

Massage therapy is the healing process by which the soft tissue of the body is manipulated by the hands of a trained therapist. Soft-tissue therapy includes the skin, muscles, tendons, ligaments, and the capsules that encase the various joints of the body.

Massage is a therapeutic technique that has been employed for many centuries in a number of cultures. Modern massage therapy has significant aspects in common with traditional Chinese medicines, including acupuncture and the use of various herbal remedies and the application of poultices, with the most important being that it is a proven aid to the enhancement of a number of physical functions.

Massage therapy is directed to a number of separate but related physical purposes. Injured muscles can be effectively manipulated to deliver pain relief in the affected areas; tight or contracted muscles can be relaxed through the application of various levels of manual pressure, especially when the muscles have been subjected to the stresses of athletic competition and training. The various massage techniques are effective in stimulating blood flow in the body. Massage is also useful in improving the function of the lymphatic system and the central nervous system.

Massage therapy is also employed for the purpose of relaxation. Stress is created in a number of circumstances for an athlete, both as a direct result of the production of the hormone adrenaline when the body perceives itself confronted by exciting circumstances, and indirectly through the accumulated effect of stressful circumstances. Diverse and critical functions such as heart rate, immune system, and the digestive tract are all adversely impacted by stress.

There are well over 50 different defined techniques used in the various applications of massage therapy. Many of these techniques are used in combination. Four common forms of massage therapy used to assist in the resolution of athletic injuries include:

- Acupressure: This therapy is closely related to acupuncture procedures, which involve the utilization of the *chi*, the inherent healing energy believed to be present throughout the body, by manipulation of the tissues at defined pressure points. These pressure points are connected to the function of the internal organs and the circulation of blood throughout the body; their stimulation is designed to aid in the direction of healing power to an affected area. A technique similar to acupressure is that of *shiatsu*, a Japanese-derived system that involves the application of finger pressure to pre determined zones of the body.

- Rolfing: This is a vigorous form of massage that involves a manipulation of the skin to effect a loosening of the underlying muscle structure. Rolfing is employed both as a preventative as well as a therapeutic treatment.

- Swedish massage: This is a technique in which the basic direction of the hands in the course of the application is toward the heart of the person. The central object of a Swedish massage is improved circulation; it has also been employed as a technique to reduce scar tissue in muscle groups.

- Sports massage: These techniques are often an amalgam of massage therapies designed to reduce injury and inflammation, to relax the athlete, and as use as both a warm up or a cool down ritual. A vigorous massage applied for up to 20 minutes, generally one hour in advance of competition, often prepares the athlete. Post-event, a massage will stimulate circulation, especially in the region of the working muscles, flushing out metabolic waste materials such as those related to lactic acid production.

Athletes seeking the benefit of massage therapy, no matter what type, will often receive the benefit of fascial techniques. These are manipulations that are intended to focus on the fascia, the general term for the connective tissues located at the joints throughout the body. In this context, the fascia may include cartilage, ligaments, tendons, and muscles in the vicinity of the joint. A well-known fascia problem experienced by athletes is plantar fasciitis, where the connective band between the heel and the forefoot under the arch of the foot becomes inflamed.

The illiol band between the hip and the knee joint is another connective tissue that may become stressed in athletic activity.

It is a testament to the legitimacy of massage as a therapeutic technique that many elite-level athletic organizations and individual athletes regularly undergo massage therapy. Many teams have a full-time athletic therapist on their staff, whose focus is as much injury prevention as it is therapy. In many jurisdictions, massage therapists are a part of a larger regulated industry, where formalized training and licensing are mandatory.

SEE ALSO Acupuncture and Eastern healing therapies; Exercise recovery; Musculoskeletal injuries; Sports medicine education.

# Mature athletes

Until the first mass participation running boom in the 1970s, the term mature athlete was an oxymoron in the United States. Mature was popularly associated with the words "old" and "deteriorated" from a sport perspective, and aside from the so-called "beer leagues" in sports such as men's basketball and ice hockey, older athletes were unorganized. Any such persons who remained fit were usually operating on an entirely individual basis. Society at large generally perceived such persons as somewhat eccentric, as opposed to being health conscious or sports minded. Competitive athletics in all forms was regarded as the preserve of the young.

Running and its mass participatory focus changed perceptions about the older athlete and their capabilities. The combination of a changing societal demographic, with the baby boom generation passing age 40, and the nature of the races themselves, with hundreds or thousands of entrants, created a phenomenon that became known as master's competitions.

In most sports, there are a set of unalterable physiological imperatives that create a limit on the age at which an athlete, male or female, can continue to perform at the highest level. Those factors will include the decline in the function of the cardiovascular system, a circumstance that is connected to both the reduced ability of the heart to pump a maximal quantity of blood, reflected by the reduced maximum heart rate, coupled with the inevitable decrease in the capacity of the athlete to utilize oxygen, known as the $VO_2max$. While training and careful attention to health may slow the decline of these essential athletic sys-

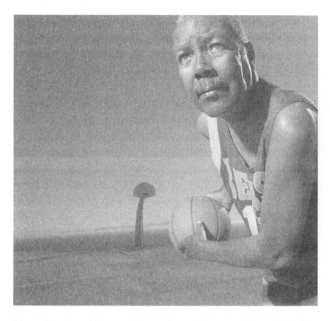

Master's competitions are now a fixture in many sports, including basketball, soccer, and rugby. © PATRIK GIARDINO/CORBIS

tems, it is impossible to maintain peak physical performance past the approximate age of 40 years.

A combination of other physiological factors contributes to the decrease in the ability of the body to build muscle and to possess the same level of muscular power and endurance. In particular sports, these physiological limits imposed by aging are accentuated by the demands of the particular discipline; it is rare to see a competitive female gymnast or figure skater active in their late 20s.

Master's competition grew from the premise that while athletes over age 40 could not reasonably compete with those in their physical prime, mature athletes could compete within their own age groups in a fashion that was both participatory and equitable. Master's competitions are now a fixture in many sports, both in individual pursuits such as tennis, squash, and athletics, as well as in team sports such as basketball, soccer, and rugby.

In most master's disciplines, the age groupings are set at five-year intervals. These divisions mirror the general progressive decline of the capabilities of the human body; just as a 45-year-old runner will have difficulty competing with a 25-year-old runner, where all other factors are equal, a 60-year-old athlete will not generally be competitive with a 45-year-old athlete. In some sports, there are rule modifications made to ensure that the safety of the competitors is preserved within a competitive framework. Examples include the popularity of non-contact ice hockey among players over age 40.

The growth of participation in sport among older athletes has propelled the growth of the World Masters Games, a celebration of the competitive aspects of master's competitions. The Masters Games are held every four years; the 2005 version, which was hosted in Edmonton, Canada, attracted over 20,000 athletes in an Olympic-style format. Studies conducted using the results of both the Master's Games track and field competitions, as well as international events with a significant master's component, such as the New York marathon and the London marathon, illustrate the rate of progression in the decline from elite performance standards as the athletes age.

The world record for races ranging in distance from the 100 m to the marathon was, on average, between 5% and 7% faster than the age group world records for ages 40 to 45. The 50-year-old age group most declined by a further 3% to 6%. To age 80, the best performances continued to decline at a rate of approximately 1% per year, while a comparable decline was noted in the comparison of various strength events such as weightlifting.

Although the actual level of performance may decline with the effect of age, the training approaches adopted by mature athletes are limited only by the decreased ability of the body to work at the same physiological level, due to the metabolic changes of $VO_2$max and maximum heart rate. Mature athletes often discover that their mental attitude towards sport, including such factors as their determination to succeed and their competitive urges, does not change in keeping with their reductions in physical ability.

SEE ALSO Age-related responses to injury; Aging and athletic performance.

# Brian Maxwell

3/14/1953–3/19/2004
CANADIAN AMERICAN
NUTRITION ENTREPRENEUR

Brian Maxwell was an elite marathoner in the 1970s, achieving third place in the world marathon rankings in 1977. Maxwell had encountered stomach cramping and problems in the later stages of marathons and he decided to seek a solution. Maxwell knew that at approximately 21 mi (34 km) into a marathon, the point in a race well known to marathoners as "the wall," the body's carbohydrate sources are severely depleted. Maxwell's wife Jennifer

was a trained nutritionist, and together they sought to create an energy source that an endurance athlete could consume before, during, and after races and training sessions to assist the body in its recovery from the depletion of its energy stores. Maxwell had initially thought that with his years of racing experience and his wife's nutritional knowledge, their ideas could simply be sold to a large food products company; no organizations expressed interest in Maxwell's ideas for an energy bar.

The original formulation of the PowerBar was developed in the Maxwell's kitchen at their home in California in 1986. The bar was designed as a high carbohydrate, low fat energy source, made entirely of natural ingredients. It was determined by testing both elite level racers and more recreational runners that a PowerBar was best consumed with water. Maxwell later developed a companion PowerBar gel that was easier to ingest if the athlete was in motion. One of the chief attractions of the PowerBar and its gel formulation was its portability and its convenience.

The PowerBar was initially sold on site at races and by mail order. It proved to be one of the most remarkably successful athletic supplements ever created. With the sustained fitness boom of the late 1980s and early 1990s producing record numbers of runners and triathletes, there was a fertile ground for the growth of the PowerBar market. Once Maxwell had established a market for the PowerBar, a significant number of competitors created their versions of sports energy bars. PowerBar also established itself with non-athletes as a healthy alternative snack food. Maxwell sold PowerBar to the Nestle company in 2000 for a reported $375 million dollars.

Maxwell, the former marathoner and health food innovator, died of a heart attack in 2004 at age 51.

SEE ALSO Carbohydrates; Dietary supplements; Exercise recovery.

# Jim McKay

9/24/1921–
AMERICAN
TELEVISION SPORTSCASTER

Jim McKay is a television sports host and commentator who became identified with Wide World of Sports, a groundbreaking weekly sports program aired in the United States between 1961 and 1998. Wide World of Sports was produced using then state of the art broadcast technologies. McKay was also the primary television commentator as the events surrounding the hostage taking and murder of 11 Israeli Olympic team members unfolded at the 1972 Munich Olympics.

Prior to his involvement with Wide World of Sports, Jim McKay had been a respected television host and personality since the late 1940s in various capacities in local and network television in the northeastern United States. In 1961, he was approached by the American Broadcasting Company (ABC) to act as host for Wide World of Sports, a program then contemplated as summer television programming that would expose esoteric and unusual sports to the American viewing public.

Wide World of Sports proved to be so popular that it was continued into the following television season. The show became one of the longest running sports programs in history, and McKay acted as the host of the program from 1961 to 1998. The producers of Wide World of Sports perceived its mandate as one dedicated to sports that were out of the mainstream of the common feature of American sports television at the time—American football, baseball, and basketball. ABC broadcast the Hawaii Ironman in 1982 on this premise, the first international media attention ever paid to the event. The rapid growth in the popularity of both the Hawaii Ironman concept and the sport of triathlon generally can be traced to this broadcast.

A signature of the Wide World of Sports program was the intonation by McKay of an introductory homage to sport, that included the phrase, the thrill of victory, the agony of defeat. This expression became one of the best-known (and often parodied) phrases anywhere in the world of sport. The program played a film montage as McKay' voice could be heard, a series of film clips that were coordinated with the words McKay spoke.

The segment played in conjunction with the words, the agony of defeat, became impressed upon the consciousness of the American public and it made a folk hero of an obscure Yugoslavian ski jumper. In 1970, Vinko Bogataj was commencing his jump in the World Ski Flying championships in Germany, when he lost control in his descent down the ramp as he neared the end of the track. Bogataj fell at a high speed from the ramp, crashing through various barriers and tumbling a considerable distance into the spectators watching the competition. Wide World of Sport was present to film the event and Bogataj's spectacular crash became forever linked with McKay's narration.

That a segment such as Bogataj's fall was captured on film is a testament to the production of Wide World of Sports, lead by then unknown television sports producer Roone Arledge (1931–2002). Arledge would later create the next ABC signature television program, Monday Night Football, in 1969. A visionary, Arledge was one of the first domestic users of the first Atlantic satellite, the means by which Wide World of Sports could provide live sports broadcasts to the United States from around the world. This technology is commonplace today. In 1965, when the satellite was first utilized by ABC, a satellite transmission of any television programming was a rarity. Arledge also made use of the relatively recent television production inventions of slow motion and instant replay in the Wide World of Sports broadcasts.

In 1972, as the Olympic hostage crisis unfolded, it was McKay who was the communicator to the world of the information concerning the crisis, an event that ABC broadcasted live. McKay became associated with Olympic coverage generally, and he was a host on subsequent Olympic broadcasts in which ABC had a broadcasting interest until 2002.

**SEE ALSO** International Olympic Committee (IOC); Track and Field.

# Medical conditions SEE Sports medical conditions

# Medical education SEE Sports medicine education

# Mental stress

Mental stress is a component of sport that is more pronounced in its effects on the athlete the more significant the event. Mental stress in the pressure brought to bear on the existing mental balance or emotional equilibrium of any person; the symptoms of mental stress will most commonly be exhibited when the demands of a situation are seen as exceeding the personal resources that the individual can bring to bear on them at that moment.

Mental stress is distinct from the broad variety of mental health conditions that are defined as illnesses, such as depression or a post-traumatic stress disorder. Stress is a more transient and focused circumstance, usually tied to well-defined and identifiable factors that are close to the subject. Stress is also a distinct psychological condition from anxiety, which is a feeling of a lack of control over one's future circumstances. Stress is usually related to the pending present event.

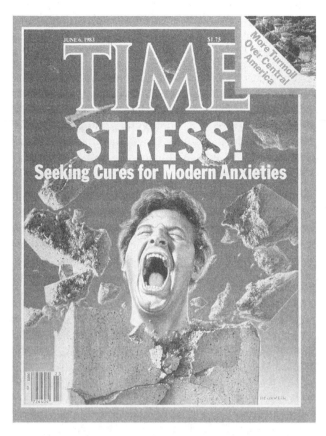

Most sport psychology techniques used to harness the energy of mental stress center on the ability of the athlete to focus on the event to the exclusion of all other thoughts and distractions.
**PHOTO BY TIME & LIFE PICTURES/GETTY IMAGES.**

Mental stress is commonly regarded as a negative circumstance in sport as well as daily living. It is often the response of the person to stress that determines how the stress ought to be characterized. Many athletes in particular train to channel their stress into positive influences on the outcome of an athletic event; this concept is better known as "healthy stress." Stress is a combination of instinctive and learned reactions. Mental stress represents a delicate balancing act for the athlete; when the athlete feels little or no stress in an important circumstance, he or she is often too relaxed and not sufficiently activated to achieve the best result. When the athlete feels the effect of mental stress in a fashion that he or she cannot control or harness for his/her own benefit, it is equally unlikely that a strong result will be achieved.

Stress arises in a number of different circumstances for an athlete, irrespective of ability level or athletic experience; elite competitors often tend to feel the effects of stress more profoundly. Stressful situations often result from a number of conditions, including: competitive pressure, the desire and the drive to succeed; training pressures, the ongoing stress of adherence to daily targets, mileages, or performance standards; the external pressures created by coaches or teammates to achieve; financial pressures created through either the cost of participation in a sport or as a career component; or the consequences of an injury, accompanied by the stresses of rehabilitation or fears of recurrence.

As a companion to the internal emotions associated with mental stress, this condition has a number of physiological reactions. Most of these consequences are triggered by the body's recognition of a dangerous circumstance, which initiates what is often referred to as the "fight or flight" response. The brain signals the adrenal gland to release the hormone adrenaline as a first-line response to a stressful circumstance. Adrenaline almost instantly creates a rise in both the heart rate and blood pressure, preparatory to any required muscle action. The body automatically raises its blood sugar level, and blood is directed to the extremities of the body, preparatory for physical action. The negative consequences of the release of adrenaline are increased excitability and a reduction in motor control skills. Controlling the impacts of stress is therefore of crucial importance to athletic success.

Of fundamental importance to athletes and their ability to separate the positive aspects of stress from the negatives is the distinction between mental stress and physiological or training stresses. Physical discomfort and fatigue associated with training are inherent in sport and must not be a source of mental stress. Increased physical fitness will act as a barrier to the negative consequences of undue mental stress.

The channeling of mental stress by the athlete from that of a limiting condition into a positive force can take a number of directions; an entire body of science, sport psychology, has evolved to assist the sports world in better understanding the principles underlying the control of mental stress in athletes. Most sport psychology techniques used to harness the energy of mental stress center on the ability of the athlete to focus on the event to the exclusion of all other thoughts and distractions. Catch phrases such as "blocking out pressure," "getting into the zone," and "positive self-talk" are tools employed by athletes to put their mind in an optimum position to assist the body.

Simulation is an important stress-defending mechanism, useful in many athletic disciplines. When athletes know the obstacles to be faced in a particular event, their stress over performance will generally be reduced. It is also important for an athlete to appreciate that the strengthening of one's abilities to counter the harmful consequences of mental stress is not an instantaneous process; stress-channeling strategies take time to develop and require experience in their execution, in the same way that an athlete develops motor skills.

SEE ALSO Hormones; Nervous system; Sport psychology.

# Metabolic response

A metabolic response is any reaction by the body to a specific influence or impact. Metabolism is a general term describing the organic process in any cellular structure. A metabolic response can occur with respect to individual cells, a gland, an organ, or a process such as the cardiovascular system. Metabolism is often understood in terms of the metabolic rate, which is the amount of energy expended by the body in a given period. Metabolic response, when stated without reference to a specific action, is a neutral term; metabolic responses occur and may be correspondingly assessed or measured in respect of a wide variety of circumstances.

Metabolism is a variable in the assessment of human performance. Metabolic function is subject to such individual factors as age, heredity, gender, level of physical fitness, and others. It is also well understood that while metabolisms are unique in every individual, there are certain generalizations regarding body types and structures that can be used in any consideration of metabolic function.

There are three general body types, also known as somatotypes, that have a specific metabolic function, namely ectomorphs, mesomorphs, and endomorphs. An ectomorph is a person with a generally slim, light build, with a faster metabolic function that makes it generally difficult to both gain weight and build muscle. A mesomorph is a more solid, muscular build, one that tends to be suited to explosive movements and contact sports. The mesomorphic build is usually associated with a moderate metabolism. An endomorph is a person with a shorter, more rounded and thicker frame, often with a higher percentage of body fat, who usually has a slower metabolic function. Most persons have a body type that is a blend of two or all three of these body types.

The body may exhibit a metabolic response to any type of external factor or change. Some common metabolic responses to different stimuli received by the body are improved physical performance, an ability to synthesize proteins, weight change, and response to injury.

Changes in diet or nutritional practices are used to achieve an improvement in a physical attribute or capability. Athletes often tinker with their diet by means of both foods and dietary supplements to assist in achieving improvements in their performance. Diet alone can significantly influence the physical performance of an athlete. As a single factor or agent for change, diet will not improve athletic performance; it will permit athletic improvement to occur through its support of more intensive physical training, while reducing the risks of both injury and illness. Diet will also facilitate changes in the manner in which the body processes particular proteins, as the effect of exercise on systems such as protein synthesis into muscle continues beyond the extent of the particular training period.

When a diet is altered from a traditional balanced ratio of approximately 60% to 65% carbohydrates, 12% to 15% protein, and less than 30% fat to one of greater fat composition, a prominent metabolic response is the generation of a greater number of low density lipoproteins (LDLs), a form of cholesterol that contributes to reduced cardiovascular function and long-term arterial disease.

The manipulation of diet may also achieve a metabolic response with respect to how the body uses its stores of carbohydrates and fats for the production of energy.

The most common desired metabolic response through diet is that of either weight gain or weight loss. A significant industry has grown around the sale of products that are described as metabolic response modifiers, all of which profess to modify the user's metabolism to stimulate weight loss. The efficacy of these products is not well established. If an athlete consumes a reduced number of calories through the diet, and the athlete does not alter his or her particular pattern of physical activity, the metabolic response will be weight loss. When an athlete seeks to build muscle and adds a protein supplement to the diet, in concert with a specific weight training routine, the athlete will expect to gain some desired muscle. An undesirable metabolic response may occur if the athlete consumes excessive amounts of protein in the training diet, causing the formation of acids that tend to interfere in normal bone function, making the athlete a long-term subject for reduced bone density and osteoporosis.

An injury or illness produces a pronounced metabolic response. A significant trauma to the body will trigger a "fight or flight" response, which will trigger the production of the hormone adrenaline. The perceived threat to the body will also initiate an increase in the body's energy demands, reflected in increased body heat and an increased rate of conversion of glucose from glycogen.

Changes in the physical intensity of athletic activity, either by training practices or competitive schedule, will generate a metabolic response. This response is particularly evident when assessing the nature of muscle composition in an athlete. When an athlete seeks to improve endurance ability, the training program will correspondingly focus on endurance exercise. The muscle groups involved in the generation of power in the exercise, each with a set pattern of distribution between fast-twitch and slow-twitch fibers, will respond by making a slight adaptation in which more fast-twitch fibers are utilized for the muscle.

Overtraining will produce the metabolic response of decreased immune system function, among other possible responses.

**SEE ALSO** Diet; Muscle protein synthesis; Nutrition.

## Middle distance running SEE
Running: Middle distance events

## George Lawrence Mikan

6/18/1924–6/1/2005
AMERICAN
PROFESSIONAL BASKETBALL PLAYER

In modern basketball, a 6 ft 10 in, 245 lb (2.09 m, 110 kg) center is something of a rarity—most National Basketball League players at that position are taller and much heavier. George Mikan, the man who revolutionized center play in the late 1940s and early 1950s, would be unlikely to succeed at his fabled position today. Like all athletes who truly changed the way in which their sport was played, Mikan, the 6 ft 10 in giant of his day, blazed a trail that all modern post players have followed.

When George Mikan first gave serious consideration to playing college basketball, many observers believed him to be too tall and ungainly for the speed and intricate passing systems then employed by most college teams. Mikan enrolled at DePaul University, where he was coached by the legendary Ray Meyer

(1914–2006). Meyer saw a potential offensive weapon in the relatively slow and ungainly Mikan, and he worked with Mikan relentlessly to build the big man's overall fitness and agility. Meyer ran Mikan through a variety of individual drills to develop his coordination. Mikan was made to skip rope, shadow box, run various distances both inside the gymnasium and out, a training program that was unheard of for large basketball players at that time. Most importantly with respect to Mikan's long term impact on basketball, Meyer had Mikan spend countless hours practicing hook shots, using both his left and his right hands. Mikan also worked on the offensive rebounding techniques that Meyer believed Mikan would be able to employ using his size and reach.

This series of shooting and footwork drills evolved into a sequence known universally among modern basketball coaches as the Mikan drill. The long hours of practice paid off as Mikan's footwork continued to improve through out his college career.

When Mikan enrolled at DePaul, the National Collegiate Athletic Association, (NCAA) of which DePaul was a member, prohibited freshmen from playing varsity sports. This three-year eligibility rule correspondingly limited Mikan to a three-year university playing career. In those three seasons Mikan established himself as the greatest force ever to play at the NCAA level until that time. In his junior and senior years, he led the NCAA in scoring. Mikan helped DePaul to an 81–17 record during the course of his university career.

Mikan's dominance at DePaul also spurred the first basketball rule amendment directed specifically at his ability to change the game. In 1945, the NCAA instituted a goaltending rule, to prohibit a defensive player from either touching the ball when shot by an offensive player at any time on its downward arc towards the basket, or from playing the ball in any way to sweep it from the basket if the ball was on or inside the rim of the basket. Mikan had been a force with his shot blocking prior to the rule change; he remained very effective at altering the manner in which the opposing player shot the ball after the new rule was instituted.

Professional basketball in the United States in 1946 was composed of a number of small and struggling leagues, each battling to survive. Mikan was the greatest possible gate attraction that any league could possibly secure at that time, as he was the best-known college player in the United States. In 1946 Mikan signed his first professional contract with the Chicago Gears of the National Basketball League (NBL); his contract provided a then astounding

$25,000 signing bonus, with a further $12,000 per season for five years. After winning the league championship in 1947, the Gears promptly folded, and Mikan was selected by the Minneapolis Lakers of the NBL in a dispersal draft.

Mikan would remain with the Lakers for seven seasons, as the Lakers joined the Basketball Association of America (BAA) in 1948, ultimately moving to the National Basketball Association (NBA) in 1949. It is a remarkable sidebar to the history of George Mikan that the Minneapolis Lakers' NBA championship in 1950 was the third title won by the Lakers in three years, each in a different professional league.

Through the 1954 season, Mikan continued to be one of the dominant players in the NBA. He regularly placed among the top five players in every scoring statistical category. Mikan was at the peak of his basketball powers when in 1954, he announced his retirement from basketball, citing a desire to quit while he was still at the top of his game. Mikan decided to pursue the practice of law.

Mikan's legacy in professional basketball includes the institution of two further rule changes. When Mikan commenced his professional career, the key, the lane that runs from the circle that encompasses the free throw line, extending underneath the backboard to the baseline, was six feet wide (1.8 m). Mikan would position himself at the edge of the key (as an offensive player was permitted stand inside the key for a maximum of three seconds), using his size to gain a significant advantage against a defender, as the tall Mikan and his remarkable hook shot ability was positioned only three or four feet from the basket. The effectiveness of this technique, known in basketball as establishing a post up position, was reduced when the NBA widened the key to 12 ft (3.6 m), to take Mikan further from the basket when he posted up.

The second rule change, the institution of a 24 second clock, was made by the NBA in 1954, in an effort to speed the pace of the game and to force teams to shoot within the prescribed period. Mikan influenced the introduction of this change, as a team lacking a large dominating center such as Mikan could slow the game to a crawl by holding the ball, controlling the tempo and keeping the big post player out of the game, as Fort Wayne did to Mikan's Lakers in a game in 1950. Fort Wayne stalled the entire game to negate the threat of Mikan. The institution of the 24 second clock was an innovation that helped establish the NBA as an exciting spectator product.

Mikan never really left basketball after his retirement as a player. He served as the Lakers general manager in the 1955–1956 season, and he unsuccessfully coached the Lakers during the first half of the 1957–1958 season. When the now-defunct American Basketball Association (ABA) organized in 1967, Mikan accepted an offer to become the league's first commissioner, a position he held for two years. The ABA was noteworthy for the development of stars such as Julius (Dr. J) Erving and Dan Issell, as well as the introduction of a red, white, and blue basketball.

Mikan was named the greatest player of the first half of the twentieth century. He was also named as one of the 50 greatest players in the history of the NBA in 1996. At the time of his death in 2005, Mikan was lauded by numerous other greats of the game for his enduring contributions to basketball. Shaquille O'Neal paid for Mikan' funeral in tribute to Mikan' influence on the career of O'Neal and other great centers. Hall of Fame players Bill Walton and Kareem Abdul Jabbar both credited Mikan in their own progression to basketball stardom.

**SEE ALSO** Basketball; Basketball shot dynamics; Basketball: Slam dunk; Basketball: Strength and training exercises.

# Patrick Miley

5/10/1958–
SCOTTISH
SWIM COACH

Patrick Miley, a helicopter pilot and amateur swim coach, developed a prototypical swim rate monitoring device that he named the Aquapacer in the mid-1990s.

One of the fixed principles of swim training is that to improve swimming speed, the swimmer must increase either stroke length or stroke rate while maintaining the other at its current level. Stroke rate improvement engages a number of possible training techniques, including methods of reinforcing fixed stroke rates through training. In a long workout, it is sometimes a difficult proposition for the swimmer to maintain a desired stroke if the athlete is fatigued or otherwise loses focus. The Aquapacer technology represented a breakthrough in training stroke maintenance.

By 2000 Miley had developed a comprehensive training aid by which a coach could program a central control mechanism to convey signals to swimmers as they trained, using a receiver the swimmer attaches to a swim cap or goggles. The receiver then signals the stroke rate to the swimmer.

The rate can be varied during the workout to permit the swimmer to engage in tempo training.

The Aquapacer's usefulness as a swimming training aid was cemented at the 2000 Olympics in Sydney, where 30% of the gold medal winners in swimming used the Aquapacer in training.

The Aquapacer is regarded as an excellent motivational tool for swim training because, much like an electronic metronome in music, the swimmer is required to keep pace. Although developed with elite level athletes in mind, the Aquapacer market has expanded to include Masters age swimmers and recreational swimmers who wish assistance in maintaining a consistent stroke pace as they complete their workouts.

In its latest version, the Aquapacer is manufactured as a multiple receiver unit, where a number of receivers can be programmed for the use of different swimmers at the same time. The Aquapacer is also available as a single unit that is programmed and attached to the swimmer's goggles or cap. In addition to its use as a stroke rate training aid, the Aquapacer can be employed to assist in assessing the fitness level of a particular athlete or the speed with which an athlete may be recovering from an injury.

SEE ALSO Biofeedback; Swimming.

## Hinda Miller

1950–
AMERICAN
FITNESS CLOTHING DESIGNER, DISTANCE RUNNER

Hinda Miller was the co-developer of the Jogbra, one of the truly iconic items in the history of women's fashion. In 1977, Miller was a Vermont clothing designer who had taken up distance running for fitness. Miller and two other women were searching for a solution to the problems they were encountering with respect to being able to run comfortably. Miller and other women found that without adequate support for their breasts, the natural rhythm of the running motion created significant strain on the supportive tissues of their breasts, as well as friction created by the outer apparel against their nipples and other sensitive skin.

Miller and her colleagues designed a bra that was modeled to a certain degree after the features of the male athletic supporter. The bra that Miller designed was fashioned with external seams only, appearing when worn as if it were inside out. In this fashion,

Miller greatly reduced the effect of friction from the outer garment to the skin of the breast. The design also permitted the breasts to be held in a much more stable position, so as to reduce the excessive movement that was cumbersome for female runners who wished to run more quickly and efficiently. The Jogbra was a design that served as an example of the dictum, "form follows function."

The Jogbra was almost an instant commercial success. Miller saw her design and the resulting appeal of the garment as a feminist statement, an article of clothing that served to empower women by making athletic participation much easier. Miller served as the president of Jogbra until 1990, when the company was sold to the multinational women's apparel manufacturer, Playtex. Miller subsequently parlayed her commercial success with the Jogbra into a political career; Miller was elected a state senator in Vermont for the first time in 2002.

A version of the original Jogbra is displayed at the Smithsonian Institute, Washington, D.C., as an example of twentieth century technology. The Jogbra was the first example of the garments now known generally as sports bras, an industry that has grown in direct proportion to the increased participation of women in athletics generally since 1977.

SEE ALSO Musculoskeletal injuries; Women's sport clothing and protective equipment.

## Minerals

Minerals are the inorganic elements that are required for a number of essential human functions. Minerals take their name from the fact that in their natural state, these are substances capable of being mined from the ground. The minerals relied on by the body in its natural processes are distinct from the organic compounds within the body, each of which has one of carbon, hydrogen, nitrogen, or oxygen, alone or in combined compositions.

Minerals are primarily absorbed into the body through the foods consumed in the typical human diet. As minerals are a part of the soil where plants are grown and cultivated, minerals become a part of the formation of the cellular structure of most plants that are directly harvested for food; plant minerals are also present in the feeds consumed by animals that are subsequently used for human food.

Minerals are utilized by the body in many different ways, both in the growth and the sustenance of the musculoskeletal structure, as well as in the effective function of the systems that carry out the operations of the body. Minerals play an indispensable role in many aspects of human function including: bone and tooth formation, construction, and maintenance; skin, tissue, and internal organ function; the transmission of messages through the central nervous system into the peripheral nervous system, the muscle function directed by the somatic and autonomic nervous systems; blood function and heartbeat regulation within the cardiovascular system; and aid to the digestion and the conversion of foods into energy sources.

Minerals are classified as one of two subtypes: macrominerals, which are those nutrients that the body requires in a minimum amount of 200 mg per day as a recommended daily allowance (RDA), and microminerals, which are often as important as macronutrients, but are required in trace amounts of a RDA less than 200 mg per day. The most notable macrominerals are calcium, chlorine, magnesium, phosphorus, potassium, sodium, and sulphur. The chief microminerals are cobalt, iodine, iron, and zinc.

Calcium is the most productive mineral in the body, essential to bone and tooth construction. It is also present in a lesser capacity in the bloodstream, where it influences the mechanism of blood clotting. Calcium is an important component in the transmission of nerve impulses and resulting muscle contractions controlled by neurons. Calcium is most commonly found in dairy products, but many green vegetables are also a source of this mineral. Calcium is absorbed into the body through the companion action of vitamin D, a fat-soluble compound. Phosphorus is found in dairy products, and it is a mineral that is also chiefly related to the development and construction of bones, possessing a similar linkage to vitamin D as that of calcium. Phosphorus is a mineral that is present throughout the entire human body by virtue of its presence in the nucleic acid that forms a part of every cell.

Magnesium is a mineral whose chemical influence is exhibited across a range of human function, as it is also present in all human cells. Ingested through plant products such as nuts and soy beans, magnesium is a necessary component in the metabolism of carbohydrates and proteins.

Sodium is a another of the omnipresent minerals. Sodium is primarily found in table salt, in the form of sodium chloride, as well as in green vegetables such as spinach. Sodium, as an electrolyte (a metal capable of transmitting an electrical charge), is essential to the body's ability to maintain homeostasis, or ongoing balance of both its fluid levels, through kidney function, as well as the ability of the muscles to respond to signals directed to them from the central nervous system and the brain. Potassium has a similar chemical composition and a companion effect on muscle function. Potassium is also an essential part of the regulation of heartbeat, as well as the metabolism of carbohydrates. Beans, whole grains, and bananas are the most abundant sources of potassium in the diet.

Chlorine is a substance found in various bodily fluids, where it assists in the maintenance of the balance between acids and bases in the body known as the pH balance. Chlorine is of particular utility in the stomach and the digestive processes through its contributions to the formation of the stomach acids used to break down foods. Chlorine is primarily obtained through the chloride component of table salt.

Sulphur is a mineral that is employed by the body as a component in the formation of the proteins used to build muscle. Sulphur is also an agent in the various detoxification processes centered in the liver. Sulphur is usually significant in foods that are a part of the protein group in the human diet, including eggs, some meats, and some varieties of beans.

The microminerals are ingested into the body in vastly smaller quantities than many of the macrominerals, but the importance of micromineral function is out of proportion to the quantities of these minerals. Iron is an essential component of hemoglobin, which permits the red blood cells of the cardiovascular system to transport oxygen. Cobalt is a vital aspect to the function of vitamin $B_{12}$, a part of the vitamin B complex. Iodine, often added to table salt, is essential to thyroid gland function and the production of growth hormone. Zinc, in addition to assisting in general cell growth, is a constituent of insulin, the hormone essential to the regulation of glucose in the bloodstream.

**SEE ALSO** Calcium; Diet; Magnesium; Nutrition.

# Modern pentathlon

The modern pentathlon is the only sport specifically invented for inclusion in the Olympic Games. The founder of the modern Games, Baron de Coubertin of France, created the modern pentathlon as an embodiment of everything demanded of a true Olympian: athleticism, strength, grace, finesse, and coordination. De Coubertin determined that this event would have five distinct components, which

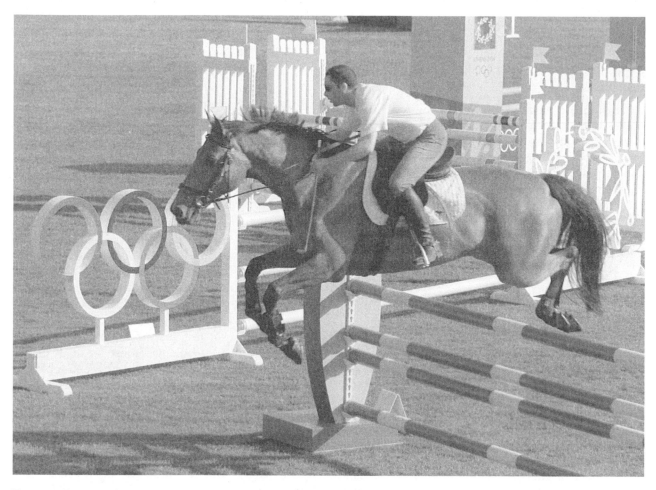

The equestrian event (horse riding) is one of the five events in the Olympic modern pentathlon. © MIKE BLAKE/REUTERS/CORBIS

symbolized the five rings of the Olympic emblem and the five corresponding continents of the Olympic movement. The modern pentathlon begins with a pistol shooting competition, followed by epee (a type of fencing), swimming, equestrian (a horse jumping competition), and concluding with a cross-country running race.

In the ancient Olympics, the pentathlon was a significantly different competition. There were a series of events within each of the disciplines that formed the pentathlon contest. The three running events ranged from a sprint of approximately 200 yd (200 m) to a race of over 1 mi (1.5 km) in length. A jumping event, discus, and the javelin were included, as was an equestrian competition. Wrestling, boxing, and a primitive form of martial arts, *pankration*, were also included in the pentathlon at various times throughout the history of the ancient Olympics.

De Coubertin, who served as president of the International Olympic Committee from 1896 until

1925, was a staunch advocate of the event, believing it to symbolize the ideals of the ancient Games. De Coubertin was successful in securing the inclusion of the pentathlon into the Olympics of 1912, strictly as a men's competition, and it has remained an Olympic event since that time. A women's pentathlon was added in 1980. The disciplines that comprise the modern pentathlon are so disparate that few modern athletes embrace the sport, relative to the popularity of most other Olympic sports; the modern pentathlon is not contested with any public fanfare outside of each Olympic Games.

The five events of the pentathlon are contested in a single-day format. The opening event, the shooting competition, is conducted by way of each athlete firing a 4.5 mm air pistol at a stationary target positioned 11 yd (10 m) away. Twenty shots are fired at 20 targets during this period, and each shot is scored relative to the center of the target. The second pentathlon event is the epee fencing event, which is conducted as a round robin tournament; every athlete fights one fencing bout with every other athlete entered in the event. A victory in each segment of the round robin is counted toward the athlete's ultimate score.

Swimming is in many respects the most important part of the pentathlon competition, as the physical techniques essential to swimming success are usually acquired at a younger age than those that can be taught to an athlete in all other pentathlon disciplines. The swim is a 200-m freestyle event, and the time achieved by each competitor is scored on a ranking system. It is common for successful pentathletes to enter the sport from a competitive swimming background.

The equestrian portion of the pentathlon requires each horse and rider to negotiate a course with 15 jumps each 4 ft (1.2 m) in height, stationed at various intervals around a course that must measure between 350 m and 450 m in length. As with a regular Olympic equestrian event, a missed jump is subject to a deduction from the overall score of the athlete. Each athlete must compete on a horse randomly selected by the event organizers.

Unlike any other multi-sport event, the cross-country running portion of the pentathlon represents both a race and an opportunity to salvage victory or an improved placing through the manner in which the race is conducted. The cross-country race is handicapped based on the standing of the athletes in the first four events. A time for the 3,000-m course that is less than the established standard gives the athlete a points bonus. The runners leave the starting line in the order of their standing going into the final event, creating the visual incentive for the trailing athletes to catch the runners ahead of them.

It was the dream of de Coubertin to create the quintessential Olympic event through the modern pentathlon. There is no question that the pentathlon is a demanding discipline, due largely to the diverse events. The five events are a classic depiction of an athletic ideal; they are also a sporting eccentricity, especially in light of the relative rarity of equestrians, fencers, and target shooters to the bulk of the modern sporting population. The modern pentathlon is in many ways the ultimate cross training challenge, from the endurance and technique of swimming and running, to the rarefied skills necessary to succeed in the shooting, riding, and fencing events.

**SEE ALSO** Cross training; Decathlon; Ironman competitions.

# Mormon tea

Herbs are a part of the plant world that have been harvested by many cultures for thousands of years. Herbal products, usually the leaves, roots, and fruit that possessed specific reviving and recuperative qualities, were processed into useful medicines and dietary supplements. The plant known as Mormon tea is one of the best known of the herbal medicines to be created by the North American native cultures and the later arriving settlers and frontiers people of the American West.

Mormon tea is a part of the family of plants known by their botanical name, *ephedra*. A green bush that grows in thin, spiky branches, ephedra grows in a number of variants across Europe, central Asia, and in pockets of both North and South America. Mormon tea is closely related in its structure and its chemical composition to ephedra, also known as *ma huang*, one of the important herbs used in the traditional Chinese medicines in use for many centuries. In every place in the world where an ephedra species has grown, an indigenous culture discovered its medicinal properties and employed them in a variety of ways.

Mormon tea exists in a number of species and it grows in reasonable abundance in the semiarid plains of the part of the North American continent that includes the states of Arizona, New Mexico, and Utah. It acquired the name Mormon tea because the beverage that was made from the steeping of the dried stems of the ephedra plant in boiling water was deemed not to violate the rules of the Church of Latter Day Saints (Mormon), whose people began to settle in what is now Utah in the mid-nineteenth century; Mormon people were forbidden from consuming caffeine. In other parts of the American West, the beverages brewed from the ephedra plant were known by equally colorful names: desert tea, squaw tea, and whorehouse tea.

The irony of the name Mormon tea is found in the chemistry of the plant and the corresponding attributes of the tea made from its leaves, which possesses stimulant properties that exceed those of caffeine. The active ingredient that made Mormon tea prized by the native cultures that came before the Mormon settlers is ephedrine and its close chemical cousin, pseudo-ephedrine. These chemicals are present in varying amounts in Mormon tea, depending on the variety of the plant. Both ephedrine and pseudo-ephedrine are stimulants that have pronounced effects on the central nervous system.

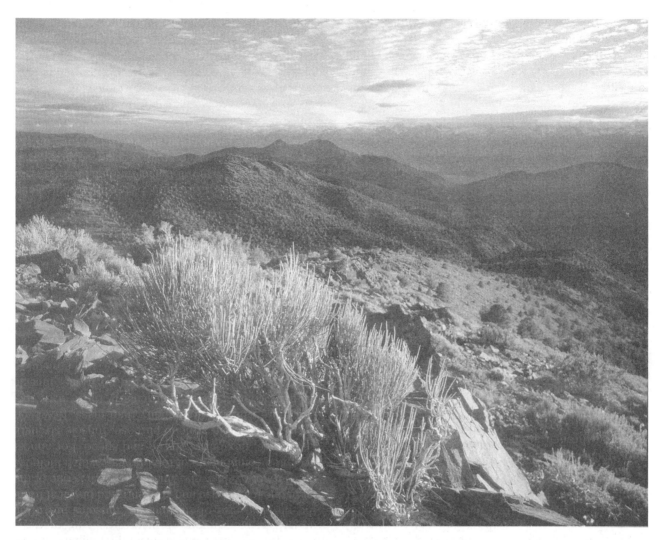

Mormon tea plant. © DAVID MUENCH/CORBIS

Ephedrine is proven to influence aspects of human function such as: increasing heart rate and blood pressure; functioning as a bronchodilator, a substance that tends to provide relief from breathing problems such as asthma through action on the bronchial passages; heightening and stimulating powers of concentration; assisting in combating fatigue.

Ephedrine and the herbal products that contain it were not well known outside of the holistic medicine community until the 1970s. Two developments cast greater public interest on the uses of ephedra products. Athletes began to consume supplements that contained ephedra in greater numbers to take advantage of the stimulant qualities of ephedrine. It was determined that significant competitive advantage was derived from ephedra consumption, and any ephedrine and pseudo-ephedrine products were banned in both Olympic as well as most international

athletic events. The World Anti-Doping Agency (WADA) bans both substances if they are present in amounts greater than 10 mcg per milliliter in the urine or the blood of an athlete when tested.

In sports leagues that have not yet placed themselves under the authority of all aspects of the WADA Anti-Doping Code, synthetic forms of ephedrine and pseudo-ephedrine, often in the form of a decongestant, are often consumed immediately prior to competition by athletes seeking its stimulant qualities. National Hockey League (NHL) players have attracted widespread attention to this practice in the years following 2000.

The second aspect to the rise in the notoriety of all ephedra products was the composition of dietary supplements, especially those promoted by the weight loss industry. As with all stimulants, the increase in heart rate and blood pressure tends to act as an appetite suppressant. After significant controversy, the United States Food and Drug Administration (FDA) banned the use of all ephedra ingredients in U.S.-manufactured supplements in 2004. The FDA concluded that ephedrine had a significant role in increasing the risk of heart attack in the users of ephedra products.

For athletes who use supplements with natural ingredients, the risk of inadvertently ingesting ephedrine or pseudo-ephedrine remains significant. Ephedra plant products continue to be mixed into supplements that are manufactured outside of the United States. The testing and third-party scientific analysis of natural diet and nutritional supplements are not usually as rigorous as that conducted in the pharmaceutical industry.

SEE ALSO Dietary supplements; Ephedra; Herbs; Stimulants; Supplement contamination.

# Motion, range of SEE Range of motion

# Motivational techniques

Motivation is the stimulus given to athletes to continue with and improve in their chosen sport. Motivation can come from a number of sources: coaches, teammates, supporters, and self-help methods can all be effective means of motivating an athlete to perform.

Motivational techniques are an aspect of the broader branch of sports science known as sports psychology. The mental aspects of sport are now understood to be essential to athletic success. Sports psychology traces its roots to the work of an Indiana University professor in the early 1900s, Norman Triplett, who made a connection between the performance of cyclists who rode alone versus those who rode in groups of two or more.

The effective motivation of athletes is an essential aspect to success in sports of every kind. The motivational requirements of every athlete are as unique as the athlete themselves. The first factor in the assessment of how an athlete may be effectively motivated is the nature of the sport played. As an example, a sport that involves repeated physical contact such as rugby or American football places entirely different stresses on both the mind and the body than does tennis or cross-country running.

The motivation of a team will often differ from that of the individual athlete; teams possess a unique collective athletic personality.

The level of athletic competition is often an important factor as to how the team or athlete can be motivated to perform at their highest level. A team that competes at an international level may possess different dynamics than those present in the members of a youth league team.

The skill level of the athlete, the gender of the athlete, and the age and the relative sophistication of the athlete are all factors as to how the subject athletes can be effectively motivated. The Hollywood style coach, screaming and neck veins bulging, who delivers a "blood and guts," "win one for the Gipper" emotional speech does not have a place in every locker room.

The nature of the training and the competitive seasons in which the sport occurs is also influences the motivational approaches to be taken. The periodization of training is the concept that provides for the division of an athletic year into components, the best known of which are the preseason, competitive season, and the off-season, all of which may be the subject of more finite divisions. The motivational techniques to successfully encourage an athlete to train effectively over an extended period of preseason work or to steer the athlete towards an upcoming competitive schedule are not necessarily the same approaches used to stimulate a best effort on race day or game day.

Motivation is rarely successful as a one-time instrument. Successful motivational techniques are built on the relationship between the athlete and the person seeking to motivate the athlete, usually a coach. If the coach does not know the athlete well, the athlete will not inherently trust the words of the prospective motivator. If the athlete senses that the motivational tools are not sincere or that they are directed to some ulterior purpose, the motivation will fall flat.

Knowledge of the athlete and the existence of a trust relationship between coach and athlete will permit the coach to understand what it is about their athlete's unique personality that will permit motivation to occur. This knowledge will take the coach and the athlete to the activation point, that region of the athlete's persona that will trigger a best effort. Through the relationship, a coach, for example, will know if the athlete (or the team) responds to a visceral challenge, or whether the motivation question is best approached on a more intellectual footing.

Long-term motivation, the practices that are emphasized day to day through the athletic season, often are based on goal setting. The ultimate goal for an athlete may be to compete at an Olympic Games

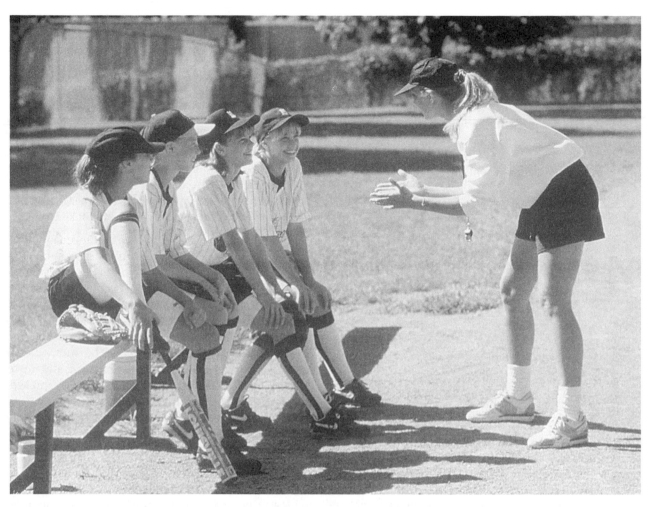

What works to motivate one team, may not work successfully for another. © ED BOCK/CORBIS

five years hence; the intermediate goals may center on intermediate competitions, and the short-term goals may involve setting a personal training best in the discipline two months in the future. Each motivational goal is a progression that bears a logical connection to the next target. Many athletes have failed to continue with sports where the goals set were either unrealistic or were ill-considered.

With the concept of goal setting comes the notion of reward as a motivator. In elite-level competitors, the pursuit of a lucrative professional career and monetary reward is often a powerful motivator. For recreational athletes, the motivation to complete a tough workout when the athlete is fatigued may result in a reward of a day off from training or an indulgence such as a rich meal that is not normally permitted in the athlete's diet.

The management of stress and its impacts on the athlete are an important aspect of motivational tech-

niques. The ability to overcome the pressures of competition, or the effects of external environmental factors such as family, educational, or employment pressures will often be determined by the ability of the athlete to be motivated beyond the stressful factors to a mental state where the athletic activity is of primary importance.

Successful athletes are able to motivate themselves to perform. For some, this is an innate part of their psychological makeup, and they might only require coaching direction as to how to keep motivated to perform. The technique of positive self-talk that reinforces with upbeat self-analysis and self-imagery is one of a number of ways that the individual athlete can strive to remain focused on training and competition.

SEE ALSO Mental stress; Sport performance; Sport psychology.

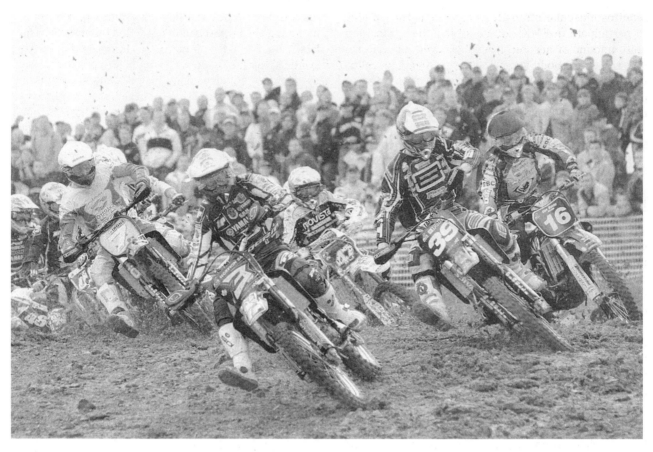

Motorbike (motorcycle) race in Belgium. JOHN THYS/AFP/GETTY IMAGES

# Motocross or Moto X

Motocross (also known as Moto X) is a form of motor cycle racing that originally took place on trails and off road venues. Motocross machines tend to be much lighter with a smaller engine displacement than conventional street motorcycles. The motocross machines are designed to be both maneuverable over rough terrain and constructed to absorb the significant forces created by the motorcycle's contact with the terrain.

Motocross races are organized according to classifications determined by the engine size of the machine. The first motocross races were held in England prior to 1930, in events known as "scrambles." The international motorcycle sports governing body, Federation Internationale Motocycliste (FIM), sanctioned the first ever motocross events in 1947. In the late 1960s, the first North American motocross events were held.

A typical outdoor motocross race course is between 1.0 and 1.5 mi (1.5 km to 2.5 km) in length. Most courses are built from a combination of natural terrain and man made alterations to the track to make it as demanding as desired by the organizer.

A modern variation of motocross is Super Cross, where the riders compete on a circuit artificially constructed inside a sports stadium. The Super Cross course is a series of irregular curves, artificial mounds and straightaways, with the riders seeking to complete a fixed number of laps in the shortest period of time.

Motocross has a similar interest in continuous technological improvement common to all sports where machinery places a key role. The largest of the motocross motorcycles have engines with a displacement of approximately 550 cc, supported by a structure that weighs less than 250 lb (115 kg). This combination of relatively powerful engine, light frame, and very strong suspension permit the machines to operate at high speeds.

Riding an FMX machine in competition is an extremely strenuous and physically demanding activity. The control of the motorcycle, both as it is operated at full speed as well as through jumps and turns requires muscular strength and stamina. The training to participate in FMX riding will include a considerable amount of aerobic fitness, as well as ensuring that the entire body subjected to stretching and flexibility training. The lumbar (low back) of the rider is particularly susceptible to strain due to the impact directed into that region through jump landings.

**SEE ALSO** Extreme sports; Motorcycle Racing.

# Motor control

Motor control is a broad term that describes the general ability of a person to initiate and direct muscle function and voluntary movements. Motor control is a concept that is distinct from the many involuntary muscle actions of the body, such as shivering when cold or flinching when an object is directed at a person without warning. A related expression, "motor skills," refers to the ability to perform specific physical movements; motor control is also the acquisition and development of a series of distinct motor skills.

Motor control is divided into two subsets. Gross motor control is the ability of a human to move a large muscle group or segment of the anatomy; the waving of an arm is an example of this type of movement. Fine motor control is the ability to manipulate precise movement, such as handwriting. All motor control is an integrated product of three aspects of the human anatomy: muscles, bones, and the central nervous system.

The voluntary motor system, also known as the somatic nervous system, is the structure that permits and creates motor control. The system takes its name from the part of the brain known as the motor cortex, from which the signals to initiate movement originate. The impulse from the motor cortex travels along pathways through the brainstem into the spinal cord. The nerve cells of the spinal cord connect to a vast and intricate network to control the skeletal muscle movement. Motor neurons, the specialized mechanisms that communicate to the muscles, are a continuation from the nerve roots that branch out from each vertebra in the spinal column to the muscle over which control is required. There are a number of pathways essential to the function of the voluntary motor system, of which the pyramidal system is the best known and the most extensive.

The voluntary, or somatic, motor system that provides the body with motor control is in contrast to the autonomic system, which begins with the regulation directed by the distinct regions of the brain, including the hypothalamus. The hypothalamus regulates the function of many of the essential bodily systems, including heart rate, blood pressure, and electrolytic balance. The hypothalamus communicates much of its direction to these involuntary structures by way of the chemical signals, hormones, that are directed to the glandular network headed by the thyroid gland.

Every healthy person will be capable of both gross motor control and fine motor control. In many sports, athletic success is measured in the fine distinctions between athletes in terms of their coordination (particularly their hand-eye coordination), balance, and overall body control. Many aspects of motor control are hereditary; others are linked to the body type of the individual. As an example, a 5 ft 10 in (1.7 m) point guard on a basketball team is expected to be able to execute complex physical movements, such as dribbling the ball with either hand at full speed under defensive pressure. The 6 ft 10 in (2 m) basketball forward is not likely to be able to move with the same grace and speed as the guard. With practice, the taller and less coordinated athlete could achieve improvements in this particular skill, but it is unlikely that he or she could surpass the smaller and quicker player.

Body type and heredity aside, all athletes have the capacity to improve their motor control through the practice and the repetition of distinct motor skills. In many sports, the drills that form the basis of improved motor control ability are collateral to the sport itself. Cross training techniques are often employed to enhance a particular motor ability that is desired for a sport in an athlete. A notable example is the use of jumping rope in sports such as boxing; the repeated coordination of the athlete's footwork and hands in the act of skipping improves the athlete's overall coordination. American football has a time-honored training technique where players are required to move at full speed while negotiating a series of tires placed in a pattern; this drill builds the ability of the body to coordinate a jump vertically with a movement laterally to avoid falling into the obstacle, a non-contact simulation of the agile movements required on the playing field.

"Muscle memory" is a muscular attribute linked to the development of motor skills. When an athlete is sidelined from an activity due to injury, the athlete will return more quickly to his or her previous level of motor ability due to the memory preserved in the nervous system as to how the motion stressed the subject muscle or structure.

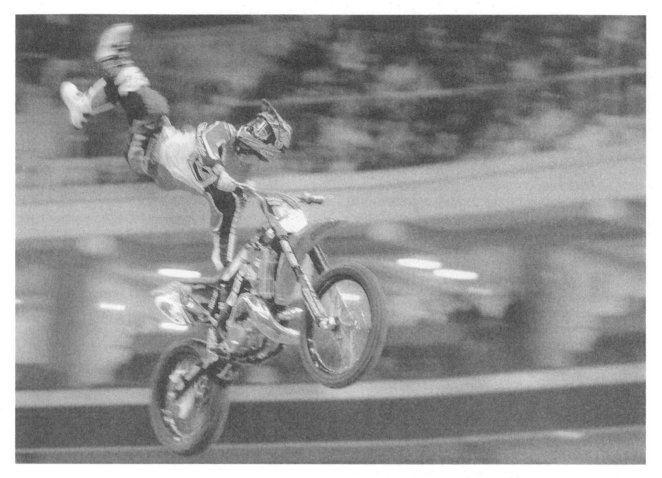

Competitor at Monster Jam freestyle motocross event. MICHAL CIZEK/AFP/GETTY IMAGES

A physical injury to any aspect of the voluntary motor system will impair motor control. A concussion or damage to the spine or spinal column is a frequent cause of such injuries. When a nerve becomes pinched or otherwise damaged through trauma, such as a carpal tunnel nerve fracture in the wrist, the pathway for the major nerve ending into the muscles of the hand, there will be similar limitations of movement.

Motor control can be significantly impaired though stresses imposed on other bodily systems. When athletes become dehydrated, they will commonly sustain an imbalance in their electrolyte levels, particularly that of the mineral sodium. A sodium deficiency will impair the ability of a nervous system transmission to be communicated to the working muscle.

**SEE ALSO** Hormones; Nervous system; Sport performance.

## Motorcycle: Freestyle

Freestyle motorcycle, or FMX, is another activity classed as an extreme sport. FMX riders do not race their machines; the motorcycles are used to perform a variety of stunts and trick riding, often at both significant speeds as well as involving an aerial component. FMX competitions became popular when this sport was added to the lineup of the annual X Games, the international extreme sports competition.

FMX is a competitive sport where riders are judged subjectively on the quality of the tricks performed. However, as with any of the extreme sports categories, the emphasis is not placed upon competition so much as it is focused upon the personal challenge to the rider of taking the activity where it had never gone previously. A leading example of the successful FMX rider is Travis Partrana (b. 1983) of the United States, who was the first FMX rider to land a back flip on a motorcycle in competition, where the motorcycle does a single revolution on its

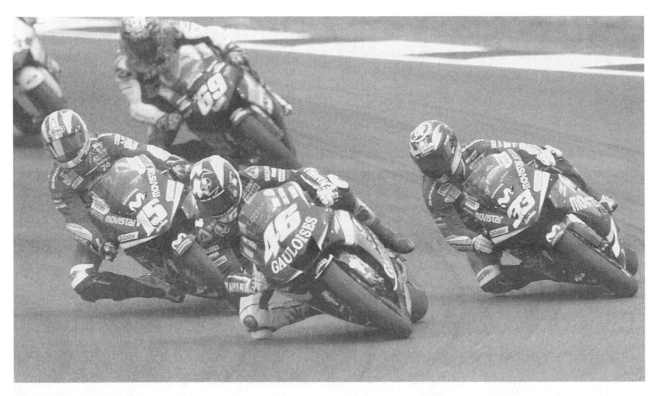

Competitors in the Motorcycle Grand Prix of Catalonia in Barcelona, Spain. **PHOTO BY FRANCO ORIGLIA/GETTY IMAGES.**

axis while traveling forward in the air. Partrana has also executed both a double back flip, as well as a back flip while taking the motorcycle in a 360° rotation parallel to the ground. Many of the FMX stunts require the rider to become airborne through the use of a ramp.

There is a significant connection between the type of tricks performed in FMX and those executed in skateboarding, BMX bicycling, and other extreme sports. To practice a stunt as inherently dangerous as a back flip while seated on a motorcycle, some clubs have constructed specialty ramps and landing areas where the rider has a reduced risk of injury in a fall.

The training on the part of an FMX rider to successfully complete a back flip is progressive. The rider will often attempt his first such stunt on a small engine machine, with a displacement of 50–75 cc. Most of the elite performers in FMX use machines of at least 250 cc or greater; the faster the rider can jump of the end of the ramp, the more time in the air the bike will remain, permitting the rider a correspondingly greater time within which to make the flip.

Protective equipment is essential to FMX riding. Riders wear helmets and face shield, as well as full body armor.

**SEE ALSO** Extreme sports; Motocross or Moto X; Motorcycle: Freestyle.

# Motorcycle racing

The history of motorcycle racing began with the development of the internal combustion gasoline engine in the latter years of the nineteenth century. The first motorcycles were bicycles to which a crude engine was attached to the rear wheel to provide power.

As with the development of early racing automobiles, the first competition motorcycles were built in a variety of styles, as racing pioneers experimented with both two and three wheel configurations. The first motorcycle race involving exclusively two wheel designs occurred at Surrey, England, in 1897. The sport quickly became popular in both Europe and the United States; the world body responsible for the establishment of motorcycle racing standards, the Federation Internationale de Motorcycles Club, now known as the Federation Internationale de Motorcyclcism (FIM) was founded in 1904.

Motorcycle racing evolved in two distinct directions—competitions organized according to the nature of the racing to be conducted, and races open to specific sizes of motorcycle engines, a determination based upon either engine displacement (measured in cubic centimeters) or the degree of customization permitted to the motorcycle. The first motorcycle races were held on open road courses, the most famous of which is Great Britain's Isle of Man TT (or Tourist Trophy) event, first staged in a number of different classifications in 1907. Hill climbing races and dirt track racing on both quarter mile (400 m) and half mile (800 m) ovals became popular in the United States in the 1930s. This form of racing has continued to the present day, on surfaces where the racers regularly exceed speeds of 100 mph (160 km/h).

Specialized closed circuit road tracks, similar in concept to the courses built for Formula 1 automobiles, were constructed in various parts of the world to accommodate the extremely high powered performance racing motorcycles beginning in the 1970s. This form of racing, organized as "MotoGP," involves motorcycles that are built for racing only, as opposed to stock motorcycles that race in other racing classifications: stock motorcycles are very similar to those available for public use through commercial sale.

The MotoGP class of motorcycles are so powerful that the engines must be de-tuned, a process where the otherwise available power of the motorcycle is mechanically restricted, to permit the rider an opportunity to control the motorcycle that has the capacity for tremendous speeds but relatively little contact between the tires on the machine and the surface of the track, when compared to a racing automobile. The small degree of tire contact restricts the amount of control that the rider can exercise over the MotoGP motorcycle by way of braking or cornering if the machine were permitted to travel at its maximum available speed.

Motor cycle drag racing, where the machines race on quarter mile (400 m) paved strips also promoted the use of sophisticated engine technologies, where modified engines 1300 cc and larger cover the distance at speeds in excess of 150 mph (241 km/h) at the quarter mile marker. Motorcycle drag racing in the United States is organized under the auspices of the National Hot Rod Association (NHRA), the organization that organizes automobile drag racing. The motorcycle drag races are known as the Pro Stock Bike series.

Motorcycle racing became a popular off road venture, from smaller scale motocross events that are staged both indoors on modified surfaces that include artificial jumps and moguls to challenge the racers, to the dangerous multi-day endurance racing events such as the Paris to Dakar, Africa event. These motorcycles are constructed with heavy suspensions to absorb the significant forces that are generated when the machine is bouncing on a dirt trail or other off-road surfaces.

Motorcycle racing requires an understanding of a number of different physical principles. One of the most dramatic of these applications is observed when a racer executes the racing technique known as cornering. On a closed course racing circuit, the riders will be observed with the motorcycle angled into the turn, with the rider's inside knee positioned very low, appearing to skim over the track surface as the motorcycle moves at high speeds through the turn.

As the rider corners, three different physical elements are at play to influence the movement of the motorcycle: the downward pull of gravity upon the motorcycle and rider, the friction between the tires and the track surface, and the centripetal force acting to the outside of the turn. The perfectly executed turn will be the product of the rider leaning the motorcycle at an angle where the force of gravity is at equilibrium with the centripetal force that is acting to force the motorcycle upright. If the lean into the turn is too acute, the motorcycle will fall over; if the lean is insufficient, the motorcycle cannot make a sharp, efficient turn. If the rider enters a turn with no lean at all, the motorcycle is likely to fall towards the outside of the turn.

One common feature to almost all types of motorcycles is the acceleration capability of the machine. If the motorcycle accelerates too rapidly, the front wheel will be pushed off the ground, a phenomenon known as a "wheelie." Some wheelies are executed by motorcyclists as a stunt; the wheelie when unexpected can flip the motorcycle over on its longitudinal axis.

**SEE ALSO** Automobile racing; Balance training and proprioception; Motocross or Moto X.

# Muscle cramps

Muscle cramps are experienced by most athletes at one time or another. Such cramps are an involuntary and usually painful contraction of a skeletal muscle, most often in a structure that is actively providing muscle power at the moment of the onset of the cramp. The surface of the affected area will present as hard and contracted, with the skin appearing as if drawn tight over the muscle. A muscle cramp will invariably occur without warning.

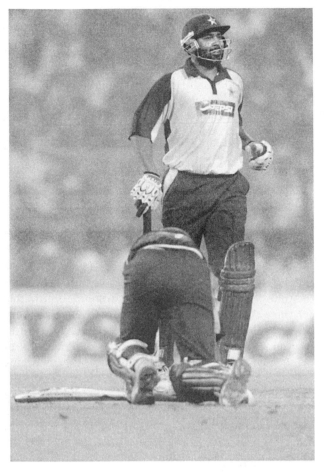

A cricket player falls due to a leg muscle cramp. AP PHOTO/BIKAS DAS

Muscle cramps are distinct from muscle twitches, another involuntary muscle action. Twitches are distinguishable from cramps by virtue of three features: their general isolation from the working muscles, an absence of pain when the twitch occurs, and the negligible impact of muscle twitching on performance. Twitches frequently occur in the eyelids and small muscle groups of the body. A twitch may be brought on by external pressures such as stress, or the excessive consumption of caffeine or other stimulants.

The cause of muscle cramps is variable, and the investigation to determine the basis for the occurrence will usually be linked to the nature of the activity and the environmental conditions in which the activity took place. The most common causes of muscle cramps, a number of which will occur in combination, include:

- fatigue
- strenuous exercise and overuse of particular muscle groups

- a failure to stretch or properly warm up prior to activity
- dehydration, and the related problem of sodium deficiency
- low blood sugar (glucose) levels
- magnesium deficiency
- calcium deficiency
- the presence of the hydrogen ion that is a byproduct of lactic acid formation in working muscles
- thyroid gland irregularity
- kidney dysfunction
- side effects of certain medications

Muscle cramps are more common is certain types of sporting activity, and the cramps tend to occur in distinct parts of the body in the course of those activities. In sports involving running, both as an event and as fundamental to team sports such as soccer, rugby, and American football, muscle cramps most frequently occur in the gastrocnemius (calf), the hamstrings, and the quadriceps (thigh) muscles. In cycling, the calf muscles are a frequent cramp location. As a general rule, muscle cramps will occur near the end of physical activity, when the body has been subjected to stress for a considerable period.

The onset of a muscle cramp is a disabling event. The first action to relieve the condition is the gentle stretching of the affected muscle. A stretch of the tissues that is slow and that does not itself create a further stress on the muscle will provide relief from the muscle contraction. At the point when the athlete can sense some reduction in the tightness of the cramp, the principles of the RICE (rest/ice/compression/elevation) treatment can be applied to the injured area. In some circumstances, the athlete can continue to gently stretch the muscle with the ice applied. As many cramps are related to the dehydration of the body, the athlete should consume fluids immediately.

Muscle cramps are a warning bell to the athlete. As the muscle cramp is often a symptom of a more serious physical issue that requires attention, the resumption of the athletic activity after the onset of a cramp must be monitored carefully. The development of a muscle cramp is an excellent opportunity for an athlete or a coach to assess the training practices, hydration, and diet of the athlete to determine what aspects of the overall sport regime may have contributed to the problem.

The prevention of a recurrence of the muscle cramp will also involve a review of the fitness level of the athlete. If the work required of the athlete exceeds his or her capabilities, the body will be more quickly fatigued. It is important that when an athlete seeks to increase a training or competitive workload, such increases are incremental, and usually no more than 5% per week.

Proper hydration and sodium levels must be maintained. When an athlete becomes dehydrated, the body will generally lose both its ability to properly cool itself as well as sustain a decrease in required levels of sodium. Sodium deficiencies contribute to an inability in the muscle to receive nerve impulses, which may contribute to cramping. Athletes must ensure that they follow a hydration strategy before, during, and after all training and competitive events, as dehydration is a cumulative condition.

Magnesium, calcium, and sodium are all minerals that are best consumed by way of food sources. The diet of the athlete should be analyzed to ensure that there is adequate provision for these minerals in the foods consumed.

A thorough and effective warm up, which includes an elevation of cardiovascular and respiratory function, combined with the stretching of all of the body muscle groups, will serve to both prepare the entire body for the stresses of the activity, as well as serve as a preventative against cramps.

SEE ALSO Cramps; Diet; Hydration; Minerals.

## Muscle fibers: Fast and slow twitch

Muscles are the instruments that power all movements made by the human body. Muscles are defined as being contractile tissues that are capable of extension and contraction to generate movement. The body uses three different types of muscles for various purposes: skeletal, cardiac, and smooth muscles.

Skeletal muscle, also known as striated muscle, is the type that constitutes most of the muscle mass within the body. Cardiac muscle is the specialized tissue found only in the heart. Cardiac muscle is activated involuntarily through the function of various impulses, including those directed through the autonomic nervous system controlled by the hypothalamus, the regulatory region of the brain. Smooth muscle is the tissue that lines the hollow organs of the body and it is also the subject of involuntary control, the autonomic nervous system.

All types of skeletal muscle are constructed from densely knit fibers, which are provided the nutrients necessary for their function by capillaries, tiny blood vessels extending from the arteries of the cardiovascular system. Muscle fibers are bound into bundles, called fascicles, to form a working unit. The ultimate control over every muscle fiber is exerted by the brain, through the transmissions that it directs to the body through the central nervous system. These transmissions emanate from the brain through the spinal cord, and ultimately through nerve pathways to neurons located within every muscle. The neuron is the local control mechanism that regulates the function of a group of muscle fibers; one neuron may control as many as 2,000 individual fibers. Given their function of the control of physical movement, these devices are known as motor neurons. The speed with which the neurons communicate with their related fibers dictates the characterization of the fiber as either a "fast twitch" or a "slow twitch."; all muscles possess both fast-twitch and slow-twitch fibers.

Fast-twitch fibers and slow-twitch fibers possess the same capacity to generate muscular power. Fast-twitch fibers are activated by their neurons at a rate ten times faster than the rate of activation for slow-twitch fibers. The distribution of fast- versus slow-twitch fibers in the muscles is primarily an inherited characteristic, determined by the genetic coding of each person. While it is common for a person to have muscles with a relatively even distribution of fast- and slow-twitch fibers, some persons inherit a tendency to a significantly greater number of one type of fiber over the other. Such persons tend to excel in the sports best suited to their muscular composition.

Fast-twitch fibers are further subdivided into two sub-categories, fast twitch (IIa) and an intermediate speed twitch fiber (IIb). Fast-twitch fibers are relied on by the body to propel it in short, intense bursts (such as those required in sprinting, weightlifting, or other short duration, explosive movements). Slow-twitch fibers are the units employed by the body to provide the power for endurance activities.

The manner in which the two kinds of fiber are utilized is tied to their construction as well as to the function of the neuron. Slow-twitch fibers possess a greater quantity of mitochondria, the portion of the human cell that acts as a powerhouse within each cell in the production of energy. Slow-twitch fiber cells can process greater amounts of oxygen to assist in the generation of adenosine triphosphate (ATP), the body's fuel for the production of energy. For this reason, slow-twitch fibers are relied on when the muscle must extend and contract repetitively, as in distance running or cycling events.

Physiological studies confirm that extensive endurance training will create an adaptation by the body, in that the intermediate fast-twitch fibers (IIa) may be converted to slow-twitch fibers over time.

The training that will assist in the development of fast-twitch fibers involves the repeated activation of the appropriate muscles. Techniques include isometric training, in which the muscle is held in a resistance-generating position for set periods. The clasping of both hands and pulling them with equal force from each arm is a simple isometric movement. A goal of isometric exercise is to ensure that the targeted muscle is contracted and extended in a disciplined fashion, which encourages an optimal relationship between each neuron and the muscle fiber group. Weight training, particularly the lifting of significant amounts with short rest intervals in each set, also stimulates fast-twitch fiber development.

The best known of the explosive training techniques aimed solely at the development of fast-twitch fiber is plyometrics. These programs that usually emphasize intense jumping and interval sprint training—which often are used by sprinters, hurdlers, basketball players, and other athletes that seek to become more explosive in their movements—are the best-known techniques to develop fast-twitch fibers in the leg muscles. The muscle becomes conditioned to respond to the stimulation provided to the neuron as dictated by the demands of the exercise. When the body senses that the number of fast-twitch fibers available to perform the movements are insufficient, neighboring fibers will be co-opted into assisting the existing fast-twitch fibers.

**SEE ALSO** Endurance exercise; Muscle mass and strength; Plyometrics.

# Muscle glycogen SEE Carbohydrate stores: Muscle glycogen, liver glycogen, and glucose

# Muscle glycogen recovery

Muscle glycogen recovery is the process through which the muscles of the body are replenished with carbohydrate sources that have been depleted through the energy expended in exercise. The muscles that are the target of this recovery to an optimal glycogen level are the skeletal muscles, those structures that are actually engaged in the movement of the body; the other muscle groups, the smooth muscles of the internal organs and the cardiac muscles do not possess a capacity for glycogen storage or conversion to fuel in the muscle.

Glycogen is the form in which the carbohydrate glucose is stored within the body; the skeletal muscles typically contain two-thirds of the body's supply of glycogen at any time, or a quantity measuring approximately 2% of skeletal muscle weight. Most of the remaining glycogen in stored in the liver, where it is released into the bloodstream for transport to cells for energy production.

Exercise by its nature places demands on the body to provide energy to power the muscles in movement. When the energy sources, particularly glycogen, are constant at the commencement of the activity, these supplies will steadily diminish, and if not replaced to any degree during the activity, the glycogen must be recovered and the supplies restored at the conclusion of the activity. Most glycogen is entirely consumed from muscle stores within 15 minutes to 30 minutes from the commencement of the exercise; in disciplines such as sprinting, where the fast-twitch muscle fibers are the components of each muscle that are of primary importance, the athlete may exhaust all of the stored glycogen reserves with 10 minutes of muscle effort. Weightlifters and other power sport competitors place similar demands on their muscle glycogen supply.

Of the glucose that is initially stored as glycogen and then converted for use in the energy-producing processes, 75% is directed to the brain and the functions of the related central nervous system; it is from the approximate 25% remainder that red blood cell production, skeletal muscle, and heart muscle functions are ultimately fueled.

Skeletal muscle glycogen depletion is a natural result of physical movement, which depletions are especially pronounced in athletic activity. Such depletion, if not corrected, carries with it risks to the structure and the function of the body. The primary danger associated with this depletion is damage to cells and muscle structures. When the body is unable to access muscle glycogen, it may trigger the breakdown of cell structures to create an alternative energy supply. Muscle glycogen depletion also places significant stress on the overall function of the immune system.

Muscle glycogen depletion is most effectively counteracted through diet; athletes who understand the demands placed on their muscle glycogen stores will plan how they shall achieve glycogen recovery through the foods ingested before, during, and after their workouts and their competitive events. There are a number of techniques employed by athletes to bolster their muscle glycogen levels, with each approach specific to the nature of the glycogen-depleting physical activity.

In sports where explosive, fast-twitch muscle movement is essential, the muscle glycogen is best restored through a post-activity meal that is rich in carbohydrates. This meal can be consumed within 30 minutes of the conclusion of the activity, as the body is most receptive to the recovery process at that time; the body's ability to ingest and synthesize carbohydrates into useful glycogen declines in the hours following the physical activity that depleted those reserves. Ideal muscle glycogen recovery will be performed through a series of small meals, as opposed to a single large meal that the body will not able to digest and process as readily. When the meals include a measure of protein replacement (the explosive muscle power activities that tax the glycogen stores often will require restoration of protein levels as well), a dual benefit is achieved.

A well-established method of ensuring that an endurance athlete has sufficient muscle glycogen is the process known as "carbo loading," when the athlete deliberately reduces carbohydrate consumption in the diet while continuing the training and energy expenditures. The athlete then loads carbohydrate-rich foods into the system, which tends to flood the muscles with glycogen. This technique, or a variation, is used after an endurance event such as a marathon race to restore muscle glycogen levels.

The development of specific sports fluid replacement products that contain carbohydrates (as well as useful electrolytes and water) has permitted athletes to more readily ingest carbohydrates during a workout or a competition. As a very general guideline, the body will process such carbohydrate sources most efficiently when the amount of carbohydrate in the fluid is between 6% and 12% by volume. This technique is effective in events that approach two hours or more in length, depending on the intensity of the athletic effort in question. For most athletes competing in events such as the Hawaii Ironman, such mid-race carbohydrate ingestion is essential.

**SEE ALSO** Carbohydrates; Glycogen depletion; Glycogen level in muscles; Overtraining.

# Muscle mass and strength

The expressions "muscle mass" and "muscle strength" are often used concurrently, but each has a separate sports science meaning. Muscle mass is the physical size of the muscle; muscles are often large due to exercise and concentrated physical training, but not exclusively. Muscle strength is one of the accepted components of total fitness, which includes endurance, flexibility, power, and speed. For almost every conceivable athletic purpose, muscle strength is a more valuable commodity than mass. However, in many contact sports, particularly those with specific roles for players in specific positions, muscle mass is important to the ability of the athlete to obtain and establish position against an opponent; the strength and sport-specific techniques employed by the athlete once that positioned is established will be the more important attributes.

The concepts of muscle mass and muscle strength are also separated from muscular power, a concept that implies explosiveness, and muscular endurance, which is the ability of the muscle to work at a steady performance rate over time.

This athletic distinction between muscle mass and strength is apparent in players such as an interior lineman in American football; a rugby forward, particularly those who play in the front row of the scrum; and a center in National Basketball Association (NBA) competition. In elite-level international rugby, the pack of eight forwards will weigh an average of 250 lb (113.3 kg); the laws of physics are immutable, for if the respective techniques of each group are equal, the pack of 250-lb players, working together, will dominate a team with 220-lb (99.8-kg) players, even when the lighter athletes have greater individual muscle strength.

In American football, where the average lineman weighs over 300 lb (136 kg), most tactics involved in line play are founded on the principle that once the player has position, he will be difficult to root out. Basketball, while nominally a non-contact sport, places a significant premium on the large center who can establish an anchored offensive position adjacent to the basket, through which his or her team will operate their sets.

In individual sports, such as wrestling or boxing, muscle mass is also an important aspect of how the competitor develops the tactics to combat the opponent. The amount of mass behind a blow delivered will be a significant factor in the ultimate force applied to the opponent.

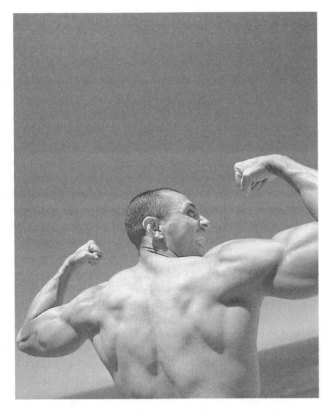

Muscles cannot become either larger or stronger through any device other than the proper application of diet and training principles. © JONATHAN CAVENDISH/CORBIS

Muscles cannot become either larger or stronger through any device other than the proper application of diet and training principles. Anabolic steroids—much publicized as a means for athletes to become bigger and stronger—are only a training aid, not a magic elixir. Steroids assist in muscular development only when the athlete is carrying out the physical training necessary to develop the muscles.

The essential components to a program that will enhance the muscle mass of an athlete will include:

- Muscles are constructed of fibers that are created within the body from the proteins synthesized in the food ingestion process. The muscle mass-seeking athlete must ensure that the diet supporting the training program has the necessary quantities of protein. A conventional balanced diet has approximately 12%–15% protein. In some configurations, the protein component may be adjusted to comprise 25% of food intake, subject to the individual needs and attributes of the athlete.
- Free weights tend to create a greater muscle mass than the muscle group-specific exercise

machines commonly used in health clubs and weight rooms. As the athlete must control a free weight through its entire range of motion, the targeted muscle and all ancillary muscle groups are also engaged in the act of lifting each weight, a process that extends the workout effect into a larger muscle region than the machines, which limit movement to the targeted muscle.

- The number of exercises performed with regard to each muscle group, defined as sets of exercises, will impact on muscle mass. As a general rule, the greater the number of repetitions, the lower the resistance, the greater the muscular endurance, the less the muscle mass. For this reason, muscle mass tends to be developed with lower numbers of repetitions per set, performed with greater amounts of weight.

Muscle mass and strength are not mutually exclusive training goals, notwithstanding the different methods by which one may seek size and strength. Muscle strength may be attained through the simplest of means—gradual increase in workload imposed on the muscles that are desired as strength increase targets. Muscles tend to get larger as they become stronger; when a strength program is accompanied by endurance training or other significant energy production and corresponding caloric output, the athlete will often possess highly defined muscles, with reduced mass but increased muscular strength.

**SEE ALSO** Anabolic steroids; Creatine supplementation; Growth; Skeletal muscle.

# Muscle protein synthesis

The synthesis of muscle protein is essential to the body's ongoing growth, repair, and maintenance of its skeletal muscle groups. The other types of human muscle tissue, cardiac muscle and the smooth muscles that are part of internal organ structure, are constituted through different cellular processes.

Proteins are the compounds comprised of amino acids—the building blocks of tissue formation within the body. The synthesis of protein is the method by which muscles are constructed. The human body synthesizes protein from diet at a rapid rate while the body is growing through adolescence and into young adulthood. The rate at which protein is synthesized slows significantly after age 20. It is for this reason that even among active, highly trained adults, the actual rate of muscle growth will be far less in relative terms to that of a healthy teenager.

In an adult athlete, the synthesis of muscle protein is also related to how the muscles are being exercised. Other than the ongoing repair and maintenance of existing muscle tissues that may be damaged through the course of daily living, human skeletal muscle will never get larger or stronger through either sedentary activities or the consumption of particular foods or supplements. Muscular activity is a prerequisite of meaningful muscle development, built on protein synthesis.

All forms of physical activity will direct specific stress into a muscle. In a sport such as distance running or cycling, the stresses are cumulative, the combined effect of repetitive movements that are at a relatively lower level of intensity. In activities that involve explosive and powerfully focused movements (such as weight training) the forces directed against the muscle are much more significant, and they occur over a much shorter time span.

In each circumstance, the muscle will naturally break down, a process known as "catabolism." The breakdown includes the physical separation of the fibers that comprise the muscle structure. The subsequent repair of the damaged muscle is "anabolism," the building up and the growth of the existing and previously damaged fiber. Anabolic steroids take their name due to their contribution to the building up of muscles. Protein synthesis is the mechanism by which the body affects this repair and muscle growth: as a very general proposition, when the body produces more synthesized protein than it consumes through its catabolic processes, muscle will be developed.

There are measurable ways to determine the balance in the body on an ongoing basis between its catabolic and its anabolic states. The essential amino acid, leucine, is used as an indicator of the state of this balance in more sophisticated sports science analyses. A positive leucine balance is evidence that this acid is present in the cells, a condition consistent with protein anabolism. Leucine is a component of numerous commercial protein supplements taken to stimulate further protein synthesis in the body.

Muscle protein synthesis is also considered in the context of sore, damaged, or overused muscles. Sports research in this area has focused not so much on whether the ingestion of protein is likely to be useful to the athlete, but at what point after the exercise should the protein be consumed so that the body can derive a maximum restorative and muscle-building effect. The combined effects of carbohydrate consumption and protein consumption have also been thoroughly considered in recent years.

The sports science community supports the usefulness of carbohydrate replacement immediately after exercise. Such replacement tends to deliver glycogen to the affected muscles more quickly; in addition, the entire body has a replenished supply of carbohydrates from which the whole of the musculoskeletal system can be restored. When proteins are consumed along with carbohydrates immediately after exercise, the catabolic process is not stopped within the affected muscles; the process of protein synthesis is immediately stimulated (a kick-start is an expression commonly employed in the research to describe the effect). This action leads to the prevention of further protein loss in the muscle. As the degradation of the muscle due to strenuous exercise will not reach its peak for approximately three days after the exercise that affected the muscle, it is important to continue the ingestion of protein. The maintenance of consistent dietary practices is essential to the body's ability to respond on an ongoing basis to the demand for muscle protein synthesis.

The body has a need to ensure effective muscle protein synthesis throughout the course of an athletic career. With the rise in masters level participation in a wide variety of sports (generally defined as competitions for athletes aged 40 years and older), older athletes are affected by catabolic and anabolic processes. The body's response to the increased consumption of protein after exercise does not significantly vary with age, for either men or women.

SEE ALSO Diet; Growth; Protein ingestion and recovery from exercise.

## Musculoskeletal injuries

Musculoskeletal injuries constitute the largest class of athletic injuries sustained in sports. Any injury that occurs to a skeletal muscle, tendon, ligament, joint, or a blood vessel that services skeletal muscle and any related tissues is a musculoskeletal injury. The musculoskeletal system is the structural movement-generating component of the body. The capacity for movement is closely allied to the relationship between the musculoskeletal and the neuromuscular systems, which is the interconnection between muscular movement and its control through nervous system impulses.

Sport participation along with a healthy and active lifestyle involve an inherent risk of musculoskeletal injury. The majority of these injuries are resolved without significant long-term consequences (or *sequelae* in medical language). The usual short-term consequences of musculoskeletal injuries will include the following limitations to physical function, irrespective of the part of the anatomy to which the injury was sustained:

- Decreased physical strength: Muscular ability will begin to decline after 24 hours of inactivity.

- Nerve impulses slow: At optimal health, the nervous system can transmit some nerve impulses, such as those crucial to coordination and reaction, at speeds of over 300 ft (100 m) per second. Inactivity through injury will reduce the overall ability of the nervous system to stimulate movement.

- Circulation and metabolic rates will slow.

- Bone mineral density decreases: Injury tends to slow the rate at which calcium and vitamin D operate in union to produce new bone cells. Collagen, the cellular protein material that provides bone with the elasticity to absorb forces directed into the otherwise hard mineral surface, is not generated at pre-injury levels.

- Collagen level decreases in the connective tissues, primarily tendons and ligaments, making these structures stiffer, less elastic, less responsive to movement, and more vulnerable to injury.

- Reduced cardiorespiratory function: The ability of the body to process oxygen, described VO$_2$max, will decline by a limited amount in the first few days of inactivity due to injury, with pronounced declines exceeding 10% of peak oxygen uptake after 15 days.

- Reduced glycogen storage: Both the musculoskeletal muscles and the liver, the primary storage sites within the body for glycogen, will not maintain peak storage levels absent muscular activity that places demands upon the body's ability to utilize glucose, converted from glycogen.

The most common cause of musculoskeletal injury is a combination of physical overloads created by overtraining or by the repetitive use of a joint or a particular muscle group. Virtually every sport has a potential for this type of injury; these injuries are more often caused by training routines than by the stresses of a single competition. Distance running is a sport that by its nature will often create conditions for both overtraining as well as leg and foot injuries that are attributable to the repetitive strains of the activity. The injuries sustained in running are rarely connected to a single event, unlike the injuries of many contact sports; running injuries commonly are a combination of the mileage covered by the athlete in a given training period, the pace with which the training distances are run, the nature of the terrain covered in training, as well as the unique physical characteristics of the athlete, such as structural deformities or imbalances and age. These overloads lead to micro fractures of the bone structure, muscle and tendon tears, and ischemia, the reduction of blood supply to an organ or tissue. In a cross-sectional analysis of the frequency of injury occurrence among athletes of all ages and ability levels, the greatest number of musculoskeletal injuries occur to males between the ages of 15 and 25 years.

The distribution of the frequency of the different types of musculoskeletal injuries is relatively equal between male and female athletes, although different types of specific injuries occurred more frequently due to the physiological differences between men and women. The most striking of these examples is the far greater risk that female athletes face regarding a prospective anterior cruciate ligament knee injury, due to the relatively wider pelvis in relation to femur length in the female anatomy.

Various sport and government organizations in North America and Europe have analyzed musculoskeletal injury rates. Approximately 25% of all athletes will expect to sustain a musculoskeletal injury in a 12-month period. The more fit and the more sophisticated the athlete, the more likely the risk of injury, due in part to the fact that such injuries often occur to athletes performing at a higher level with greater physical stresses and risks.

The research on such injuries also confirms that foot and ankle injuries are the most common of musculoskeletal injuries, constituting approximately 25% of these occurrences. Knee injuries of all types are the next most common, representing 22% of musculoskeletal damage. Back injuries are the next most prominent occurrence, at 11%. Injuries to the lower leg, thigh, hip, shoulders, and the hand/forearm structure each occur at frequencies of between 5% and 10%.

**SEE ALSO** Ankle sprains; Back injuries; Hand injuries; Knee injuries; Shoulder injuries.

# Myostatin

Myostatin is a gene, one of the units of heredity consisting of a sequence of deoxyribonucleic acid (DNA) that determines the inherited characteristics of every individual. It is a gene that contributes to the differentiation in growth factors, including physical size, and regulates muscle development. Unlike those factors that spur the growth of human structures, myostatin prevents muscles from growing too large. It is protein-produced in the skeletal muscle cells, interacting with the production of myocytes, the cells that ultimately form muscles.

Interest in myostatin is a relatively recent phenomenon. While the function of myostatin within the human body is a biological research frontier, the ability of certain cattle breeds to grow to enormous, well-muscled stature, particularly the Belgian blue, is well understood, as it is a breed that inherently possesses less of the myostatin gene.

Muscle size is both an inheritable trait as well as an attribute that may be altered through physical training, coupled with diet. A large number of proteins, referred to as growth factors (GFs), operate in different ways within the body. A GF will generally signal a cell as to its rate of growth and any differentiation from other cells. Some of these proteins, such as insulin-like growth factor-1 (IGF-1), influence cell growth throughout the entire body; myostatin has a specific impact restricted to muscle cell development.

In a healthy human, the effects of how the various GFs operate is best understood in the context of how the body recovers from a muscular injury. When a cyclist sustains a tear to the gastrocnemius, one of the two calf muscles, the repair of the torn segment commences almost immediately after the injury is sustained. IGF-1 controls the creation of the cells necessary to enable the damaged muscle fibers to be rebuilt and repaired. Depending on the nature and the extent of the damage to the muscle, the repairs triggered through the action of the IGF-1 hormone will continue over time.

It is a central principle of weight training and muscle development that the creation of tears in the fibers of the muscle are necessary to build a larger muscle. It is for this reason that weight training programs should provide for rest intervals that will allow the repairs to be affected at the cellular level and for the muscle fibers to grow. Acting alone, IGF-1 would be the facilitator of unchecked muscle growth and development. Myostatin appears to act as a counterbalance to the stimulation of muscle cell growth, as it serves to slow and ultimately limit the number of new cells created to build new muscle.

As muscle size is inheritable, there exists the potential to create a variable gene, where the increase in muscle size in an athlete could be achieved through a decrease in the action of the myostatin. The precise details of how myostatin operates within the muscle cells are not yet known to sports science, as myostatin first became the subject of published scientific commentary in 1997. The principles of myostatin function are sufficiently understood to support the significant research undertaken to develop a myostatin inhibitor. Such research is directed not only at the athletic advantages that are believed to flow from such a product, but also to combat muscle-wasting diseases such as muscular dystrophy, various cancers, and AIDS. Research directed at both cattle and poultry, both of which have myostatin-type genes, have confirmed that, in theory, a myostatin inhibitor will permit greater muscle growth in human athletes.

Supplements known as myostatin blockers have become prominent in the weight training and bodybuilding markets. These products are widely advertised throughout the health and fitness industry, with seemingly countless variations available through the mass marketing of the Internet. The products that make the claim as possessing myostatin-blocking or inhibiting capabilities have not been the subject of scientific verification.

Further research on myostatin will focus in part on the risks of the wide-scale use of this prospective inhibitor. The impact of a myostatin blocker on the function of the heart and cardiovascular system is unknown. With greater muscle size through the administration of myostatin blockers, the risk of additional strain on tendons and bone structure through increased muscle mass must also be considered.

The prospect of genetic doping with respect to the limitation of the action of the myostatin gene is one that has been considered by international sport. The fear of agencies such as the World Anti-Doping Agency (WADA) is the development of a technology where a myostatin inhibitor could be injected into a specific tissue, permitting the enhanced development of the subject muscle.

In a more benign fashion, testing for the presence or extent of the myostatin gene in an individual has other potential applications. Testing for the extent of the myostatin gene would be useful in determining which persons would be best suited to sports involving significant muscular development.

**SEE ALSO** Anabolic steroids; Genetic prediction of performance; Genetics; Nandrolone.

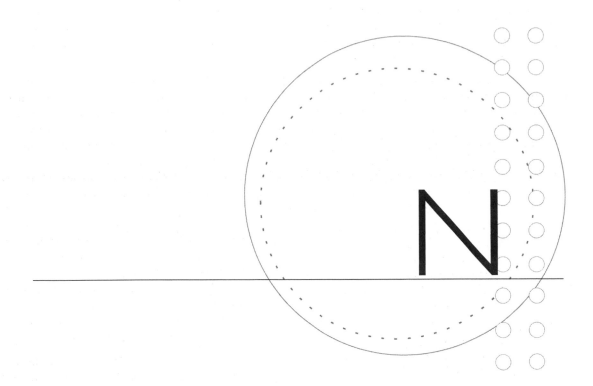

# James A. Naismith

11/6/1861–11/28/1939
AMERICAN
PHYSICAL EDUCATION INSTRUCTOR

James Naismith invented basketball in 1891 to provide an outlet for some energetic male students at the Young Men's Christian Association (YMCA) Training School (now Springfield College) in Springfield, Massachusetts. The simplicity and the athleticism inherent in Naismith's creation remains the essence of modern basketball, one of the true world games.

Naismith's roots extend into both Canada and the United States. Born at Almonte, Ontario, a small village located near the Canadian capital of Ottawa, Naismith's first athletic success was achieved while he was a well regarded undergraduate student at Montreal's McGill University, beginning in 1883. Naismith was a classic all round athlete, a success in sports as diverse as rugby, gymnastics, and lacrosse. Naismith played for McGill in at least one of the early rugby football games against Princeton University, contests that were the forerunners to modern American football.

When Naismith beganed graduate studies in theology, Naismith's professors disapproved of his active athletic career. However, Naismith advocated that it was possible, and even desirable, to encourage young men to pursue both an athletic and a spiritual life. This philosophy was central to much of what Naismith accomplished throughout his later career in athletics.

While attending university in Montreal, Naismith became acquainted with the YMCA, an organization that had been founded in London in the early 1800s. The YMCA established branches in Montreal and Boston in 1851. At the Montreal YMCA, Naismith approached the Association administrators regarding his desire to become a physical education instructor who combined spirituality and physical training in a program for young athletes.

It was as a result of these discussions that Naismith joined the faculty at the international YMCA training school located at Springfield, Massachusetts in 1890. In the winter of 1891, during his second year at Springfield, Naismith was placed in charge of the indoor physical education program. His students consisted primarily of bored but otherwise active older teenagers and mature men who had tired of available winter indoor sports options, primarily gymnastics. The senior physical education instructor directed Naismith and his colleagues to develop a new indoor game to occupy their students; two weeks was the timeline permitted to create the new game.

To create a new sport, Naismith sought inspiration from the outdoor sports with which he was familiar, such as soccer, lacrosse, and rugby football, with modifications to suit an indoor format. As the new game would be played on an unforgiving hardwood floor, a new sport that involved tackling or excessive physical contact was not feasible. As Naismith considered other ideas, he recalled a childhood game called 'duck on the rock', where the players threw balls into empty boxes or baskets. Naismith's first creative step towards the invention of basketball was to place peach baskets placed at opposite ends of a court. To pose a greater challenge to the players, Naismith raised the goals above the height of the court. As the gymnasium at Springfield had an indoor running track situated 10 ft (3 m) above the floor of the gymnasium, Naismith selected this height as the position of his basket goals, goals that Naismith attached directly to the facing of the indoor track.

It is one of the legends associated with Naismith and the development of basketball that the gymnasium janitor became very upset with Naismith for having the bottom of the janitor's valuable peach baskets removed to save Naismith's players the time and the trouble of climbing a ladder to retrieve the ball.

With his concept now given a rudimentary physical structure, Naismith, with the assistance of several colleagues, devised a set of 13 rules to govern the play of the created game. Among the first rules were several important concepts, each of which has survived in one form or another in the modern game. These fundamental concepts were: (1) no running with the ball in hand (a rule which that lead to the codification of the rules respecting dribbling the ball); (2) no tackling or rough body contact; (3) the freedom of any player to obtain the ball and score at any time.

In December 1891, Naismith's students were the participants in the first ever game of basketball. The score was 1-0, and the new sport was an instant success.

Basketball quickly spread to other countries through the national and international structure of the YMCA. Basketball was played in at least 12 countries within two years of its invention. On a local level, Naismith passed along his knowledge to Senda Berenson Abbott, the head physical education instructor at near by Smith College, a female institution, where Abbott modified the rules of the game for her female students, with the first games played at Smith in 1893.

Naismith was humble regarding the success of basketball. He was pleased that he had created a popular and beneficial sport. Naismith was apparently content to let his game evolve as it might, and he left Springfield to obtain a medical degree at the University of Colorado in 1898. Naismith soon after became the assistant athletic director at the University of Kansas. He left Kansas to serve as a captain and an Army chaplain with the United States forces in World War I. In 1918 he served as the YMCA Secretary in France, before returning to the University of Kansas as its Director of Athletics from 1919 until 1937.

Naismith was a part of two important developments in the history of basketball in his tenure at Kansas. The first was his influence on the career of Forrest (Phog) Allen (1885–1974), the legendary University of Kansas coach, a member of the Basketball Hall of Fame, and one of the great college coaches, innovators, and tacticians in the early development of basketball.

The second development occurred shortly before Naismith died at age 78 in 1939. Naismith was on hand to witness the introduction of basketball as an official Olympic sport at the 1936 Summer Games in Berlin. Although he generally shied away from public acknowledgement with respect to his role in the creation of basketball, Naismith accepted an invitation to the Games' inaugural ceremony, and he agreed to throw the ball up for the opening tip-off at the first Olympic basketball game.

Naismith has received considerable posthumous fame for his creation of the sport of basketball. His game has evolved dramatically since 1891, but basketball, with its freedom of movement and its emphasis on skill and execution, has remained true to the spirit of Naismith's creation. He was the initial inductee into the Basketball Hall of Fame in 1959.

SEE ALSO Basketball; International Olympic Committee (IOC); Sports coaching.

# Nandrolone

Nandrolone is an anabolic steroid, one of the class of muscle-building chemicals often employed by athletes to improve their strength and durability. Steroids are substances composed of carbon, hydrogen, and oxygen molecules, constructed in rings. Nandrolone occurs naturally in the human body in extremely minute quantities. It has a chemical composition that is very similar to testosterone, the male hormone, which is also a steroid and essential to the growth and development of the male body. Nandrolone is also a similar composition to that of progesterone, the equivalent female hormone. For these reasons, nandrolone has been valued as a training aid since it was first developed.

The application of anabolic steroids to sports was discovered by accident in the 1930s; steroids became the subject of systematic testing by Russian and Eastern Bloc sports scientists in the 1950s when weightlifters were provided the substances in controlled circumstances and significant performance gains were measured. Nandrolone was an anabolic steroid created in the course of the experimentation that arose in the 1960s regarding general steroid use. Nandrolone became popular in the 1980s as a preferred steroid choice as it was perceived as having fewer side effects than other anabolic steroids, particularly those of increased growth of body hair and sudden, unpredictable outbursts. As with all other steroids, nandralone was proven to reduce fatigue, and increase the rate at which muscles and overall strength could be developed while permitting athletes to train harder.

Nandrolone is obtained through injection. It is marketed in North America under the trade name Winstrol; in England and Europe, it is marketed as Deca-Durabolin.

Although anabolic steroids were established as a performance-enhancing drug in the late 1960s, the capacity of sports science to provide athletes with them far exceeded the ability of sports regulatory agencies, such as the International Olympic Committee (IOC), to police their usage. The IOC declared anabolic steroids illegal for all Olympic competitions in 1976, but effective and scientifically verifiable steroid testing methods did not exist until the early 1980s. As science progressed in its ability to detect steroids, in most cases through the presence of trace evidence known as metabolites detected in urine samples, that progress was a defined compound at one time. The ability to detect one variety of steroids was not proof of the detection of a compound of similar chemical composition. The IOC did not have access to reliable testing for nandrolone until the late 1980s.

Once the science was available, the testing for nandrolone was further complicated by the fact that nandrolone is a naturally occurring substance in the body. The test procedures would be required to take into account this fact; for this reason, the legal limit of nandrolone permitted in the body was fixed at 2 mcg per ml of urine. It was established through significant rounds of scientific testing that, for athletes who consumed nandrolone, they would be expected to produce metabolites excreted in urine at levels 100 times the natural level of nandrolone present in the body.

In the 1990s, world champion sprinters Linford Christie of Great Britain and Merlene Ottey of Jamaica were the subject of positive tests for nandrolone, as was Czech tennis player Petr Korda. In 2006, National Hockey League player Brian Berard tested positive for this steroid as well. The involvement of these high profile athletes in nandrolone use is a testament to its popularity and perceived usefulness as a training supplement.

Nandrolone positive tests have attracted further controversy from the scientific perspective, as further study has been directed to the issue of whether intense exercise, combined with a high protein diet and the use of the supplement creatine, is capable of increasing the natural production of nandrolone within the body, so as to generate a false-positive steroid test. The most common defenses proffered by athletes in cases of a positive nandrolone test have been either that the positive test was due to a dietary supplement that was unwittingly consumed by the athlete that contained nandrolone, or that the body naturally produced nandrolone in the course of the processing of the proteins contained in the diet or supplement.

As with every other anabolic steroid, there are proven long-term health risks associated with the use of nandrolone. In the short term, nandrolone will usually stimulate the production of acne on different parts of the body. All steroids will tend to make the user more edgy and irritable, prone to mood changes, and short tempered; the extent of this side effect is variable. In the medium term, the body of a male nandrolone user will undergo physiological changes that may include the development of breasts, as well as reduced sexual drive and ability. For female users, an interruption or cessation of the regular menstrual cycle is a common consequence of all forms of steroid use.

The most dangerous consequences of steroid use are long term. Because nandrolone and other anabolic steroids mimic the effect of testosterone in the body, as well as stimulating its release, the excess quantities of the hormone must be broken down; this is the function of the liver, the organ primarily responsible for cleansing and cleaning functions in the body. An increased risk of the development of liver tumors is a well-established consequence of steroid use.

The other serious long-term effects of nandrolone usage include a generalized greater risk of cancer, as well as the potential expansion of the heart muscle, leading to cardiac arrest.

**SEE ALSO** Anabolic steroids; Creatine supplementation; Supplement contamination.

## Nasal sprays

Nasal sprays are a common method by which various types of medications are delivered into the body. Nasal sprays are powered by either a gas-

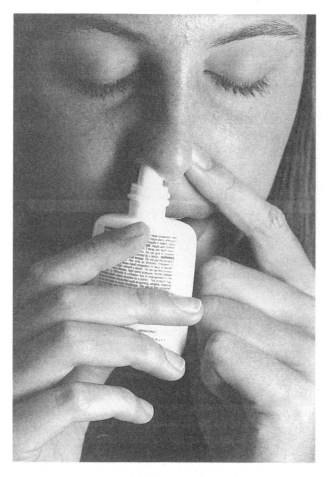

Nasal sprays are often used as a medium by which medications can be delivered into the body. WILL & DENI MCINTYRE/PHOTO RESEARCHERS, INC.

pressurized device (often carbon dioxide), or by a pump mechanism. The contents of the nasal spray are delivered into each nostril by the insertion of the spray nozzle and the compression of the spray device.

Nasal sprays are most often employed to counteract breathing-related ailments, including allergies, the effects of air pollution, and infections of the upper respiratory tract such as sinusitis, an inflammation of the tissues in the sinus passages.

Allergies are caused when the body detects the presence of an antigen, a foreign substance that the body determines to be harmful when it makes contact with the body's immune system. In the case of airborne antigens, the response by the body includes the production of histamine, a chemical that creates the watery eyes and excess mucous production that is typically associated with an allergic reaction. Many persons find breathing difficult in these circumstances; athletes are generally not able to function at a

peak level if their body produces histamine at its natural response rate.

Nasal sprays containing an antihistamine compound are often effective in reducing the level of histamine produced by the body. As a result, the nasal passages remain clearer. The sprays, depending on their formulation, are fast-acting; cromolyn sodium is a well-regarded allergy nasal spray for this purpose. Antihistamine sprays are available both as a prescription medication and as an over-the-counter (OTC) product. Nasal sprays are also used to deliver allergy medications that are designed to address allergic reactions that occur in other parts of the body, as the blood vessel structure of the nasal passages is an effective entry point into the cardiovascular system for the ultimate transport of the medication to the targeted cells.

Corticosteroids are also delivered into the body by way of nasal sprays. These substances are synthetic derivatives of the body's naturally produced anti-inflammatory hormone, cortisone. Corticosteroids are particularly effective in countering the swelling and inflammation of sinusitis. In severe cases of this infection, an athlete will experience sinus pain through the heavy breathing of vigorous exercise as air rushes in and out of the upper respiratory system, as well as any sudden changes in the position of the head that result in variations of pressure in the sinus.

Commercially available decongestants often include ephedrine or similar stimulants in the composition. Ephedrine acts to stimulate the dilation of the blood vessels in the nasal passages. There are risks associated with long-term use of these types of nasal sprays because the user may feel dependent on the spray, promoting an unnatural dilation of the vessels.

A simple saline solution is sometimes employed by athletes as an aid to washing out the nasal passage, clearing excess mucus and permitting easier breathing. The saline aids in simply cleaning the passage in a sanitary fashion. Athletes who are performing in dry, less humid conditions often employ these sprays; the body's ability to process the air inhaled is most effective in slightly humid conditions, which the nasal passage can replicate if a saline spray is administered from time to time.

**SEE ALSO** Bronchospasm, exercise-induced; Cardiorespiratory function; Nonsteroidal anti-inflammatory drugs (NSAIDs); Prescription medications and athletic performance.

# NASCAR auto racing

The National Association for Stock Car Auto Racing, or NASCAR, was founded in the United States in 1947. Throughout its early years, NASCAR was a series of automobile races that involved vehicles that bore a very near resemblance to the vehicles then being produced for commercial purposes in post World War II North America; the typical NASCAR race vehicle was a factory manufactured sedan.

"Stock" is the term employed throughout all motor sports to signify vehicles that have not been significantly modified in terms of the size and displacement of the engine, suspension, or transmission. Stock is often employed in the same circumstances as the expression "street legal," a phrase meaning that the vehicle in question complies with the rules respecting highway operation in a particular jurisdiction.

The first NASCAR races in the late 1940s and early 1950s attracted a significant following, particularly in the southeastern United States. Many of the races were often contested on dirt track ovals, where the competitors raced 0.5 mi (0.8 km) for each lap. NASCAR racing took a significant step forward with the construction of its super speedways, the most notable of which was built at Daytona, Florida in 1953. NASCAR racing gradually moved away from its stock format to vehicles built for the specific demands of racing in to the late 1950s; the development of the 355 cubic inch displacement V8 engine by General Motors was one of the early landmarks of that progression.

Modern NASCAR is a sport that enjoys a strong following in North America, and a steadily growing international fan base. NASCAR successfully marketed its racing product on a combination of the vehicle performance, the nature of NASCAR racing (which requires the drivers to operate the vehicles at very close quarters to one another at speeds that frequently exceed 150 mph (241 km/h), which sometimes leads to relatively frequent and spectacular collisions), and the personalities of the successful drivers. "King" Richard Petty became a NASCAR icon, especially as he was followed into racing competition by a son and a grandson. Junior Johnson, Dale Earnhardt, and Rusty Wallace attained similar levels of public acclaim. North Carolina and the adjacent southern states have remained the epicenter of NASCAR, as a number of highly regarded tracks are located in the region; many of the prominent racing teams are also headquartered in the vicinity.

The modern NASCAR race vehicles have a silhouette similar to the production vehicles built for commercial sale by their sponsors. Beneath the outer shell of the vehicle, the NASCAR race car is a combination of high technology and older styled automotive features that are mandated by NASCAR rules. These machines are capable of speeds in excess of 200 mph (322 km/h) on a race track straight away. The driver is secured within a roll cage through a series of safety mechanisms, designed to deflect the forces of collision away from the driver's body. With the rise in the television appeal of NASCAR, most of the vehicles are equipped with on board television cameras that provide a view both of the driver as he operates the vehicle, as well as a vantage point on both the movements of opposing drivers and any the collisions that occur during the race.

The typical NASCAR race car is powered by a V8 engine, built to run at high speeds in warm weather conditions without failure for several hours at a time. Each engine is capable of producing as much as 750 horsepower, with an engine design that forces much larger quantities of air into the engine for combustion than does a conventional engine design. The carburetor, the mechanical device that mixes the required amounts of air with fuel in an internal combustion engine, is a "low tech" instrument in the face of modern technology such as fuel injectors; NASCAR rules prohibit fuel injector use. As a result, large amounts of air and fuel can be mixed, increasing the potential power to be generated by the vehicle.

A NASCAR team will employ two different body types in a racing season, depending upon the length of the track. On short tracks, where the circuit is fewer than 0.75 miles (1.2 km) in length, the racing teams seek a vehicle that will handle the tighter turns and the shorter straight-aways in an optimal fashion. In such conditions, vehicles handle best when they are able to generate down force, the physical quality achieved where the aerodynamics of the vehicle force it closer to the surface of the race track when traveling at high speeds. Down force permits greater handling characteristics in the tires while cornering, which allows for greater vehicle speed on these shorter courses.

NASCAR places technical limits on engine capability at the longer, super speedway courses, where there are longer straight-aways and a consequently greater risk of high speed collisions. The most prominent of these tracks are Daytona and Talladega. The most effective of the limitations is the mandatory use of restrictor plates on the super speedways. The carburetor mixes fuel in vapor form, with air directed

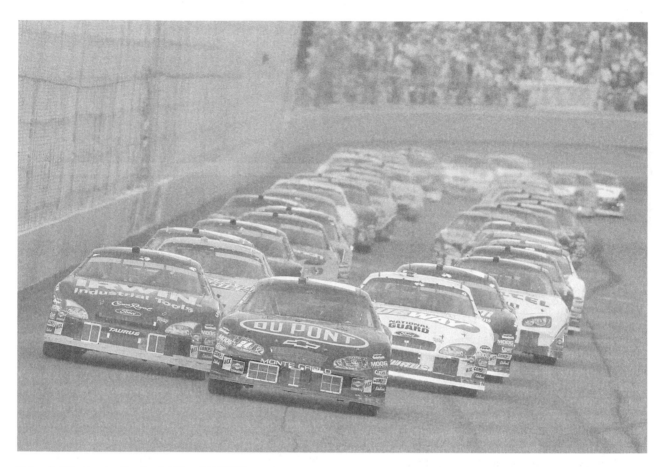

Driver Jeff Gordon leading the field in a NASCAR race. © SAM SHARPE/THE SHARPE IMAGE/THE SHARPE IMAGE/CORBIS

into the carburetor through an intake manifold. The greater the flow of air from the intake manifold into the carburetor, the greater the amount of fuel drawn into the carburetor. The more fuel available to be mixed in the carburetor, the greater the volume of combustible mixture to be consumed by the engine, resulting in more engine power and greater potential for speed.

The restrictor plate is a metal barrier with a pattern of holes drilled through it that is placed between the intake manifold and the carburetor. The plate restricts the flow of air into the carburetor, creating a smaller available volume of fuel and air to be mixed and combusted in the engine, reducing available engine power and speed.

All NASCAR racers are constructed with a number of aerodynamic features. The most obvious of these are such items as the air dams (the skirting that extends from the body of the vehicle encircling the structure except for the wheels) and rear spoilers (the wings attached to the rear of the vehicle to assist in producing down forces that push the vehicle closer to the road surface and enhance stability, especially

when moving through a corner at high speeds. In addition to these features, standard NASCAR race tactics include drafting behind a lead vehicle. Drafting is the procedure where a driver positions his vehicle directly behind the lead vehicle, so as to take advantage of the partial vacuum created by the lead vehicle movement through the air. By positioning the second vehicle on the bumper of the first, the second vehicle is essentially pulled through the partial vacuum by the lead vehicle. It is common in NASCAR races to see multiple vehicles drafting, one after another.

In contrast to open wheel racing such as Formula 1 Auto Racing, the driving tactics of NASCAR are usually less complex, as the NASCAR circuits are almost always an oval with all vehicles heading in an identical fashion for between 200 and 600 mi (322-966 km). Drafting at very close quarters, the bumping of vehicle ahead to gain an advantage, and very daring passes at high speeds on banked turns are standard driver practice.

**SEE ALSO** Automobile racing; Formula 1 auto racing; Motorcycle Racing.

# National Collegiate Athletic Association (NCAA)

The National Collegiate Athletic Association (NCAA) is a governing body unique in the sports world. The NCAA is an organization that blends athletic governance, academic regulation over its participants, and revenue generation under one tightly structured umbrella. While primarily a body that is devoted to the advancement and supervision of sport in an amateur setting, the NCAA methods regarding the stewardship of intercollegiate athletics are consistent with classic corporate organization models.

The NCAA was founded over 50 years after American intercollegiate sport established a niche in the public consciousness. From the first truly intercollegiate football games in the 1870s, football rivalries grew in the universities of the eastern United States. The rules of the game were not fully formalized until 1906, when the forward pass became legalized. The early contests were both hard fought and dangerous, including "gang tackling" and tactics such as the "flying wedge," a device by which the ball carrier was shielded by his ten teammates in a wedge formation that was thrust full-speed into the opposition. Serious head injuries and skeletal fractures were relatively common, and after a number of football player fatalities in the early 1900s occurred during intercollegiate contests, the then-president of United States, Theodore Roosevelt, was subject to considerable public pressure to ban football from intercollegiate athletics.

At the urging of Roosevelt, representatives of 13 universities met in 1905 with the intention of making football safer. From these meetings came the formation of the Intercollegiate Athletic Association of the United States (IAAUS), which was constituted with 62 members in 1906. The IAAUS became the National Collegiate Athletic Association in 1910. The membership of the modern NCAA is an aggregation of over 1,000 institutions. In the nomenclature of American intercollegiate athletics, the expression "college sports" includes colleges, which are four-year degree-granting institutions often specializing in liberal arts programs, as well as universities, which tend to offer more comprehensive academic programs, including postgraduate and doctoral studies. Junior colleges are not a part of the NCAA framework; these are two-year institutions that offer associate degrees. Junior colleges have their own national governance and structure. It is not uncommon for junior college student athletes, particularly in basketball, to transfer to a college or university program after completion of their two-year program; such players are often referred to as a "juco transfer."

While the initial focus of the IAAUS and the successor NCAA was the regulation of football safety, intercollegiate sports of all types experienced a dramatic expansion after the end of World War I. The NCAA provided governance over the men's intercollegiate sports of its member institutions only until the late 1970s, offering no championship opportunities for women until that time. The first collegiate track and field championships were organized by the NCAA in 1921, and through the succeeding years the NCAA expanded its sanctioned championships to include team sports such as baseball, whose first College World Series was held in 1947, ice hockey in 1948, soccer in 1959, and lacrosse in 1971.

The history of the national collegiate basketball championships highlights the rise of the NCAA in contrast with other bodies that have been a part of competitive college sports landscape throughout the history of the NCAA. Created in 1901 by James Naismith at what is now Springfield College in Massachusetts, basketball enjoyed a remarkable growth at a collegiate level. In 1901, a group known as the Helms Committee determined the national champion through a vote of its members. In 1937, a business group based in Kansas City organized a national basketball championship, with an emphasis on small college participation. This organization later became known as the National Association of Intercollegiate Athletics (NAIA); the NAIA exists today as a distinct governing body with a membership of over 250 academic institutions.

In 1939, the NCAA assumed control of the Helms Committee, and it convened its first tournament that year. At the same time, the National Invitational Tournament (NIT) was born, a tournament where college teams were invited to play in a single knock-out elimination format at Madison Square Garden in New York City. For many years, the NCAA and NIT competitions were not mutually exclusive, (City College of New York won both events in 1950, the only institution to do so) and the NIT had equivalent prestige to that of the NCAA championship. By the 1960s, the NCAA basketball tournament had become the premier college postseason tournament, and by the 1980s, the NIT was relegated to an event for teams that could not qualify for the NCAA championship. In 2005, the NCAA acquired all rights to the NIT competition, which is now operated under the NCAA auspices.

The growth of all NCAA sports prompted the creation of different competitive divisions in the early

1970s. It had become evident that in many sports, smaller institutions had difficulty competing against larger and better-funded schools that offered better and more comprehensive forms of athletic scholarships, thus attracting better athletes. The tension between the academic purposes of postsecondary education, and the corresponding attention paid by admissions directors to College Board results and high school grades, and the value accorded athletic success at many institutions has been an undercurrent in the work carried out by the NCAA in its regulatory capacity since the 1930s. In modern America, where the cost of university education will commonly range from $20,000 to $50,000 per year of study, a "full-ride" athletic scholarship is a significant prize, as it is common for students to graduate from university with student loan debt in excess of $50,000.

As an attempt to standardize the practices of the institutions, the NCAA created competitive divisions in 1973. All NCAA member schools must comply with the rules with respect to their division in order to compete within the sports championships offered at each division. The divisions include:

- Division 1: Schools are permitted to offer full athletic scholarships, in accordance with both NCAA rules regarding entrance grades and the recruitment of athletes. Division 1 schools tend to be the larger academic institutions, although not exclusively so. There are over 350 Division 1 schools in the NCAA.

- Division 2: Schools are permitted to offer both full athletic scholarships, partial athletic scholarship (often the value of tuition or a similar component of the full academic costs), or scholarships that combine both academic and athletic components. There are 25 different sports championships contested in Division 2 by approximately 200 member institutions.

- Division 3: Members tend to be smaller, academically centered colleges and universities. Athletic scholarships are prohibited among the approximately 430 NCAA institutions at this level.

For the sport of football only, the NCAA created the subdivisions of Division 1A and Division 1AA in 1978.

Since 1973, the NCAA has created an extensive regulatory framework regarding the structure of each division. In addition to the rules with respect to the availability of athletic scholarships, each division has requirements for its participating institutions. In Division 1, all members must provide seven varsity sports

for each gender, with each sport having a minimum number of games required in each season. In revenue-generating sports such as football, Division 1A schools must comply with minimum stadium seating requirements, and all such Division 1 institutions are capped regarding the amount of financial aid that they may offer to prospective student athletes. A significant feature of many Division 1 sports programs is the ability of the school to recruit its prospective athletes on a national and international basis.

Division 2 schools are required to offer a minimum of four varsity sports for both men and women. Division 2 schools are not bound by the facility requirements of Division 1. Division 2 student athletes are often recruited on a regional as opposed to a national basis.

Division 3 schools offer no financial aid based on athletic ability, as the athletic departments at these institutions are funded as with any other aspect of the institution. While highly competitive, Division 3 athletics emphasizes the athlete over the nature and the quality of the facilities.

The NCAA imposes standard rules regarding participation in its championships, including minimum academic averages and a power to test athletes for prohibited substances such as anabolic steroids.

Almost all NCAA institutions are organized into conferences for the purposes of competitive play. Each conference is a regionally based entity, and conference play between the member schools comprises the bulk of a school's competitive schedule in a season. Conferences such as the Big Ten began as football leagues. The Big Ten, whose most famous members include Ohio State and University of Michigan, was first organized in 1896. It is an irony in the formation of the Big Ten that it was created for the express purpose of "restricted eligibility to athletics for bona fide, full-time students who were not delinquent in their studies." This sentiment has bothered college and university administrators to the present day across the United States.

Although most conferences have an extensive tradition, which has served to create passionate inter-school rivalries, some athletic conferences came into being to take advantage of increased television revenues that flow to the conference and ultimately to its member institutions. The most successful of the relatively recent conference formations has been the Big East Conference, created in 1979 to both increase the level of competition for its member schools and to take advantage of a media market centered in the

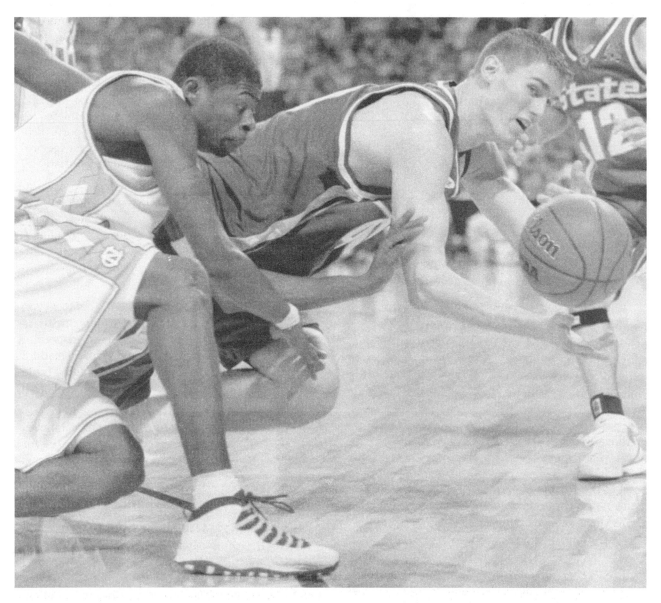

Michigan State and North Carolina battle during the semi-finals round of the 2005 NCAA men's Final Four Tournament. © PETER JONES/REUTERS/CORBIS

basketball hotbeds of New York, Philadelphia, and Washington, D.C.

The NCAA governed men's sports exclusively until 1979; the organization of women's intercollegiate athletics had begun on an ad hoc basis with a golf championship in 1941; other championships in a number of sports were convened throughout the 1960s, to little national attention or acclaim. The Association for Intercollegiate Athletics for Women (AIAW) was founded in 1971, as a separate governing body from the NCAA. With the passage of the federal U.S. legislation known as Title IX, which provided a number of guarantees regarding women's sport and its funding relative to male sports, women's sports of all types enjoyed an unprecedented growth in American colleges and universities; by 1980, the AIAW had over 900 member institutions. The NCAA organized its first women's basketball national championship in 1982, and this action prompted the disintegration of the AIAW. From 1982 forward, the NCAA has organized its women's championships along the same lines as those in male sports.

A large portion of the current work of the NCAA is with respect to its generation of revenues from the major championships held in the Division 1 men's sports of basketball and football. March Madness, as national basketball championship is popularly known, attracts a huge television audience; each of the conferences to which the 64 successful qualifiers belong receives a share of the monies from the tournament, as does the individual team and their athletic department. The BCS, the corresponding football championship series for Division 1A teams, also generates hundreds of millions of dollars in television revenues for the NCAA.

The concept of the student athlete has been one of constant attention from the NCAA throughout its history. The chief criticism of college sports in the United States has been the perception that in many sports, particularly those where the athlete has the potential to move on to the professional ranks, have been rife with abuses. The most common criticisms are with respect to recruiting students who do not have the grades that would qualify them for admission to the institution from high school, the payment of illegal monies or gifts to student athletes while they are attending the college or university, or the failure to vigorously monitor the academic progress of student athletes while they are in attendance at the institution. The NCAA has in place a number of very specific rules concerning each of these areas, the violation of which carries significant sanctions. These penalties include the suspension of the sports program from NCAA competition, the disqualification of the individual athlete, the loss or restriction of future scholarships to the program in question, and similar penalties. Critics of NCAA governance often point to the companion rules regarding the manner in which teams may train, with up to 20 hours per week in practice, additional weight room and personal training obligations, and extensive in-season travel as conditions that entirely contradict a student athlete model.

The most prominent of these initiatives has been the attention paid to student athlete graduation rates, particularly among black athletes. As of late 2005, the NCAA states that 62% of all student athletes graduate within six years of their commencement; the graduation rate among the student body as a whole is 60%.

**SEE ALSO** Basketball; National governing bodies; Title IX and United States female sports participation.

# National Football League (NFL)

The National Football League (NFL) is one of the most successful professional sports organizations anywhere in the world. The NFL successfully marketed a game that has no significant participatory base outside of North America to global prominence through the media frenzy of the Super Bowl, its annual championship game.

The NFL was founded in 1920, a league that was a progression from the semiprofessional clubs that had sprung up in the working-class towns of the eastern United States, particularly in the states of Ohio and Pennsylvania. The NFL's birth took place against the backdrop of the higher profile competitions and rivalries that were developing between the university teams of the era. The Big Ten Conference, which included such noted football institutions as Ohio State University, the University of Michigan, and Northwestern University, was located in the same region as many of the new professional franchises. Each school had an established fan base, both as a result of the glamour attached to college sports, as well as through the loyalty that college alumni possessed for their former schools.

The NFL began its existence as the American Professional Football Association (APFA) with a membership of 22 teams in 1920. Olympic decathlon champion and accomplished footballer Jim Thorpe was named the first president of the association. Many years before the racial makeup of NFL coaching staffs became a controversial issue, in 1921 Fredrick "Fritz" Pollard (1894–1986) was the first African American to lead an NFL team. After two years of play and a number of reorganizations among the membership, the APFA changed its name to the NFL in 1922. By 1925, the NFL had established tentative roots in small cities such as Canton, Ohio, Green Bay, Wisconsin, and Buffalo, New York, as well attracting franchises to New York and Chicago. In an effort to stimulate a broader public interest in the game and to build the credibility of the new league, collegiate All-Americans Ernie Nevers and George "Red" Gramge, the most famous football players of the era, were signed to NFL contracts.

The Great Depression of the 1930s and World War II combined to blunt the ability of the NFL to grow; the NFL did not have a franchise in the western United States until the 1940s. During this period, the NFL remained a distant third choice in the popularity of the American team sports public, far behind baseball and college football.

The end of World War II was accompanied by the return of servicemen who had played high level football in the armed forces. The All-America Football-Conference, established as a rival to the NFL, signed many of these players, and by 1950 the franchises from the All-American Football Conference were absorbed into the NFL. More importantly, the 1950s

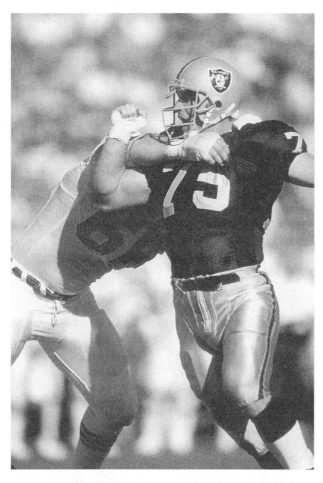

In 1922, the American Professional Football Association changed its name to the National Football League and fielded 18 teams. Today, it boasts 30. **PHOTO BY PAUL SPINELLI/GETTY IMAGES.**

spawned a revolution in American society—television sports, to which NFL football was ideally suited.

With television coverage came an unforeseen bonanza for the NFL team owners; where the survival of franchises had previously depended on gate receipts, television revenues, which the NFL owners agreed would be divided equally among the member clubs, were crucial to the stability of the league. Teams from relatively small media markets such as Green Bay had essentially the same available resources to spend on their teams as did large-market centers such as New York or Los Angeles.

A group of football entrepreneurs who had sought to take advantage of the increases in the growth of football had formed the rival American Football League (AFL) in 1960. It was the merger of this league with the NFL in 1967, initiated by NFL commissioner Pete Rozell (1926–1996) that created the championship known as the Super Bowl. From a rather pedestrian merger game in its first two years,

the Super Bowl took its first step as a media event in 1970 when an AFL team, the New York Jets, defeated the heavily favored NFL team, the Baltimore Colts.

By 1990, the Super Bowl was one of the top three rated television broadcasts on North American television; single 30-second commercial spots were sold for over three million dollars each, with the public reaction to the commercials a media subject by itself. The quality of the game, which was often significantly below the level of play during the NFL regular season, was often secondary to the Super Bowl spectacle.

With increased television exposure, a collateral force drove the popularity of the NFL: the wagering industry. The "Vegas line," the established odds on every game played each week in the NFL, became a part of North American slang. Fantasy (or "rotisserie league") football became a popular pastime by the year 2000; fantasy leagues are created by participants who each select mock teams comprised of actual NFL players, with the week-to-week statistics accumulated by the chosen players representing the method of scoring in the fantasy league.

The NFL has continued to expand its revenue base, in the face of a number of issues that carried with them negative publicity. Anabolic steroid use is regarded by the public as an ever-present feature of NFL life, yet the occasional positive test for these performance-enhancing substances has evidently not diminished public appeal. The NFL is one of very few sports leagues anywhere in the world that does not have to spend significant monies on player development. The NFL, other than through the maintenance of the franchises of NFL Europe, a developmental league, has the benefit of the successful National Collegiate Athletic Association (NCAA), whose college football program supplied virtually all of the players who compete in the NFL. "Free agency," the ability of players to sell their services to the highest bidder, has altered the competitive landscape in the NFL, as franchise owners are driven to achieve immediate success, as opposed to building a team with a consistent player base.

**SEE ALSO** Football (American); National Collegiate Athletic Association (NCAA); National governing bodies.

# National governing bodies

National governing sports bodies are found in every country of the world. These organizations may exist in relation to a single sport, such as the

United States Soccer Association, or with respect to a group of sports that are traditionally treated as aspects of one sporting discipline, such as the Canadian Ski Association. On a broader basis, the national sports bodies may regulate a wide range of individual sports, such as the national track and field associations, or a sport concept, such as participation in the Olympic movement.

The first and the most durable of the national governing bodies has been the Football Association (FA), the governing body of English soccer. The FA was created in 1863 to provide structure to fast-growing sport of soccer; the FA regularized the rules for the size of the field, dimensions of the goals, permitted equipment, and the rules of play. Once the FA had established itself credibly as the ultimate authority in the English game, it was in a position to sponsor and convene a national championship: the FA Cup, the world's oldest domestic sports championship. The first FA Cup was awarded in 1872, and the modern Cup Final remains a powerful symbol of English sport.

National governing bodies in sport are at the apex of the sport in their country. The national body is supreme within a particular country in the following aspects of the sport, including:

- The leadership of the national body will generally be created by through the election or appointment of persons from smaller, subordinate regions or states within the national framework.
- The national body in turn will be the official representatives of the country to the appropriate international sport authority. The various national Olympic Committees that exist in every country of the world are supreme in Olympic matters within their own nation, but are from a part of the hierarchical pyramid below the Olympic apex, headed by the International Olympic Committee.
- The national body is the supreme authority for the interpretation and the application of the rules of the sport within the country. In many sports, such as track and field, the rules applied by a particular country in its competitions are universal. In other sports, the national body enforces and administers a set of playing rules that may vary from the international standard. Notable examples of rule variation being permitted by a national governing body are in basketball, where the game as played at the amateur level and administered by the United States Basketball Association differs from that

supervised by the international body FIBA, and ice hockey, where the North American game is played on ice surfaces smaller than those sanctioned for international competition.

- The national body supervises all national championship competition, including the selection of a national team.
- The national body will provide the means by which competition venues are selected; the national body will certify courses, approve stadiums, or otherwise ensure that all standards for the convening of a competition are met.
- The national body will be responsible for all coaching certification within the sport. In many countries, to coach at a regional or national level, the coach is required to pass such testing as may be determined by the national body. The certification process often involves both technical knowledge of the sport as well as a more generalized expertise in sports theory.
- Many national sport bodies take the lead in their culture in the promotion of healthy sport practices, often in conjunction with government agencies. Sport education will also include the dissemination of information concerning international rules and competition standards for items such as performance-enhancing drugs.
- The national body will be the sole liaison in the sport to any companion international body; the national body will also deal directly with international organizations such as the World Anti-Doping Agency (WADA).

There are a number of sports organizations that have significant control over a particular sports activity on a national level, but which are not a governing body. The professional sports leagues, such as the National Football League (NFL) or the various national soccer leagues in existence throughout the world are professional associations, distinct from national governing bodies in that they do not regulate the sport on a national level. The professional leagues are for profit entities that do not have any influence or authority over the regulation of the sport beyond the bounds of the league members. Conversely, such national leagues are not bound by the authority of the governing body for the sport established within the country. It is common for professional sport leagues to have a relationship with a corresponding national governing body, such as that existing between the National Basketball Association (NBA) and the United States Basketball Association (USBA).

SEE ALSO International Federations; International Olympic Committee (IOC); National Collegiate Athletic Association (NCAA).

## NCAA SEE National Collegiate Athletic Association (NCAA)

## Neck injuries

Injuries to the neck may originate with the bones of the cervical spine, the disks present in the spinal column, the spinal cord, the nerves that extend into the neck, or the muscles that work with the cervical spine to create movement.

The neck is generally described as the region of the human anatomy that extends from the base of the skull to the top of the shoulders. It is supported by the cervical spine, a portion of the backbone that is a series of seven vertebrae, semicircular bones that are assembled into a column. Between each vertebrae is a disk, a ring-shaped fibrous structure that is designed to assist in the absorption and cushion of the shocks received by the spine.

The vertebrae are connected to one another by facets, ligaments that permit the various vertebrae to flex in movement. The cervical vertebrae are constructed to permit the head and the neck to move the head forward, backward, and in rotation. Vertebrae are designated in accordance with their position in the spine; the cervical, or neck, vertebrae are numberd C1 through C7, with the C1 vertebrae being the structure that supports the skull.

The vertebrae are shaped to provide bone protection to the spinal cord, which extends from the brain through the length of the spine; the brain and the spinal cord are the components of the central nervous system. From the spinal cord emanate nerves from individual openings in each of the vertebrae, extending into the body to create the network of muscular control and direction that is the peripheral nervous system. A serious injury to the spinal cord has the potential to ultimately compromise the entire peripheral system.

The muscles that work most closely with the cervical vertebrae to provide movement are the splenius capitis, which is positioned on both sides of the neck along the spine, and the trapezius, the muscles that connect the base of the neck to the shoulders.

The neck is subjected to a number of direct traumas in many different sports. The most common types of sport injuries that involve either the neck of the cervical spin include:

- Fracture of the cervical spine: This serious injury most commonly arises when the athlete has the neck driven forcefully into the shoulders. Common mechanisms of this injury are a football tackle, when either the ball carrier or the tackler has his/her head driven in a compressive fashion into the cervical vertebrae, which are forced into one another. This fracture may also occur when a diver strikes his/her head upon either the bottom of a swimming pool, or if he/she is diving from a significant height, where the diver's head collides with the water surface at an acute angle.

- Whiplash: This is an injury that may occur in similar circumstances to those of a cervical fracture. Whiplash most commonly is the result of the body moving and then coming to a sudden stop, with the head and neck continuing to move forward in a violent motion. Whiplash is a common outcome of collisions in sports such as auto racing, ice hockey, American football, and other contact sports. The reverse of the whiplash mechanism occurs, to the same physical effect, when a boxer is punched to the head, causing the skull and neck to be forced backward, while the rest of the body is relatively stationary. Unlike a fracture, whiplash is a soft tissue injury.

- Pinched nerve: This is the generic term used to describe a circumstance when one of the components of the nerve network that extends from the spinal cord becomes the subject of pressure, often from physical contact. The pressure prevents the nerve from functioning correctly, which may create a loss of function in the muscle serviced by the nerve.

- Disk injury: As with any other part of the back, the disks that separate the cervical vertebrae may become irritated, or the disk may become herniated, where its gel content leaks out and creates pressure upon the adjacent nerves. The herniated disk can occur as a result of a single movement, such as a strenuous lift, or the condition may arise over time through repeated stresses to the neck or poor posture.

- Spinal cord: An injury to the spinal cord is usually the most serious neck injury. Spinal cord damage usually occurs along with a significant force or impact. When the spinal cord becomes

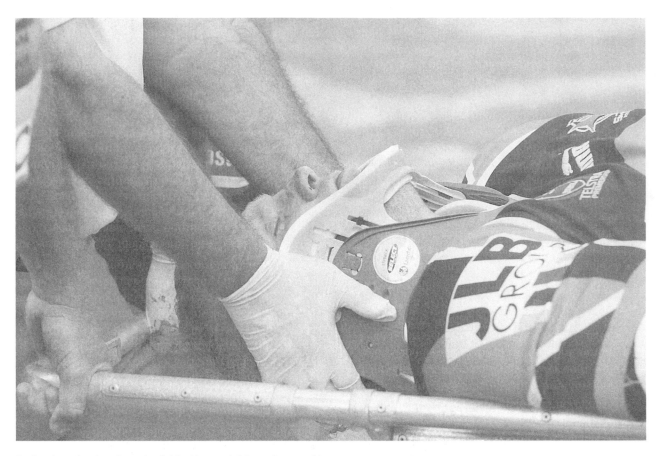

Rugby player is taken from the field with a neck injury after a tackle. **PHOTO BY MATT KING/GETTY IMAGES.**

severed, the person will almost always lose the function of either the lower limbs (paraplegia), or all of the the limbs, (quadriplegia).

Improper technique in contact sports is the leading cause of cervical spine and neck injuries in sport. When the athlete is either instructed to initiate contact with the head, or when they are reckless in the manner in which their head is exposed to such contact, neck injuries are a far more probable outcome. American football, where all players wear a helmet that in some circumstances accentuates this risk, and ice hockey, where the athletes are subject to being driven into a the barrier surrounding the playing surface, are each higher risk sports for a neck injury.

**SEE ALSO** Back injuries; Head injuries; Musculoskeletal injuries.

## Nervous system

The sophistication and the incredible dimensions of the human nervous system are the basis for the infinite range and subtlety of human movement. The nervous system, centered by the brain, generates every impulse that is directed into the musculoskeletal system for the stimulation of both muscular movement and reaction. The brain is the organ that operates the body; the human mind is the more intangible concept, connected to the physical organ and the nervous system, but extending into the aspects of intelligence, reasoning abilities, and human perception.

The brain is the most far-reaching organ in the body, with its influence and its control over every aspect of human function extended by way of the network that is the nervous system. Physical abilities that are at the essence of athletic ability, including muscular control, hand-eye coordination, reaction time, and the utilization of the body's composition of fast-twitch versus slow-twitch fibers, are all determined by the brain.

As the chief component of the nervous system generally, the brain is positioned at the top of the first branch of the nervous system, familiar as the central nervous system (CNS). The CNS has two parts, the

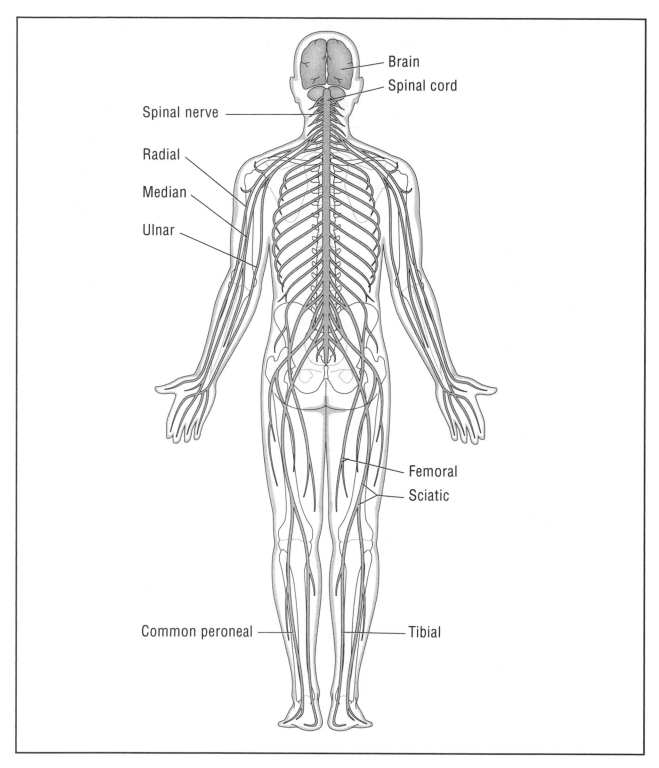

Brain

Spinal cord

Spinal nerve

Radial

Median

Ulnar

Femoral

Sciatic

Common peroneal

Tibial

The human nervous system. THE GALE GROUP

brain and the spinal cord, that extend from the region of the brain known as the brain stem, located at the base of the skull. The spinal cord runs through the spinal column, a bony protective structure, to the base of the spine at the pelvis. The spinal cord is primarily composed of nerve cells, known as neurons.

The brain is divided into a series of regions, each of which has a distinct responsibility for a function of the body. The cerebellum, located near the base of

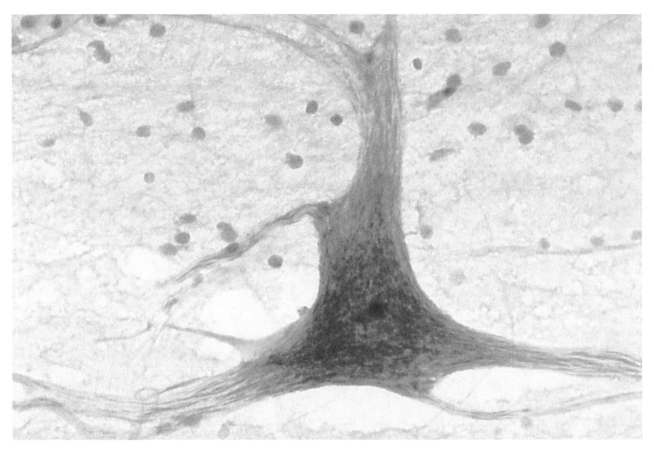

A nerve cell. © ROYALTY-FREE/CORBIS

the brain, is the learning center of the brain. The hypothalamus, connected to the pituitary gland, regulates body temperature and other functions that are a response to external stimuli. Whenever any of these control centers seek to transmit a message to another part of the body for action, the message begins it travel along the spinal cord.

The central nervous system is connected to a far more extensive nerve network. This structure is the peripheral nervous system. Unlike the central nervous system components, which are protected by the bone of the skull and the spine, the elements of the peripheral nervous system are not protected, extending through the tissue in pathways. The peripheral nervous system is a highly complex series of nerves and neurons that extend to every part of the body. The peripheral nervous system is itself subdivided into two major operational systems: the somatic (or voluntary) nervous system and the autonomic nervous system. The somatic system directs movement and the control of the skeletal muscles. The nerves that extend into the muscles ultimately terminate in a motor neuron, the device that transmits the particular

instruction to the adjacent muscle fibers. The speed with which the particular neuron is designed to direct its impulses into the muscle fiber will dictate whether the fiber is a fast-twitch or slow-twitch fiber.

The other branch of the peripheral nervous system, the autonomic system, has three further subdivisions. As the name implies, the autonomic system is responsible for the regulation of a number of bodily functions that are either involuntary, or where the body generates an initial response that may be the subject of further voluntary action. The sympathetic nervous system includes the management of the body's "fight or flight" response, triggered when the brain, after receiving stimulation of a threat or other challenge, directs the production of adrenaline, the hormone that stimulates heart rate, respiratory function and the expansion of blood vessel capacity.

The counterpoint to the sympathetic nervous system is the parasympathetic nervous system, whose function is often summarized as the "rest and digest" response. After stimulation, the parasympathetic system acts to calm the body, through stimulation of the salivary gland to encourage eating and slowing the heart rate.

The third aspect of the autonomic system is sometime regarded as a separate nervous system, due to the nature of the organs that it controls. The enteric nervous system regulates the stomach and colon.

The nervous system functions as an entity, with the brain providing the ultimate direction. Although many nervous system functions are involuntary, damage to the central nervous system in particular can dramatically alter nervous system function as a whole. Much of the response of the nervous system to injury or impairment is one directional, for if the body senses damage to a lesser aspect of one of the subordinate components to the nervous system, it will endeavor to compensate; brain or spinal cord injuries do not permit alternate paths or compensatory routes.

SEE ALSO Motor control; Muscle fibers: Fast and slow twitch; Neck injuries.

## NFL SEE National Football League (NFL)

# Nonsteroidal anti-inflammatory drugs (NSAIDs)

Nonsteroidal drugs take their name from the class of compounds created to act as an anti-inflammatory and analgesic (painkiller). A steroid is a compound that may occur both in a natural form as well as through synthesis. Steroids are defined chemically as substances that possess 17 carbon atoms, arranged in a series of four rings. Many of the natural steroids are hormones, the chemicals that are involved in the control of many physical processes. The most notable of these steroid hormones are the male hormone testosterone, the female hormones estrogen and progesterone, vitamin D, and adrenalin. The naturally generated anti-inflammatory cortisone is also a steroid.

Anti-inflammatories are those agents that are intended to reduce the pain and swelling caused when a joint becomes irritated, often through overuse. Ice is a common treatment for an inflammation or swelling of a muscle tissue or joint. Nonsteroidal anti-inflammatory drugs (NSAIDs) also tend to reduce fever. NSAIDs function by neutralizing the cyclooxgenase (COX) enzyme that is produced at

the site of a musculoskeletal injury. Enzymes are proteins that act as a catalyst in specific types of biological reactions; at the injury location, the COX enzyme will naturally generate inflammation. COX enzymes are present in the body in two forms, COX-1 and COX-2.

COX-1 is present in cells throughout the human body. It plays an important role in the regulation of the protection of the stomach lining, the regulation of salt and fluid balances, and the flow of blood to the kidneys. COX-2 is found primarily in the immune cells and the cells of the central nervous system (CNS). Each produces prostaglandins, the actual cause of inflammation and pain. NSAIDs function by inhibiting these enzymes that otherwise produce prostaglandins.

The most well-known of the NSAID class of medications is aspirin, or acetasalicylic acid, first synthesized in 1899. The history of this active ingredient of aspirin as an analgesic and as an anti-inflammatory is much longer. More than 3,000 years ago, the use of extract of the myrtle plant, which contains salicylic acid was used to relieve joint pain and inflammation. Willow bark, which also has salicylic acid in its chemistry, was used by Hippocrates, the founder of modern medicine, as a pain reliever more than 2,500 years ago. The use of boiled willow bark as a pain reliever and as a general aid to muscle and joint pain continued through the Middle Ages. Felix Hoffman (1868–1946), a scientist employed by the pharmaceutical company Bayer, modified the salicylic acid extracted from plant sources to produce aspirin, which became the largest selling pharmaceutical product in history. Aspirin has been a generic drug, not the subject of a corporate patent, since the 1930s, and it continues to be marketed by Bayer and numerous other pharmaceutical companies.

Aspirin was found to be effective as an anti-inflammatory, although the actual mechanism of how it acted on the COX enzymes was not determined until the 1970s. The second most famous of the NSAIDs is ibuprofen, approved for use in the United States by the Food and Drug Agency (FDA) in 1974; it is marketed under trade names such as Advil and Motrin. Both aspirin and ibuprofen are regarded as milder formulations of NSAIDs, with generally fewer side effects and a less pronounced anti-inflammatory action than more recently developed products. The current generation of NSAID medications are sometimes referenced as COX inhibitors.

It is a testament to the familiarity of these agents within the sports world that NSAIDs are consumed by all manner of athletes to help them manage minor pain. In the long-distance running world, aspirin and ibuprofen are commonly taken by recreational athletes before a marathon to anticipate the anti-inflammatory effects desired.

There are a number of physical advantages to the use of NSAIDs over other steroid-based anti-inflammatories, all of which must be assessed against their demonstrated risks to the user. These advantages include:

- There are fewer adverse reactions noted in NSAID use.
- Low-dose NSAIDs such as aspirin and ibuprofen have the additional demonstrated benefit of enhancing circulation; there is significant scientific data supporting aspirin and ibuprofen as inhibitors of excess blood clotting and reducing the risk of heart attack.
- NSAIDs are effective in the ongoing management of the pain associated with osteoarthritis.
- The use of NSAID, especially over the long term, presents risk of gastrointestinal tract bleeding, with risks of stomach, liver, and kidney disease.
- There are well-known interactions between NSAIDs of all types and other medications. As all NSAIDs have a blood-thinning capacity, the use of NSAIDs in conjunction with blood-thinning medication as used by some persons to lessen the risk of stroke may be dangerous.

SEE ALSO Glucocorticoids; Herbs; RICE (Rest/Ice/Compression/Elevation) treatment for injuries; Topical corticosteroids.

# Nordic skiing SEE Skiing, Nordic (cross-country skiing)

# Nutrition

Nutrition has two separate but related meanings when considered in relation to sports science. Nutrition is the course of academic or scientific study directed to the relationship between diet and the health and function of the human body. Nutrition is also the actual nourishment of the body, the supply of the substances that sustain it.

As with many of the overarching concepts that often affect nutrition, the broadly applicable areas of diet, exercise and fitness, health, and longevity will often come into play; nutritional practices never exist in the abstract.

For the athlete, proper nutrition is as essential as the training that underlies a sports program. It is impossible for an athlete to reach the physical potential unless those efforts are supported by healthy food, vitamin, and mineral intake. Health scientists have determined that a balanced diet, one that provides proper amounts of carbohydrates, proteins, and fats, is the foundation to good overall nutrition. Although the proportions may vary from person to person, the usual guidelines are approximately 60-65% carbohydrates, 12-15% proteins, and less than 30% fats.

The governmental authorities in many countries publish scientifically based guidelines concerning optimal nutritional practices that mimic the carbohydrate/protein/fats ratio, using descriptions that employ quantities of each food group as opposed to finite measurements. Governmental attention to the concept of healthy nutrition, coupled with more active lifestyles, has increased throughout the Western world as populations have become demonstrably more overweight and obese since 1960. Weight gains have been accompanied in dramatic rises in related health conditions such as diabetes and cardiovascular problems.

In the United States, the federal Department of Agriculture is the agency responsible for the promotion of healthy diet and nutritional practices through the publication of the *Food Guide Pyramid*, first released in 1992. The successor guide, known as *MyPyramid*, was revised and published in 2005. MyPyramid illustrates the balance between healthy food consumption, activity, and rest, with information concerning other general nutritional issues. The MyPyramid rendering breaks the traditional carbohydrate, proteins, and fats divisions into six parts: grains, vegetables, fruits, oils, milk, and meats/beans. The user-friendly divisions of MyPyramid contemplate healthy consumption as a part of a strong nutritional practice in the same approximate ratios as the traditional divisions.

Devices such as MyPyramid emphasize the interrelated nature of health as achieved through diet and nutrition. How the individual moderates consumption of each component of a diet will determine how nutritional his/her dietary practices are likely to be. The components of a typical diet include:

- Carbohydrates are essential to the production of energy within the body, particularly through the processing of foods into glucose and its stored form, glycogen.

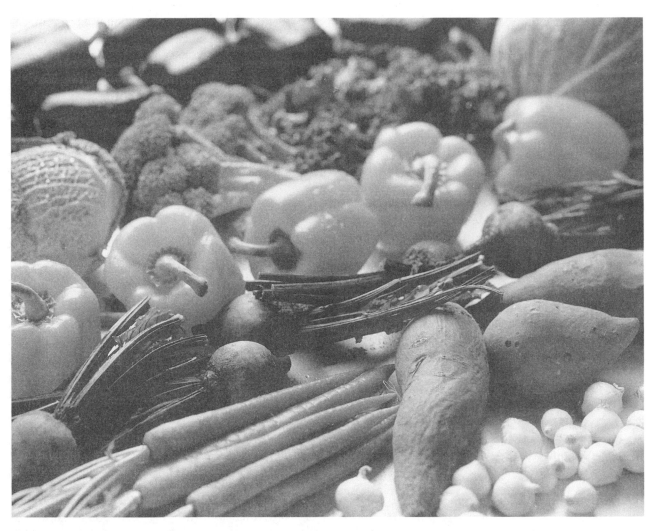

Vegetables play a key role in maintaining balanced nutrition. © ENVISION/CORBIS

- Proteins are containers of amino acids, essential to the formation, development, and maintenance of muscles and tissues.
- Fats are stored within the body as triglycerides, released as glycerol and fatty acids, which are essential to both energy production and the absorption of numerous vitamins.
- Minerals are required for both bone construction and the efficient functioning of hundreds of various human systems, including fluid levels and the effective transmission of nerve impulses in the body.
- Vitamins are the chemicals responsible for both healthy function of the digestive and absorption processes, as well as the function of bone construction.
- Athletic supplements, such as creatine, have a pronounced impact on the body during training,

which will necessitate careful monitoring of the consequences of training on both the body and its dietary and nutritional needs. Supplements must correspond to athletic need, such as the use of creatine in training for explosive, anaerobic sports.

- Caffeine, euphemistically referred to as a food group due to its large consumption, has no nutritional value; the effects of caffeine as both a stimulant as well as a diuretic require careful attention to be paid to its impact upon the body.
- Alcohol is technically a carbohydrate, as its active compound breaks down into sugar and carbon dioxide when digested, although it is a poor nutrient. Alcohol also must be very carefully regulated as a healthy nutritional aspect, given its impact on the central nervous system and the effect of alcohol as a diuretic.

Alcohol also impacts the thermoregulatory system, making its ingestion even more subject to scrutiny in cold weather exercise.

One important benchmark of success in nutritional practice is the formulation of the pre-event and post-event meals that are nutritionally sound. As a general rule, subject to the individual needs of the athlete or the dictates of competition, the following meal pattern will support the nutritional needs of the athlete, including:

1. A regular meal that has a carbohydrate emphasis, between four hours to six hours prior to the event. For a morning competition, this meal can be taken the night before.
2. A small, carbohydrate-rich meal can be taken two hours prior to the event.
3. A very low fat snack can be taken 30 minutes to 45 minutes prior to the event.
4. A small carbohydrate-rich meal can be taken within one hour of the event.
5. A further, larger carbohydrate-rich meal can be taken within three hours of the event.

Each of the post-event meals is intended to immediately replace lost stores of both carbohydrates and nutrients; the body absorbs these replacement foods best closer in time to the event. Proper nutrition will always include adequate rehydration.

**SEE ALSO** Carbohydrates; Diet; Fat intake; Growth; Minerals; Vitamin C.

# Nutrition and athletic performance

The relationship between nutrition and athletic performance is as certain as the connection between physical training and athletic success. The physical demands of all sports necessitate the consumption of healthy foods, with the correct proportion of carbohydrates, proteins, and fats. The types of foods consumed must also contain optimal amounts of vitamins and minerals, all supported by appropriate and consistent hydration levels in the body.

Athletic performance is an expression that is distinct from many of the broader sports science concepts, such as health, fitness, or longevity. Athletic performance describes the efforts made by an athlete to attain specific performance objectives over a period of time. The natural talent or fitness of the athlete will impact the level of performance; all ath-

letes ultimately measure performance by their own standards. Performance is usually regarded as an aggregation of individual results, such as performance over a month, or a season of competition, as opposed to a single or isolated activity. Athletic performance includes not only the assessment of a particular result, but also the concept of recovery; how quickly an athlete can return to the regular training or routine is an important performance factor, as recovery will dictate how the athlete is able to prepare for the next event. Nutrition places a vital role in the improvement of every aspect of performance.

There is no single wonder food or miracle supplement that will guarantee perfect nutrition for an athlete. Science has determined that while there are many ways to nutritionally enhance a diet that is deficient in respect of one or more components, the best approach for athletes and non-athletes alike is to consume a traditional balanced diet, variations of which have been promoted by most governments in the world for over 40 years. There is also strong scientific support for the proposition that subject to modification of caloric intake, due to the energy requirements of sport, the type of diet that provides nutritional value to athletes is very similar to that consumed by the healthy non-athlete.

The balanced diet is usually expressed in one of two ways: as a ratio of the carbohydrate, protein, and fat food groups, or as a food pyramid, where the recommended daily consumption of different kinds of food within the three food groups is defined by portions or quantities. The Canada Food Guide and the formulation named *MyPyramid*, developed and published by the United States Department of Agriculture (USDA), are two examples. In each recommendation, daily amounts of whole grains, dairy, vegetables, fruits, fish, and meat products are specified, as are suggested methods for cooking and food preparation that will maximize the nutritional value of each food.

It is a central premise of the balanced diet, whether viewed from the apportionment of carbohydrates, proteins, and fats, or by food type and portion, that if the right kinds of foods are consumed, the person will invariably obtain the other crucial nutritional benefits, including the necessary amounts of vitamins, minerals, fiber, and fluids. Carbohydrates such as whole grains, fruits, and vegetables are all excellent vitamin and mineral sources; examples are whole grains, which provide both the vitamin B complex and dietary fiber to aid in digestion, and citrus fruits, all of which are rich in vitamin C.

The development of a specific nutritional plan for an elite-level athlete will represent variations, as opposed to any wholesale changes, to basic nutritional approaches. A common belief among strength athletes, such as weightlifters or those seeking to build muscle, is that their diet must reflect their training through a greater consumption of protein, essential to muscle building and repair, through both foods and dietary supplements. While in short-term situations an athlete might increase protein to assist in a weight program, as a general proposition these athletes require only minimally greater amounts of protein on a daily basis to support their training levels than do other athletes.

Some athletes share the same misconception concerning the fat component of the balanced diet; fats must be reduced, in the belief that the body will be leaner. This approach overlooks that fats are themselves an excellent energy source for the body, released from their storage in the adipose tissues as fatty acids, which are utilized by the cells to produce energy, and glycerol, which is processed by the liver into glycogen. As importantly, when athletes seek to reduce the quantity of fats from that suggested in a balanced diet, they potentially impair the ability of the body to absorb fat-soluble vitamins, including vitamin D, critical to the ability of the body to use calcium in bone construction and repair.

The one class of athlete who may require a more significant deviation from the patterns of the healthy diet is the young athlete, whose body will be experiencing normal growth increases and be subject to the demands of athletic activity. The nutritionally sound diet for this athlete will often require both greater quantities of each food group, as well as careful attention to the levels of minerals such as calcium and magnesium, which are essential to the growth of the musculoskeletal system.

**SEE ALSO** Carbohydrates; Diet; Minerals; Nutrition.

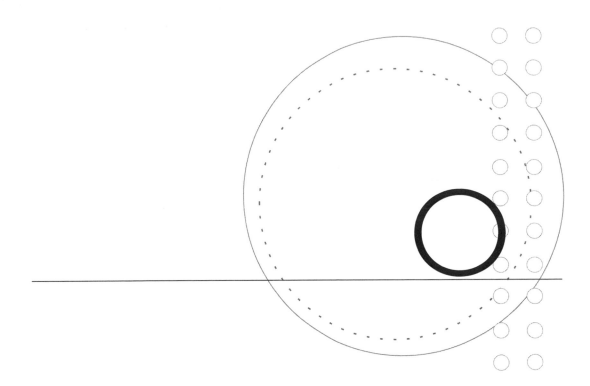

# Obesity

In its simplest expression, obesity is a physical condition where the amount of fat stored within the cells of the body significantly impairs the overall health of that individual. Obese persons are visibly overweight, with their physical ability to move without strain significantly reduced. Obesity is a designation that is a part of a body mass continuum that begins with the term underweight, or skinny, continuing through ideal weight, overweight, obese, and an ultimate condition, morbid obesity. Obesity is a significant health problem throughout the industrialized world, and in many countries it has replaced smoking and the illnesses related to that habit as the most important societal health concern to be addressed, especially among young people.

Obesity has become so prevalent that, in the last 30 years, the study of obesity and its causes has evolved into a distinct medical specialty, bariatrics, a term derived from the Greek word *baros*, meaning weight.

There is no unanimous agreement as to how obesity should be defined in terms of the physical size, the percentage of body fat, or physical capabilities of a person. A common tool used in the assessment of obesity is the formula known as the body mass index (BMI). The BMI was developed as a method to assist in the determination of a particular person's weight relative to a range of ideal weights, calculated in reference to height. BMI is determined by dividing the weight of the person by their height squared. Subject to a number of physical variables, BMI defines the positions on the index using the following reference points: ideal weight, 18.5–25 BMI; overweight, greater than 25 BMI; obese, greater than 30 BMI; and morbidly obese, greater than 35 BMI.

The BMI definitions are subject to significant individual factors, as a person's body type and other genetic features may influence weight without necessarily creating the adverse health concerns of obesity. An example is the large, muscular athlete who will often possess a ratio of lean body mass to fat that is far higher than the average sedentary person; the BMI may otherwise categorize this athlete as overweight or obese. Conversely, a sedentary female adolescent may be tall and appear very slim, but due to the combination of an unhealthy diet and little exercise, she may possess a significant amount of body fat.

An alternative definition of obesity is determined through the determination of body fat percentage, the relationship between stored fat and overall body mass. Body fat can be measured with some degree of precision, using tools such as skin calipers, to measure skin folds at the places on the body where fat-storing adipose tissue are most concentrated, such as the chest, abdomen, triceps, and upper thighs. Water displacement machines can also accurately determine body fat percentage. While there is no strict consensus in the medical community on what amount of body fat will render a person obese, most definitions set 20% or greater as a baseline.

Whatever measure is employed as yardstick to determine whether a person is obese or is significantly overweight, the body and its ability to function are severely compromised, both in the immediate term and with respect to the longevity of the person. The most common health problems that arise as a direct result of obesity are cardiovascular disease, diabetes, and various forms of osteoarthritis.

Cardiovascular function is the first casualty of a body whose weight is far in excess of the ideal. The heart is required to pump blood through an oversized structure, which places significant stress on overall cardiac function. The typical fat-rich diet of the obese person leads to the creation of low-density lipoproteins (LDLs), a form of cholesterol that forms plaque within the blood vessels, resulting in narrower arterial passages and a greater risk of stroke.

The incidence of diabetes in the Western world has risen by over 50% since 1970; the prevalence of juvenile diabetes has climbed even more dramatically. Diabetes is generally caused through the inability of the body to generate insulin, the hormone produced by the pancreas that regulates the glucose levels within the bloodstream. The onset of diabetes is often due to a combination of factors, with obesity and a sedentary lifestyle chief contributors.

Osteoarthritis and other diseases of the joints and the connective tissues are a common result of obesity. The mechanisms are very simple—if the body is genetically designed to support a particular mass, the body will eventually break down as it is not be able to adequately support the excess weight.

The health risks and the limitations of obesity are not restricted to the observable examples. Bariatric science has established that the overall health risks associated with being persistently overweight, if not clinically obese, are far higher than those for the balance of the population. Numerous medical studies, including those of the American Medical Association, confirm that persons who were overweight through their middle age (approximately 40 years to 60 years of age), were at a significantly greater risk of dying from heart disease or diabetes by age 65.

The obvious cure to obesity is to restrict the number of calories consumed and to adhere to an exercise program. As obesity so often carries with it a host of psychological and physical health problems, many obese people undergo bariatrics surgery, which involves either restricting the size of the stomach to limit intake through the insertion of a gastric band, or physically stapling the stomach to create a smaller-sized organ.

SEE ALSO Diet; Health; Juvenile obesity; Obesity and insulin resistance; Weight gain.

# Obesity and insulin resistance

Obesity is a condition that is defined by a range of physical factors, the most important of which is the excess amount of fat stored within the body of any person. Obesity is the most extreme form of excess weight; the greater the excess, the more limited the person will be in physical capabilities, and the more significant the corresponding strains placed on the bodily processes such as the cardiovascular system. Obesity carries with it an inevitably greater risk that the person will develop and die from a serious disease.

One of the most common physical consequences of obesity is the development of insulin resistance. Insulin is a hormone produced by the pancreas as a part of the body's mechanism of processing and regulating the level of glucose in the bloodstream. After food has been consumed, insulin acts as a chemical-signaling device to maintain glucose levels at a steady rate. The countervailing hormone to insulin is glucagon, which will signal the body to correct a glucose level that is too low through the release of glucose, stored as glycogen, from the liver.

In a synthetic form, insulin is used as a medication, injected directly into the bloodstream of persons who suffer from type 1 diabetes (also known as juvenile diabetes), the disease caused when the body is not able to produce any, or enough, insulin. These insulin injections are essential to the survival of patients in these circumstances. The discovery of synthetic insulin by Frederick Banting (1891–1941) and Charles Best (1899–;1978) of the University of Toronto in 1921 is regarded as one of the great advances in the history of medical science. Insulin is essential to the health of millions of diabetics throughout the world.

Insulin resistance arises where the ability of insulin to regulate and to signal changes to glucose levels in the blood is decreased. When the cells of the body become insulin resistant, the message that should otherwise be conveyed to the cells by the presence of insulin is not the subject of an immediate response from the body. When the cells do not respond to the insulin signal for glucose balance, ever-increasing amounts of insulin are produced in the pancreas, which treats the lack of cellular response to the presence of insulin to mean that more insulin is required. Insulin resistance is a form of biological misinformationthe body believes that it must increase the amount of glucose. When the insulin message is finally acted on by the cells, there is a flood of glucose into the cells from the bloodstream, which creates a condition known as a hypoglycemic reaction, more commonly stated as low blood sugar. Insulin resistance produces a cycle of repeated spikes in blood sugar level will eventually exact a toll on the pancreas and its ability to produce insulin. When the body is not protected by its blood sugar-leveling mechanism, it is vulnerable to the opposite condition, hyperglycemia, excessive blood sugar. When insulin resistance is untreated, death is a likely event.

The risk of becoming diabetic, or insulin resistant, is genetic in origin for some persons, creating a greater likelihood of becoming diabetic no matter what environmental factors are involved, including diet and lifestyle. There is, however, no question that all persons who are overweight or obese are at far greater risk. As an obese person gains excessive weight, they subject their pancreas to long-term stresses in insulin production.

Insulin resistance has other serious consequences, as it will often lead to the progressive illness known as the metabolic syndrome, which is the combination of a series of distinct physical conditions. Each component of the metabolic syndrome is potentially dangerous to human health when present alone: type 2 diabetes (diabetes mellitus), hypertension (high blood pressure), hyperlipidimedia (the production of excessive levels of low density lipoproteins, a harmful cholesterol that causes plaque to form inside the blood vessels, which causes a narrowing and the potential for restricted blood flow), and obesity, characterized by the presence of a "beer belly," the presence of fat deposits that are more pronounced along the abdomen.

The onset of type 2 diabetes creates a further series of health risks. Type 2 diabetics have a proven greater risk of cardiovascular disease, renal (kidney) failure, and the risk of various infections, particularly when the skin is cut or a sore develops. Type 2 diabetes can often be controlled through a comprehensive program of proper diet (with careful attention to the amount of carbohydrates consumed), weight management, and an exercise program, coupled with medication, chiefly insulin or those of the thiazolidinedione type. The diet formulations required for persons with insulin resistance will involve a consideration of the glycemic index, a food-ranking system that assists in determining which types of food are absorbed more slowly and steadily into the body, and which are absorbed quickly. As glucose levels in the blood are never constant, due to variable impacts of environment, exercise, illness, stress, or similar factors, an effective

program to counter insulin resistance must be flexible and responsive to the effect of these variables.

Insulin resistance is an irreversible and progressive condition; once the body's cells do not respond to insulin, the glucose levels must be controlled through human intervention and monitoring. In obese persons, insulin resistance is another stressor on the body that heightens the considerable risk of early mortality.

**SEE ALSO** Carbohydrates; Hormones; Juvenile obesity; Obesity.

# Obesity, juvenile SEE Juvenile obesity

# Patrick O'Grady
6/7/1936–
AMERICAN
GOLF EQUIPMENT DEVELOPER

Patrick O'Grady is a golf equipment sales executive and equipment developer who was responsible for the promotion of several equipment innovations in both North American and international golf, most notably with respect to golf shoe technology.

O'Grady's early employment career had little bearing on his subsequent professional success in the golf industry. He was a soldier in the United States Army until 1955, and upon his discharge into civilian life, O'Grady worked in a variety of businesses until his entry into golf merchandising in 1961.

O'Grady had become a respected member of the golf equipment industry when he joined the Etonic shoe company in 1985. Etonic was a respected manufacturer of golf shoes and related golf equipment. Between 1985 and 1997, O'Grady was a key figure in the development of three distinct technical advances with respect to golf shoe design—the waterproof golf shoe, the first biomechanical golf shoe insole, and the spikeless golf shoe (known as soft spikes).

Golf is both an international sport and one of the world's most popular recreational activities. The nature of the activity is one that attracts both elite professional talents as well as those persons of almost any age who play golf for its own sake. Golf is one of the few sports that can be played by any healthy person to their own ability. The golf handicapping system, where a lesser player can compete with a better player through the provision of a stroke advantage to the lesser player, is one of golf's attractions.

It is the nature of golf that its players will seek any competitive advantage, however slight, through improvements to equipment. Golf club and golf ball technology alone is an international multi-billion dollar sub-industry. It is that light that the developments with respect to golf shoe technology as championed by O'Grady should be examined.

Early golf shoes were constructed from conventional footwear; these shoes were as much a fashion statement as they were intended to assist the player. The early spiked shoes were made from wing tip styled Oxford shoes with small steel spikes inserted through the soles of the shoe. The conventional golf shoe as it was marketed by 1980 had a number of ongoing design problems. As golf is an outdoor activity, the shoes did not always stand up to wet weather; the golfer's feet would be exposed to the wetness of the ground for extended periods of time.

Golf shoes at that time were not manufactured with any particular design attention given with respect to how the golfer's foot was supported by the shoe, particularly at the insole. As a function of biomechanics, the more secure the foot could be positioned with in the golf shoe the greater the prospect of an effective swing. Where the foot is secure, the golfer's body will be more stable as the forces of the golf swing are directed into the ball. Where the foot was subjected to an unequal force, such as those caused by excessive pronation (where the ankle and foot rotate inwards on contact with the ground), or supination (where the foot and ankle rotate outwards), the ability of the golfer to maintain stability throughout their entire swing is affected.

The spikes fitted to golf shoes were viewed as essential to assisting golfers with stability in their swing; the cost to golf course maintenance due to the damage caused by metal spikes to the surfaces of greens was a significant issue at many golf clubs. Further, the fundamental enjoyment of golf was seen as compromised when players were subjected to a playing surface that had been chewed up by the metal spikes of preceding players.

As one with a leadership role in the merchandising of golf equipment, O'Grady received significant feedback from recreational golfers and club professionals regarding the quality of the equipment sold by Etonic. O'Grady worked with Etonic technical personnel in each of these three areas of golf shoe technology to improve the product. To assist golfers in achieving biomechanical efficiency, golf shoes were constructed to accommodate an orthotic if the player required additional stability. Modern waterproofing fabrics such as GORE-TEX were incorporated into the linings of the shoe to repel water. The spikeless shoes were constructed with a series of studs made from various rubber compounds. The studs were often configured into individual and removable cleats. The spikeless design was proven to provide the golfer with stability equal to that of the conventional metal spikes while preserving the surfaces of greens.

It is a testament to O'Grady's understanding of the golf market that each of the developments in which he had a role in 1985 had became the standard in the golf industry by 2000.

In recognition of his contributions to the development golf equipment, O'Grady was recognized for his contributions to American golf by the United States Professional Golfers Association (PGA) in 2004.

SEE ALSO Golf; Recreational sports.

# Older athletes SEE Mature athletes

# Scott Olson

3/9/1959–
AMERICAN
INVENTOR

Scott Olson, along with his brother Brennan, are credited as the first developers of a commercially viable inline skate.

In 1979, the Olson brothers came across a pair of old inline skates in Minneapolis. They were competitive ice hockey players and each possessed a strong understanding of how skaters propel themselves across ice. The Olson brothers acquired the skates and they began to experiment with the configuration of the skate wheels and the construction of the boot. As hockey players, they saw the potential of inline skates as an off-season training aid.

The notion of using wheeled skates to travel on dry land was not a novel one in 1979, as roller skates, with a box shaped wheel configuration, had been available for decades in the United States. The concept of inline skates, where three or four wheels were positioned in a straight alignment, had been patented many years prior to 1979, but the concept had never been commercially marketed.

In theory, an inline configuration would provide the user with greater maneuverability and the wheels would present less rolling resistance than conventional roller blade wheels, and consequently permit the user to travel at greater speeds on paved surfaces. Where the user desired speed, the wheels on the inline skate could be of greater circumference, as larger wheels provide produce as they travel further in each revolution (there is also a correspondingly greater amount of energy required to initiate the movement of the larger wheels). Smaller circumference wheels will permit ease of stopping for the user and are preferred for the performing of tricks. The inline skating motion is one where the skater will naturally shift their center of gravity to a point above each leg as it drives the respective skate forward. In doing so, there will be a greater efficiency of motion, as the full weight of the body will be hind each stride.

Scott Olson ultimately added four wheels made from urethane (ethyl carbamate), a hard rubber compound, to a boot obtained from an old ice hockey skate. Olson added a rubber toe brake to assist the user in stopping, positioned in a similar fashion to the toe picks that assist a figure skater in stopping and performing jumps. Olson argued that a boot such as that used in ice hockey was required to provide the user with both flexibility and ankle support. The urethane wheels provided efficient, reduced friction movement in relation to one another as well as a measure of traction not available between metal roller skate wheels and pavement.

A rubber heel brake was subsequently added to the design, a device that permitted a skater to depress their heel and stop quickly and remain in a stable position.

Between 1979 and 1983, Scott Olson directed the research and development of the inline skates that he had created. Olson formed a company, Rollerblade Inc. to further the production of the product.

The initial Rollerblades were popular, but as with many new products, there were flaws in the original design that limited performance. The most common difficulty occurred in the wheels and their tendency to not run smoothly due to the build-up of dirt inside the ball bearing mechanism within each wheel. However, Olson's initial belief as to the utility of the Rollerblade as a off season hockey training aid was also embraced by the cross-country skiing community. The natural motion required to propel oneself on inline skate permitted the off season skiers to approximate the skiing motion on pavement.

In 1983, Olson sold the Rollerblade company. In the late 1980s, the Rollerblade product became extremely popular with recreational users who sought fitness. Rollerblades also became the basis of competitive inline skating hockey competitions popular in various parts of North America. Inline speed skating races, conducted both on indoor tracks as well as on road courses, became one of the earlier recognized extreme sports. The success of Rollerblade prompted a number of corporate competitors to enter the inline skating market after 1990.

Inline skating has also become a performance art, with tricks and various stunts performed at skateboard parks. The skaters use fixed structures such as half pipes and ramps to generate both speed and the hang time necessary to complete complex aerial routines.

It is a testament to the foresight of the Olson brothers that the terms Rollerblade and blading are cemented into everyday North American language; the generic term for any inline skate is a rollerblade.

Scott Olson continued his career as a developer of fitness products after selling the Rollerblade company. Olson patented a design called the RowBike a two-wheeled machine that is configured like a bicycle, but one that is powered by the rider who employs a rowing motion. The action of the rider is similar to that of the railroad hand carts in use in the early days of railroading in North America.

**SEE ALSO** Recreational sports; Roller hockey; Roller skates.

# Olympic Committee (IOC) SEE International Olympic Committee (IOC)

# Olympic Committee, U.S. SEE United States Olympic Committee

# Olympics, Special SEE Special Olympics

# Open water swimming SEE Swimming: Open water

# Orthotics

Orthotics include a broad range of physical aids used primarily to correct structural problems in the feet, knees, lower back, neck, and wrists. An orthotic may be any orthopedic device that is external to the body. Orthotics is also the name given to the medical field that provides specialized consultation and advice concerning corrective devices. Orthotics are distinguished from prosthetic devices, which are artificial or mechanical devices that replace an absent limb.

An orthotic may have one or more purposes, including to provide support to a limb or joint; to protect and prevent a part of the body from exposure to a particular range of motion; to assist in a particular function or movement; and to correct a specific structural weakness or imbalance, particularly through the realignment of the joint or structure.

The most common orthotic devices are foot orthotics, which are designed to correct the irregularities in the runner's gait that lead to both uneven foot strikes on the ground and consequent injuries; neck braces, which are primarily to restrict neck movement when the person has sustained a neck muscle sprain or similar injury; a back support, often referred to as a truss or girdle, designed to provide additional support to the lumbar vertebrae and muscle structures; knee braces of various kinds, all of which are structured to provide support to the joint where it has sustained a structural injury such as ligament damage, as well as to restrict it from being bent or twisted; and wrist supports, which are designed to maintain the strength of the wrist, in conjunction with the thumb joint.

For athletes, the most common reason for orthotic use is the desire to correct an inherent structural or alignment problem, most often in the manner in which the athlete runs. When the athlete has one leg longer than the other or the arch of one foot higher than the other, the running motion will naturally generate unequal forces from the moment the foot strikes the ground. This force radiates into the sole of the foot, particularly the plantar and heel, through the ankle joint, along the lower leg, into the knee, and is ultimately absorbed by the hip joint. Each of these points is vulnerable to the repetitive nature of the running motion, causing damage to its structure. An orthotic, typically a lightweight molded insert, will be custom designed for the runner to be worn on the inside of each shoe to create a more even footfall and correspondingly equitable distribution of the forces. These shoe insert orthotics have become quite popular and are not restricted to correction of alignment of the structures of distance runners. The efficiency and the ultimate performance of athletes in every running discipline will be influenced by structural misalignment, including track running and all field sports.

Brace orthotics perform a different role for the athlete. Neck and knee braces, the most common of these appliances, are intended primarily to restrict the ability of the subject joint to move in a fashion that might cause a re-injury. Neck braces, modified to fit even an American football player while wearing other protective equipment, are sometimes worn by players who have either sustained a minor neck muscle strain or who have a history of neck problems. The neck brace will assist in the prevention of the neck being extended. In a similar fashion, knee braces are almost always worn by athletes who have sustained a previous injury, often to the medial or anterior cruciate ligament (ACL), the connective tissues that essentially hold the femur (thigh bone) to the tibia and fibula (shin bones). When the athlete has had reconstructive ligament surgery, the brace serves to prevent the knee from being forced from one side to the other, which places undue stress on the repaired joint.

To provide the maximum degree of desired support, an orthotic brace must extend beyond the target joint. Knee braces that are the most supportive will extend from the calf muscles, with a hinge at the joint, to the quadriceps. Effective ankle braces will often be designed to extend from the top of the Achilles tendon, secured at a point near the forefoot.

The best orthotics are those custom-made for the individual. A foot orthotic will be constructed from a casting made of the foot of the athlete; the relevant medical specialist, often a podiatrist, will often utilize a video image of the gait to best determine how to customize the device to suit the particular needs of the athlete.

SEE ALSO Knee: Genetic and non-athletic conditions affecting performance; Musculoskeletal injuries; Running injuries; Running shoes.

# Osgood-Schlatter disease

Osgood-Schlatter disease is described as osteochondrosis of the tuberosity of the tibia (also known as the shinbone). With this condition, there is pain about 2 to 3 in (5 to 7.5 cm) below the kneecap, where a tendon inserts into a bony protrusion called the tibia tubercle. In about 25% of cases, the pain can also exist on both sides of this area.

First described in 1891, Osgood-Schlatter disease is named for Robert Bayley Osgood and Carl B. Schlatter. Since the condition tends to disappear with age without treatment, Osgood-Schlatter disease is more correctly considered to be a symptom.

Whether described as a condition or disease, and even though it usually persists for only a few years at most, the hallmark knee pain is disruptive and painful for adolescents.

Rapidly growing active boys and girls between 11 and 15 years of age are most commonly affected. Boys are approximately three times more susceptible than girls. This may reflect the past tendency of adolescent boys to participate more in physical activities than girls. However, those times have changed. With girls increasingly being part of the game, rather than being on the sidelines, the incidence of Osgood-Schlatter disease in adolescent girls may well rise.

The pain can arise from a single event such as a blow to the knee. More often, however, the pain arises from the repeated flexing of the knee against a quadriceps muscle that has become abnormally tight due to rapid body growth during adolescence. This strain aggravates the tibial area. So, typically, Osgood-Schlatter disease is an overuse injury.

For some sufferers, the pain is mild and periodic and occurs after athletic activity. For others, the pain can be severe and constant. Usually, only one knee is affected, although for a small percentage of people, both knees become painful.

When pain is mild, it is possible to continue with sports activities by following some or all of the treatments. However, severe pain can cause an athlete to stop engaging in sports entirely until the problem is resolved.

Because flexing of the knee aggravates the injury, adolescents who are involved in certain athletic activities are especially prone. Sports that involve a lot of knee motion, jumping, and rapid side-to-side movement, such as soccer, gymnastics, basketball, figure skating, and distance running, can lead to Osgood-Schlatter disease.

Swelling of the area below the kneecap and pain that is accentuated when the area is gently pressed are diagnostic hallmarks of Osgood-Schlatter disease. Once a diagnosis is made, treatment can involve curtailing athletic activity, applying heat before the activity to increase circulation, applying ice after activity to help prevent inflammation, taking regular doses of an anti-inflammatory such as ibuprofen, and even wrapping the knee to restrict movement. Some or all of the treatments are continued until there is little or no discomfort or pain following exercise. This may require several months.

Stretches that strengthen the bone, tendon, and cartilage in the knees can help lessen the chances of a reoccurrence of pain. One exercise involves stretching the quadriceps (the muscles in front of the thigh) by grasping a foot with the hand on the same side of the body and pulling the foot up until the heel touches the buttock. This can be done standing up or lying stomach-down on the floor. The stretch is held for about 30 seconds.

Another useful stretch focuses on the hamstring, the muscle located in the back of the thigh. For this stretch, a person sits with one leg straight out in front and the other leg is bent so that the sole of the foot touches the other leg. Leaning forward and keeping the extended leg straight produces stretching in the back of the thigh. The stretch is held for about 30 seconds.

Other stretches can be done as well. It is advisable to consult with a physician or a physiotherapist before starting a stretching program. With their guidance, a diligent stretching routine can help get an athlete back into action.

The symptoms of Osgood-Schlatter disease can persist for several years. However, most typically, symptoms disappear within 12 to 14 months, soon after the end of the growth spurt experienced by many adolescents (generally around the age of 14 for girls and 16 for boys).

**SEE ALSO** Bone mineralization patterns; Bone, ligaments, tendons; Osteoporosis; Recurrent stress fractures.

# Osteoarthritis

Osteoarthritis, also known as degenerative arthritis, is a disease which may arise in any human joint. Over 100 specific types of arthritis have been identified by medical science. Osteoarthritis is classified as a rheumatic disease, meaning that it is an affliction that is isolated to the particular joint structure without attacking any other organ or bodily system.

Osteoarthritis is the general description of the progressive breakdown and loss of cartilage in the joint: there are a number of factors that may contribute to both the origin and the development of the condition. Joints are created in the human musculoskeletal system where two or more bones meet. All bones consist of hard mineral compounds, primarily those including calcium, the mineral that gives bones their hard surface and density, with a measure of the protein collagen present to provide a measure of elasticity to the bone surface to permit the structure to absorb impact. At the joint, the epiphysis (the area at the end of every bone), is coated with cartilage, a protein substance that provides both cushioning and a reduced friction surface on which the other joint bones can move more readily. These coverings are known as articular cartilage.

There are two general types of osteoarthritis. Primary osteoarthritis does not have a specific cause and is generally attributable to the aging of the body. For many people, the wear and tear to their joints from the repetitive nature of human movement causes the cartilage in the joints to thin over time. Pieces of cartilage fiber tend to peel away from the surface of the bone structure, and where the cartilage thins bone spurs may occasionally develop, further limiting joint movement. Primary osteoarthritis is also known as rheumatism.

Secondary osteoarthritis arises from specific and definable physical circumstances. Hereditary causes occur in people born with unequal leg length or similar structural imbalances that tend to create unequal stresses on weight-bearing joints during movement. These stresses will often cause damage to the cartilage in the affected joint. These alignment or structural deficiencies particularly contribute to the formation of osteoarthritis in the joints of the foot, knee, hip, or lower spine.

Another circumstance the leads to secondary osteoarthritis is sports injury, in which excessive force is directed into a joint and will often cause the cartilage to tear or to partially tear. The most common cartilage tear injuries in sport occur in the knee. A torn knee cartilage often occurs in conjunction with other injuries to the knee structure, such as the patella (knee cap) or one of the ligament structures.

Secondary osteoarthritis also occurs in the obese, those persons who are overweight, which places a significantly greater strain on all weight-bearing joints, rendering the joint more vulnerable to injury.

The symptoms of secondary osteoarthritis are pain in the affected area, accompanied by swelling and limited mobility in the joint. Persons who have sustained longer term cartilage loss in the knees often appear bow legged, due to the fact that the cartilage, having thinned on the epiphysis, has created a narrowing in the space between the femur and the tibia and fibula. The bow-legged appearance is the result of the bones meeting at a different angle than when the epiphysis had optimal cartilage covering. The loss of knee cartilage is the most common basis for total knee replacement surgery in North America.

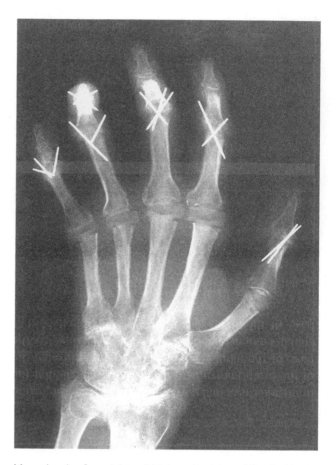

X-ray showing finger joints which have been immobilized with pins to remedy severe osteoarthritis. © LESTER V. BERGMAN/CORBIS

Osteoarthritis often occurs in the regions of the spine that support movement, particularly the cervical spine, the seven vertebrae that support the neck and the skull, and the lumbar spine, the lower back region located above the pelvis. In the joints formed by the individual vertebrae in these areas, when cartilage is reduced, bony spurs, which are composed of the same calcium and mineral material used to build and repair bones, will tend to form on the surface of the vertebrae. These spurs interfere in the natural motion of the spinal joints, and the spurs will sometimes irritate the spinal nerves that emanate from the spinal cord, causing significant pain.

Other than the history communicated by the patient to an examining physician, the primary diagnostic tool available to determine the extent of osteoarthritis is x-ray technology. The x-ray results will reveal where there is either an observable loss of cartilage, a narrowing of joints spaces, or the presence of bone spurs.

The treatment options for the relief of osteo-arthritis are limited. If the cartilage is capable of being repaired, arthroscopic surgery may be employed to both suture the damaged cartilage as well as to remove free-floating particles of carti-lage in the joint, that may further impair its move-ment through becoming lodged in the space between the bones of the joint. There have been a number of successful, yet experimental surgeries performed in recent years where new cartilage was successfully cultivated outside of the body and then injected into the joint to encourage a re-growth in the damaged area.

In many cases, the subject will obtain relief from over-the-counter medications such as acetaminophen, or nonsteriodal anti-inflammatory drugs (NSAIDs) such as ibuprofen, or the more powerful NSAIDs, Cox-2 inhibitors, that block the development of the inflammation-causing enzymes at the site of the injured cartilage. A more immediate anti-inflammatory procedure is the injection of a corticosteroid such as cortisone directly into the affected joint.

As there is no certain restorative treatment for cartilage that has been thinned away from the interior of the joint, athletes who suffer from the affects of osteoarthritis often must reduce both the frequency and the intensity of their activities to manage the pain of this condition.

SEE ALSO Bone, ligaments, tendons; Calcium; Minerals; Osteoarthritis.

## Osteochondritis dissecans

Osteochondritis dissecans (OCD) is the general heading given to a series of degenerative joint dis-eases, all of which center on the inflammation or detachment of cartilage from the joint surface.

All joints in the human body have a number of common characteristics. A joint is created by the meeting of two or more bones. The joint is stabilized and supported by ligaments, which connect the bones of the joint together; the nature and extent of the movement of the joint is determined by the configu-ration of the bones in the joint; a hinge joint such as the elbow will move differently than the hip, which has a ball and socket construction.

At the epiphysis, or end, of the bones that form joints, there is usually a condoyle, a rounded segment on the bone surface that makes the movement of the bone against the opposite side of the joint easier. The condoyle portion of the epiphysis is covered by artic-ular cartilage, a layer of slick, frictionless material that both provides ease of movement for the joint as the bones move against one another, as well as a degree of additional cushion to absorb the forces directed against the end of the bones.

OCD arises when a fragmentary piece of carti-lage, most often with a piece of bone attached, sepa-rates from the surface of the condoyle. The fragment may remain on the surface of the articular surface, where it appears, if observed by way of x ray, as a lesion. Most often, the fragment will float loosely within the joint space, which is filled with synovial fluid. When the fragment moves into the space between the bones of the joint, the fragment will often prevent the full extension and consequent range of motion of the joint. The result is both a loss of full movement and significant discomfort. The per-son will often experience significant pain during an athletic activity, and a corresponding stiffness in movement at other times. In some circumstances, due to the position and the size of the loose fragment, the joint, particularly a knee or elbow joint, will seem to "stick" as the athlete attempts to fully extend the structure, much like a sensation experienced when the transmission on a motor vehicle that does not function properly when moving from gear to gear.

OCD is caused most often by a trauma or series of traumas absorbed by the affected joint. A related cause is ischemia, the restriction or loss of blood supply to a part of the body. When the bone to which the cartilage is attached has its blood supply inter-rupted, the fragmentation of the cartilage may occur. The most common site for the onset of OCD is the knee; the condoyle located on each side of the bottom of the femur (thigh bone) are the areas where cartilage and bone fragments most frequently become dis-lodged. The elbow is the second most likely structure to sustain an OCD occurrence; OCD in the elbow is sometimes referred to as bone chips. A less common location for OCD is the ankle joint, at the talar dome, the rounded portion of the talus (ankle bone).

Athletes account for approximately 60% of all diag-nosed cases of OCD. OCD often occurs in athletes whose bones have not yet reached full maturity, as the articular cartilage and underlying bone in the epi-physis is not developed. Athletes engaging in contact sports, gymnasts, and baseball players form the largest group of persons injured through OCD. Research con-firms that over 40% of the athletic injuries involved one or more significant traumas to the knee.

The diagnosis of the injury and the determination of the most appropriate treatment options depends on the elimination of all other possible causes. In the knee, the OCD symptoms are similar to those of a fracture and a serious sprain. A partial tear of the meniscus (the cartilage-like cushioning device on each side of the interior of the knee joint) can also result in loose cartilage pieces being present in the joint. Both x-ray images and magnetic resonance imaging (MRI) technology can isolate the precise location of the fragment. In many cases, arthroscopic surgery can remove the offending object. In some circumstances of elbow OCD, young athletes, often injured through baseball pitching, have successfully had the damaged portion of the articular cartilage grafted onto the bone surface. When the fragment is surgically removed, the typical recovery time from procedure to full resumption of sports is a minimum of three months.

OCD is of particular long-term concern to athletes. OCD carries the additional risk of the development of osteoarthritis, the chronic inflammation and deterioration of the cartilage in the affected joint, at a rate of incidence that is far higher than that of the general population.

**SEE ALSO** Bone, ligaments, tendons; Elbow injuries; Knee injuries; Osteoarthritis.

# Osteoporosis

Osteoporosis, the degeneration of the bone structure through a progressive reduction in bone mass and bone density, is one of the leading bone diseases, whose prevalence in most countries of the industrialized world has increased dramatically over the past 20 years. In the United States alone, it is estimated that 1.5 million fractures per year are directly attributable to osteoporosis. Osteoporosis is a skeletal condition that is tied almost exclusively to the life style, dietary, and exercise habits of its subjects. Osteoporosis most frequently affects the hip, spine, and wrist, making the bones fragile and less able to absorb a shock or a blow. The progress of osteoporosis is not forecast by the development of specific symptoms; it is painless, first manifesting itself with a fracture, often in the course of a fall or other accident.

An understanding of the causes of osteoporosis begins with the formation and the growth of bones. Bones begin their development in the body at birth, and continue until full maturation at the approximate age of 20. The mineral calcium is the most important element in the formation of the cells that are used in bone construction. Calcium is found in many food products, particularly milk and other dairy products.

Calcium requires the presence of vitamin D in the body to be properly absorbed into the various systems where it plays a role in human function; even when a person is otherwise consuming appropriate amounts of dietary calcium, a vitamin D deficiency will contribute to a calcium deficiency. There is no substitute within the human biology for calcium in bone construction, and when the bone does not receive the proper amount of this mineral, the bone cannot be either as dense or as hard as it must be to function properly.

Collagen is another component of bone formation. Collagen is the protein-based substance that gives the otherwise inflexible bone some measure of elasticity on impact. Although far less important to lifelong bone health, a deficiency in this protein during the adolescent period will contribute to the potential for bone disease later in life. The mineral potassium is also an essential but less substantial part of the bone development process.

The healthy formation of bones during the period prior to physical maturity also requires a healthy and active lifestyle. Exercises and sports that require the bone to bear resistance, such as running, jumping, cycling or any other movement where forces are directed into the bone structure, assist in the development of both bone mass and density. Later in life, bone mineral density is the indicator relied on by the medical community in assessing the health of older bones. There is considerable sports science evidence that confirms that young people who participate in sports or other regular and structured physical activities are far more likely to have healthy bones in their later adult years.

While the foundation of healthy bones is established as a young person approaches physical maturity, the issue of lifestyle continues to be operative in bone health through adulthood. Participation in activities that provide resistance continues to assist the body in the maintenance of bone density. While it is an unalterable genetic fact that adult bone mass will begin to decrease after age 40 in most persons, the rate of this decrease is significantly slowed by the combined attention to diet and exercise.

Post-menopausal women are the largest single group of persons afflicted by osteoporosis, which generally is most often diagnosed in persons who are over the age of 50 years. Menopause tends to cause a reduction in levels of estrogen, the female hormone. As many women breastfed one or more children, there exists a potential limitation on the amount of calcium that such women received into their own bodies during such periods. For other affected persons, the most common factors identified

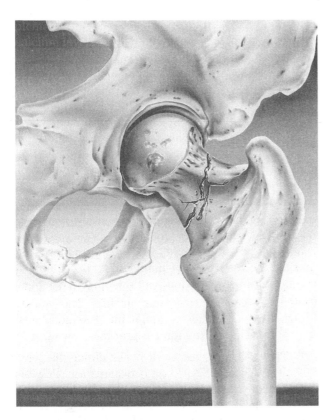

Illustration showing a hip fracture due to osteoporosis. JOHN BAVOSI/PHOTO RESEARCHERS, INC.

as contributing to osteoporosis include a bone fracture of any type that occurs after age 50, insufficient intake of calcium and vitamin D, low testosterone levels in males, sedentary lifestyle, excessive alcohol consumption, smoking, and the use of corticosteroid medications, such as cortisone, for extended periods.

Osteoporosis is an almost entirely preventable disease. It is also an incurable and progressive condition, as once bone mass is decreased, it cannot be increased, but simply maintained. If aggressive steps are not taken to address the identified causes of the condition, the bone mass will continue to deteriorate, with the bones being prone to fracture more readily. The approaches to healthy bone development over a lifetime are the same techniques to be employed in countering the effects of osteoporosis. These approaches include a balanced diet (with emphasis on calcium and vitamin D consumption), weight-bearing, resistance exercises that require the bones to respond to force, and abstinence from smoking. In some circumstances, a physician may prescribe supplements to assist with the maintenance of proper calcium levels in the body.

SEE ALSO Bone, ligaments, tendons; Calcium; Minerals; Osteoarthritis.

# Out-of-competition testing

Out-of-competition testing is the second of the two major components in the conduct of comprehensive testing of athletes for the presence of performance-enhancing substances. This type of testing is generally known as doping tests. Irrespective of the particular national or international sport federation that might be responsible for the athlete in question, in-competition testing is conducted on an athlete selected for a specific competition, such as an Olympic event or at a World Cup match. Out-of-competition testing is any such testing of an athlete not in competition, or in any way associated with the athlete's immediate participation in an event or match.

Since the advent of in-competition scientific testing for performance-enhancing substances, particularly processes aimed at the detection of anabolic steroids, stimulants, and blood doping hormones such as erythropoietin (EPO), uncertainty had existed as to the effectiveness of a testing process where the fact of an upcoming test was known to all participants. Many performance-enhancing substances could be consumed by an athlete until a date in advance of competition; the athlete would then suspend the taking of the product to permit the testing to take place, and resume consumption after the test. Alternatively, the presence of such substances might be chemically masked, or the processing of the illegal substance assisted with the consumption of other pharmaceutical products such as diuretics. The challenge for sports organizations was to develop a comprehensive model to permit the investigation of illegal substance use throughout the entire year.

This challenge was long in being remedied, as the difficulties faced by sport organizers to detect anabolic steroids best illustrates. Steroids were first used in a systematic fashion by Eastern Bloc weightlifters, wrestlers, and other strength-event athletes in the 1950s. American competitors, having observed the success of their Eastern rivals, began to employ steroids in their own training. The sports science community was well aware of the performance-enhancing power of anabolic steroids, but there existed no reliable and efficient method of physical testing for these substances.

Anabolic steroids were first declared to be illegal by the International Olympic Committee (IOC) at the 1976 Summer Olympics in Montreal. Testing methods were crude and uncertain by modern standards. When science began to develop certain tests that identified steroid metabolites, the substances produced by the body as a byproduct or breakdown of steroids within the body, testing at the Olympic level began to take on a meaning and an immediacy that it previously lacked.

A serious of high-profile positive doping tests, including that of sprinter Ben Johnson at the 1988 Summer Olympics, which resulted in the disqualification of his world record race in the 100 m, created a sense of urgency in the international athletics community regarding performance-enhancing substances of all kinds. It was in this culture that various international sports groups took affirmative steps to counter doping. The rise to prominence of the World Anti-Doping Agency (WADA) in the late 1990s was a significant stimulus to the development of established and transparent out-of-competition testing practices. With the acceptance by the IOC and its member countries of the WADA Anti-Doping Code, the sports bodies that were aligned primarily to the Olympic movement or the International Amateur Athletics Federation (IAAF), moved their constituent national memberships to adopt the same out-of-competition procedures provided by the WADA Code.

At a national level, amateur athletes who receive government funding must comply with their home federation rules regarding out-of-competition testing.

With the sophistication of doping science keeping apace with the ability of sports federations to access scientific developments in test procedures, the random out-of-competition test is a powerful weapon.

The broader world of international sport now has three different types of comprehensive doping testing being utilized: the WADA regulated model, the testing conducted in professional sports leagues where the testing procedures are negotiated between the league and the players association through a collective bargaining agreement (CBA), and athletes participating in sports where the testing is conducted on an ad hoc basis.

The procedures created by WADA regarding both in-competition and out-of- competition testing were intended to be comprehensive in their scope. The signatories to the WADA Anti-Doping Code include the national Olympic committees of virtually every nation, major world sports bodies such as the IAAF, FIFA, FIBA, as well as the national anti-doping agencies in each country; the United States Anti-Doping Agency, the Canadian Center for Ethics in Sport, UK Sport (Great Britain), the Australia Sports Drug Agency, and the Anti-Doping Commission of India are examples. By adopting the WADA Code, each sports body agrees to conduct all doping tests in accordance with its procedures. WADA does not determine which athletes should be subjected to out-of-competition testing, as this is a matter for the national and sports bodies on an individual basis; WADA provides the procedure to be followed where such tests are administered.

As a general rule, sports agencies will make known whether an athlete will at any time be subject to an out-of-competition test. In addition to compliance with rules with respect to ongoing financial aid, testing creates a track record of its own—when an athlete is subsequently tested at competition in circumstances that may raise issues as to the quality of the test procedures, series of "clean" tests may establish a measure of credibility to a protest to the result. Further, the administering association, through transparent out-of-competition testing of its members, establishes its own credibility.

Out-of-competition doping testing under the WADA Code may take one of two forms: a random test, or a test conducted on a predetermined date, known as an advance notice test. Random testing is organized on the basis that the athlete provides sufficient data that he or she might be reached at any time. Most organizations will permit one unexplained failure to contact the athlete; it is common for a second such problem to initiate a process where the athlete may be deemed to have failed the test unless he or she exhibits complete cooperation to the testing authority.

When the athlete has no advance notice of the test, he or she will be chaperoned continuously from the moment of contact from the testing officials until the sample is provided. The test is usually a urine sample, as this is the easiest and least intrusive means of obtaining bodily fluids for testing. WADA has detailed protocols about the manner in which the sample is physically placed into a test container, the sealing of the container, and its secure transport to an accredited test facility. The test must usually provide for a designated A and B sample, with the B acting as the basis for a second test if the A sample tests positive. The athlete is deemed to have tested positive when both the A and the B samples generate that result.

The prescribed standards for what actually constitutes a positive sample are published by WADA on an annual basis. With many prohibited substances, there are permitted levels to be present in the body; the test is aimed at detection of illegal levels of the substance. An example is the anabolic steroid nandrolone; it is a prohibited substance, but as nandrolone naturally occurs in the human body in minute quantities, a positive test for the steroid is not the discovery of the presence of nandrolone in the subject urine sample; a positive test results when the nandrolone metabolite is present in amounts exceeding the prescribed level of 2 mg per liter in urine.

When the athlete is subject to advance notice of a test, he or she will be directed to attend a designated Doping Control Station at a fixed time and date. As with the athlete who cannot be located for the purposes of a random test, the failure of an athlete to attend an advance notice test may trigger consequences that include the test being deemed to have a positive result. In such circumstances where the test is conducted under the auspices of the WADA Code, the athlete will be suspended for a period of time from competition; in most national governing bodies, a deemed failure of a doping test will generate a two-year suspension. Repeat offenders will often face a lifetime ban from the sport.

Although uneven in its application in some sports, the high-profile efforts of first the International Olympic Committee, and later WADA, to create a worldwide anti-doping protocol produced an undoubted domino effect. An example is large amateur sport organizations such as the National Collegiate Athletic Association (NCAA) that have drug testing regimes both in-competition and out-of-competition that mirror the WADA approach.

Professional sports organizations across the world were much slower to adopt comprehensive anti-doping procedures than were the Olympic movement and international multi-sport associations such as the IAAF. The interest of professional sports, the generation of profits for the ownership of teams, and the desire of players to achieve often exceedingly lucrative professional status, took a clear precedence over concerns regarding fair play or the significant health concerns surrounding performance-enhancing substances.

The Tour de France, the world's foremost cycling road race, is sanctioned by the International Cycling Union (ICU). In the period prior to 2004, the ICU conducted its own anti-doping tests for the Tour; the Tour had a history of athletes who used various stimulants. In 2004, the ICU became a signatory to the WADA Code, making the Tour a professional event that has bound itself to the same standards as the international athletic community. Professional soccer leagues that are sanctioned by FIFA, whose leagues include the high-profile English Premiership, the Serie A of Italy, and the German Bundeslega, another party to the WADA Code, are also subject to the same rules with respect to out-of-competition testing.

North American professional leagues have long been resistant to a WADA-styled out-of-competition testing protocol. In the case of professional American football, ice hockey, and baseball, each sport and its players association have negotiated a CBA governing all aspects of their relationship, including drug testing. As a general rule, each CBA provides that there will be out-of-competition and in-season testing at designated periods.

The penalties imposed for illegal substance use in North American professional sport are typically more lenient than those imposed in WADA-style testing. A first offense for the use of a banned substance in American football is a four-game suspension; a similar violation of the Major League Baseball policy is a 10-day suspension. The professional leagues have a seemingly far greater *laissez faire* attitude to this issue. The ice hockey public has never expressed significant concern over the widespread practice among NHL players in the pre-game consumption of decongestants that contain ephedrine or pseudoephedrine, prohibited stimulants under the WADA Code. Steroid use among baseball sluggers became well known in the late 1990s, but it was a revelation that did little to affect the overall popularity of the sport.

SEE ALSO Doping tests; EPO; Prohibited substances (competition bans); U.S. Anti-Doping Agency (USADA); World Anti-Doping Agency (WADA).

# Overtraining

Overtraining is the description given to a particular athletic approach to the physical development required in a sport, when the training workload or volume of the athlete exceeds their present ability to perform. This general understanding of what represents excessive training is defined more comprehensively in the recognized sports medicine condition, overtraining syndrome.

Overtraining syndrome is a neuron-endocrine disorder, when the function of the hormones, the chemical messengers that stimulate a wide array of functions within the body, are disrupted. This condition leads to a wide range of physical, emotional, and behavioral consequences for the athlete. While the syndrome most commonly affects high-performance or elite-level athletes, overtraining can result in any circumstance where the athlete's current training workload exceeds present abilities. Overtraining can affect athletes in any sport.

Simply, overtraining is excess. No athlete has ever achieved competitive success without taxing the body in training to a point very close to the physical limit. Successful athletes are often intense, driven people who ignore certain physical signs of injury or other dangers to their health in the pursuit of their competitive goal. It is this athlete who most commonly falls victim to the overtraining syndrome.

Overtraining can also impair more recreational athletes, who through inexperience, may not understand what their body is telling them as they increase their training volume in pursuit of a personal goal. Overtraining syndrome occurs most often among recreational athletes who are training for a marathon or similar event.

Athletic training is founded on the fundamental principle of workouts followed by rest; as the workouts intensify, a rest interval consistent with both the intensity and the duration of the workout becomes crucial. In this cycle, the rest period is the means by which the body becomes stronger, because while at rest, the body restores the cardiovascular system and the glycogen stores to greater levels than existed prior to the workout. While at rest, the body also enhances the enzymes utilized by the mitochondria in each cell to produce adenosine triphosphate (ATP), the ultimate energy fuel source. If the body has sustained periods of insufficient rest, the restoration processes do not occur and the body is not able to repair itself.

When the balance between workouts and rest is not sustained, the body becomes fatigued, leading to a cumulative exhausted state that is the overtraining syndrome. Overtraining is distinct from the natural and day-to-day variables that occur in training; one or two poor workouts because the athlete feels tired may be a signal as to workout practices, but are not evidence of the overtraining syndrome.

The overtraining syndrome is also referred to as staleness or "burnout." It often presents with a number of physical and emotional indicators, including:

- decreased performance levels, including an inability to properly complete regular workout assignments
- rise in resting heart rate to 10% or greater than usual rate
- depressed mood
- heightened feelings of mental stress, often arising from performance expectations, or coaching or team pressures
- reduced immune system function and greater vulnerability to infection; lymph glands (a component of the immune system) often swell; the production of lymphocytes, the cells manufactured by the immune system to fight infection, is reduced
- lower testosterone function and reduced sexual desires
- generalized muscle and joint pain
- insomnia
- gastrointestinal problems

The treatment to resolve an overtraining syndrome is rest. The amount of rest required will usually be proportionate to the period of overtraining; as an example, if the athlete has been overtraining for two months, he or she may require a two- to three-week period of rest before resuming training. The bodily systems most affected by the syndrome, especially the immune system, must be restored to full capacity or the syndrome will likely return. The return to training must be gradual, with careful attention paid to both the intensity and the volume of the workouts. When an athlete has been afflicted with the overtraining syndrome, a training log will often assist in reminding the athlete and any support personnel to keep the workouts within the physical capabilities of the athlete.

There are no pharmaceuticals or dietary supplements that will serve to cure overtraining syndrome. If in the course of the overtraining period the athlete had not been eating a balanced diet or otherwise consuming all necessary foods, vitamins or minerals, these points can also be addressed in the rest period. A plant extract, *Eleutherococcus senticosus*, has been tested in Eastern Europe as a potential aid to assisting the body in overcoming the fatigue associated with overtraining syndrome, with some success; it is not marketed commercially.

**SEE ALSO** Carbohydrate stores: Muscle glycogen, liver glycogen, and glucose; Fatigue; Muscle glycogen recovery; Recurrent stress fractures.

# Oxygen

The element oxygen is essential to all human life. It is the most abundant element in the Earth's crust, and it is the second most abundant element in the air, constituting approximately 21% of the Earth's atmosphere. The human body ingests oxygen primarily through the respiratory system, with the cardiovascular system the vehicle by which oxygen is then transported for uses throughout the body.

Oxygen is also a constituent part of such vital energy sources as the carbohydrates that are converted to glucose, which in molecular form is composed of carbon, hydrogen, and oxygen atoms aligned as $C_6H_{12}O_6$. Oxygen is also essential to the structure of the dietary fats absorbed and stored in the body. Triglycerides represent the storage form of such fats; when released from the adipose storage cells, these molecules break down into fatty acids and glycerol, which is a substance with a carbon/hydrogen/oxygen structure similar to glucose. Oxygen is an agent in virtually all metabolic processes. Oxygen also is a part of most organic molecules in the body, the building blocks for all living things.

The importance of oxygen to an athlete is most obvious in the healthy function of the respiratory system, without which competitive athletics would be impossible. Air is inhaled through the mouth or nose and ultimately passes through the bronchial tubes into the lungs. Within the lung cavity, there are tiny, thin-walled alveoli, air sacs that are connected to the wall of the lung and which are each a part of a dense network of capillaries, the blood vessels that act as exchange mechanisms. Inhaled oxygen passes through the sac wall to directly enter the cardiovascular system, and waste carbon dioxide passes out into the lung.

Once the oxygen enters the bloodstream, it is transported by a component of the red blood cells, hemoglobin. The oxygen is taken to the cellular sites within the body where energy is being generated. While the body can produce energy without the presence of oxygen, through its two anaerobic systems, for limited periods of time, ultimately the aerobic system will be required. It is the presence of oxygen that permits the release of energy for long-term physical needs from the body's ultimate physical fuel source known as adenosine triphosphate (ATP). ATP is the product of a complex process that involves the breakdown of glucose or fatty acids.

Sports performance is impossible without the supply of oxygen in an uninterrupted fashion. When supplies of oxygen are restricted, the body must make adaptations to correct the shortage. The most common environmental change that limits the body's oxygen supply is as a result of the body performing at an increased altitude. As altitude increases, the atmosphere is described as becoming "thinner." The molecules in the air are less dense as the effect of gravity is less pronounced, and the amount of oxygen present in the elevated atmosphere is reduced. From the sea level percentage of approximately 21% oxygen, at Denver, Colorado's famous Mile High Stadium, located at 5,500 ft (2,400 m), the oxygen percentage is reduced to approximately 18%, and at the soccer stadium in Quito, Ecuador, with an elevation of 9,300 ft (2,850 m), oxygen is only 15% of the available air.

There are only two mechanisms available to counter the reduced amount of oxygen entering the body at those altitudes. The first is the process known as acclimatization, where the athlete spends a period of time in the oxygen-reduced environment prior to the anticipated event. Research confirms that the adaptations required by the body will be complete within two to three weeks of living and training in the thinner air.

Acclimatization spurs the production of a hormone in the kidneys known as erythropoietin (EPO), which is the chemical signal to the body to produce a greater number of erythrocytes (red blood cells) to counter the effect of less oxygen; if there is less oxygen available to be transported, the greater number of red blood cells can more efficiently acquire what available oxygen there is to be consumed.

In a related way, the goal of enhanced oxygen transport has been the reason for the development of synthetic versions of EPO, used as the primary blood-doping agent.

It is common in sporting events to see oxygen being administered on the sidelines to athletes. It is evident that there is a belief that such practices will aid athletes in their recovery and permit them to return to play more quickly. In events contested at sea level, such oxygen aids are not anything more than a placebo to the athlete; the lungs cannot absorb oxygen any more readily than if supplied by the air. At elevation, where the athlete is not acclimatized to the thinner atmosphere, the portable oxygen supply may be a modest assist to recovery.

**SEE ALSO** Blood doping; Cardiorespiratory function; EPO; Glycogen depletion.

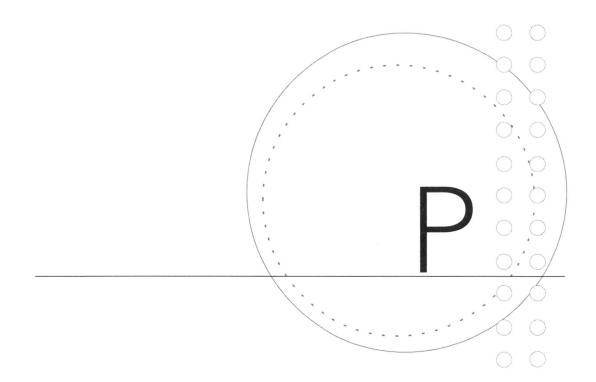

## Paralympics

The Greek word *para* is a suffix commonly employed in medical and scientific usage in reference to disciplines or circumstances that are stand beside or are comparable to a preexisting condition. The Paralympics are the disabled athletes version of the Olympic Games in both summer and winter, each conducted in the same competitive venues with similar competitive structures as the Olympics.

The Paralympians and many of their Olympic counterparts share another common athletic attribute—their Games are the only true showcase of their talents in a sports world otherwise dominated by exploits of teams and players competing in professional leagues.

When the modern Olympics grew from the stewardship of Baron de Coubertin (1893–1937), who sought to emulate the ancient Olympic ideals of "higher, faster, stronger," the Paralympics have taken a direction that is in many ways a symbol of the inclusivity and the respect that disabled persons are now accorded throughout the world; the motto of the Paralympics, "Spirit in Motion" is an extension of the broader vision of the Paralympics movement, "Empower, Achieve, Aspire," an encapsulation of the stated purpose of the Paralympic Games, to enable Paralympians to achieve sporting excellence and inspire and excite the world.

The roots of the Paralympics stem from the carnage and the human suffering caused by World War II. Sports clubs for disabled persons had existed since the late 1800s, but these groups were not a part of any national or regional organizational structure. In 1944, the British government opened a treatment facility for badly injured armed forces personnel at the town of Stoke Mandeville. The chief physician at the facility, Dr. Ludwig Guttmann (1899–1980), instituted sport programs for the wheelchair-bound patients as a part of their overall physical therapy. By 1948, the programs had evolved from purely therapeutic applications to recreational sport, and the first Stoke Mandeville Games were held for wheelchair athletes.

In 1952, the inaugural effort was expanded when a Dutch group of disabled persons joined the British facility to create the first disabled athletes sports organization, the International Stoke Mandeville Games Committee. By 1960, the Stoke Mandeville initiative had evolved into the forerunner of the modern Paralympics movement. The Paralympics are now contested in the same years as the Olympics. The Paralympic movement is headed by the International Paralympics Committee (IPC), which is representative of over 160 national Paralympics committees, as well as four distinct international sports federations, each formed to advance and regulate the interests of specific athletic interests: cerebral palsy, vision impaired, intellectually disabled, and wheelchair/amputee athletes. The IPC is a member of the Olympics movement, and it is a signatory to international sports protocols such as the World Anti-Doping Agency's Anti-Doping Code. The Paralympics are a distinct athletic avenue from the Special Olympics movement, which is a global organization devoted to athletes with intellectual disability.

Paralympic events are largely traditional individual and team Olympic sports that have been modified to accommodate the physical limitations of the competitors. Sports developed specifically for disabled athletes include *boccia*, a sport designed for persons afflicted with cerebral palsy that requires balls to be directed toward a target, with the competitor seated in a wheelchair, and goalball, a competition where vision-impaired athletes react to the sound of a ball being directed toward an opponent's goal.

The classification of athletes is a process at the root of the rules of competition in both the Summer and Winter Paralympics. Disabilities are often unique to each athlete, and to ensure fair competition, the IPC developed rules regarding the manner in which athletes would be classified in each sport. The classification process involves both technical and physical assessments of each athlete, in concert with observations of the athlete both in and out of competition. The key tool in the determination of an athlete's classification is the degree of function. There are six general areas of classification, which include:

- Amputees: These are athletes who have had a minimum of one major joint in a limb removed, often a knee or an elbow. In some classifications, an amputee will compete using a wheelchair.

- Cerebral palsy: This classification refers to athletes who suffer from one of a group of motor disorders that impair movement and motor control. Cerebral palsy athletes often compete in wheelchairs.

- Vision impaired: This classifies athletes with all manner of sight limitations, from those whose sight ranges from correctable vision problems to those are experience 100% blindness.

- Spinal cord injuries: This classification is for athletes whose spinal cord has been damaged so as to limit movement in arms, legs, or both. Parapalegia and quadrapalegia are the most common conditions.

- Intellectual disability: This classifies athletes who have either lower functioning mental abilities or who suffer from a specific limiting disability. The intellectual function of the athlete is assessed through the determination of a number of factors considered as a whole, including self-care, community use, home living, level of social skills, and leisure and work pursuits. The intellectually disabled athlete must have been so disabled prior to age 18.

- Others: This classifies athletes whose disability limits their ability to move but does not fit into one of the first five headings. Dwarfism, the genetic disease whereby growth is severely stunted, is an example.

The wheelchair is a common denominator to many of the athletes in the six general classifications. As a general rule, an athlete must have at least 10% loss of function in their lower legs to be permitted into the wide range of wheelchair-based events. The modern wheelchair is a sophisticated piece of athletic equipment, with each type of machine designed for a specific application. The wheelchair basketball athletes, whose sport involves significant contact between the competitors while on their machines, are significantly different than the ultra-light, very sleek racing versions used both on the track and on the roads for distance racing. The progression in the development of racing wheelchairs mirrored the technological advances in the design of racing bicycles, as each relies on light metals such as titanium and carbon fiber composites in construction.

Within this framework, each of the Paralympic sports develops its own event specific classifications. As an example, Paralympic alpine skiing has three visually impaired classes (to differentiate between varying levels of sight), seven amputee classes (to encompass the ranges of amputee and prosthetic usage), and three seated ski divisions, for different types of quadriplegia. Athletes compete only against competitors who fall within their designated range of disability.

Athletics, or track and field, provides the opportunity for the greatest range of competitions at the Summer Paralympic Games. When possible, given the purpose of the Paralympics, the rules of the International Amateur Athletics Federation (IAAF) are employed in competition. Various athletics events, such as wheelchair racing, are the subject of significant competition at annual international events as well as venues such as the Boston Marathon and other international races. The IPC maintains an active world record databank in all of the disciplines.

The particular interest of both the Paralympic movement and its member athletes is the continued research and development of more effective sports science applications to assist the disabled. Known as the VISTA conferences, the IPC convenes a biennial event to further the science of disabled sport. One focus of the VISTA conferences has been the enhancement of physiological testing methods to further refine the classification of disabled athletes.

The IPC became a signatory to the WADA Code with an appreciation that doping could be as serious a matter in Paralympic competition as in any able-bodied one. In 2004, the IPC instituted, with WADA, an out-of-competition testing program, providing for both random drug tests and those conducted with a measure of advance notice to the athletes. In further

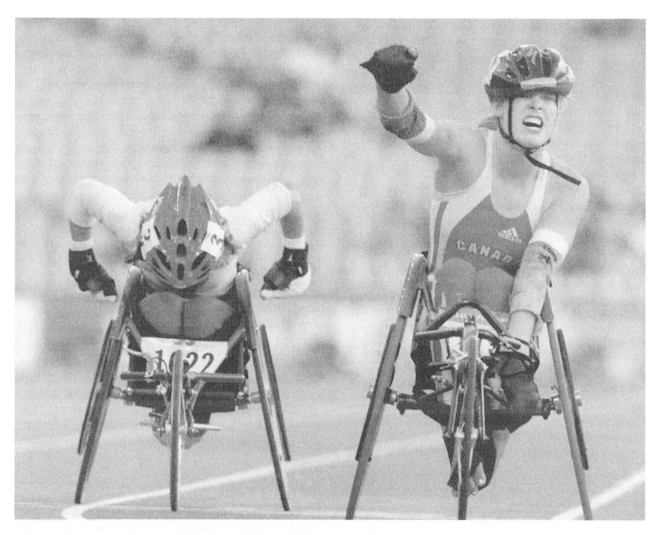

Winners at Paralympics Games in Sydney, Australia, 2000. © REUTERS/CORBIS

recognition of its athletic constituency, the IPC maintains a Therapeutic Use Exemption list, where athletes may apply to the IPC to use an otherwise banned substance for treatment purposes. A common example of such a medication is any member of the corticosteroid class of anti-inflammatory.

Most Paralympic athletes have trained and competed in obscurity throughout the history of disabled athletic competition. The Olympics are the most publicized sports event in the world; the Paralympics, which follow every Olympic festival, garner a very small fraction of the media attention. The world at large may respect and admired these Paralympic athletes for their efforts in their achievements in overcoming disability, but it is a respect that is muted, especially in the global sport media. The perception of the Paralympic athlete as one performing in the shadows of the able-bodied was altered to a considerable degree in Canada in 2004 by Chantal Petitclaire,

winner of five gold medals in various wheelchair events at the 2004 Athens Paralympics, the greatest ever Paralympic performance. Petitclaire spoke out publicly about her concerns of being cast as an athletic second-class citizen, not capable of having the magnitude of her accomplishments measured on an equal footing against those of able-bodied athletes in the voting for Canada's female athlete of the year. Petitclaire asserted that any other consideration of her achievements in the Paralympics denigrated the efforts of all disabled athletes. Petitclaire's crusade was endorsed by the Canadian sports media, and she was ultimately the recipient of the national female athlete of the year for 2004. Petitclaire was the first such disabled athlete to be recognized for a mainstream athletic award in North America.

SEE ALSO International federations; International Olympic Committee (IOC); National governing bodies.

# Pedometers

A pedometer is a device that is capable of measuring the distance traveled by a person for a given period. A pedometer is the size of a pager or cell phone, and it is worn on the hip or secured by way of a belt to the person's body. The pedometer is calibrated to the user's stride length to provide an approximation of distance traveled; pedometers are most accurate when used to determine distances walked as opposed to running.

As a pedometer is a digital instrument, it may be readily integrated into other forms of biofeedback, including a heart monitor. The pedometer can also measure average rates of speed. Some models of pedometers also have a feature that determines the number of calories consumed by the user through the time period in which the pedometer is worn.

While a pedometer is not a device commonly used by serious or elite-level athletes, it is a powerful motivational tool for many recreational athletes or persons interested in improving the general standard of their personal fitness. When people do not have an interest in conventional exercise programs, such as team sports, running, or fitness classes, or where they have impediments to participation as a result of lifestyle or employment commitments, the pedometer can serve to provide an ongoing incentive to incrementally boost the amount of physical activity in which they engage on a daily basis.

Pedometers have become sufficiently popular that research has determined some rough guidelines for the person seeking improved fitness. Ten thousand steps per day is now cited as a target for those who seek to maintain a base level of cardiovascular fitness and weight control; for the average person, 10,000 steps is approximately 5 mi (8 km) of total daily movement. When a person seeks to lose weight and obtain enhanced cardiovascular risk reduction, the suggested targets are 12,000 steps to 15,000 steps per day (6-8 mi [10-13 km] of total daily movement). For additional cardiovascular fitness, it is recommended that the user walk 3,000 of the target step distance at a quick pace without stopping (1.5 mi or 2.5 km).

In recent years, formal walking programs have gained popularity, especially among people with a history of heart problems. "Mall walkers" is a generic term that is frequently applied to walkers who use indoor shopping malls to walk in a controlled environment.

**SEE ALSO** Biofeedback; Heart rate monitors; Treadmills.

# Pelé

10/23/1940–
BRAZILIAN
SOCCER PLAYER

Edson Artantes do Nascimento, more famously known by his childhood nickname of Pelé, is one of the best soccer players ever to play the game. Nearly three decades after his retirement from competitive soccer, he is still idolized in his home country of Brazil. His "bicycle kick" started not only a movement in aggressive play but spurred sports scientists to break down the mechanics of previously simple actions such as striking the ball.

Pelé was the son of a soccer player. His soccer skills were evident early in his life, despite the lack of training facilities and equipment that were the result of poverty. By the time he was 11 years old, he had caught the attention of Waldemar de Brito, a famous Brazilian soccer player of the time. Invited to play for de Brito's amateur team, Pelé's talent soon brought him a professional contract offer from the Santos football club.

He joined Santos in 1956, when he was just 15 years of age. Pelé's professional debut was an auspicious four-goal performance. Later the same year, now 16 years old, he was a regular player for Santos, led the league in scoring, and joined the squad of the Brazilian national team.

Pelé played for Santos from 1956 to 1974. During that time, he scored over 1,200 goals (the most by any soccer player to date) and assisted on over 1,100 others in 1,360 games. His career on the Brazilian national team spanned 15 years, from 1956 until 1971. In international competitions, he averaged one goal per game.

Playing at midfield, Pelé had offensive and defensive skills that made him the best player in the world of his era, and debatably the finest player ever to play soccer. He was an exceptional attacker, whose speed and exceptional passing ability with either foot allowed him to move the ball quickly and accurately upfield. When given the opportunity to score, he seldom missed. He could direct the ball, with power and precision, using his head. He was also a skilled defender, and thus able to hinder the advance of the opposition players.

Of all his prodigious skills, Pelé is most famous for a move dubbed the "bicycle kick." In this move, he would leap into the air, somersaulting during flight, so that his feet moved above his head. In a coordinated motion that looked similar to the pedaling motion of bike riding, he would kick the ball with one of his feet. The move was performed with his back to the net; the kick would send the ball rocketing toward, often into, the net.

Two years after joining the national squad, Pelé led his team to victory in the World Cup. Only 17 years old, he was a dominant player, especially in the team's victory match, in which he scored twice. He played in three more World Cups, in 1962, 1966, and 1970. Brazil was victorious in the 1962 and 1970 campaigns.

During his career, Pelé was coerced to join European soccer clubs with tremendously lucrative offers. However, to ensure that his career would not take him away from Brazil, the government officially declared him to be a national treasure.

After his retirement from Brazilian soccer competition in 1974, Pelé resumed his professional career in 1975 by joining the New York Cosmos of the fledgling North American Soccer League. His salary—reportedly $7 million for three years—was the highest at that time. His presence helped popularize and legitimize soccer in North America.

He retired from competitive soccer in 1977. In his two-season career with the Cosmos, he scored over 100 goals and had 65 assists. Since then, he has been an active participant in activities of the United Nations, including UNICEF and U.N. environmental initiatives. The honors he has received include an honorary British Knighthood in 1992 and recognition as Athlete of the Century by the International Olympic Committee in 1999 (although he never played in Olympic competition). In an age when video games have become universally popular, Pelé is also noteworthy for being the first sports figure featured in a video game, a product of the Atari company that was called *Pelé's Soccer*.

Pelé remains an internationally recognized personality and soccer ambassador.

## Pentathlon SEE Modern pentathlon

## Pentathlon (women's)

The women's pentathlon is a part of a continuum of multi-event competitions, the roots of which extend to the athletic traditions of the ancient Greeks. Pentathlon is the Greek word for a five-part competition, and in ancient times, the pentathlon was often used by Greek governments to assess the potential of men for military service.

The ancient pentathlon blended strength, speed, and agility. The five events were a short footrace (the distances varied depending on the place of the competition), wrestling, a long jump in which the athlete was weighted down, the javelin throw, and the discus. As with all athletic events at that time, the contest was restricted to men.

The pentathlon for women was first introduced into the Summer Olympic Games in 1964. The International Olympic Committee (IOC) had been slow to add women's events to the Olympic Games; there was a lingering belief that women could not physically perform certain strength and endurance sports. In 1964, the women's pentathlon had the requisite five events, but with a different focus; the events were conducted over a two-day period, with the first three events contested on the first day, the remaining events the next day. The first women's pentathlon included 80-m hurdles, the shot put, the high jump, the long jump, and the 200-m sprint.

Preparation for the pentathlon is a variation of the cross training principles employed by athletes in many sports, with less emphasis on endurance training than would be a part of a triathlon or a decathlon program. Explosive muscular movement, such as is developed through interval sprints and plyometrics training, as well as the flexibility and agility required for the high jump and the long jump are crucial. Shot put training is a further extension of muscle power and the coordinated approach required to combine technique and strength.

The women's pentathlon was included in the Summer Olympics from 1964 to 1980. In the era of the political Cold War that existed between Western nations and the Soviet Union-led Eastern Bloc, success in the pentathlon was primarily with the Eastern Bloc nations; their athletes captured 10 of the 15 medals awarded during the time period that the women's pentathlon was an Olympic event. As with many of the sports that did not enjoy a high profile in Western nations—of which the hammer throw, a traditional field event, and team sports such as handball, are examples—the Eastern Bloc nations and their state-based, systematic approaches to athletic training targeted the women's pentathlon as one where success could be achieved on the Olympic stage.

Due to increasing demands from many nations within the Olympic movement to have consistency and equality between all male and female sporting competitions, not only in the quantity of the events, but also in the maintenance of the balance between running and field events, the women's pentathlon was replaced in 1984 by the heptathlon, an expanded version of the women's pentathlon. The transition from the pentathlon to the heptathlon (a seven-event, two-day discipline) was generally welcomed, as the heptathlon presented greater athletic challenges for the female competitors. Yet there remained critics of the IOC who argued that the only proper female multi-sport event should be a female decathlon to create prefect symmetry between the male and female competitions.

The women's pentathlon is now something of a historical footnote, a bridge in the history of women's athletics at the Olympics between the days of limited female participation and a far broader range of women's events. The women's pentathlon was the first multi-sport women's event to be included in the Olympic Games. The 1984 Olympics were also significant in this respect for the inclusion of the marathon as a women's event for the first time.

Since 1912, another pentathlon event had been contested at the Summer Olympics, the modern pentathlon. This five-event discipline, comprised of pistol shooting, fencing or epee, swimming, equestrian (horse) jumping, and cross-country running, was a designated men's event until 2000, when the IOC created a women's modern pentathlon competition. To further involve multi-sport competitions in the Olympics, the IOC added the triathlon for both men and women in 2000.

The women's pentathlon has not disappeared as an international athletic competition. The International Amateur Athletics Federation (IAAF) sanctions the heptathlon as a women's world championship event, and the pentathlon is the equivalent indoor track and field championship, typically during in the winter track and field season. The IAAF pentathlon was introduced at the world indoor track and field championships in 1993, with the 60-m sprint, 800-m run, high jump, long jump, and shot put as the constituent elements. The IAAF standard pentathlon is also a national indoor track and field championship in many countries, and in collegiate competition such as the American National Collegiate Athletic Association (NCAA).

SEE ALSO Decathlon; Ironman competitions; Modern pentathlon.

## Performance SEE Sport performance

## Chantal Petitclerc

12/15/1969
CANADIAN
PARALYMPIC ATHLETE

Chantal Petitclerc is one of the most dominant athletes in the history of both the Paralympic movement and all wheelchair sports. Petitclerc is one of

the few athletes in any sport to hold multiple world track and field records at one time.

Petitclerc was raised in a rural area near Quebec City, Canada. At age 13, she sustained an accident where a barn door fell on her, damaging her spinal cord and rendering Petitclerc a paraplegic. Soon after she had recovered sufficiently to resume such activities as she could, Petitclerc discovered wheelchair racing. Petitclerc has been actively engaged in wheelchair sports since that time.

After completing her university studies, Petitclerc qualified for the 1992 Paralympics in Barcelona. At those Games, Petitclerc demonstrated some of the talent that would later propel her to the peak of wheelchair sports, winning bronze medals in both the 100m and the 800m events. In 1996 at Atlanta, Petitclerc established herself as the most dominant female wheelchair racer in the world, as she won two gold and three silver medals in the various wheelchair track events. Petitclerc followed this powerful result with a two gold, two silver performance at the 2000 Paralympics in Sydney.

At age 34, Petitclerc entered the 2004 Athens Paralympics as a favorite to win multiple medals. She captured an unprecedented five gold medals, winning every wheelchair event in the event distances from 100m to 1,500m, establishing three world records in the process.

Wheelchair racing is a demanding sport at any distance. In the shorter events of 400m or under, the racer seeks to combine an explosive start by driving their arms powerfully to rotate the wheels on the chair, combined with a sustained, high tempo rhythm to generate as many revolutions of the wheels as possible. As with all sprinters, sprint distance wheelchair racers employ interval training techniques as an essential component of their preparation, incorporating high intensity intervals and recoveries.

Fifteen hundred meter events generally involve different training approaches for the wheelchair racer. The interval work carried out for sprinting is secondary in preparation for these events to training at longer distances that build aerobic fitness in the athlete. An explosive start is of lesser importance in the 1,500-m event than is the ability to maintain a steady pace and then utilize a finishing kick.

Petitclerc's ability to win at every distance between 100m and 1,500m in wheelchair events is a testament to her ability to incorporate these disparate training requirements into one overall athletic program.

With her considerable success, Petitclerc has enjoyed the benefits of various sponsorships in recent years. The most prominent of these benefits is the wheelchair used by Petitclerc in her races. Petitclerc uses state-of-the-art three-wheeled machine. The wheels are sloped inwards towards the athlete at an angle of 13°, with the frame specially configured to suit the build of Petitclerc. The wheelchair frame is constructed of tubular aluminum, and the entire machine weighs less then 14 lb (6 kg).

The wheels on the Petitclerc wheelchair are constructed from carbon rims. Each wheel is very thin to create a highly aerodynamic profile. The wheels are inflated to an air pressure of 180 psi (pounds per square inch), to ensure that the rolling resistance of the wheel against the track surface is minimized. The steering mechanism is adjustable to permit the angle of the machine to correspond with the lane in which Petitclerc will be competing.

In Canada, controversy arose after Petitclerc had achieved her successes at the Athens Paralympics. Athletics Canada, the government sponsored agency involved in the supervision of Canadian sport, determined that Petitclerc would be named the disabled female athlete of the year for 2004, with 2003 world 110-m hurdler Perdita Felicien, the female athlete of the year. This decision touched off a significant public debate about the importance of disabled sport in society as a whole, and how an athlete such as Petitclerc should be regarded in comparison to other athletes. Petitclerc indicated that she believed that she was being treated as a second class athletic citizen by Athletics Canada, and that her accomplishments at Athens must be weighed on their own terms; she refused the Athletics Canada award.

The Canadian sports media voted Petitclerc the female athlete of the year in 2004. Petitclerc is active as a spokesperson for a number of charitable organizations.

**SEE ALSO** Paralympics; Track and field; Wheelchair sports.

# Phosphate

Phosphates are an essential aspect of the function of the human body, particularly in the systems relied on in the production of energy, as well as in bone formation. A phosphate is a molecule created by the combination of one phosphorus atom, and four atoms of oxygen, stated in the chemical form $PO_4$. Phosphorus is one of the elements listed in the Periodic Table, and it is a substance well known beyond the processes of human biology as a powerful component in applications as diverse as munitions manufacturing and fertilizers. If consumed in its pure form, phosphorus is highly toxic. Phosphorus is also flammable in the air.

In its phosphate form, phosphorus is a significant presence in the body, comprising approximately 1 lb (0.5 kg) of the total mass of the average adult. Phosphates are present in a wide variety of food groups; it would be highly unlikely that a person consuming a typical balanced diet of carbohydrates, proteins, and fats could ever experience a phosphate deficiency. A healthy adult will have phosphates present in the blood. The phosphates that are most important to human function are adenosine triphosphate (ATP) and calcium phosphate.

ATP is the crucial energy storage and transportation mechanism present in the muscles of the body. ATP is the ultimate fuel produced and consumed in the production of the cellular energy necessary for the contraction of muscles. Adenosine is a product of nucleic acid, an essential building block in cell formation. Nucleic acid is the portion of the cell that contains hereditary and other related information; deoxyribonucleic acid (DNA) is the best known of these nucleic acids. To create ATP, adenosine combines with three phosphate molecules. ATP also has an important role in the synthesis of proteins within the body. The portion of each cell that acts as the powerhouse for the utilization of ATP by way of chemical reaction is the mitochondria.

ATP is used by the cell to produce energy both anaerobically (without the presence of oxygen) and aerobically (with oxygen). The ATP molecules contain very high amounts of energy potential, and the breakdown of the ATP molecule in the mitochondria releases very large amounts of energy relative to the size of the molecule, a characteristic due to the presence of phosphorus in the ATP molecule.

The primary means by which ATP is created within the body is through the processing of glucose, itself a product of the carbohydrates consumed through food. When processed by the body for the production of energy, one glucose molecule will ultimately render two molecules of ATP. Once formed, ATP is replenished and recycled within each cell indefinitely; ATP is a partner to a reversible reaction that involves a series of conversions involving phosphocreatine (creatine phosphate) that are at the hub of the energy production process. The creation and the reduction of ATP is continuous, as ATP is not stored within the cell in the fashion that glucose or fats can be retained for periods of time in the body. ATP and phosphocreatine are a part of an ongoing recycling process that creates and produces approximately one kilogram of ATP per hour within the entire population of cells in the body. For athletes who have higher energy demands than the general population, the consumption of appropriate carbohydrates is one method of ensuring that the ultimate ATP capacity of the body remains intact. Without glucose, the manufacture of ATP will be limited.

Calcium phosphate is the compound that is essential to the formation of the bone cells. An imbalance in the optimal levels of calcium and phosphates will result in an inability of the body to maintain a strong bone structure. Persons with kidney disease are particularly vulnerable to the effects of such an imbalance. When the kidney fails to maintain the healthy ratio of calcium to phosphorus, usually though a shortfall in its release of vitamin D, the compound that permits the absorption of calcium into the bloodstream, phosphate levels with in the blood rise. This increase in phosphates itself initiates a release of a hormone from the parapituitary gland (PTP), which chemically signals the bones to release stored calcium into the bloodstream to restore the balance between calcium and phosphorus. Over time, the release of calcium from the bones to the bloodstream in the disturbed vitamin D/calcium/phosphate balance can lead to osteoporosis, a loss of bone mass and density that causes a irreversible weakening of the bone.

When phosphate levels rise, the condition is commonly treated by extra supplements of vitamin D to ensure proper calcium absorption. High phosphate levels in the bloodstream are also a powerful indicator of the presence of ketones, the byproduct of excessive fat products in the blood, caused by ketoacidosis. This condition is a symptom of type 2 diabetes, the adult-onset version of this disease.

In recent years, there has been significant sports specific research into the effectiveness of phosphates as a training supplement. Research with the compound sodium phosphate, which involved athletes in controlled conditions engaging in a form of phosphate loading, where predetermined amounts were consumed for a number of consecutive days in training for endurance events, suggested, without concluding, that there could be a reduction in the buildup of lactic acid, accompanied by a slight increase in VO$_2$max, the maximum of oxygen the

athlete was capable of processing. Given that there are no adverse impacts known in the ingestion of sodium phosphate, the loading practice is, at worst, neutral.

**SEE ALSO** Dietary supplements; Minerals; Phosphocreatine.

# Phosphocreatine

Phosphocreatine is a substance that, in its chemical partnership with adenosine triphosphate (ATP), is fundamental to the ability of the body to produce muscular energy. Phosphocreatine, which is also known as creatine phosphate is a compound constructed of carbon, hydrogen, nitrogen, oxygen, and phosphorus, in the molecular structure $C_4H_{10}N_3O_5P$.

Phosphocreatine is formed naturally within the body, with over 95% of the compound stored within the muscle cells. Approximately 5 oz (120 g) of phosphocreatine is present in the body of a healthy adult; the levels of the compound do not fluctuate to a significant degree. When phosphocreatine stores become reduced, the body replenishes its supply from one of two sources. The first source is amino acids, the muscle- and tissue-building blocks present in all proteins. The liver produces phosphocreatine from amino acids. The body also receives dietary creatine primarily through the consumption of meat.

The role of phosphocreatine in the production of the energy required to produce muscular contractions must be understood in the context of the three pathways or systems through which the body produces energy, and the circumstances that dictate which pathway will be relied on at any given time. The aerobic system is the primary means by which muscular energy is produced, where the activity involving muscle movement lasts longer than approximately 90 seconds. The anaerobic lactic system responds to demands of between approximately 10 seconds and 90 seconds. The anaerobic alactic is the system employed where the energy need is short and intense, up to 10 seconds in duration.

In each of these systems, the cells engaged in energy production will utilize ATP, itself the ultimate product of glucose stored in the body. ATP is essential to the life of the cell. Phosphocreatine is not an energy source itself, like ATP, but it is crucial to the cyclical chemical reaction that is repeated in the mitochondria of each cell to continue the availability of ATP. When the need for energy is immediate and of short duration, as with weightlifting or a short sprint, ATP will provide the energy; phosphocreatine is available in the cell to be immediately broken down into its phosphate component, to provide further materials for the recycling of greater amounts of ATP. This recharging process can occur with tremendous speed during the 10-second period that the body utilizes the anaerobic alactic system, creating an indefinite cycle of energy generation and replenishing ATP, through the agency of phosphocreatine. The rate at which phosphocreatine is broken down depends almost entirely on the intensity of the muscle contraction required. Once other sources of fuel, through the aerobic system, are made available, the phosphocreatine stores will be restored.

The amount of phosphocreatine available to restore ATP through periods of intense muscle exercise are small. It is for this reason that muscle fatigue will be noticeable to the athlete through this process, even when the activity is of short duration.

The essential role of creatine phosphate in the ATP generation and restoration process spurred significant interest in the use of creatine as an athletic supplement. By virtue of the energy system that is primarily influenced by phosphocreatine, most interest in this compound as a training aid has come from athletes in sports where explosive power is of critical importance, including weightlifters, velodrome sprint cyclists, and race sprinters.

Creatine supplementation has been proven to assist athletes in extending their maximum ability to work. As with most minerals otherwise available in through a balanced diet, such supplementation is not required to address a deficiency, but to seek optimal performance. The body has difficulty absorbing phosphocreatine, and it is for this reason that the common creatine supplement is in the form of creatine monohydrate. The body can readily produce the necessary phosphocreatine once the creatine has been ingested; phosphocreatine is manufactured in the liver, pancreas, and kidneys. Studies also demonstrated that when creatine supplements were combined with a carbohydrate component, the ability of the body to retain phosphocreatine was significantly increased. As the period within which the cell is working and will require phosphocreatine to assist in the ATP cycle, the greater the amount of creatine phosphate to be retained, the greater the likelihood that the ATP cycle can be extended.

When phosphocreatine in the muscle breaks down, it is not reprocessed into a working form. Phosphocreatine metabolizes into a substance known as creatinine, which is excreted through the kidneys and passed as urine. The level of creatinine in the blood is a useful indicator in the determination of kidney function; high levels of creatinine are a symptom of an inability of the kidney to filter the creatinine wastes.

**SEE ALSO** Creatine supplementation; Glycogen depletion; Phosphate.

# Physics of banks and curves

A bank in a racetrack is an upward slope toward the center of the track that is designed to hold objects such as cars and people on the track at high speeds and, thus, reduce the chance of the object going off the track. A curve is a bend in a track that has no upward slope, as in the case of a bank. Banks and curves within, for instance, the sport of auto racing are especially challenging because of the principles involved in classical physics.

English physicist and mathematician Sir Isaac Newton (1642–1727) stated within his first law of motion that any object of mass at rest will tend to stay at rest and any object in motion will tend to stay in motion at the same speed and direction unless acted upon by a force. The first law is often called the law of inertia because the term inertia means the resistance to motion. Because of inertia, the race car and driver, when coming upon a bank or a curve, would normally continue on a straight line on a racetrack if some force were not applied to them. Thus, the car and driver would miss the bank or curve and crash into the outside wall of the track or leave the track entirely.

In order for the race car to change direction—that is, to navigate through a bank or curve on a racetrack—a force must produce a change in direction (but not necessarily a change in speed) toward the center of the bank or curve. This type of force is called centripetal force (or center-seeking force), and it acts perpendicular to the car's velocity. It is defined as $mv^2/r$, where, in this case, $m$ is the mass of the race car traveling in a circular path of radius ($r$) at a constant velocity ($v$). (The equation changes if the racing track is not circular in shape; that is, if $r$ is not constant.)

When the driver changes the direction that the tires are moving by rotating the steering wheel, friction is produced between the car's tires and the racetrack—that is, centripetal force is produced. As the equation implies, it is directly related to the square of the speed (the magnitude of the velocity) of the car. In the worst-case scenario, if the car is traveling too fast, the frictional force is not strong enough to hold the car on the racetrack. The centripetal force is also inversely related to the radius of the banking or curving track. The larger the radius of turning, then the less force needed to make it through the bank or curve.

SEE ALSO Automobile racing; Formula 1 auto racing; NASCAR auto racing.

# Physiology of exercise

The physiology of exercise is a broad concept that addresses the central issue as to how the body adapts itself to the demands of physical activity.

Physiology is the academic study of the various processes, systems, and functions of the human body as influenced by the performance of physical activity. Exercise is a term that has a variety of possible meanings, each dictated by circumstances. In a sports context, exercise is the performance, conditioning or training undertaken in respect to a particular athletic or sporting purpose. Exercise may also be directed to improvement of a person's general health, physical fitness, or as physical therapy, to augment an existing treatment to remedy or to ameliorate the effects of a disease or illness upon the body.

The term exercise physiology is used to identify the corresponding course of academic study offered at universities around the world.

The human body undergoes adaptations on a continuous basis. Sport tends to heighten the power of the body to adapt to training, competition, or other circumstances, as sport is often the most profound stress experienced by the body. As an example, when the body is subjected to a fever, where the subject's temperature becomes significantly elevated above its usual range centered at 98.6°F (37.7°C), the body's metabolism (the overall rate of activity in the body's processes) increases; the running of a marathon may increase metabolic rates to many time their normal level.

Virtually every process and organ within the body is affected by exercise. As an example, the skin, the largest human organ, undergoes physical changes when exposed to the environmental factors encountered in sport, such as increases and decreases in external temperatures. The physiology of exercise is tends to center upon the most important physical systems to athletic performance: the cardiovascular system, the cardiorespiratory system, the thermoregulatory system, body composition and the musculoskeletal system. It is these aspects of human function that tend to have the greatest impact upon the ability of an athlete to maintain or improve their level of performance in any sport.

The cardiovascular system is the physical network composed of the heart and its connected arteries, veins, and capillaries. The cardiovascular system is the vehicle through which the oxygen and fuels required by the cells within the body are supplied; the cardiovascular system removes all waste products from the cells and organs for disposal. When the body is subjected to exercise, and its increased physical demands, the cardiovascular system is forced to work more quickly and more efficiently to fulfill bodily needs. A number of physiological changes occur over time to this system through exercise.

The first and the most fundamental change to the cardiovascular system is with respect to the function of the heart. The cardiac muscle of the heart will grow stronger over time, as the heart becomes adapted to working harder during exercise. A stronger and more efficient heart reduces the resting pulse of the subject; as the heart strengthens, it does not have to beat as frequently as when at rest to achieve the same effect in the pumping of blood through the cardiovascular system. The greater flow of blood available to a person who regularly exercises tends to reduce the amount of low-density lipoproteins within the blood vessels that can form a harmful blockage known as plaque, a condition that tends to narrow the passage within each artery. Exercise does not make the arteries larger, but these vessels become more elastic through exercise permitting a greater and more beneficial blood flow through out the body.

The second important physiological change experienced by the cardiovascular system due to exercise is the reduction of blood pressure. Blood pressure is defined as the force of blood being pushed against the walls of the arteries of the cardiovascular system. High blood pressure has two components; systolic pressure is that measured during a heartbeat, and diastolic pressure is that present between heartbeats. Blood pressure is measured as the relationship of systolic to diastolic levels. High blood pressure, expressed as a measurement greater than 140/90 mmHg (millimeters of mercury, a unit of atmospheric pressure), is a condition where the heart is forced to work harder than it was designed in order to direct blood through the entire system. High blood pressure raises the risk for heart attack and stroke. Subject to other genetic factors or environmental impacts such as smoking, exercise will tend to reduce blood pressure. Athletes almost always possess a blood pressure reading significantly lower than that normally found in the regular population.

The most profound impact of exercise upon the cardiorespiratory system also affects the function of the cardiovascular system. The maximum volume of oxygen that an athlete can consume during exercise is known by the expression $VO_2$max. Particularly in the endurance sports, where the athlete is fueling their body by way of the aerobic energy system, endurance training will increase the athlete's $VO_2$. The ability of athletes to increase their maximum oxygen capacity is universal; female athletes will generally possess a $VO_2$max ranging between 60% and 75% of that of a similarly conditioned male, due to the greater muscle mass present in a male athlete which must be serviced through the delivery of oxygen to the energy producing cell. Female athletes are as strong as a male counterpart when muscle strength is measured per unit, as per cubic inch of muscle ($cm^3$).

Exercise improves the ability of the cardiorespiratory system to take oxygen from air inhaled into the lungs, and then load and transport it more efficiently. Greater efficiency in the movement of blood through the cardiovascular system permits greater amounts of oxygen to be transferred from the respiratory system; lung size does not increase due to exercise by any appreciable degree.

Thermoregulation is the ability of the body to maintain the optimal internal temperature levels for the function of all organs in different external environment conditions. Where the athlete is unaccustomed to warm weather exercise, the body will adapt through the process of acclimatization to the new conditions. Within a period of approximately 14 days, the positive physiological changes typically noted through heat acclimatization include expanded blood volume (corresponding greater blood capacity), reduced heart rate (making the heart more efficient), increased direction of blood to the skin surface and the capillaries (greater cooling effect on blood through directing the blood to the cooler skin surface), and an increased conservation of sodium to promote more effective hydration (to preserve the optimal proportion of sodium to water, a part of the body's osmoregulatory system).

Body composition is the most visible of the physiological changes often observed to have occurred through exercise. The body is constructed from body fat, lean muscle mass, and the organs and skeletal bone, the dimensions of which are not altered through exercise. Body composition is affected by two distinct exercise mechanisms—through a reduction in the percentage of body fat in a subject, and through the increase of lean muscle mass developed through specialized exercise. Body fat is the storage form of the triglycerides that are processed by the body from the fats consumed through diet. These fats may be stored for indefinite periods in the adipose tissues located in the region of the abdomen, pelvis, buttocks, and chest. Exercise, when combined with proper attention to diet, will result in a weight loss in any subject where the amount of caloric energy required to fulfill the body's needs, including exercise, exceeds the amount of caloric energy sources ingested as food. One pound of body fat (0.4 kg) represents approximately 3,500 available calories of energy.

Muscle development through exercise programs often occurs in conjunction with the reduction of body fat that results from the difference between energy intake and output. In the early stages of weight reduction where the subject is participating in muscle building resistance exercise, it is common for the subject to experience frustration in terms of their desired weight loss, as the body fat that is available to the body as fuel is countered by the gain of denser muscle tissue.

The musculoskeletal system undergoes a multitude of physiological changes, in addition to the additional muscle produced through particular types of training. Stretching and flexibility exercises tend to create a greater range of motion in all of the joints that are subjected to these stresses. Where the joints of the body are able to move more dynamically, the related structure will generally be capable of both faster, more powerful and more stable movement. A joint with an improved range of motion is less likely to become overstressed and injured.

The bones of the musculoskeletal system also undergo structural changes that result from exercise. Resistance, either through weight training, or in activities that require running or other forces to be directed into the body, generally tends to increase bone density.

In addition to creating greater muscle mass, exercise will have an effect upon existing muscle structures. All humans possess specific kinds of muscle fibers, each of which is distributed relatively evenly throughout the muscles of the body according to the genetic makeup of the individual. The two general muscle fiber types are fast twitch and slow twitch fibers. The designation between fast and slow is determined by the frequency with which the neuron that governs the impulses that control the contraction of the particular fiber. Fast twitch neurons fire at a rate of approximately 10 times greater frequency than does a slow twitch neuron. The effective function of fast twitch fibers is essential to anaerobic sports such as sprinting and jumping. Specialized exercise, such as plyometric programs, can enhance the performance of fast twitch fiber. The proportion of slow twitch muscle fibers, the backbone to the muscle function in endurance sports such as marathon running and cycling, will increase in proportion to fast twitch fibers when the athlete undergoes vigorous endurance training.

SEE ALSO Endurance exercise; Fitness; Metabolic response; Sport performance.

## Physiotherapist

A physiotherapist is a healthcare professional whose work is directed to the improved movement and function of persons who have sustained a musculoskeletal injury. The physiotherapist is most often a part of a larger healthcare team, as physiotherapists work closely with the physicians who provide a diagnosis with respect to a particular physical condition, which the physiotherapists seek to either correct or improve through treatment. In a sports setting, physiotherapists work closely with athletic trainers and sport coaches to assist injured athletes.

The general role of the physiotherapist is the treatment of physical disorders through the manipulation of the joints and other components of the musculoskeletal system. Physiotherapy is now recognized as a distinct branch of the medical sciences. In most countries, the academic training required for a career in physiotherapy is a course of university study, where the physiotherapy school is most often affiliated with a medical faculty. The chief components of a physiotherapy curriculum are biology (including anatomy and kinesiology), psychology, biomechanics, and pharmacology (the study of how drugs interact with bodily function). In many jurisdictions, physiotherapy is a freestanding and accredited profession, with independent control over its membership regarding licensing, education, and professional standards.

In a sports setting—particularly with respect to elite competitive programs—the physiotherapist plays a key role with respect to the development of preseason training programs, especially for those athletes who have previously sustained a particular injury, as well as acting as an ongoing training and educational resource for athletes and coaches. High-level athletes, in conjunction with their coaches, will

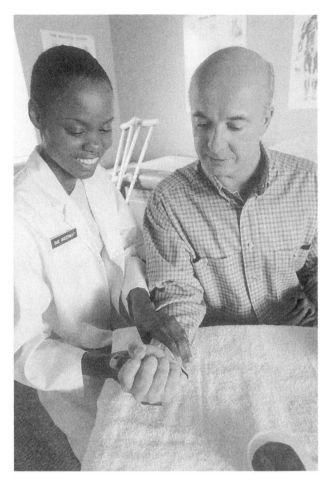

Physiotherapists treat physical disorders through the manipulation of the joints and other components of the musculoskeletal system. © LWA-STEPHEN WELSTEAD/CORBIS

develop a year-long segmented training regimen, a process often referred to as the periodization of training; the physiotherapist will often have significant input as to how the periods should be structured.

The role of the physiotherapist is also vital in terms of collecting data about a recovering athlete regarding performance and the ability of the athlete to achieve defined results during rehabilitation. The overriding objective of the physiotherapist extends beyond the recovery of the athlete into the broader concepts of restoration of physical health and the prevention of a similar occurrence. The progress made in the athlete's rehabilitation will often dictate what other professional steps are taken to preserve recovery, such as the use and design of orthotics or other protective equipment.

SEE ALSO Disabled individuals and regular physical exercise; Fitness; Massage therapy; Musculoskeletal injuries.

# Phytochemicals

Phytochemicals are an important aspect of human diet and consequent athletic performance. "Phyto" is a Greek work for plant life, and the phytochemicals are a very broad range of substances that are ingested through food, but that do not themselves possess any nutritional value, in terms of energy, vitamin, or mineral contribution. Most foods, except those that are heavily refined such as sugar, contain one form of phytochemical or another. The primary sources of these substances are fruits, vegetables, whole grains, and most beans.

The phytochemicals are substances that influence the function and the outcome of various bodily systems, as opposed to directing or dictating that function. The phytochemicals that are of most interest to humans are those that act to protect the body from illness or disease.

Phytochemicals have long been recognized by various cultures throughout the world as possessing special qualities in relation to human health. The ancient system of traditional Chinese medicine (TCM), and its reliance upon herbs such as ginseng, is an example of the extent to which various phytochemicals have been used. A more recent phytochemical medicinal application was the synthesis of salicylic acid, first extracted from the bark of a willow tree, in the manufacture of the most commonly used of aspirin, the nonsteroidal anti-drugs (NSAIDs), created in 1899.

As phytochemicals enter the body as the components of a broad range of plant products consumed as food, each with its own chemical complexity, the action of the various phytochemicals on the human systems is equally diverse. No phytochemical is believed to be essential to optimal body function as, in many cases, the action of the phytochemical is a counteraction of an unrelated environmental impact on the body. The following are the more common types of desirable actions and related food sources for each phytochemical:

- Antibacterial agents: Allicin, the active ingredient of garlic and other plants that provides this vegetable with its characteristic strong odor, is well known as a substance that acts as an effective agent against harmful bacteria entering the body.
- Antioxidants: This term is broadly and often incorrectly applied to a variety of plant sources. An antioxidant is a substance that tends to act against molecules in the body that have an unpaired electron, known as free radicals, which

themselves tend to form cells that often contribute to the formation of cancer-causing cells. The phytochemicals present in items such as fruits, carrots, onions, and other vegetables are well-regarded antioxidants. Lycopene is the phytochemical compound found in the skin of tomatoes, and it is a powerful antioxidant, particularly with respect to preserving the health of the cells in the cardiovascular system.

- Alkaloids: The most important alkaloid is caffeine. Caffeine is the world's most consumed stimulant, possessing a powerful effect on the central nervous system. In excess amounts, caffeine is counterproductive to the health of the body.
- Digoxin: This is found naturally in the foxglove plant, which grows in various parts of North America and Europe. It is a well regarded as a medication in the treatment of heart failure, as it acts to regulate and to strengthen a failing heart rate.
- Flavanoids: The flavanoid group, which are present in a number of fruits, such as cranberries, raspberries, grapes, and blueberries, often act as antioxidants. Flavanoids also work to inhibit the progress of low-density lipoproteins in the cardiovascular system, the form of cholesterol that causes plaque and contributes to the narrowing of arteries and the development of arteriosclerosis. Red wine has been long regarded as possessing this antioxidant quality.
- Beta-sitosterol; This substance is found in peanuts, wheat germ, and various rice products; these agents tend to reduce cholesterol levels, especially in men with prostate problems.

While phytochemicals can be added to an existing diet by way of supplements, the best and most absorptive fashion that such chemicals can be introduced into the body is through a balanced diet that has significant fresh fruits and vegetables. As a general rule, the closer to the natural or whole food state, the more likely the food is to possess phytochemicals. An example is whole grain products; much of the phytochemical presence is contained in the grain or kernel shell. When the grain is removed during processing, a large measure of the phytochemicals in the grain are removed.

Two food types that are sometimes overlooked by those seeking the advantages of phytochemicals are dried fruits, which lose little of their natural phytochemical effect in this state, and various herbs and spices commonly employed in food preparation.

Most dried herbs such as basil, thyme, and oregano are rich in various phytochemicals. The active ingredient in many types of red pepper, capsicum, is an effective antioxidant agent.

SEE ALSO Caffeine; Diet; Nutrition.

# Pilates

Pilates refers to an exercise regimen that emphasizes stretching and balance. A series of specific movements is performed while breathing in a focused way. In contrast to more vigorous workouts such as aerobics, Pilates does not need to be strenuous to the point of sweating. Nonetheless, Pilates is a strenuous activity that increases flexibility, strength, and cardiovascular capacity.

Pilates is named after its originator, Joseph Hubertus Pilates. In the decades prior to World War I, he studied the physical aspects of yoga, Zen, and exercises practiced in ancient Greece and Rome. During the war, when he and other German nationals were interned in a camp in Lancaster, England, he taught other detainees these exercises. As well, he incorporated these exercises into an original series of exercises that were done while lying on the floor. Pilates called these exercises "contrology"; today, they are called "matwork."

Later in World War I, Pilates was transferred to another internment camp on the Isle of Man, where he helped in the medical care and physical rehabilitation of sick and injured detainees and soldiers. He modified his exercise regimen for those who were too infirmed to get out of bed by using bedsprings to create devices that offered resistance when pulled.

Today, Pilates is done essentially the same way. Instead of bedsprings, participants use elastic cords that can be gripped and slipped over the feet to provide resistance in the stretching movements.

The resistance-based exercises that form Pilates are directed first at the core area of the body, which include the muscles in the stomach, buttocks, lower back, and thighs. These muscles are strengthened before exercises that involve other areas of the body are introduced, the idea being that a stronger core will enable the expanded series of exercises to be done with a lesser risk of injury.

Pilates consists of a flowing series of connected movements. Although different from tai-chi in execution, Pilates is similar in that movements are rarely held for long. Rather, each movement should flow gracefully into the next. Pilates is also similar to tai-chi in that correct form is essential to attain the benefits of the exercise.

In each Pilates exercise session, the core muscles are worked on first, followed by exercises directed at other muscles in the arms, legs, and neck. Movements are performed slowly, always with the emphasis on maintaining form.

Focus is on the abdominal muscles. When done correctly, the abdominal muscles are pulled slightly upward toward the navel and slightly inward, and the spine is kept straight. This posture is maintained while breathing, which is done by expanding the rib cage rather than the stomach. This style of breathing can be challenging for those beginning a Pilates program, requiring concentration. Once mastered, however, the concentration required in rhythmic breathing pattern, combined with the flowing exercise movements, can be meditative, providing an added benefit to the exercises.

Resistance is another key of Pilates. Instead of modified bedsprings, a device called the Reformer is now used. The Reformer, which is similar in appearance to a low table, uses various cable, springs, pulleys, and sliding boards to provide the resistance. Pushing and pulling will move the sliding platform in a motion similar to that of a conventional rowing machine.

Another piece of equipment resembles a half barrel attached to a short ladder. By positioning the feet under a low rung of the ladder and lying at an angled, stomach-down position on the barrel, the back can be gently arched forward and backward. A large air-filled ball called a Swiss Ball can also be used to achieve the same effects.

Smaller exercise balls can be positioned between the feet and the groin while sitting on the floor. By pushing against the ball, gentle resistance is provided to the inner muscles of the legs and the groin.

Another, more exotic, piece of equipment is called the trapeze table (or Cadillac). A low-slung table forms the base for a horizontal end supports and vertical parallel bars. Springs and supports positioned on the horizontal and vertical bars permit a variety of acrobatic stretches and movements to be done.

A device called a Chair resembles a bench with handles positioned near the ground. Users press down on the handles while in a sitting or lying position, to stretch muscles on the sides of the body.

When done correctly, Pilates is claimed to restore the proper equilibrium between various muscle

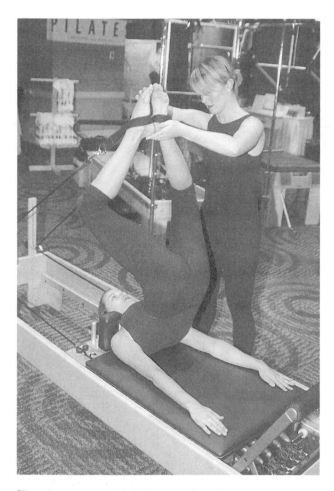

Pilates instructors and their class members demonstrate proper form. PHOTO COURTESY OF THE PILATES METHOD ALLIANCE FOR BUSINESS WIRE VIA GETTY IMAGES.

groups, which reduces stress on over-utilized muscles. Restoration of equilibrium can prevent injury or speed recovery from injury. Because these benefits can be attained in a low-impact workout, Pilates has become a popular part of the training regimen for athletes as diverse as dancers, rugby players, soccer players, runners, and track and field competitors.

SEE ALSO Aerobics; Balance training and proprioception; Yoga and Pilates.

# Ping pong SEE Table tennis

# Piriformis syndrome

The piriformis muscle is a structure that lies beneath the larger gluteus maximus muscle in each buttock. The piriformis extends from the base of the

spine where it connects with the top of each femur (thigh bone). The sciatic nerve is a major nerve pathway that extends from the spine to the pelvis and travels directly beneath the piriformis, as it continues into each leg and foot. The piriformis is a part of the muscle complex that permits the hip to rotate.

Piriformis syndrome is characterized by pain that is experienced deep in the buttock, often radiating into the lower back and the legs, occasionally as far as the foot on the affected side of the body. Until recently, piriformis syndrome was not widely accepted as a distinct physical condition within the sports medicine community, as it was believed to be a type of sciatica, the well-known inflammatory condition of the sciatic nerve. Sciatica has a cause distinct from that of piriformis syndrome in that it occurs due to pressure on the nerve canal where the sciatic nerve exits the spine at the top of the pelvis. The piriformis syndrome is most evident to an affected person when walking, running, sitting for extended periods of time, climbing multiple sets of stairs, or performing any movement involving a squat or deep knee bend.

Piriformis syndrome results from either a tightness developing in the muscle structure itself, or through the combined effects of muscle tightness and pressure being applied to the underlying sciatic nerve. A number of other musculoskeletal conditions may exist concurrently with piriformis syndrome, the most common of which are unequal leg length, which directs unequal pressures into each leg, and weak abductor muscles, which control the ability of the legs to spread apart.

When piriformis syndrome is identified, the first course of treatment prescribed to an athlete is usually rest for a period of two to three weeks. During the rest period, specialized stretches will often be recommended, movements that are designed to reduce the tightness of the piriformis in relation to the surrounding muscle structures. On a permanent basis, athletes often find that a commitment to a rigorous stretching and flexibility program is essential to prevent a recurrence of piriformis syndrome. Yoga and Pilates are two exercise systems that emphasize a number of different stretches that specifically target the buttocks and hips. In more severe cases, a corticosteroid may be injected directly into the affected piriformis to provide an anti-inflammatory effect. Ultrasound therapy may also be engaged. Surgery is a procedure that is rarely employed, given the position of the muscle and its proximity to the sciatic nerve.

SEE ALSO Back anatomy and physiology; Back injuries; Hip and pelvis anatomy and physiology; Nervous system.

# Pitching machines and related devices

Baseball is a sport in which success is built on the ability of the athlete to replicate specific movements. Many baseball drills are situational; throwing, fielding, and batting practice are directed toward the player being conditioned to react to specific defensive and offensive situations. The physical attributes of hand-eye coordination, reaction time, and agility may be more important to success in baseball than in almost any other sport.

Pitching machines are a training aid designed to permit players to practice, hone, and refine their batting stroke without requiring the presence of a pitcher, or otherwise requiring a catcher to receive the batting practice pitches. Pitching machines are similar in their purpose to the simulators used in other sports, such as computer-supported bobsled trainers. The pitching machine is more limited in its application than some other sports simulators because the athlete is focused on one narrow aspect of baseball training in facing pitches thrown by the machine. The pitching machine does not require the athlete to engage in the entire sport skill set as would be required in an actual competition.

The history of the automated pitching machine suggests that there are a number of contenders for the title of inventor of the world's first such device. Many authorities confirm that Lorenzo Ponza (1918–2004) was the developer of the first portable on field pitching machine; Ponza created his machine in 1952 to assist in the development of Little League players (age 14 and under).

Baseball is a game with the fundamental objective of scoring more runs than the opponent. Two means to meeting this objective are batting practice, to enable players to hit the ball more effectively, and pitching, to limit the hitting of the opponent. No sport depends to a greater degree on the repetition of the elements of both pitching and hitting. The physical requirements of pitching are such that pitchers are the most injured players in baseball. At the youth level, when the pitching arm is not fully developed, serious injuries that result from overuse are common. The strain created by the forces directed into the pitcher's throwing elbow and shoulder, from the twist necessary to deliver a curve ball or a slider, restrict the number of pitches that should safely be thrown in any given training period at any age.

The striking with a bat of a round ball thrown at a significant velocity with spin imparted to it is a difficult task; at a major league level, a batter is deemed to be competent if he or she is able to hit safely three times out 10. For this reason, the most important feature of batting practice is the ability to replicate the game day swing of the bat as many times as possible. Pitching machines safely permit this replication without wear and tear on the pitcher's arm.

A pitching machine is typically employed with a related piece of equipment—the batting cage, an enclosed area usually forming a 90° angle with the apex behind the batter. The cage is entirely enclosed so as to prevent any batted balls from striking other persons. The pitching machine is positioned at precisely the same distance from the batter as would be the pitcher, to precisely simulate the pitched ball. Pitching machines are constructed as one of two types: a machine with an overhand arm delivery or one constructed with two horizontally opposed wheels, with the ball delivered by their rotation effect. The machine may be configured to simulate a baseball pitch, delivered overhand, or a softball delivery, delivered underhand.

Pitching machines permit both the speed and the spin imparted to the ball to be varied. For youth players, the ball might be delivered at speeds in the vicinity of 40 mi (64 km) per hour; for a professional player, the ball would be thrown at the speeds expected in major league play, a range from 80 to 100 mi (129–160 km) per hour. The machine can also be configured to throw fastballs, curveballs, sliders, and screwballs, the most common pitches thrown in the game. The practicing batter can face the same pitch for an indefinite period, practicing against it and endeavoring to remove any perceived flaws in the batting stroke.

The pitching machine and the companion batting cage are also an excellent venue for the batter to combine the physical work on the batting stroke with the mental sports training known as visualization. As each pitch is delivered by the machine, the athlete can imagine being in various game situations and attempt to strike the ball thrown by the machine in the same fashion as he or she would react to each pitch. The athlete can also visualize where various base runners might be at that point in the game, the number of outs, or the ball and strike count, to make the batting practice more realistic.

SEE ALSO Computer simulations as a training tool; Cross training; Visualization in sport.

# Plantar fasciitis

Plantar fasciitis is a condition of the foot that results from the repetitive overstretching and irritation of the plantar tissue, a relatively stiff, fibrous material that connects the calcaneus (heel bone) to the ball of the foot. The term plantar fasciitis is often used interchangeably with another foot and heel condition, heel spurs, and while the two have a similar origin, they are not always the same ailment.

Plantar fasciitis occurs during athletic activity as a result of how the foot responds to the stresses of either walking or running. During either motion, movement begins with a pushing off from the pads at the ball of the foot and a lifting of the heel. The heel is connected to the calf muscles (the gastrocnemius and the soleus) through the Achilles tendon. If the lower leg structure is overly tight, the plantar cannot move easily and it becomes more rigid along its length. The repetitive nature of this tension imbalance between the calf muscles and the plantar is the most common cause of plantar fasciitis. The condition will often cause significant pain, which is chiefly experienced on the sole of the foot closest to the heel. In many cases, the pain is sufficiently acute to limit the training of an athlete, as full intensity running is not possible.

Other factors that may contribute to plantar fasciitis are poor support for the arch of the foot (combined with either high arches or low arches in the subject foot), inadequate cushioning in the footwear used for running on hard surfaces, a sudden increase in either training intensity or workloads, and being overweight. Each of these factors acts on the plantar structure in the same fashion as the lower leg muscle imbalance.

In as many as 70% of plantar fasciitis cases, heel spurs will develop on the affected foot. A heel spur is a deposit of bony material that accumulates on the surface of the heel; in most cases the heel spur is not the cause of pain in the affected foot.

Once the condition of plantar fasciitis has been determined, the person will often notice that the pain is more pronounced in the early morning than at any other time. This is due to the fact that, at night, the plantar tends to contract during sleep, and the tissue takes time, through movement and stretching, to become more pliable and less restricted.

The most effective manner of dealing with plantar fasciitis is a modified version of the RICE (rest/ice/compression/elevation) treatment. The first and most important component in the treatment of plantar fasciitis is to rest from the activities that have contributed to its formation. Runners and other athletes for whom the striking of a surface with their foot is the essence of their training often cross train through swimming, a sport that does not aggravate the plantar tissue, until the condition has resolved itself. Ice on the affected area will assist in management of the condition, and should be applied as soon as there is pain, with the icing repeated up to eight times per day, for a maximum of approximately 15 minutes per session (the ice pack should be applied so that the skin is not at any risk of freezing, but the pack should be cold enough to promote the reduction of swelling and to reduce the risk of scar tissue formation.

As plantar fasciitis is commonly caused by calf muscles that are too tight, a daily stretching program involving those muscle, the Achilles tendon, and the foot is an excellent rehabilitative and preventive step. Also, pressure, or compression, by applying athletic tape or compression bandages over the affected area provides both support for the plantar tissue but also assists in keeping the foot stable through movement. The application of pressure will also combat any lingering tightness present in the calf muscles that tends to counter the rehabilitation of the plantar. The foot and heel can be taped so as to provide one contiguous support structure.

There are measures to be taken once the plantar fasciitis has been controlled. In some cases, an investigation of how the person's foot moves during athletic activity will suggest that either an arch support or an orthotic be crafted to stabilize the motion of the foot when it strikes the ground. Only in the rarest of circumstances will surgery be recommended to correct plantar fasciitis. This procedure involves making an incision into the plantar tissue, with a goal of making the plantar less rigid; such procedures are not a guarantee of improved, pain-free motion.

SEE ALSO Bone, ligaments, tendons; Foot: Anatomy and physiology; Heel spurs; Musculoskeletal injuries.

# Joseph Jacques Plante

1/17/1929–2/27/1986
CANADIAN
ICE HOCKEY PLAYER, GOALTENDER

Joseph Jacques Plante, who was more commonly called Jacques Plante, or by his nickname of "Jake the Snake," was a professional ice hockey goaltender from 1947–1975. A solid journeyman goaltender, Plante is best remembered for his influence on the style of goaltending and most especially for his use of the facemask and protective gear to reduce facial and head injuries.

Like many of his generation who were born in the Canadian province of Quebec, Jacques Plante grew up playing hockey. Before he left high school his talent as a goaltender was considered of professional caliber, and after his graduation in 1947 he joined the Quebec Citadels of the Quebec Junior A League. He played for the Citadels and the Montreal Junior Canadians for two years. In 1949, he joined the Montreal Royals of the Quebec Senior Hockey League. He played for the Royals into the 1952–1953 season, when he joined the Montreal Canadians of the National Hockey League (NHL). With the exceptions of a few brief stints playing for the Buffalo Bisons in the American Hockey League, Plante remained with the Montreal NHL squad through the 1962–1963 season.

Prior to the 1963–1964 season, Plante was traded from Montreal to the New York Rangers. Then 34, he was judged by the Montreal coaching staff to be too old to be a reliable starting goalie. As well, his hockey skills had seemingly begun to diminish.

Indeed, the next two seasons with the Rangers proved to be difficult and his play was substandard. This prompted his retirement in 1965. The retirement proved to be short–lived, as the following year he was convinced to return to the NHL. He reported to the preseason training camp of the newly formed California Golden Seals. However, he left training camp early and retired once again.

Plante's second retirement was also short–lived. Two seasons later, he accepted an offer to join the St. Louis Blues. In the 1968–1969 NHL season, he shared goaltending duties with another veteran, Glenn Hall. Plante's play was splendid, and he and Hall led the Blues to the league finals. The goaltenders jointly received the Vezina Trophy that season, an award recognizing the best goaltending in the league.

After another solid season with the Blues, Plante was traded to the Toronto Maple Leafs, with whom he enjoyed two good seasons. In particular, during his first year with the team, he led the league in allowing an average of less than two goals per game.

Late in the 1972–1973 season, Plante was traded to the Boston Bruins. At the conclusion of the playoffs, he officially retired from the NHL, though not yet from professional hockey.

In 1974, Plante played one final season of competitive hockey, this time for the Edmonton Oilers of the newly formed World Hockey Association. At the season's conclusion, at the age of 45, he retired for the last time.

Plante's accomplishments as a goaltender were significant. For five consecutive seasons beginning in 1955, he won the Vezina Trophy. He was named to NHL All-Star teams in seven seasons, three of these as the starting All-Star goalie. These and other accomplishments as a player led to his admission to the Hockey Hall of Fame in 1978.

As impressive as his play was, Plante's greatest impact on hockey came during the 1959–1960 season when, after being hit in the face by a shot, he donned a goalie mask. While he had been wearing the mask during team practices, the attitude of players and coaches at that time was that such protection had no part in a real game. By continuing to wear the mask in subsequent games, even despite the early disapproval of his coach, he convinced other goaltenders to try out the protective face gear (which Plante designed for them).

Plante's continued use of the face mask changed the nature of hockey. Before then, wearing a protective mask was unheard of, and was considered to be unmanly. Players and coaches began to realize that protective gear could enhance the game, rather than detract from it after watching Plante in action. This change in attitude led to the acceptance of helmets as required playing gear.

Other goaltending innovations that Plante introduced included skating behind the net to retrieve the puck and initiate another play, and a stand-up style of hockey in which he would move out of the net as an opposing puck-carrier neared, making it more difficult for the player to shoot the puck into the net ("cutting down the angle"). Prior to Plante's career, goalies tended to stay within the zone of the goal and would sprawl on the ice to make a save.

Plante's innovations, which gave his teammates an offensive advantage, are now a standard part of hockey.

Jacques Plante died of stomach cancer at the age of 57. Posthumously, his Montreal Canadians jersey number was retired. As well, the award for the leading goaltender in the Quebec Major Junior Hockey League was renamed the Jacques Plante Trophy.

# Gary Player

11/1/1935–
SOUTH AFRICAN
PROFESSIONAL GOLFER,
GOLF COURSE ARCHITECT

Gary Player is a professional golfer, golf course designer, and marketer of golf-related products. During the peak of his career from the 1950s to the 1970s, he was one of the best golfers in the world. His golf career is also notable because the American Professional Golfers Association (PGA) was dominated by Americans during these years. Player was one of the first non-American and non-European golfers to both play and dominate on the PGA tour. Player was also one of the first to emphasize general fitness exercises for golfers and devoted parts of his golf lesson videos to general training and fitness.

Throughout his career, Player has been a global golfer, traveling an estimated 14 million miles to compete in tournaments and conduct golf exhibition matches all around the world. This globetrotting produced at least one tournament victory each season for 27 years in a row. Now 71 years old and with his tournament-level golf behind him, Player's career victory tally over five decades of competitive golf stands at 166, the best of any golfer.

Nicknamed "The Black Knight" for the intimidating all-black golf attire he typically wore, Player brought a fiercely competitive nature to his golf. This approach enabled Player to become one of golf's elite despite his small size of 5 ft 8 in and weight of 150 lb (1.7 m and 68 kg).

Player became a professional golfer in 1953, at 18 years of age. He joined the PGA tour in 1957. From then until 1985, when he began to play regularly on the Champion's tour (a PGA-sanctioned tour reserved for professional golfers aged 50 and older), Player won numerous PGA events. As well, he was victorious in nine of the so-called "Majors," including three Masters championships (1961, 1974, and 1978), three British Opens (1959, 1968, 1974), two PGA championships (1962 and 1972), and a U.S. Open (1965). The last major victory was especially memorable, as Player came from seven shots behind in the beginning of the final round of the 1978 Masters to win by a single stroke, recording a birdie on seven of the final 10 holes. A birdie is one shot less than par (the number of shots a hole is designed to be played in).

He is the first non-American to win the Masters; is one of a handful of golfers to have won more than one major in the same competitive season; and is one of only five golfers to have won all four of the major tournaments during their careers. Player's career grand slam was achieved by the time he was 29 years of age. Only Jack Nicklaus and Tiger Woods have won more major golf tournaments. He is also the only golfer to have won the British Open in three different decades.

On the Champion's tour, Player proved to be no less competitive, winning his first senior tour event and going on the win 19 in total. He has amassed nine Senior Major titles, including the Senior Players Championship (1987), and three each of the Senior PGA championships (1968, 1988, 1990), Senior U.S. Opens (1987, 1988), and Senior British Opens (1988, 1990, 1997).

He was able to maintain a high level of play into his senior career, exemplified by his qualification for the final two rounds of the British Open (in 1995 at 59 years of age) and the Masters (in 1998 at 62 years of age). In a golf tournament, players who shoot better than a set score during the first two rounds "make the cut" and can participate in the final two rounds. Player made the cut at the Masters for 23 consecutive years.

His career earnings exceed $12 million. In 1961, he was the leading money winner on the PGA tour.

Player is now known more for his golf course design than for his tournament play. Over the past several decades, he has designed more than 200 courses around the world. He is also a breeder of racehorses.

Having grown up in South Africa when racial disparity was the norm, Player uses his recognition and international celebrity to promote racial equality in South Africa. He established The Player Foundation, which promotes education for underprivileged South Africans, in 1980. The foundation has raised in excess of $100 million. The foundation-built Blair Atholl School, located in Johannesburg, provides education to more than 500 students each year.

Among the honors he has received, Player was one of the original inductees to the World Golf Hall of Fame on its founding in 1974.

SEE ALSO Golf.

# Plyometrics

Plyometrics is the science examining the explosive movement generated by muscle power, with particular application to sport training and performance.

As power is the product of speed plus strength, the ability of an athlete to generate force in a short period of time is at the root of developing greater explosive effect.

It is an anatomical fact that muscles in the human body contract in order to generate force, a process known as concentric contraction. Further, if the muscle is lengthened in the period immediately prior to contraction, the muscle will develop greater power. The lengthening process is known as an eccentric contraction. The shorter the time period between eccentric and concentric muscle contractions, the greater the power capable of being generated by the muscle.

Plyometrics training is designed to develop rapid alterations of eccentric and concentric contractions, while constant resistance is applied to the target muscle or muscle group.

Plyometrics was first popularized by the former East Germany state sport trainers in the 1970s, as a method of building the myotactic reflex, the term used to describe this stretch reflex in the muscle that enhances the power of contraction. As an example, when a person performs repeated forward jumps, there will be stretch of the quadriceps (located on the front of the thigh) muscles in the first jump. The subsequent contraction of this muscle will make the jump immediately following more powerful.

Sports in which explosive speed and power are at a premium are those in which plyometrics training techniques are often employed—the delivery of an effective punch in boxing, various positions in American football, basketball, and volleyball are examples.

A typical plyometrics workout for a sport in which explosive lower body power is key might include ground-level jumping on soft surfaces such as padded mats or grass, with a progression to jumping over cones or foam barriers. As a general rule, lower body plyometrics are performed on semi-resilient surfaces. Advanced plyometrics jumping often involves bounding exercises, both in straight lines and in patterns. The exercise routines emphasize speed, not endurance, with a number of repetitions typically performed quickly. When accompanied by both an active warm up, designed to elevate the athlete's core body temperature, as well as a stretching program and other weight training to build an overall strength base, there is considerable evidence that plyometrics will improve the explosive movement capabilities of an athlete.

However, plyometrics training has generated debate regarding athlete safety in the sport science community. A number of experts have criticized plyometrics as being compared to high-impact aerobics, a fitness activity that fell into disfavor due to the risk of injury to participants' lower body joints from excess stress on the musculoskeletal system. There is little question that some athletes, because of their physical structure, fitness level, and related factors, are poor candidates for a plyometrics training program.

Any training method that builds strength through an explosive movement, such as a plyometrics jump program, carries with it an greater inherent risk of injury. This danger can be minimized if the athlete incorporates the plyometrics drills into a broad-based weight training and stretching program. The strength of the muscles of the lumbar (lower) back, the gluteal muscles (the buttocks and pelvic muscles), and the abdominals is important in providing stability to the body both at the moment of moving explosively into a jump, as well as upon the body landing.

These long-term injury concerns underscore a number of critical safety factors to be applied to all plyometrics training programs. Given the intensity of the training techniques, extreme caution should be employed before a young athlete participates in plyometrics. The stresses of the exercises create a potential for injury to a young athlete's skeletal growth plate (the epiphysis).

Further, an introduction to and maintenance of a plyometrics regime must be progressive in nature. Even where there is little by way of equipment, and the exercises appear simple, the stresses on the body must be introduced over time. In this regard, an athlete must also assess the effect of any previous injury or physical condition on the ability to benefit from plyometrics.

Other critical safety factors that should form a part of any plyometrics program are the use of foam or other soft barriers, boxes or jumping surfaces that will not twist on impact, and the provision for built-in rest periods of at least 48 hours between training sessions.

The ultimate measure of the success of any athletic training program is directly related to an athlete's success in competition. However, to directly assess the benefits of a plyometrics program, as well as planning further training, the athlete or the coach must determine an appropriate baseline through periodic field testing.

SEE ALSO Ankle: Anatomy and physiology; Foot: Anatomy and physiology; Lower leg anatomy; Muscle fibers: Fast and slow twitch.

# Pole vaulting

The pole vault is a sport where the successful competitor must combine a high level of athletic prowess with the development of unerring and fluid technique. Pole vaulting also involves a consideration of the advanced technologies used to construct the pole; the physical characteristics of the pole will be critical to the generation of the lift necessary to take the athlete over the bar.

As with many of the disciplines that are predominately in the public eye only during Olympic competition, the pole vault is a relatively simple event. The vaulters must clear a bar, positioned above a landing mat, using a long pole with which to propel themselves upward for leverage to assist in the clearing of the bar. The event commences with a run up along a track. The athlete runs as fast as possible, holding the long pole. The pole is thrust into a pre-positioned box on the track surface, and the athlete converts the forward motion along the track into vertical lift. The pole provides considerable flexion, as it absorbs and then releases the energy of the athlete generated by the approach as the pole is straightened. As the vaulter nears the bar, the pole is used for balance as the vaulter angles his or her body across the bar, falling onto the landing mats below.

In international and Olympic competition, each athlete is provided with three opportunities to clear the determined heights. The winner of the competition is the last vaulter to have cleared a height; in the event of a tie, where one or more competitors have each missed three jumps at a height, the tie is broken through determining the least number of misses at the earlier heights.

The pole vault has been an Olympic sport since the inaugural modern Games of 1896. It is also an event at the World Track and Field championships, held every two years. Women have competed for their pole vault championship at the Olympics since the 2000 Games. The pole vault is also one of the 10 disciplines that make up the Olympic decathlon, often referred to as the competition that determines the world's greatest athlete.

The object of the pole vault is to clear the greatest height possible; this object may also be

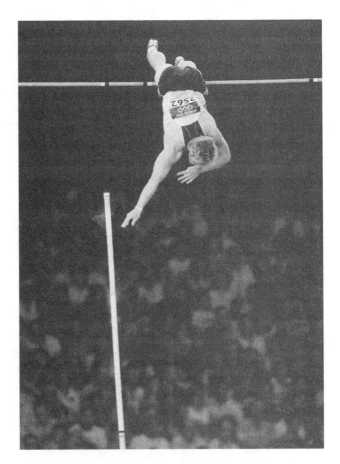

Rens Blom of Netherlands competes in the men's pole vault final during the Athens 2004 Summer Olympic Games. PHOTO BY DONALD MIRALLE/GETTY IMAGES.

stated as how to best optimize the energy of the athlete created by the run up and the planting of the pole prior to take off. The technology of the pole has been central to the progression of vaulters in achieving greater heights in the past 100 years. As a physical proposition, the greater the amount of energy that can be released from the pole as it is flexed by the athlete on the path up toward the bar, the further the athlete will be able to travel. This property of the bar is known as its coefficient of restitution; similar considerations apply to how far a golf ball will travel when struck by a club. In 1896, the Olympic champion used a pole constructed of bamboo; he jumped 10 ft 6 in (3.2 m). With aluminum poles in the early 1950s, vaulters could achieve heights of 15 ft 6 in (4.7 m), due in part to the more flexible nature of the aluminum construction, one that absorbed greater amounts of energy when struck into the ground by the vaulter, and which then released the stored energy to the body of the vaulter as the pole uncoiled. In 1994, Sergey Bubka of Russia set a pole vault world record of 20 ft 1.75

in (6.15 m), using a pole constructed of a carbon fiber/fiberglass composite, materials that are both lighter and possessed of a greater coefficient of restitution than the aluminum model.

For safety reasons, the poles are rated for use by athletes of a minimum weight to prevent a larger than rated athlete falling as a result of a pole that snaps under an excess weight. Vaulters use as light a pole as possible to ensure that they carry as little weight as possible on the run up, permitting the fastest approach possible, and the corresponding greatest amount of energy to be directed into the pole.

Most high jumpers, who are also attempting to leap as high as possible over a stationary bar, are tall and very slim and lithe. Pole vaulters tend to be heavier and much stronger athletes. The world-class pole vaulter will often possess sprinting capability not far removed from that of an elite sprinter, as the more speed the vaulter can develop on the runway approaching the jump, the more energy can be directed into the pole and then transferred into the vertical movement of the athlete to the bar. The vaulter must also have a strong upper body, particularly in the shoulders, to generate additional forces on the push of the pole into the ground on takeoff. The vaulter must also be extremely coordinated, able to contort their body in midair on the approach to the bar.

**SEE ALSO** Cross training; Decathlon; High jump.

## Polo, water SEE Water polo

## Popping joints SEE Joint noise: Popping and cracking

# Richard W. Pound

3/22/1942–
CANADIAN
CHAIRMAN OF THE WORLD ANTI-DOPING
AGENCY, MEMBER OF THE INTERNATIONAL
OLYMPIC COMMITTEE, LAWYER

Richard (Dick) Pound is the chairman of the World Anti-Doping Agency (WADA), which is responsible for monitoring athletes for the use of banned substances. Pound is an outspoken advocate of fair play in sports and the need to detect and punish those who use illegal drugs to increase their competitive advantage.

Pound was born in St. Catharines, a small city in Ontario located between Toronto and Niagara Falls. The area is well known as a competitive rowing center. However, Pound pursued swimming. He became the Canadian champion of freestyle in 1958, 1960, 1961, and 1962, and in the butterfly in 1961. Pound was a member of the Canadian Olympic swimming team that competed at the 1960 Summer Olympics in Rome. There, he was a finalist in the 100-m freestyle, where he finished sixth, and a member of the 4 x 400 m relay team that finished fourth. Two years later, at the Commonwealth Games held in Perth, Australia, Pound was victorious in the 110-m freestyle, captured silver medals as a member of the 440-m and 880-m relay teams, and was a member of the bronze medal winning 440-m medley relay team.

These swimming accomplishments were recognized by his induction in the Canadian Swimming Hall of Fame.

Following his retirement from competitive swimming, Pound became involved in the administrative side of sports. By 1968, he had become Secretary General of the Canadian Olympic Association, a post he held until 1976. During this time, he acted as the chef de mission of the Canadian team at the infamous 1972 Munich Olympics. From 1977–1982, he served as President of the Canadian Olympic Association. Finally, when WADA was created in 1979, Pound began as its first President, a position he continues to hold as of early 2006.

Pound is also well known for his involvement in the highest levels of the International Olympic Committee (IOC). He was elected to the IOC in 1982 as a member of the executive board. His first term expired in 1991. He served another term from 1992–1996. He also served as vice president of the IOC from 1987–1991 and 1996–2000.

While on the executive board of the IOC, Pound was responsible for negotiations of the broadcast deals for several Winter and Summer Olympics. The lucrative television and sponsorship deals he secured helped transform the IOC into a powerful and influential sports organization.

Pound unsuccessfully pursued the presidency of the IOC in 2001. His outspoken views regarding drugs in sports and the need to reform the IOC proved unpalatable with some delegates, and he finished third in the voting. He subsequently resigned as vice president to devote his energies to his post at WADA. As of 2006, he is still an IOC member.

In his everyday life, Pound is a partner in the Montreal-based law firm Stikeman Elliott LLP, where he practices tax law. Since 1991, he has also been Chancellor of McGill University, his alma mater, where he graduated with a Bachelor of Commerce degree in 1962.

As the chairman of WADA, Pound is responsible for the agency that monitors urine and blood samples for the presence of drugs that have been banned from use, according to the World Anti-Doping Code. This includes the random, unannounced testing of elite athletes outside of competition, and the testing that takes place during competitions such as the Olympics. As well, WADA provides funding to develop or refine technologies to enable the detection of substances that are currently undetectable. The organization is also involved in determining which drugs will be banned from use by athletes, and which substances are permissible.

Under Pound's leadership, WADA has changed the face of sports. Efforts to restrict the illicit use of drugs as a boost to athletic performance have become popular. Despite this turnabout in society's attitude toward drugs in sport, Pound's often blunt criticism of "doping" continues to be provocative. As one example, his public comments in late 2005 on the prevalence of performance-enhancing drugs in the National Hockey League have been harshly denied by league executives and player representatives.

In recognition of his accomplishments as an Olympian athlete and executive, Pound became an Officer of the Order of Canada in 1992 and an Officer of the National Order of Quebec in 1993.

SEE ALSO Anabolic prohormones; Cortisone steroid injections; Nasal sprays; Therapeutic use exemption.

# Pregnancy and exercise

Pregnancy is a physical condition that brings with it profound changes to the function of the female body. The growth of another living being within the uterus creates a remarkable organic partnership between the mother and the developing fetus. The maintenance of physical health in the mother, both through adherence to strong dietary and nutritional practices, as well as through exercise consistent with the physical changes brought by pregnancy, are the most important factors in the corresponding healthy development of the unborn child.

Pregnancy begins the moment that the female ovum (egg cell) has been fertilized by a male sperm cell; this fertilization is the act of conception. The cell division that propels the growth of the embryonic fetus begins approximately 30 hours after conception. The cell division and growth continue from the embryonic stage until the fetus (as the unborn child is often referred from the fourth month of pregnancy until birth) is delivered into the world as a newborn infant. From the moment that cell division begins, any environmental impacts on the mother, such as exercise activities, will impact how the fetus will develop within the uterus.

In many cultures throughout the history of the world, pregnant women were expected to carry on with their daily chores in both the home and the community. Any physical work that was usually required of women continued through their pregnancy, almost until the moment that birth was imminent. Many industrialized societies adopted a different view of the capacities of pregnant women in the later 1800s; in the middle classes of England and North America, it was common for pregnant women to be virtually confined to their homes for the duration of the pregnancy, with pregnancy regarded with the same precautions as would have been taken with an illness.

Modern medical science clearly endorses the proposition that both the health and the overall well-being of both mother and unborn child is enhanced by exercise, so long as the physical activity is proportionate to the physical condition of the mother. The general benefits gained by a pregnant woman through a structured exercise program include:

- A healthy body is better prepared for the possible difficulties of the labor and delivery process.
- In the same fashion that aerobic training is a recovery tool for athletes who participate in anaerobic sports like boxing or sprinting, exercise assists a mother in her recovery from the birth of the child.
- Exercise, which has positive, stress-relieving capabilities, will also assist a new mother in successfully assuming the demands of motherhood.
- Exercise will aid a pregnant woman in maintaining a strong lumbar (low back) structure, which will assist her in the support of her abdomen as it grows through the course of the pregnancy.

Exercise places energy and overall nutritional demands on the body, as does the growing fetus; by the fifth week of pregnancy, the embryonic fetus has its own heartbeat and it is receiving nutrition directly through the wall of the uterus. As the fetus grows, its own nutritional demands on the mother's reserves of

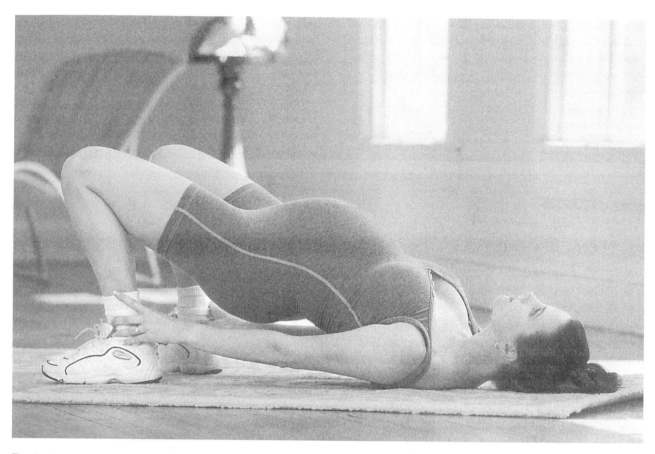

The health and the overall well-being of both mother and unborn child are enhanced by exercise. © ARIEL SKELLEY/CORBIS

vitamins and minerals increase. The mother must be conscious of these two separate demands on her system and structure her diet accordingly.

The exercise selected by the mother must be comprised of activities that avoid any significant physical risk. Sports where a fall is possible are important to avoid, especially as the female center of gravity while pregnant will affect normal balance. The generation of or exposure to excessive heat is also dangerous for both mother and fetus, as activities that cause dehydration will often trigger such dangerous conditions as lower blood volumes. A pregnant woman's resting pulse is elevated from her normal resting rate, which creates a further reason to avoid excess heat.

As a general rule, the more stable the body of the pregnant woman during exercise, the better the activity. Due to the hormonal changes that occur during pregnancy, ligaments and other connective tissues become softer and more prone to joint injury if the tissue absorbs a trauma or if it is subjected to overstretching. The additional weight gained as the pregnancy progresses also can impact joint health.

The intensity and the volume of the exercise undertaken by a pregnant woman can be moderated to suit her personal medical circumstances and her previous level of fitness. Activities such as walking, yoga, Pilates, and stationary cycling are generally safe. Swimming and a variant of aerobic exercise, aquarobics, are both excellent exercises for pregnant women.

SEE ALSO Diet; Female exercise and cardiovascular health; Stretching and flexibility; Yoga and Pilates.

# Prescription medications and athletic performance

Prescription medications are those drugs that are only capable of being obtained by way of a written order from a physician or other medical professional. Prescription medication is an expression that is commonly used as a contrast to over the counter medications that may be purchased without restriction at pharmacies and other commercial outlets.

Athletic performance is defined as the physical ability of the athlete to perform in a desired way. The physical abilities of an athlete may often be impacted by non-physical factors, such as the psychological state of the athlete.

There are a variety of different ways that prescription medications can impact upon athletic performance. In many cases, medications are prescribed to assist an athlete in overcoming an identified physical limitation. In other circumstances, the medication is intended to counter a non-athletic condition, but the medication has either known or unforeseen consequences upon performance.

Insulin, prescribed to counter diabetes in some persons, is an example of a medication that impacts upon an athlete. In many cases the athlete who is prescribed insulin must carefully adjust their dosage to ensure that the body's natural response to exercise does not interfere with the intended effect of the insulin.

In all circumstances, the fact that a medication was prescribed by a licensed doctor is not a defense to a charge against an athlete for using a banned substance. International athletic organizations are bound by the rules of the World Ant-Doping Agency (WADA). The agency requires athletes to obtain therapeutic use exemptions in circumstances when medication is required for an athlete to maintain his or her normal health.

Of the medications prescribed to specifically assist an athlete, the various types of asthma medications are most readily associated with improved athletic performance. There are many different asthma medications that may be prescribed, all having bronchodilator effects, serving to open the otherwise constricted passages of the airways. Corticosteroids are available as an asthma medication; these are steroid formulations that assist in reducing the inflammation of the airways that often occurs in conjunction with an asthma attack. Beta 2 agonists are another common group of asthma drugs. These substances act to relax the muscles in the vicinity of the affected areas of the airways.

For millions of people around the world, physical exercise would be difficult if not impossible but for these prescribed medications.

In a similar fashion, prescription anti-inflammatories aimed at relieving the effects of joint pain are often the only means by which an athlete can continue to compete pending either surgical intervention or retirement from the activity. Steroid based cortisone and nonsteroidal anti-inflammatory drugs (NSAIDs) are prescribed for this purpose. These anti-inflammatory med-

ications are sometimes taken in conjunction with prescription analgesics (pain killers), particularly among professional or elite level athletes. These medications, as they do not treat the underlying cause but address only the symptoms, may permit the athlete to perform in the short term. Prescription painkillers have become a frequent source of addiction. National Football League quarterback Brett Favre was one of many athletes in recent years to become addicted to prescription painkillers, initially prescribed to assist him in his play. OxyContin (oxycodone hydrochloride) is a very powerful prescription painkiller where dependency is a risk if the athlete is attempting to compete and "play through pain."

The prescription of painkilling medication can, in some circumstances, lead to more significant injuries for the user. Painkillers tend to entirely mask the normal pain signals that are produced by the body when a tissue or structure experiences pain. Particularly in cases of soft tissue injury that has been the subject of an analgesic treatment, an athlete can do significantly greater damage to their body while the pain sensors are masked. In intricate structures, such as the groin muscles, or ones that are subjected to significant ongoing stress, such as the knee, serious tears of the tissue can be masked by the administration of a pain killer.

The number of prescription medications that are likely to impair performance or otherwise present a risk to an athlete is almost endless. Many of the medications are seemingly innocuous in a non-athletic context. Examples of a common prescription medication with possible athletic ramifications are oral contraceptives prescribed to women. In some women, the contraceptive tends to regulate menstrual periods, which can be an advantage to competitive athletes who wish certainty as to the extent and timing of their menstrual cycle.

SEE ALSO Beta-2 agonists; Cortisone steroid injections; Glucocorticoids; Sport performance.

# Preseason strength training

For all competitive athletes, whether they participate in a team sport, or whether they are active in an individual sport, the competitive season is composed of a number of distinct but related segments. Persons who enjoy sport on a purely recreational or fitness level may approach their training regimes in the same fashion day to day and week to week; the goal of the recreational athlete is often a mixture of personal enjoyment and general fitness. When the athletic goal is to achieve the highest possible competitive standard, the sport season will be approached from the perspective of maximizing the training benefit of each segment to enhance overall competitive success.

Competitive athletic training is usually divided into training periods, an approach known as the periodization of training. Every sport will have its own distinct approach to how the length of each period is determined; the length and the extent of the competitive season, the fitness level of the athlete, and the personal and team goals are all factors in this determination. As a general rule, an athletic calendar year will be divided into three training periods: the preseason (the preparatory period), the competitive season (with its own sub-periods timed around key competitions), and the off-season (a period of rest, recovery, and rebuilding).

Preseason strength training will have a different purpose than the work carried out in the other two seasons of the athletic year. Depending on the sport, preseason weight training will include aspects of buildup (increasing overall physical strength) and a special emphasis (weight training that is isolated to develop a particular sport-specific maneuver or application).

As with the other elements of athletic training, the preseason is a bridge from the off-season to the competitive season. Prior to the advent of specialized sports science approaches in the 1960s, it was common for athletes to use the preseason period as their primary conditioning period; the off-season was usually a time of complete inactivity on the part of the athlete. Today, periodization means that the off-season is when the athlete will establish a weight training foundation, the preseason will usually be a period of increased intensity, if not weightlifting volume, and the competitive season lifting is designed to maintain, not necessarily build, strength.

The preseason weight training must also be periodized; the coordination of workouts versus rest periods is essential to preseason development. In most cases, the preseason training period is not a time to experiment with different lifting techniques or dietary supplements; those are matters for the off-season, when the athlete is not bound by a particular or finite training schedule.

Preseason is often one where the athlete must take his or her body in a number of different directions. The preseason program of a competitive 200-m and 400-m sprinter is an example. The athlete knows that to achieve success, the technical aspects of this discipline must be executed with the utmost precision, or the hundreds of a second that may determine a race will be lost. In these races, the explosive start, a powerful drive from the blocks, the ability to reach top speed, stride length and form, the approach to each bend or turn, and the finish are all matters that demand intense practice and attention to detail. None of these crucial techniques can be executed to the highest standard unless the athlete is very strong. One of the great challenges of the preseason weight training program is to maintain the same high level of training intensity in the weight room as will be required of the athlete in the track work that is directly related to the actual competition.

The intensity of all aspects of preseason training makes the inclusion of a well-planned and integrated stretching and flexibility program most important. In the preseason training period, it is common for the athlete to be subjected to the stresses of activity in addition to that provided in the weight room. A musculoskeletal system that is flexible and limber will respond more favorably to these diverse physical requirements.

In many sports, the preseason is the time when coaches make decisions about the composition of a particular team for the coming competitive season. The mental pressure that athletes either impose on themselves or absorb from the preseason environment will often compel them to put specific weight training goals ahead of overall body fitness. Athletes who feel compelled to impress a coach with their commitment to weight training could risk injury unless they have laid the appropriate foundation for the preseason in the off-season period.

**SEE ALSO** Muscle mass and strength; Range of motion; Skeletal muscle; Strength training; Weightlifting.

# Prohibited substances (competition bans)

Athletes have employed different substances throughout the history of sport to improve performance. Doping is the term universally understood to describe the use of performance-enhancing drugs by athletes. While certain doping practices were first seen as more unsportsmanlike than illegal, the ingestion of performance-enhancing drugs or dietary supplements was not a significant part of the science of sport until the 1950s, when anabolic steroids were

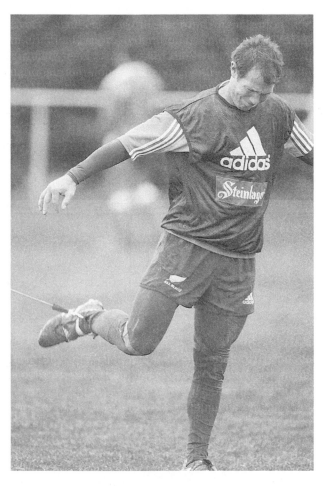

Preseason strength training is imperative. **PHOTO BY ROSS LAND/ GETTY IMAGES.**

first determined to provide significant benefits to strength athletes.

In 1963, the International Olympic Committee (IOC) first prohibited the use of a wide range of substances in Olympic competition. It took approximately 30 years for the combination of scientifically indisputable testing methodology and global support in the athletic community for comprehensive legislative anti-doping frameworks to be erected. This convergence led to the creation of the World Anti-Doping Agency (WADA), which has fostered a unified approach to the battle against the use of illegal performance-enhancing substances in athletic competition. WADA is the supervisory organization that develops and enacts the regulations to be followed in the administration of its anti-doping practices. Every significant world sporting organization and international sports federation is a member of WADA. Virtually every nation in the world has its own national anti-doping agency with membership in WADA, of which the U.S. Anti-Doping Agency is an

example. A key objective of the WADA anti-doping initiatives is the harmonization of global approaches to doping detection and sanctions.

A cornerstone of the WADA based approach is its Anti-Doping Code, which sets out the Prohibited List, the precise summary of all prohibited substances, updated on an annual basis. The Prohibited List is well publicized in the international athletic world to ensure that all athletes know precisely what substances will be the subject of doping tests, both in competition as well as through out-of-competition testing. A prohibited substance is a broader concept than that of a prohibited drug, although in sport the two expressions are often used interchangeably. A drug is any substance that is not a food that produces or induces a change in the body; a substance is any element, compound, or mixture. WADA expresses in its Code the underlying philosophy to the prohibition as "The use of any drug should be limited to medically justified indications."

The broader expression "substance," as opposed to the narrower term "drug," is illustrated by the prohibition against the use of erythropoietin (EPO), the hormone that stimulates erythrocyte (red blood cell) production and aids in the better transportation of oxygen in the body. EPO is a naturally occurring substance, but it is the method in which this substance is employed by athletes that leads to the prohibition.

Generally, all governing bodies in sport have enacted their own specific rules regarding the consequences for a violation of the prohibited substances rules. A competition ban, also known as a suspension, is a specific penalty imposed on the athlete as a consequence of a positive test for a prohibited substance. The length of the ban will depend on a number of factors, some of which tend to mitigate the penalty, others of which may be perceived as an aggravating circumstance. Those factors include:

- Evidence that the prohibited substance may have been ingested on an innocent basis, such as a contaminated supplement.
- Evidence that the athlete took the prohibited substance at the direction of a coach or trainer while being provided assurances of the legality of the substance.
- When the athlete is a first-time violator of the substance rule.
- When the athlete is a previous offender.
- When the athlete has been deemed to have failed the doping test because the athlete failed or refused to attend for an out-of-competition test.

Professional sports leagues generally enforce their respective prohibited substance policies within the framework of a collective bargaining agreement (CBA) with a players association. Such CBAs uniformly provide for appeals of any decision respecting a suspension from play. Professional sport substance testing will often extend to substances generally regarded as recreational drugs, such as marijuana and alcohol, drugs with limited athletic performance applications.

Professional sports have become much more sensitive to its collective public image in relation to the enforcement of all rules regarding prohibited substances. In the United States, a notable example was the Congressional hearings convened in 2004 regarding the use of performance-enhancing substances in major league baseball. One of the players who testified before the Congressional committee, Rafael Palmeiro, vehemently denied his personal involvement in any steroid use in the course of a successful playing career; Palmeiro later tested positive for the substance and was subject to both a competition ban and broad public scorn. Major league baseball enacted its own rules regarding prohibited substances in 2005, banning not only steroids and similar substances, but also the stimulant amphetamine, whose use had been an accepted part of professional baseball culture for decades.

**SEE ALSO** Blood doping; Doping tests; Out-of-competition testing; Stimulants; World Anti-Doping Agency (WADA).

## Proprioception SEE Balance training and proprioception

## Prosthetic research and sport

A prosthetic device is an artificial replacement for a part of the body that has been removed. A prosthetic may be a limb or a joint; the purpose of the prosthetic may be entirely functional, cosmetic, or both. The term prosthetic is derived from a Greek word, meaning to add to or to add on.

Prosthetics have existed throughout history. In earlier times, when a leg or a hand was lost through war or misadventure, the artificial limb was a simple peg leg or a hand hook. The U.S. Civil War (1861–1865) was the first great impetus to prosthetic research; the Union army had over 30,000 amputations in the course of conflict.

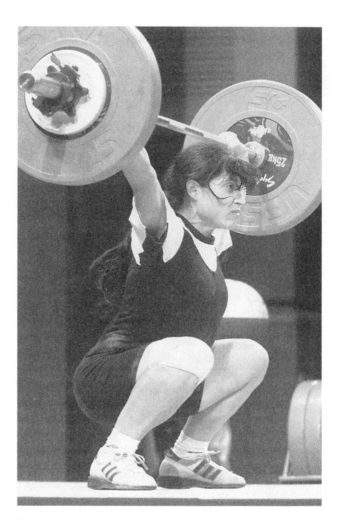

Bulgaria's Izabela Dragneva won the gold 2000 Olympic Games, but was later disqualified and stripped of medal after traces of a banned substance were found in a urine sample.
© REUTERS/CORBIS

A prosthetic is closely related to another common sport device, the orthotic. While a prosthetic is a replacement device for a component of the musculoskeletal system, an orthotic is designed to support a weakened area or to correct a structural misalignment. For example, foot orthotics are designed to equalize leg length.

Research has taken modern prosthetic devices far beyond simple peg legs and hooks. The development of effective prosthetic devices for use in sport engages a number of scientific disciplines, including kinesiology (the science of human movement), biomechanical engineering (the relationship between the mechanisms and the living function of the body), structural engineering (design and construction principles), materials and fabrication experts (optimal metals and composites), coaching input (regarding the specific demands of the sport), and the athlete. Once operative, a prosthetic used in sport will involve the ongoing support of experts from the sports medicine, orthopedic medicine, physical therapy, and athletic therapy disciplines.

The design and construction of a modern above-the-knee prosthetic device illustrate the science that supports the application. Where the residual limb of the person ends, the prosthesis begins. A socket, with its fit adjustable to the wearer by means of an inflatable pouch, is the component that connects to the leg. Below the socket, encased in a protective lightweight plastic structure, is the artificial knee, constructed of aluminum, titanium, and other metals. The knee is connected to the lower portion of the prosthesis through a device that both reduces shock and suppresses torque, which is the force generated by the turning of the knee during running motion, which would otherwise be absorbed by the person. The prosthetic is supported by an artificial foot constructed from polyurethane, with the foot carefully oriented to ensure that the individual is not misaligned during a running or walking motion so as to direct unequal forces into the opposite leg.

Such prosthetics have benefited from the development of materials that are both lighter and stronger. The artificial leg used by Terry Fox, the cancer patient who endeavored to run across Canada in 1981 before succumbing to his disease, was approximately 50% heavier than modern prosthetics, which also have sophisticated cushioning that the Fox version lacked.

The Paralympic movement has fostered many technological developments in sports prosthetics. The Paralympic competitions each have separate classification rules, with the degree of the disability of the athlete determining the competition class. The lighter and more functional the prosthetic is, the greater the ease of movement experienced by the athlete. Athletes now benefit from prosthetic devices such as the gait-adaptive knee, an artificial limb that can be modified to suit the particular variations and idiosyncrasies of its user.

One testament to technology is found in the results achieved by Paralympic athletes who use prosthetics in the 100-m sprint. In the various classifications based on the degree of limitation, the slowest of the winning times at the 2004 Athens Paralympics in the men's categories was 12.1 seconds, a result that compares favorably to the able-bodied elite time of slightly under 10 seconds.

In addition to the advances made in the material composition of sport prosthetics, significant research has been carried out on the development of devices that are hardwired into the nervous systems of the athlete. The connection between the user and the machine is referred to as the neural linkage. The ability of science to develop the necessary interface between user and machine depends to a considerable degree on the nature of the amputation: the more extensive the loss of limb, the more difficult the proposition to connect the artificial component to the body, as there will be a greater degree of connectivity required. Both direct connections of existing muscle to machine and those of bone and machine have been attempted, with limited success. The best success in achieving a true interface between the prosthesis and the body have been with respect to artificial hands, where very simple muscular commands have successfully been obeyed through the prosthetic.

**SEE ALSO** Musculoskeletal injuries; Orthotics; Paralympics.

# Protein ingestion and recovery from exercise

Proteins, carbohydrates, and fats are the three food groups that comprise the human diet. For a healthy and active person, with no specialized dietary needs, protein should be approximately 12-15% of the total food consumed every day. The ingestion of proteins, both in terms of the timing and the quantity consumed, is critical to an athlete's quick and efficient recovery from the stresses imposed on the body by exercise.

The ingestion of proteins is the first step in the conversion of these foods into a form that the body can utilize. Ingestion is the act of physically consuming food; digestion is the conversion of the food to a form that the body can assimilate and absorb; and synthesis is the process of using the absorbed protein to create a functional substance. The key components of proteins are various amino acids, which are the building blocks for the construction and repair of muscles within the body. Protein is also an essential aspect of the ability of the nervous system to transmit impulses. They are also a part of the chemistry of many hormones secreted by the endocrine system and are essential to the functioning of the immune system.

The ingestion of dietary proteins is important to the health of the skeletal muscles, one of the three different types of muscle in the body. The other muscle types, the cardiac muscles that power the heart and the smooth muscles that work within the interior portions of many of the internal organs, are maintained and restored by other internal means.

A healthy athlete should consume protein in the diet on a relatively steady basis throughout the day. Steady consumption usually ensures an equally steady and continuous protein synthesis. All forms of exercise will place demands on the body that deplete the levels of proteins and their constituent amino acids; the intensity of exercise, particularly resistance exercises such as weight training and other explosive movements, will have a correspondingly greater effect in the reduction of protein levels. Muscles cannot grow in either mass or strength unless they are stressed and then provided the opportunity to be repaired. As a very general guideline to how much protein a healthy person should consume on a daily basis, one gram of protein per pound (0.5 kg) of lean body weight (the total body weight less body fat) is an accepted figure.

A blood test can assist in determining precisely how much protein should be consumed by a specific athlete. The blood urea nitrogen test is a measurement of the amount of urea on the blood. Nitrogen is one of the elements present in all forms of protein; nitrogen will exist in its elemental state as a byproduct of protein breakdown. Urea is also a byproduct of protein synthesis, in which excess proteins will lead to the generation of excess amino acids that must be broken down and processed by the liver for ultimate excretion from the body by the kidneys as urine. If protein consumption is too high for the body to use in the synthesis process, this fact is revealed through an elevated urea level. Long-term excess protein consumption may place significant stress on the liver and kidney functions.

Amino acids made available to the body from digested protein also require significant amounts of water to become metabolized in the liver; amino acid molecules require twice as much water to be broken down as does a glucose molecule. High protein consumption can easily lead to dehydration for this reason.

When the amount of protein consumed into the body is too low to meet the needs of repair and restoration of muscles, these tissues will ultimately break down, without any corresponding build up. This process, known as muscle catabolism, is dangerous to the long-term health of the musculoskeletal system, as the body does not have an alternative means with which to sustain these structures.

Research studies with respect to the optimum timing of protein replacement suggest that proteins should be ingested between 30 minutes and one hour after the muscle resistance or other strenuous activity. It is generally agreed that a series of smaller meals, each with a protein component, will be digested more agreeably by the body than one large meal. A number of amino acids necessary to human function must be obtained through food, and certain types of foods are superior protein sources in this regard: eggs, most fish, milk, and other dairy products are known as complete protein sources for this reason. Incomplete or complementary proteins are found in beans, nuts, and many vegetables.

**SEE ALSO** Diet; Exercise recovery; Muscle protein synthesis.

# Protein supplements

Protein supplements have gained favor with athletes as a means of increasing their body's ability to develop and maintain skeletal muscle. Protein is one of the three essential components of the human diet, along with carbohydrates and fats. Protein, which is composed of various types of amino acids, provides the raw material for both muscle construction and repair, as well as playing an important role in the immune system, the endocrine (hormone production) system, and the transmission of nerve impulses throughout the nervous system. A supplement is any addition to an athlete's regular diet to achieve a particular nutritional goal; a supplement may be a natural or a synthetic product. Supplements are available in fluid, powder, and solid food formulations.

The issue of whether an athlete requires protein supplements is hotly debated in the sports nutrition industry. Many nutritional experts contend that the best way to ingest protein is by way of a properly constituted, well-balanced natural food diet. This position is supported by the fact that the body is well suited to receive proteins through natural digestive processes, and that supplementation is never as strong a dietary option as whole food sources of any nutrient, including protein. Whole foods will often contain phytochemicals, the components of food that do not possess any caloric or other nutritional value, but that act as important trace substances to promote healthy functions within the body, such as anti-oxidization and the bolstering of the immune system.

Protein supplements were first popularized by bodybuilders, weightlifters, and strength athletes. One appeal of the supplement was the fact that the quality of the proteins contained could be consistently high; the second appeal was the ability of the supplement to shore up any protein deficiencies that might arise after a particularly demanding workout or if the athlete was not able to consume requisite amounts of dietary protein at a given time. The third appeal of the supplement is that an athlete may be limited by lifestyle pressure, such as school, employment, or family, in the preparation of protein-rich foods in the best possible fashion. Supplements offer a quick and nutritionally effective alternative; some protein supplements are marketed as meal replacements, a nutritional concept that is a further extension of protein supplements.

The pro-supplement constituency also advances the argument that high quality, concentrated protein products will repair the muscles stressed from a demanding workout more quickly than proteins consumed through food. Among the proteins that are popular for this reason are whey protein (a byproduct of cheese), and soy protein, extracted from the soya bean. Glutamine, a specific type of amino acid, is another well-regarded component in many protein supplements.

There is no question that from a biological perspective, if the body has a shortage of protein, a supplement will assist in the correction of the deficiency. Protein deficiency will prohibit the body from affecting the repairs necessary to maintain muscles structure. The consumption of additional amounts of protein, over and above the amount necessary to promote healthy muscle development, must be approached with caution.

Many approaches to protein supplementation have been advocated on the premise that if a little extra protein is beneficial to muscle repair and growth, greater amounts of protein supplements must be even better. The error in this premise is revealed by the chemistry of how the body processes excess amounts of protein. Unlike carbohydrates, which have a particular series of storage mechanisms, such as muscle glycogen and liver glycogen, or the fats ingested in the body, which are stored in the adipose tissues designed for fat storage, excess proteins are broken down into their amino acid components for elimination. The deconstruction of amino acids produces several byproducts, particularly urea which must be subjected to further processing in the liver before it can be excreted through urine. The process of filtering additional amounts of urea from the body creates the potential to place a significant strain on renal (kidney) function.

There are particular times when the body is better equipped to digest and utilize nutrients of all types. Proteins are best provided to the athlete's body nearer a competitive or training event that resulted in muscle stress. As a general rule, the ingestion of a protein supplement is likely to be more effective if consumed 30 to 60 minutes after the event, rather than at a later time. Protein supplements will always serve to address a deficiency, but optimal absorption through the digestive processes of the small intestine occurs in a timeframe closer to the activity.

In sports such as the triathlon, where the athlete requires significant carbohydrate recovery at the end of competition, as well as the need for muscle repair and recovery, competitors will often consume a carbohydrate/protein mix of supplements to achieve this dual purpose. The effect of the supplement, taken immediately or within 30 minutes of the end of the event, is to "jump start" the bodily process of restoration.

There are further issues regarding the use of protein supplements and the precise method by which the supplement is consumed. The human digestive tract is constructed to most efficiently process foods into useable substances when the particular material reaches the digestive system in a food-like condition. The consumption of amino acid pills and similar formulations, a product that essentially bypasses the digestive process, as amino acids are a product of protein digestion, do not speed the absorption of these substances into the system.

**SEE ALSO** Diet; Muscle protein synthesis; Nutrition and athletic performance; Protein ingestion and recovery from exercise.

# Psychological disorders

A psychological disorder is a mental health condition that disrupts the normal feelings, mood, or ability of one person to interact with others. A psychological disorder may be caused by genetic or inherited characteristics, or it may result from environmental factors. Psychological disorders are distinct from physical illnesses or injury, although a physical condition may be a contributing factor to the progress of a psychological condition.

A healthy relationship between mind and body is fundamental to optimal athletic performance. Any disturbance in the equilibrium between physical and mental performance will usually create a cause and effect relationship: impaired mental health will lead inexorably to an equivalent physical result. A body of science, sport psychology, has grown dramatically in recent years as the demand to better understand the mind/body relationship in all sports has increased.

There are common psychological disorders that influence athletic performance. These conditions are not limited to sports, but are frequently the source of problems for athletes. Some of the disorders are interrelated in that they may occur concurrently in the athlete. Others exist alone, but are found to arise when more generalized factors such as the mental stress of competition also exist. The athletic environment is a fertile breeding ground for many disorders, as traditionally, an athlete who failed to maintain the level of training or competitive skills due to psychological reasons was perceived as weak and unsuited to high-level sports. For this reason, athletes would often keep secret any psychological problems they found themselves experiencing.

There are common psychological disorders affecting athletes. Overtraining syndrome is a condition that affects athletes who appear to overreach with their training, attempting either to gain too much, too fast, or who otherwise fail to maintain a healthy balance between workout intensity, workout volume, and rest. In its initial phases, this condition manifests itself as one of simple physical or mental fatigue, circumstances that are often dismissed as correctable through the athlete either reducing training or competition loads. Overtraining syndrome is separated from simple physical fatigue by the mindset of the athlete toward the condition: the athlete tends to lose all interest in even basic fitness. The athlete will invariably feel lethargic about both athletic activities and other social aspects of life. This syndrome is also known as "unexplained underperformance syndrome," where the athlete quite suddenly loses interest in attaining performance goals.

Depression is another very common and debilitating condition in athletes. Depression as a clinically diagnosed illness does not simply describe a person who is sad or otherwise in poor spirits for a brief period of time. Depression is defined as a disorder where the person experiences the symptoms of depressions for two weeks or longer. Mental stress, a loss of self-esteem, or similar events can trigger a depressive episode. The disruption in the levels of serotonin, a neurotransmitter, or conduit of signals in the brain, is a physiological contributor to this illness. Depression will significantly reduce the mental outlook of the subject; athletes suffering from depression often are uninterested in training or competition, they sustain a loss of appetite, and they often present as anxious. Anxiety is a sense of fear, upset, and dread, and is a condition that is often closely related to depression.

Eating disorders are the most common of psychological disturbances in athletes and include anorexia nervosa and bulimia. Both anorexia and bulimia are more prevalent among female athletes, particularly those participating in sports where one's weight and personal appearance are important components of competitive success. Figure skating and gymnastics are the prime examples of sports where eating disorders can arise. Anorexia is a condition where the athletes believe themselves to be too large or otherwise overweight, while to an objective observer, such persons are usually at least of normal build and sometimes quite slim. Bulimia is motivated by the same psychological belief, but it is characterized by the binge/purge cycle, where the bulimic athletes will eat, often to excess, and then deliberately vomit or use laxatives to empty their body.

Substance-induced psychological disturbance is the most common disorder precipitated by the use of a training substance, as in the infamous "roid rage," the well-documented side effect from the consumption of anabolic steroids. Steroids have the potential to become psychologically addictive; once the athlete has developed a larger and more muscular body, the athlete will regard the steroid consumption as a psychological crutch. Steroids can contribute to violent mood swings and uncontrollable bursts of anger.

The desire to relieve physical pain can sometimes create a dependency, or addiction, in the athlete for painkillers and anti-inflammatories. Alcohol, marijuana, and various stimulants are common substances that are abused by athletes, consumed as stress-relieving substances.

**SEE ALSO** Eating disorders in athletes; Mental stress; Sport psychology; Sports medical conditions.

# Psychology SEE Sport psychology

# Pulls and strains, groin SEE Groin pulls and strains

# Pulmonary edema SEE High altitude pulmonary edema

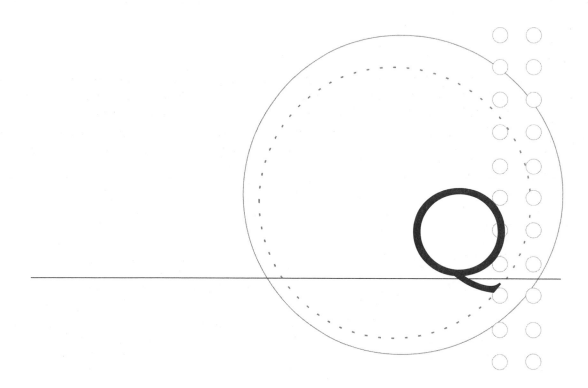

# Quadriceps pulls and tears

The quadriceps, the short-form reference for the quadriceps femoris, is the group of four muscle structures positioned at the front of the thigh that are commonly described as the "quads." The quadriceps extends from below the patella (kneecap) on the tibia (shin), over the entire length of the thigh. The quadriceps is also connected to the patella by way of the quadriceps tendon. Three of the four quadriceps muscles originate at the top of the femur and the fourth, the rectus femoris, is connected to the pelvis. The quadriceps is a large, stable muscle structure whose function is to permit the extension of the knee, and as a result the quadriceps is crucial to the movement of the leg.

The quadriceps is so integral a part of human movement that it is frequently injured, although rarely in a fashion that causes permanent muscle damage. The exposure of the quadriceps to sports injury is governed by two separate factors: the stability and structure of the entire leg structure, and the nature of the athletic activity.

The action of the quadriceps, powering the extension of the leg from the front of the thigh, is countered by the hamstring tendon and muscle complex at the back of the thigh. The hamstrings are attached to the pelvis underneath the gluteal muscles of the buttocks, and like the quadriceps, the hamstrings extend past the knee joint to the tibia. The hamstrings provide flexion to the knee, permitting the lower leg to bend as well as facilitating the ability of the hip to be extended. All movement of the leg, whether walking, running, or jumping, require the harmonious and balanced action of the quadriceps and the hamstrings.

Imbalances between the relative strengths or flexibility of the hamstring versus the quadriceps are a major contributing factor in quadriceps injuries. It is a generally accepted proposition of sport science that the relative strength of the quadriceps to the hamstring should be a ratio of 3:2. This balance ensures that neither muscle group dominates the other; one of the chief causes of knee injury generally, and anterior cruciate ligament (ACL) injury in female athletes in particular, has been the structural imbalance between these muscle groups. When the hamstring is unable to counter the power of the quadriceps, the ACL is subjected to excessive stress.

In the quadriceps itself, such imbalances are manifested as a pull or a tear to the muscle fibers. A pull, also known as a muscle strain, is an over-extension of the muscle fibers, which may involve tiny or micro tearing of the structure. A tear is a progressive injury from that of a pull, where the muscle structure sustains a significant separation of the fibers and a resultant loss of muscle function. The most serious form of a muscle tear is a rupture, which is the complete severing of muscle fibers.

Overuse and repetitive motion are the most common causes of quadriceps pulls or tears. All running, cycling, and kicking sports athletes such as soccer and rugby often experience quadriceps tears or pulls. Weightlifting is another sport where quadriceps pulls and tears are common, especially in the lifting of

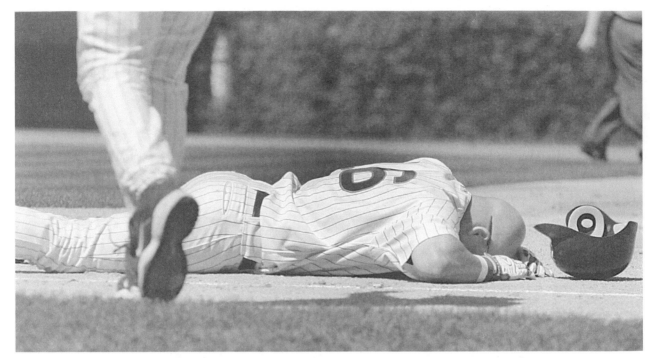

Chicago Cubs' Aramis Ramirez lies face down in pain after stumbling trying to beat out a throw at first base; he was forced to leave the game with a strained left quadriceps muscle. **AP PHOTO/JEFF ROBERSON**

free weights, when the ability of the legs to support the explosive lifting movement is an integral part of the activity.

Another common injury of the quadriceps occurs in jumping sports such as basketball or in athletics events such as the high jump, where the athlete repetitively places stress upon the quadriceps in the generating of lift. The quadriceps tendon, the connective tissue between the quadriceps muscle and the patella, and the patella tendon, leading from the patella to the tibia, are the frequent sites of the tendinitis known as "jumper's knee." This condition causes significant and often immobilizing pain to the athlete. Jumper's knee may also cause swelling in and around the tendon.

The most serious tear that can be sustained to the quadriceps is that of a quadriceps tendon rupture. This form of injury can occur as a progression from an existing pull or tear that an athlete sustains, or it may occur spontaneously when the quadriceps sustains a sudden overloading force, such as a effort to drive the leg forward with as much power as possible. The loss of the connection between the quadriceps and the patella creates a buckling effect in the knee, because the leg cannot be straightened. The only treatment for such an injury is surgical repair, where the quadriceps tendon is physically reconnected to the patella.

Most quadriceps pull or tear injuries are resolved through the application of RICE (rest/ice/compression/elevation) treatments, initiated immediately after the onset of any pain. For more serious occurrences, nonsteroidal anti-inflammatory drugs (NSAIDs), such as ibuprofen, or more powerful prescription medications may assist in the recovery process.

The recovery from a quadriceps pull or tear should be a gradual one. The return of the athlete to regular training must be managed to ensure both the compete recovery of the injury, as well as an emphasis on flexibility, stretching, and the balance between the relative strengths of the quadriceps and hamstring structures.

**SEE ALSO** Musculoskeletal injuries; Sprains and strains; Thigh and upper leg injuries.

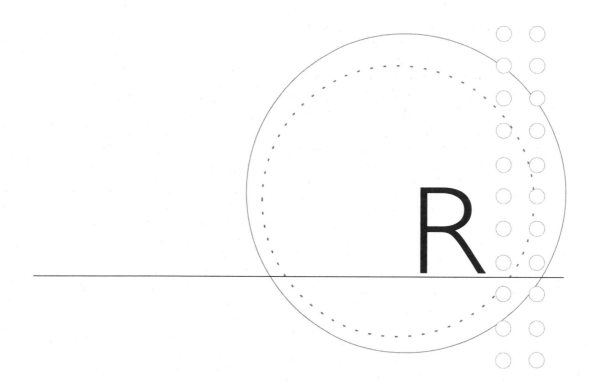

# Racquetball

The sport of racquetball is one of recent origins in comparison to most athletic activities that enjoy a popular following. Joseph Sobek (1918-1998), a tennis professional with the Greenwich, Connecticut, Young Men's Christian Association in the late 1940s, is recognized as the inventor and the developer of racquetball. Sobek, who was also an active four wall handball player, sought to create an indoor activity that would save his hands from the significant stresses of competitive handball, while preserving handball's fitness benefits. Sobek used the available YMCA handball courts to create what he referred to as "paddle racquets," a game that combined many of the features of squash and handball.

The paddle racquets concept gained significant measure of popularity in the northeastern United States, with a governing association created in 1952. The modern name for the sport, racquetball, was confirmed with the formation of the International Racquetball Association in 1968. The sport sustained explosive growth in the late 1970s in the United States, as racquetball became a fashionable recreational sporting activity. In addition to a biennial world championship, racquetball is a medal sport at the quadrennial Pan-American Games; it is also a recognized National Collegiate Athletic Association (NCAA) sport. The country with the greatest participation in racquetball remains the United States, where approximately two thirds of the world's 15 million racquetball players reside.

The rules of racquetball are relatively simple. Played in a four-walled court, the object of the sport is to strike the ball to create a rebound from the front wall (or by a combination of a front wall and side wall carom, or angled rebound), that cannot be returned by the opponent after the first bounce from the floor. The court dimensions are identical to those used in the sport of four wall handball, an enclosed area 40 ft long, 20 ft wide and 20 ft high (6 m by 12 m by 6 m); the rear wall of the court must be at least 12 ft high (3.5 m).

Racquetball may be played in a singles (two player) or doubles (four player) format. In racquetball clubs, players will often play an unofficial version known as "cut-throat," where one player serves against the other two players, with the serve rotating among all three players. Racquetball players use a racquet that is constructed from a combination of lightweight composite materials that is strung with a mesh similar in appearance to a tennis racquet. The ball is constructed from a rubber compound, with a hollow center that makes the ball capable of being compressed and generating a resultant velocity on a hard serve or a strong forearm shot at speeds that may exceed 150 mph (250 km/h) when struck by an elite player. The speed of the ball, and not its spin, is the most important characteristic of the racquetball both in flight and after a carom from the walls of the court.

The ball is put into play through a serve, delivered by the serving player from a designated service zone. The opposing players station themselves behind a receiving line. A legal serve is one that

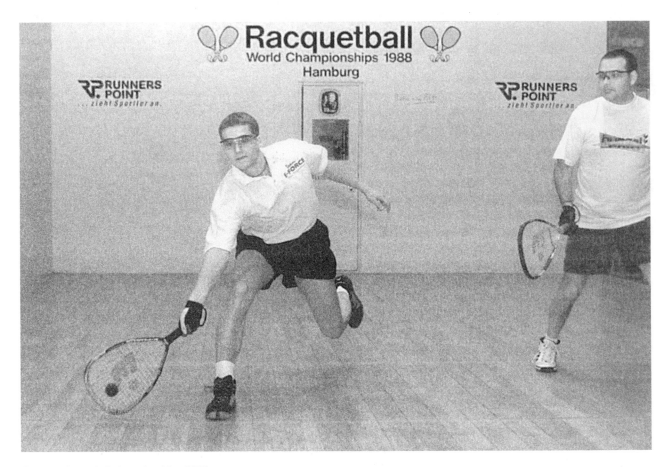

German racquetball championships, 2002. PHOTO BY ANJA HEINEMANN/BONGARTS/GETTY IMAGES.

strikes the floor of the court before making contact with the front wall; the ball must then bounce into an area marked by the "short line," where it may be played by the opponent. A legal serve may also strike one of the walls, including the back wall of the court, prior to being returned by the opponent. Points are scored on the serve only, with a game concluded when the first player achieves a score of 15 points.

Once the ball is put in play with a legal serve, both players may use all of the walls in their shot making. As a general proposition, the ball remains in play until the ball strikes the floor of the court twice. Racquetball is a game played with one hand on the racquet; players are not permitted to change their hands on the racquet during a rally. Where one player unintentionally impedes the movement of an opponent in making a shot, the opponent may call a "hinder," which results in the serve being replayed without penalty to either player. Deliberate obstructions (in competitive racquetball a referee is empowered to make such determinations) usually result in a point being awarded the hindered party.

The fundamental tactic employed in racquetball is to obtain the control of the center of the court. From the center position, a player can best react to shots struck by the opponent. The center is the position from which the angle of the carom of any shot that strikes any of the walls may best be judged. The player with center position will force the opponent to travel a longer distance to get to shots, as the center positioned player presents a legal obstruction to the opponent.

Rcaquetball is a fast paced sport, with an anacrobic fitness emphasis. A rally often continues with intense physical effort for periods of between 5 seconds and 20 seconds; the interval between rallies is also short, averaging approximately 10 seconds. Aerobic fitness assists in the body's recovery mechanism, especially after long games or during multigame tournaments. Most racquetball shots are executed by players who assume a low, crouched position, from which they can both move dynamically in all directions on the court, and which permit them to strike the ball with power from a stable physical platform.

For these reasons, muscle strength and an ability to strike the ball with great power is sometimes helpful, but it is not an essential element of racquetball success. Lateral quickness, flexibility, and core body strength (the inter-related function of the abdominal, gluteal, lumbar (low back), and groin muscles to provide stability) are important fitness considerations.

SEE ALSO Handball; Squash; Tennis.

## Paula Jane Radcliffe

12/17/1973–
BRITISH
LONG-DISTANCE RUNNER

Paula Jane Radcliffe is a British long-distance runner who, as of 2006, is still in the prime of her running career. In early 2006 she held the women's world record for the marathon (a running race that is 26.2 mi, or 42 km, in length) in a time of 2 hours, 15 minutes, 25 seconds. The record, set at the 2003 London Marathon, represents an average pace of 5 minutes, 10 seconds per mile.

Born in Northwich, England, in the county of Cheshire, she grew up in Bedfordshire, and is still a member of a local running club in that community. She attended Loughborough University, graduating in 1996 with first-class honors in French, German, and economics. During this period, competing in distances ranging from 5,000 m to 10,000 m, she won the 1992 World Junior Cross County Championships. She also placed seventh at the 1993 World Championships at the age of 19.

In 1995, Radcliffe returned to form after a lengthy recuperation from a foot injury, placing fifth in the 5,000-m competition at the World Championships. The next year, she was fifth at the Atlanta Olympic Games 5,000 m. In the 2000 Summer Olympics held in Sydney, Australia, she was a finalist in both the 5,000-m and 10,000-m events, but failed to win a medal. In the latter event, she finished fourth after leading the race until the final lap of the track.

The late race fade was the result of Radcliffe's race strategy. She is not known for her blazing speed in the closing stages of track races. Indeed, at the 1999 World Championships, she finished second in the 10,000 m after being overtaken in the final 200 m of the race. Thus, her strategy has been to surge to the front of the pack right from the start of a race and, by establishing a sizable lead, attempt to hold off the other competitors. As a result, scientific analysis

of hydration and endurance strategies are a key element of Radcliffe's race planning.

Prompted by the knowledge that her competitive strength as a runner lay in her endurance, Radcliffe began to train for the marathon following the 2000 Olympics. The effort was worthwhile, as she was victorious in her first marathon, the 2002 London Marathon. Her time was over four minutes faster than the existing women's record for the course, and she finished over three minutes ahead of the second place competitor.

In her next marathon in Chicago, she set a new women's world record with a time of 2 hours, 17 minutes, 18 seconds. Her 2003 London Marathon victory chopped nearly two minutes off this record Chicago time.

As of 2006, Padcliffe has won six of the seven marathons she has run, and has compiled four of the five fastest recorded women's marathon times.

A blemish on this exemplary record came in the 2004 Summer Olympics in Athens. She was forced to end her run after 22 mi (36 km), suffering from the effects of the high temperature and, it was revealed later, the lingering effects of both a leg injury and the anti-inflammatory therapy for the injury. The therapy had upset her stomach and affected her diet in the weeks preceding the marathon. The lack of food energy proved to be her undoing. Later in the Olympic Games, her weakened physical condition forced her to withdraw from the women's 10,000-m final.

Her disappointment at these performances has been tempered by subsequent victories in the 2004 New York Marathon, 2005 London Marathon, and the 2005 World Championships.

In addition to her marathon prowess, Radcliffe is the holder of the women's world records for road races of 10, 20, and 30 km (in contrast to track events, road races are run on varying terrain and surfaces). She also won the World Cross-Country Championships held in 2001 and 2002.

For her athletic accomplishments, Radcliffe was made a Member of the Order of the British Empire in June 2002.

Radcliffe is a staunch advocate of drug-free competition and has been a vocal critic of the use of illicit performance-enhancing drugs. As an example of this resolve, at the 2001 World Athletic Championships held in Edmonton, Canada, she publicly protested the reinstatement of a Russian competitor who had previously tested positive for the banned substance erythropoietin (which increases the number of red blood cells, and so

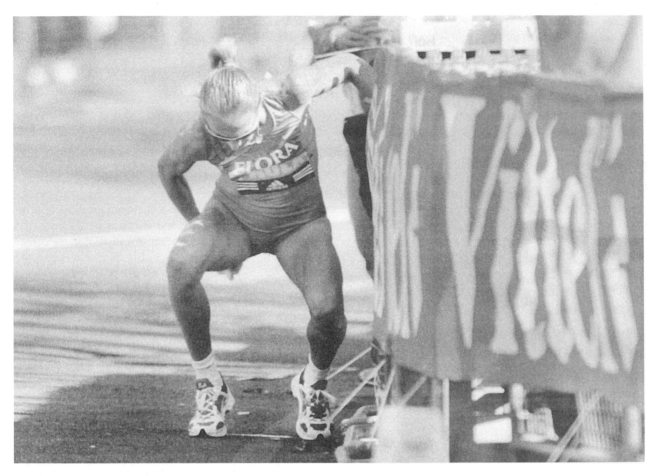

Paula Radcliffe. © KIERAN DOHERTY/REUTERS/CORBIS

the oxygen-carrying capacity of the blood). She competes with a red ribbon attached to her racing singlet, a symbol of her support of blood testing of athletes.

As of 2006, Radcliffe is still training and competing. She intends to compete in the women's marathon at the 2008 Summer Olympics to be held in Beijing.

**SEE ALSO** Exercise and thermotolerance.

## Range of motion

Range of motion (ROM) is an aspect of sports science that assists in the determination of how far a particular joint can move. Joint flexibility as defined by the ROM of the particular structure is essential to both injury prevention, as well as measuring rehabilitative progress after an injury. Joints that are capable of an additional range of motion typically permit the athlete to move with greater grace and power. The archetypal "loose-limbed" athlete is the person who possess a greater ROM than the average individual.

ROM is measured by the number of degrees that a joint can be moved without the application of external force from a determined position. The common tool used to perform the measurement is a double-armed goniometer, an instrument used to calculate geometric angles. Each joint, by virtue of its unique structure, has a different optimum ROM. Particular attention is paid by sports scientists to the ROM of the shoulder, elbow, wrist, hip, knee, and ankle; all joints in the body are capable of ROM measurement.

The measurement of shoulder ROM is a complex one, due to the variety of ways that the shoulder is called on to move in different sports. The ROM of the shoulder of a baseball pitcher will bear different considerations than the ROM of the shoulder of a cross-country skier. The forces directed into the shoulder joint in each sport are significantly different, both in terms of the degree of the force as well as the direction that the shoulder is required to move. For this reason, the shoulder ROM will be determined from a variety of perspectives: abduction, with the arm extended from the body; adduction, with the arm pulled in toward the body; flexion, in a bending motion; extension, in a straightening or extending motion; hyperextension, extending the joint past 180° of motion; and rotation, the movement of the joint in a circular motion, in both clockwise and counterclockwise directions.

With the ROM determined in each of the aspects of shoulder movement, a definitive picture can be drawn regarding the laxity or flexibility of the joint.

In a hinge joint such as the elbow or the knee, the ROM measurement is simplified. The key determination in these joints is the relationship between the flexion (bending) and the extension (stretching). In the elbow, a normal person can bend the elbow sufficiently back that the wrist approximately reaches the ear. If the wrist is moved from a position with the arm extended parallel to the floor, the angle created by the flexion is approximately 140°. If the person is able to extend the wrist past the point where the arm is parallel to the floor, this is described as a hyperextension of the elbow. A small degree of hyperextension is common; any further flexibility in the joint is often described as "double-jointed."

A hyperextension of a joint can also occur through physical contact and result in an injury to the joint, particularly to the ligaments. A hyperextended position is generally an unstable position for a joint, one where the ability of the joint to sustain the forces of movement or a direct blow is much reduced. Given the structure of the knee joint, with six sets of ligaments providing support to the joint, a hyperextension of the knee is often one that compromises the strength of the ligament structures, as the joint is forced through a ROM that the ligaments cannot sustain.

Wrist ROM, like that of the shoulder, is measured in more than one direction. The flexibility of the wrist is assessed first from the perspective of wrist flexion, the degree by which the wrist can extend and flex from a position where the wrist is palm down, parallel to the ground. The joint is also observed from the same position, with the movement measured on the ulnar side (the side opposite the thumb, the location of the ulnar bone), and the radial side (the thumb side).

The ROM in the foot is assessed in terms of the joint's dorsi flexion, the amount by which the front of the foot may be flexed upward, and the plantar flexion, the corresponding measurement of how far the toe may be pointed downward.

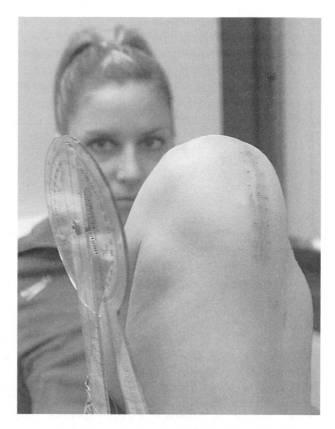

Physical therapist examines range of motion of an athtlete's knee. **PHOTO BY EZRA SHAW/GETTY IMAGES.**

ROM will be improved in all joints through a focused and dedicated stretching and flexibility program. All athletes will suffer tightness and reduced joint laxity if muscles are subject to forces but the connective tissues to the joints are not adequately stretched. Reduced ROM will tend to limit both the explosive ability of the athlete as well as the agility in the execution of an athletic movement.

In strength training, greater ROM is achieved through work with free weights as opposed to those carried out with stationary machines that limit the ROM required to carry out the exercise. Free weights, used properly, will compel the athlete to value form, which is an alternative expression of greater ROM.

**SEE ALSO** Musculoskeletal injuries; Skeletal muscle; Strength training; Weightlifting.

# Recreational sports

Recreational sports are those activities where the primary purpose of the activity is participation, with the related goals of improved physical fitness, fun, and social involvement often prominent. Recreational sports are usually perceived as being less stressful, both physically and mentally, on the participants. There are lower expectations regarding both performance and commitment to the sport in the recreational sphere. In theory, there is a clear demarcation between purely recreational pursuits and competitive sports, where emphasis will be centered on the achievement of success and the attainment of physical skills through rigorous training. Competitive sport involves not only contests, but it also advances as a central tenet that the athlete or team will continually seek progress and advancement to a higher level. Professional, international, national, and regional championships and university competitions are exclusively competitive activities. In practice, the division between the concepts of recreation and competition at all other levels is often blurred.

Recreational sports are the most popular type of athletic activity undertaken throughout the world. While elite professional leagues and glamorous international sport festivals are the events on which the media focuses its attention, for every professional athlete there are thousands of participants who use the same sport for the satisfaction of their personal fitness needs. Recreational sport enthusiasts include individual athletes, such as persons who run, cycle, or participate in aerobics; this sport category also extends to those who play a sport as a member of a community-based league, such as master's (over 40 years) age soccer or mixed (male and female) slow-pitch baseball.

Recreational sport is the aspect of overall fitness often promoted by government health agencies in the larger societal quest for better health and consequent reductions in the strain on public health care costs. Recreational sports, at both youth and adult levels, is advanced as a component of the healthy lifestyle that leads to less incidence of serious disease (particularly diabetes and cardiovascular diseases associated with obesity), and greater longevity in the population generally.

The distinction between competitive and recreational sport is more often a matter of degree, as opposed to the application of a descriptive label. Competitive sport is not always an elite athletic activity; the attitude of the individual athlete toward the sport is an important aspect of how to define it. The best examples of this categorization are found in the mass participation sports such as marathon running and the triathlon, which are invariably further subdivided into age group classifications. These age group distinctions, in contrast to the elite, often professional, competitors, are where the recreational/competitive boundaries are challenged. If a marathoner runner, who has achieved a four-hour time for the event at age 40, decides that he would like to qualify for the prestigious Boston Marathon, that runner must improve to the Boston standard in his age group, 3 hr 15 min. A four-hour marathon time is faster than the approximate median time of most mass participation marathons (those races with over 5,000 participants); the four-hour runner could take some justifiable pride in that accomplishment. The reduction of 45 minutes from the previous personal best will require an improvement of over 1.7 minutes per mile; the winner will conquer the hilly Boston course in approximately 2 hr 10 min or faster, approximately two-thirds the time the prospective qualifier must run. There is a huge competitive gap between the winner and the qualifier; most objective observers would classify the qualifier as a recreational runner.

To improve his qualifying time by 45 minutes, the recreational runner will be required to make significant changes to his training workload, training intensity, and perhaps diet. This athlete will have to consider the tactics of running the racecourse most effectively and economically, with special attention to hydration and supplementation. At his athletic level, the prospective Boston Marathon qualifier must increase the level of his competition, even if that competition is essentially with himself.

The Football Association (FA) of England organizes the annual FA Cup, the world's oldest soccer championship. Unlike the professional league championships, the FA Cup is open to any registered man's team, amateur or professional. The teams are drawn at random in the first number of rounds to play a home and home series. It is not uncommon for a "minnow," the English expression for an entirely unheralded side, to advance deep into the competition. The minnows are often teams composed entirely of amateurs. From the heights of English football, such teams would be seen as no more than recreational players when compared to the elite, multimillionaire professionals of the sport. When a team or an athlete seeks to compete at their highest level, the recreational aspect becomes secondary to the competitive dimension.

An aspect of recreational level sport that is often overlooked is the importance of a proper warm-up and cool-down period. While the body may not be put to the same degree of muscular stress in a recreational event as in a high level competition, the nature of demands on the musculoskeletal system in recreational sport are similar. A failure to properly stretch the muscles, joints, and connective tissues often

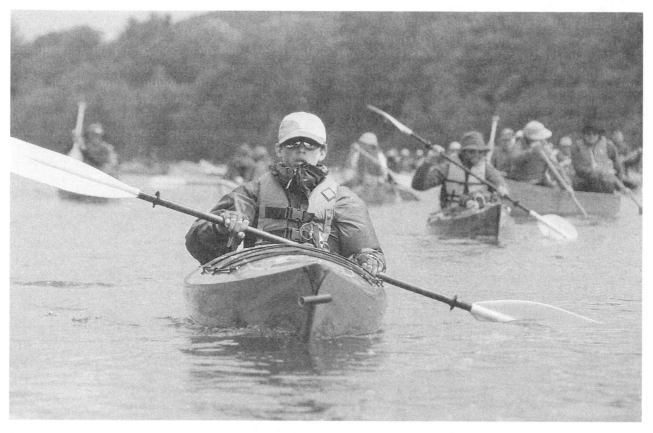

Recreational sports, such as kayaking, are an important component of the healthy lifestyle. RAYMOND K. GEHMAN/NATIONAL GEOGRAPHIC/ GETTY IMAGES

leads to serious injury for the recreational athlete. In a related way, when there is a failure to wear proper footwear or protective gear in an environment where the activity is seen as being "for fun," preventable injuries are common.

SEE ALSO Diet; Fitness; Health; Longevity; Warm up/ Cool down.

# Recurrent stress fractures

A stress fracture is a localized breakdown of a bone, that occurs when the forces directed into the bone tissue exceed the ability of the bone to repair itself. A stress fracture is distinct from the fractures caused by the direct, one-time application of a force to the bone, such as created by a fall or a blow. When bone sustains damage, it mobilizes its reserves of minerals, primarily calcium and phosphates, to repair the bone damage; repetitive stress prevents the repair effort from being effective. Stress fractures occur most often in the tibia and fibula (the bones of the lower leg), the ankle, and the foot. Stress fractures

are less common in other parts of the body, but may occur in any sport where repetitive motion isolates forces into a specific skeletal region. Distance running, running-oriented sports, and traditional track and field events such as the high jump and the long jump are the most common activities leading to the development of stress fractures.

Stress fractures recur for a number of reasons, some of which are caused by the structure of the athlete's body, others of which are related to the athlete's preparation, equipment, and attitude toward training. Sports science research confirms that approximately 60% of all athletes who have sustained a single stress fracture will later sustain at least one other. Female athletes are somewhat more likely to suffer a stress fracture than male athletes.

Unlike a direct fracture, stress fractures are more often a progressive condition, identified by the onset of pain while participating in the sport, a sensation that disappears when the athlete is at rest. Stress fractures are observable on an x ray; bone scans and magnetic resonance imaging (MRI) are also commonly employed diagnostic techniques. The recovery from a stress fracture is will primarily require rest, with appropriate stretching or activities that do not direct forces or apply resistance into the fractured bone.

There are two general sets of factors that are typically present to cause a stress fracture. The structure and manner of movement of the body, often referred to as biomechanical factors, will significantly influence how the forces directed into the skeletal structure are distributed and absorbed. The risk of an athlete developing a stress fracture in the lower leg will be increased when different factors are present, such as any sport that requires repetitive leg movement that places stress upon the lower leg. Also, unequal leg length in which the difference in the length of legs of the athlete are greater than 0.25 in (0.5 cm), causing the forces generated by the strike of the foot on the ground to be uneven. The greater force will be repeatedly directed into a region of the foot or the lower leg, causing the formation of the stress fracture.

Another structural factor is a high-arched foot that causes the forces directed into the foot on impact with the running surface to radiate unevenly. High arches are a key contributing factor to stress fractures of the metatarsal bones (the connective bones between the ankle and the toes).

The different manners in which the foot contacts the surface during running are other structural problems. Athletes are generally classed as either "forefoot strikers," where the ball and toes of the foot strike first, or "rearfoot strikers," where the force is first absorbed by the heel, and the foot rotates forward to generate force to push off from the forefoot. Forefoot strikers tend to direct greater amounts of force through the foot into the lower tibia and fibula, in a region located above the ankle, often to the medial (inside) aspect of the lower leg.

Biomechanical deficiencies are unlikely to cause stress fractures alone. A recreational runner who enjoys an easy 3 mi (5 km) run four days per week, will most likely not be affected by any one of these structural factors. It is the combination of greater workout and competitive intensities, training methods, and equipment that elevate the biomechanical factors from the background to prominence.

Stress fractures recur as a result of both a failure on the part of athlete to counter the biomechanical factors, as well as through the imposition of factors personal to the athlete. When an athlete has sustained a stress fracture, aggressive steps must be taken to ensure that the footwear is sufficient protection. An orthotic is often prescribed to correct leg length imbalance of high arch irregularity; a failure to take such steps is often a guarantee of a recurrent

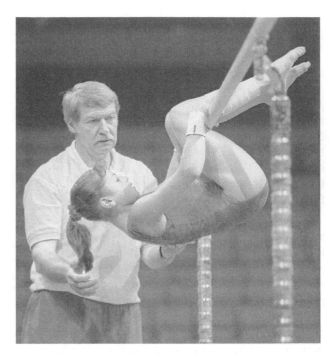

Gymnast Dominique Moceanu was not expected to participate in the 1996 Olympic Team Trials because of a stress fracture in her right tibia. AP PHOTO/SUSAN WALSH

injury. Many athletes, especially those with competitive aspirations, feel significant pressure to return to high level training too quickly. The body, after an injury of this nature, is not equipped to bear the stress of high training volume and is more prone to break down again in the same physical area.

Other training basics must be addressed to prevent a recurring stress fracture. The overall nutrition of the athlete must be examined to ensure that the proper daily intakes of calcium, its companion vitamin D, and related bone-building materials are being ingested. The athlete must ensure that stretching, flexibility, and general warm-up procedures are followed; poor flexibility will create biomechanical problems of its own. In the initial recovery stages from a stress fracture involving running, the athlete must select the training surfaces with care, as uneven or angled ground and roadways creates uneven distribution of forces into the feet and lower legs.

Extreme caution must be exercised in the treatment of a stress fracture that occurs in a young athlete. The long bones, such as the femur, tibia, and fibula, are constructed with a growth plate, located next to the end of the bone, known as the epiphysis. Any damage to the growth plate by way of a stress fracture may compromise the ability of the bone to grow to maturity.

SEE ALSO Growth plate injuries; Lower leg injuries; Overtraining; Running injuries; Stress fracture of the foot.

# Renal function

Renal function is the assessment of the health and the viability of the kidneys, with a particular focus on the kidneys' ability to filter out waste products and toxins from the blood system. When the kidneys are functioning in an optimum fashion, there will generally be electrolytic balance in the body (sodium and potassium levels will be constant), and fluid levels will be balanced between blood volume and urine production by the kidneys for the excretion of wastes.

The body has two kidneys that perform equal and identical functions within the body, each located on either side of the spine; one kidney is positioned next to the liver, the other adjacent to the spleen. The adrenal glands, important in the production of the hormone adrenaline, are positioned at the top of each kidney. Humans possess an overcapacity of kidney function, in that a person may live a normal and healthy life with only one functional kidney. The kidney is an integral part of the urinary, or excretory systems, part of a continuous process that extends from the kidney to the bladder to the urethra.

Renal failure is the condition that arises when the kidney is unable to filter wastes; when this inability becomes irreversible, end stage renal failure is the consequence, which results in the need for dialysis treatment to mechanically perform the required toxin filtering. End stage renal failure will ultimately necessitate a kidney transplant, or death will result. The study of the various diseases that impact on renal function is nephrology, named for the portion of the kidney where the filtering function is carried out.

In their function as a filter, the kidneys receives all of the circulating blood within the cardiovascular system. There are a number of methods to assess whether the kidneys are adequately filtering wastes and toxins from the blood. The two most prominent of these tests are the blood urea nitrogen test, sometimes referred to as the BUN test, and analysis to determine the levels of the substance creatinine within the body. Both tests involve a chemical analysis of the person's blood.

The BUN test centers on the presence of urea in the blood stream. Urea is a compound composed of nitrogen, hydrogen, carbon, and oxygen, described by the chemical equation $(NH_2)_2CO$. Urea occurs in the bloodstream as waste produced by the body through the digestion of protein and

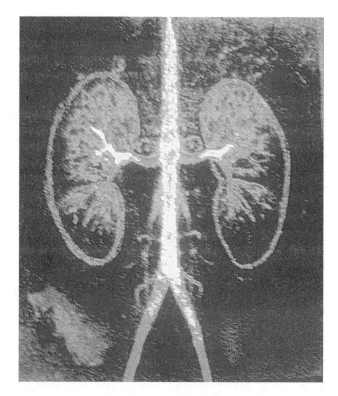

Angiogram of kidney. © HOWARD SOCHUREK/CORBIS

its constituent amino acids. The normal range of urea in the bloodstream is well established to be between 7 mg and 25 mg/100 ml of blood. When the test reveals significant excess in the urea level, a reading in excess of 100 mg/100 ml of blood, there are three possible causes. The first is renal failure, with its very serious physical consequences.

The second possible cause of a excessive urea reading is dehydration, which occur during sport when the athlete has failed to properly hydrate either during the workout or the competition. When a person is dehydrated, the ratio of normal urea presence in the blood volume is disturbed. This condition is usually one that may be remedied through the improvement of fluid levels in the body.

The third possible cause of excess urea is the consumption of excess proteins, such as occurs with weightlifters and other strength athletes who are seeking to develop greater muscle mass and strength. As with dehydration, this condition is remedied through correction of diet. Prolonged excess protein consumption tends to place a greater strain on renal function.

Creatinine is a byproduct of the metabolism of phosphocreatine (creatine phosphate), the compound essential to the production of energy in skeletal muscles. Creatinine is a waste product that is of no use to the body once it is created, and it must be eliminated through the kidneys. As phosphocreatine is present in all skeletal muscles, and creatinine is produced at a relatively constant rate through muscular activity, creatinine levels are a reliable indicator of renal efficiency. Males have a greater amount of skeletal muscle than do females, and the normal creatinine level for men varies between 0.7 mg and 1.4 mg per 100 ml of blood; the corresponding range for women is 0.5 mg to 1.0 mg per 100 ml of blood. Readings in excess of those levels indicate an inability in the kidneys to carry out normal filtration of the blood.

The reasons for diminished renal function are many. When a kidney becomes enlarged, it will not properly function. Due to the continual exposure to the blood system and all of the potential toxins that are transported through it, the kidney is vulnerable to the development of tumors, both benign and malignant. The kidney is also vulnerable to infections that originate in the urinary tract, which may diminish its filtering capacity.

**SEE ALSO** Diuretics; Hormones; Hydration; Sodium (salt) intake for athletes.

## Resistance exercise SEE Variable resistance exercise

## Resistance exercise training

Resistance exercise is that which focuses on the development of musculoskeletal strength. This type of exercise includes weight training or strength training, as a resistance program seeks the enhancement of muscle strength, endurance, and power. A well-rounded and well-balanced athlete will incorporate resistance exercises, aerobic conditioning, and flexibility exercises into an overall training program. Resistance exercise commonly, although not exclusively, utilizes weight training to generate the forces necessary to create resistance against which the working muscles can act; weightlifting, as a competitive sport, is distinct from resistance exercise.

The essence of resistance exercise is the principle of overload. The progressive increase of the load (or the resistance) applied to a muscle, will cause the muscle to become fatigued. Through the combination of overloading during workouts and the repair initiated by the body on its muscle fibers when at rest, the muscles grow stronger. Resistance training, in addition to being an essential component of total fitness, is a specific contributor to stronger and denser bones. A body with a greater percentage of lean muscle mass will consume greater amounts of energy at rest, as muscles place greater demands on the body's metabolism than do fat cells.

Resistance exercise training can be started at almost any age, although considerable caution must be taken with young athletes (persons under the age of 18 years). As the bodies of these persons are not yet mature, the growth plates present on the long bones of the juvenile athlete are not yet ossified, or hardened into their final adult form. Overly vigorous resistance training can place unhealthy levels of stress on these structures, causing the bone to either grow incompletely or to become vulnerable to later bone damage. Any resistance exercise training program must be accompanied by a comprehensive stretching and flexibility routine, both as a part of the warm up/cool down aspect to a particular workout, as well as those stretching exercises conducted on a daily basis.

Resistance training, especially those exercises involving free weights, will emphasize a complete range of motion to obtain the maximum resistance benefit. The more flexible the joints of the athlete, the greater the range of motion is achieved. The types of stretches that are central to yoga and Pilates are a very effective counterbalance to the stresses placed on the body in resistance exercise training. Conversely, when the range of motion in the athlete is more limited, the desired form necessary to execute the particular routine may be absent, which will both limit the effectiveness of the exercise and increase the risk of musculoskeletal injury.

Successful resistance exercise depend upon a number of factors, including the level of fitness of the athlete at the beginning of the program. When a person is new to resistance training, or otherwise does not possess a moderate level of general fitness, the resistance program must be advanced gradually. Also, the warm up should involve both stretching and flexibility exercises as well as a light aerobic workout, such as an easy run or a short session on a treadmill, elliptical machine, or other stationary trainer.

Resistance training will ultimately require the involvement of all muscle groups. For this reason, the workout should begin with the larger muscle groups, such as the back and chest muscles, and

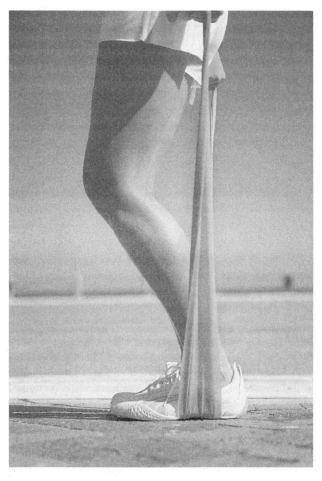

Resistance and strength training can be done with free weights, for example, or with an exercise band, as shown here.
© BROOKE FASANI/CORBIS

repetitions, or decreasing rest, will contribute to the overall intensity and volume.

As all resistance training is anaerobic in nature, the efficient production of muscle energy is important to training success. Adenosine triphosphate (ATP) is the ultimate fuel used to generate energy in working muscles; ATP functions in an energy cycle with phosphocreatine (creatine phosphate). Persons engaged in serious resistance training often consume creatine supplements to assist in this energy process.

While resistance training most often involves the use of weights to provide the necessary resistance, other training aids can be effective. Sprinters use either parachutes or similar devices to create additional drag on their bodies to increase the resistance to their leg muscles; the blocking sleds used for many years in American football by linemen to simulate line play against an opposing team are a similar device.

SEE ALSO Cross training; Exercise, high intensity; Free weights; Muscle mass and strength; Variable resistance exercise; Weightlifting.

## Rest treatment for injuries SEE RICE (Rest/Ice/Compression/Elevation) treatment for injuries

## Restricted substances

The concept of placing restrictions upon the use or possession of certain substances is a familiar one in many countries in the world. Restricted is a term that is generally applied in the sense of a limitation, as opposed to a prohibition.

In the criminal law context, many countries have regulated the possession and consumption of certain drugs by restriction as opposed to prohibition. In Holland and Canada, cannabis marijuana possession is not the subject of prosecution, when it is possessed in small quantities or where required for medicinal purposes. Alcohol is the most popular restricted drug in the world, as most countries tend to regulate the age and places where alcohol may be consumed, with significant penalties for a breach of such rules.

It is with these notions in mind that the regulation of certain substances in an athletic context should be examined. In sport, restricted substance is a broad concept. A restricted or prohibited

progress to the smaller arm and shoulder muscles. The first several resistance sessions should be devoted to the development of proper form; the training should cover all of the muscle groups of the body. Once the person is comfortable with the movements to complete the exercises, the training should become more focused, with planned sessions that move from one exercise to another with defined recovery periods between each set. Finally, the cooldown phase should involve the easy stretching of the entire body, as well as a gentle aerobic exercise.

Like any form of training, resistance exercises develop greater muscular strength, endurance, and power by virtue of their progressive nature. The training progression is accomplished through increases in both training intensity and training volume. The variables in any resistance program are the amount of resistance (often the weight to be lifted), the number of repetitions, and the rest period between exercise; increasing resistance or substance also includes certain practices undertaken by athletes. Restrictions and prohibitions have a potential application to any substance that might be ingested by an athlete to enhance performance.

Restricted substances may include conventional drugs and narcotics used by society as a whole, such as alcohol. Drugs specifically manufactured to achieve improved athletic performance are almost invariably prohibited substances; anabolic steroids are a prominent example. Naturally occurring substances that can be consumed without resort to any chemical process, such as caffeine (through coffee, tea, and guarana among other sources) or ephedra (present in a wide variety of herbs) are proven stimulants and are regulated at most levels of international athletic competition.

The general classes of restricted drugs for the purpose of international sport are: local anesthetics; asthma and respiratory ailment/breathing dysfunction drugs; glucocorticosteroids, usually prescribed to treat arthritis or other osteoinflammatory diseases; caffeine; beta blockers, prescribed as heart medication; alcohol; cannabanoids such as marijuana.

The definition of what substances will be classed as restricted as opposed to prohibited is never closed. The World Anti-Doping Agency (WADA), in consultation with both its own national anti-doping agencies and the scientific community, reviews its definition of both restricted and prohibited classifications on an annual basis. In 2006, WADA embarked upon a review of the technology used by athletes known as hypoxic tents to determine whether these devices should be classed as a form of restricted or prohibited substance. Hypoxic tents create an artificial atmosphere that simulates the lower percentage of oxygen found in the air at higher altitudes. In these conditions the body's production of the hormone erythropoietin (EPO) is stimulated, triggering the production of a greater number of red blood cells. The increase in red blood cells will permit the athlete to transport greater amounts of oxygen during exercise. WADA embarked on its investigation regarding the hypoxic tents to determine whether they were a performance enhancing practice that ought to be restricted or banned.

Conversely, naturally occurring hormones manufactured within the human body, such as testosterone and EPO, are invariably used in furtherance of illegal purposes in sport (muscle development and oxygen transport) and are prohibited substances.

The modern regulatory regimes promulgated by the World Anti-Doping Agency (WADA) and administered by the national anti-doping agencies throughout the world recognize that athletes may require certain substances to preserve and maintain heir own health, with very little if any true competitive advantage gained. The most prominent example of such substances is the various asthma and respiratory medications available by prescription through a medical professional. For an otherwise healthy person competing in an aerobic sport, medication that tended to open the airways might produce a competitive advantage for that athlete. However, a healthy, asymptomatic person could not legally obtain such a medication.

The WADA-sanctioned approach concerning restricted substances is known as the Therapeutic Use Exemption, or TUE. Most sports now administer a schedule of out of competition testing for their national team athletes, in conjunction with the national anti-agency (in the United States the national agency is the United States Anti-Doping Agency, USAGA); in some sports the testing is administered to a broader classification of athletes by the sport governing body. As out of competition testing may occur at any time, athletes are required to make a formal declaration in advance of the testing year as to what medications if any they may be taking and whether that medication is prescribed for a particular physical or mental health condition.

In every year, or so often as the national anti-drug agency may determine, every athlete is required to apply for a TUE for any prescribed substance that they are taking or that they may take in future (if known); if the TUE is approved, any subsequent test that reveals the subject substance is a deemed negative test. If the athlete fails or refuses to apply for a TUE, and fails a doping test as a result, the general approach of WADA is to treat the result as one attracting a competition ban.

SEE ALSO Doping tests; Prohibited substances (competition bans); Therapeutic Use Exemption; World Anti-Doping Agency (WADA).

# Retro running

Retro running is a lesser known term for a well-established athletic activity: running backward. Retro running has a number of significant applications throughout sport, both as a training aid and as a rehabilitative tool in the management of various leg injuries. In some sports science commentaries, the broader expression "retro locomotion" is used to describe both retro running and the gentler version, retro walking.

The value of retro running in training is rooted in the mechanics of the running motion. The development of an optimal running stride depends on the ability of the athlete to power the quadriceps (thigh) muscles forward to create extension in the knee joint. As the knee extends, the lower leg muscles respond through the contraction of the calf muscles, which in turn direct the Achilles tendon and the muscles of the foot to complete the stride. The counter movement, the flexion, or bending, of the knee, is a movement that originates with the hamstring muscles and tendon located at the back of the thigh behind the knee. To generate an efficient and powerful stride, the strength of the quadriceps relative to the hamstrings should be in approximate ratio of 3:2; when the quadriceps is too powerful, the knee will sustain forces it is not constructed to bear, a circumstance that may lead to overstress and ultimately damage to the anterior cruciate ligament (ACL), the connective tissue essential to knee stability. If the quadriceps is weak, the hamstrings tend to dominate the running muscle motion, often becoming overstretched through the repetitive movement of running. This circumstance will often result in hamstring pulls or tears. Distance runners are often susceptible to an overly strong quadriceps structure and resultant hamstring injury.

Other injury sites created by the structural imbalances that are accentuated by the natural running motion are lumbar (low back) region, hip, and groin. Shin splints, compartment muscle injuries of the lower leg, and Achilles tendon injuries are all most often connected to either structure or muscle imbalances created by running programs that provide insufficient stretching and flexibility exercises in relation to the distances covered in training.

The first benefit of retro running is that it tends to counteract the forces that produce musculoskeletal pain. The body is designed to move more efficiently forward than backward; the maximum speed of the retro runner is no more than 80% of maximum forward speed. When the retro running is performed on a treadmill or stationary exercise machine, the muscles of the legs are required to move in coordination with the abdomen and lower back without risk that the structural imbalances of the body will cause the forces of movement to be misapplied. When the athlete is recovering from an injury such as a stress fracture

or knee damage, retro walking can be substituted to eliminate any additional degree of impact being directed into the injured area.

Retro running is a powerful sport specific training tool. Athletes such American football cornerbacks, basketball players, and tennis players must all be able to move powerfully and decisively through backward motion. Maximum speed in a retro position is essential to success in each of these sports. Training programs such as shuttle run drills, where the athlete is required to move backward and forward at a high speed within a short period of time, are effective in developing retro running skills specific to the sport.

When retro running is incorporated into a training program, the athlete can expect to obtain the musculoskeletal benefits: higher leg turn over (increased stride rate); increased stride length due to the better strength ratio between the hamstrings and the quadriceps muscles; an improved range of motion in the knee joint, which permits freer and more powerful movements in both running and jumping; creation of optimal balance between the function of the knee in the generation of the power necessary to create running motion, and the ankle/foot as the absorber of the forces generated through the running motion. Retro running requires more energy than does forward running motion; and both the ability of athlete to utilize oxygen, the $VO_2max$ as well as the heart rate of the athlete are increased through retro running training.

The incorporation of retro running into an interval running or intermittent exercise program places positive stresses on both the musculoskeletal and cardiovascular systems. Additionally, retro running stimulates the fast-twitch fibers present in the muscles of quadriceps, hamstrings, and calf. Sports science research confirms that the introduction of movements that represent a variation from regular training tend to reduce training injury rates.

**SEE ALSO** Cross training; Exercise, intermittent; Hamstring injuries; Running strength training and exercises.

# RICE (Rest/Ice/Compression/ Elevation) treatment for injuries

RICE (Rest/Ice/Compression/Elevation) treatment is a system of soft tissue injury treatment that is both a first aid application as well as an ongoing approach to injury management. The individual components of RICE have been well recognized for many years as effective in managing athletic injury; since the 1970s, sport science has endorsed the RICE method as the most effective method to deal with ankle and knee sprains, muscle and tendon pulls or strains, and the bruising that results from the physical contact of sport.

The component of rest of RICE begins at the time of the injury. The injured player must be removed from competition to permit an assessment of the nature and extent of the injury; many types of musculoskeletal injuries become worse if the athlete is permitted to play through the problem. In many cases, the use of topical painkillers to permit continued play will deaden the athlete's ability to sense further physical injury. When the injury is determined to be sufficiently serious that continued play would likely cause further structural damage, the athlete should immediately be subjected to the second part of RICE, the application of ice or a similar cold product to the site of the injury is recommended.

Damage to the soft tissues of the body will invariably create swelling in these structures. Swelling is caused by the release of intracellular fluid at the point of the injury, coupled with an increase in blood flow to the site. Swelling will slow the healing process, as it is the body's natural mechanism to impair joint movement as a signal to the body not to use the injured joint. If these natural healing processes took priority, the recovery from injuries such as an ankle sprain or a twisted knee (a sprain of the knee ligaments) would be slow. The application of ice to the area of swelling serves to constrict the flow of blood to the affected area, thus reducing swelling. The ice has a secondary effect of deadening the pain receptors in the area of the affected structure.

There are considerable differences in scientific opinion as to how and for how long ice may be applied to a soft tissue injury. The nature, location, and the extent of the injury are significant factors; ice applied to a bony area such as the knee has a less insulating soft tissue beneath the skin than a contusion (bruise) sustained to the thigh. As a general guideline, the less soft tissue that is present at the injury site, the shorter the period that the area should be iced; 10 minutes would be a minimum application, with 25 to 30 minutes representing the upper end of a safe icing range. The application of ice for too long a period can cause permanent damage to the underlying tissue not unlike that caused by frostbite. Further, some chemical ice products available for sports first aid purposes are colder than ice, and the application time must be adjusted accordingly.

Ice can be applied on a regular basis after the onset of the injury. For a tendinitis injury such as jumper's knee, a strain often experienced by jump sport athletes and basketball players, the injury site might be iced three times per day. When the athlete has sustained a more serious ankle sprain, the joint could be iced every two hours throughout the day. Ice will typically be most effective within the first 72 hours of the occurrence of a soft tissue injury.

The third RICE element, compression, is the physical application of pressure to the location of a soft tissue injury. Compression is useful as a first aid treatment, as the application of pressure will reduce the effect of any internal bleeding or swelling that may result from the injury. Compression has two separate roles in the course of RICE treatment: first, as a companion to the icing of the injury, and second, as the day-to-day maintenance of the injured structure. Elastic bandages and athletic tape are both used to provide compression, as are sleeves that are designed to fit over an entire joint and surrounding limb, such as in knee or elbow injuries.

In ideal circumstances, the injured portion of the body will be maintained at an elevation above that of the heart. Such elevation serves to both reduce swelling as well as to promote the healthy action of the veins of the cardiovascular system to return blood from the injured area to the heart (a process known as venous return), which counters the pooling of blood near the injury.

RICE works best when it is implemented immediately from the time of injury. However, even the delayed application of the treatment (for example, the day after the injury occurred) will promote better healing than if the injury is untreated. Various studies of recovery time experienced by athletes who sustained ankle sprains suggest that RICE treatment reduces time lost to injury by over 40%, as well as contributing to a reduction in scar tissue formation.

**SEE ALSO** Ankle sprains; Calf strain or pull; First aid kits for sports; Knee injuries; Musculoskeletal injuries; Quadriceps pulls and tears; Sprains and strains.

# Road rash

Road rash is the slang term used to describe the abrasions and small cuts that often result from a crash or other accident involving the skin of an athlete and an unforgiving asphalt or road surface. Road rash is most common in cycling, with similar injuries also occurring to in-line skaters and skateboarders who lose their balance and fall on a hard surface. Virtually every cyclist or in-line skater will sustain at least one fall that produces road rash at some point in their career; given that impact between the cyclist and the road surface may occur at speeds in excess of 30 mph (50 km/h), the extent of skin damage can be considerable.

There are three general kinds of skin injuries sustained by athletes: abrasions, cuts, and lacerations. Road rash is usually an abrasion, an injury that will appear as a bright red series of blotches or marks caused by the body being dragged across rough pavement as the athlete falls. Road rash will impart a bumpy, cracked texture to the damaged skin that will be tender to the touch, due to the fact that many nerve endings over a relatively wide area of skin are exposed through the rash.

In more serious falls, the athlete may sustain a cut to the skin that involves damage to the blood vessels beneath the surface of the skin and an accompanying loss of blood. The most serious of skin injuries, a laceration, is a deep wound that damages both the skin and a significant portion of the underlying tissue.

Road rash most commonly occurs in the sport of cycling when a rider miscalculates the angle of approach entering into a corner of a roadway or race course, causing the bicycle to slide out from under the rider's body. In this angled position, the rider and the bicycle slide together on the road surface, often at significant speed. Road rash will result on the exposed position of the cyclist's body; the most frequent injury sites are the outside portion of the lower legs, the knee, the outside of the quadriceps and ilio band (thigh), the palm of the hands, the arm, and the shoulder. The hip is also subject to road rash, even where it is usually covered by the cyclist's clothing; the abrasion created on the hip is usually caused by the clothing being pulled across the skin surface during the slide along the road surface. When the force of striking the paved surface is severe, the road rash may overlay a more serious bruising or fracture.

While road rash is most common to cyclists who experience a fall on a paved road surface, mountain bikers who fall on gravel road ways and trails can also sustain this injury; given the greater cushioning of an unpaved surface, the consequences tend to be less severe that those on a paved road. In-line skaters tend to sustain their road rash in the same general regions of the body as the road cyclists.

The skin is the largest human organ. It has two major components: the epidermis, the outer layer, and the dermis, the underlying layer. The epidermis is the protective shell for the body, repelling harmful and infectious organisms from entering the muscles or internal organs. The epidermis has no blood vessels within its structure; it is nourished through its proximity to the denser dermis, which contains the nerves, hair follicles, blood vessels, and sebaceous and sweat glands of the skin. Most road rash is damage to the epidermis; where a cyclist sustains significant bleeding as a result of a fall, it is likely that the skin has been cut or lacerated into the dermis.

Road rash carries with it three major potential consequences. The first is that continued riding may be painful until the injury is treated; road rash often affects one or both of the legs, where the repetitive extension of the limb through pedaling is painful. A first aid kit with appropriate cleansing and antibiotic products should be immediately available to treat this injury. The other consequences are longer term, such as the potential for the skin to be come scarred as a result of the fall and the risk of infection developing in the affected area.

Road rash has a greater potential for long-term damage to the body than do other types of sports abrasions such a skinned knee that results from a fall on the basketball floor. The road surface has various kinds of loose dirt, small pieces of gravel, engine oils, and chemicals, all of which may enter the skin on impact. The careful cleaning of the injury is essential to the long-term health of the skin. The time-honored remedy for road rash was the cleaning of the affected area with mild soap or an antiseptic, with the area kept dry; more modern treatment options favor the physical cleaning of the rash, including a gentle scrubbing of the injury, followed by the application of a nontoxic cleaner (where the active ingredient is sodium chloride), with the area covered by a semipermeable bandage. A more serious road rash injury, especially where there is any degree of bleeding, should be attended to by a physician. Tetanus and other infection diseases can occur as a result of an improperly treated road rash injury.

Simply permitting the road rash to "scab over," without properly cleaning, abrading (removal of debris), and protecting the injury is an invitation to the promotion of infection.

**SEE ALSO** Abrasions, cuts, lacerations; Cycling; First aid kits for sports; Roller skates.

# Rock climbing and wall climbing

Rock climbing is the sport of climbing sheer rock faces and outcroppings, using specialized equipment and climbing techniques. The principles of rock climbing are similar those of mountain climbing; rock climbing is not directed at an ascent to the peak of a mountain, and the suitable rock formations for sport climbing can occur in any elevation. Wall climbing is a sport that is a man made creation; wall climbing is a miniaturized form of rock climbing, where the participants climb artificial surfaces constructed from wood or other materials and built either indoors or outdoors. Both rock climbing and wall climbing are a part of the growing group of activities often classed as extreme sports.

Rock climbing first began as an organized activity in the hills of England's Lake District in the 1880s, with the climbs attempted on the face of the sheer 115 ft rock (35 m) outcropping called "Nap's Needle." The sport also became popular as a training aid for mountaineers intent upon climbing various peaks in the European Alps in the later part of the nineteenth century, as the mountaineers sought out very difficult individual sections of boulder or rock face upon which to train for their expeditions.

The primary object of both rock climbing and wall climbing is simple—to move safely from the ground to a desired objective on the climbing surface, and return. The techniques employed to achieve the climbing objectives vary according to the difficulty of the climbing surface (including the presence of overhangs and crevices) and the skill level of the climber.

In rock climbing the essential equipment includes specialized shoes to provide extra grip on the rock surface, a harness to attach the ropes that will be used in the climb, and various types of anchors to be inserted into the rock face into which the ropes are secured or the climber's body may be positioned. All climbers carry a chalk manufactured from magnesium carbonate, a chemical that dries a climber's hands and fingers from the perspiration generated during a climb.

Rock climbs are divided into two general categories, free climbing and aid climbing. Free climbing is performed without assistance, as the climber ascends a particular section of rock using their hands and feet only, which entirely support their body weight. The climber is usually secured to a safety line, known as the belay line. The belay line is secured at a point on the rock face to prevent the climber from falling more than a short distance in the event of an accident or misadventure. In an aid climb, the climber uses artificial devices such as extra ropes, slings, pulleys and other hardware to assist in the movement of both themselves and any other equipment upwards along the rock face. The sling permits the climber to rest as they move along the climbing route.

As with any sport, rock climbing has developed a number of systems to grade the level of difficulty that a climber may encounter from a particular climb. The degree of difficulty attributed to a climbing route is determined both in terms of the decimal ratings, scored between 5.0 and 5.14 (easiest to most difficult), and the commitment rating, a measure of how long a climber of a particular level of ability would take to finish the climb.

Wall climbing involves the ascent of a structure that is generally smaller than the typical rock climb. The climbing wall used also has pre drilled holes and grips built into the surface for ease of use by the climbers.

The fundamental movement in rock climbing is the pull up, where the climber pulls their body weight upwards using the fingers and arms above, and the legs positioned below. The position of the climber's center of gravity (the place in the body where its mass is equally balanced) is a fundamental element to rock climbing. As a general proposition, the closer to the rock face the climber positions their body, the greater the importance of the larger leg muscles below the body in support, as the center of gravity is positioned over the climber's feet. As the climber moves away from the rock face, the smaller muscles of the arms and shoulders will be required to provide a greater amount of the necessary support to the body.

Brute muscular strength is not as important to rock climbing as is excellent over all fitness, well developed endurance capabilities, both aerobic and muscular, and a combination of balance and flexibility. In rock climbing, the concept of strength to weight ratio is especially important, as the larger the body mass of a climber the greater the muscular effort required to successfully ascend the obstacle. The constant demands that climbing places upon the fingers, wrists and forearms require specialized training for these muscle structures. A periodized approach to training is necessary to assist the climber in building each of these fitness areas; each period is directed to a specific climbing fitness need, and the subsequent periods build to the establishment of the necessary base to climb safely.

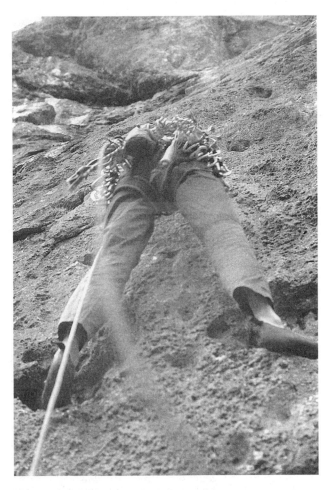

Rock climber on ascent. © LINDA/ZEFA/CORBIS

The first training period is directed to climbing endurance. In addition to cardiovascular training such as running, the climber seeks to build over all fitness by performing repetitions up and down a particular segment of a climbing wall. These segments have the same physiological effect as any other interval training.

The second training period builds upon the first by developing exercises specifically aimed at the climbing motion. These exercises include finger and wrist strength grip actions, pushups, and squats performed without extra resistance, to take the hips, thighs, and abductor muscles through a range of motion similar to that to be encountered on a climb. The athlete also extends the degree of training difficulty through the addition of a weight belt to the climber when using a climbing wall.

The third phase is a blending of power and endurance concepts, replicating the sport itself. Using the methods of the first two phases, the climber incorporates further core strength training (abdominal, lumber [low back], and groin muscles), the muscle groups essential to the maintenance of balance during the climb.

The final training stage is that referred to by athletic trainers as active recovery, where the climber continues with vigorous workouts that avoid undue stress on the muscles subjected to repetitive strain during rock climbing, such as the fingers and forearms. Swiss ball training and other abdominally focused exercises are useful. The four periods of training can be used as a training cycle in preparation for an actual outdoor climb.

SEE ALSO Balance training and proprioception; Extreme sports; Wrist injuries.

# Knute Kenneth Rockne

**3/4/1888–3/31/1931**
**NORWEGIAN AMERICAN**
**COLLEGE FOOTBALL COACH**

In the over 75 years since his death, the name Knute Rockne remains synonymous with both Notre Dame University and football coaching excellence. Rockne combined innovative approaches in both game strategy and practice techniques to become the best known college coach of his era.

Knute Rockne's legendary coaching career was founded upon a number of remarkable and almost improbable sequences. Born in Norway, Rockne immigrated with his family to the United States at age 7. Rockne was a very proficient high school athlete, but he did not graduate from high school in the usual course; he left school at age 17 to work in a series of different jobs in the Chicago area. It was only at the urging of friends that Rockne enrolled at Notre Dame University in South Bend, Indiana in 1910, when Rockne was 22 years old.

Rockne joined the Notre Dame football team, know as the 'Fighting Irish' in 1911, where he played both running back and offensive end. Rockne captained the Notre Dame team during his senior year in 1914, helping the team to its third undefeated season. The Fighting Irish were one of the first college teams to incorporate the forward pass into their regular offensive strategies (a tactic that had only be legalized in 1909), as the Notre Dame offence was described in the national media as possessing football's first all out air attack.

Rockne was 26 years old when he graduated from Notre Dame magna cum laude in pharmacy.

When his application to enter medical school was rejected, Rockne took an assistant professor position in chemistry at Notre Dame, where he also worked as an assistant football coach.

Rockne assumed the Notre Dame head coaching duties in 1917, and by the 1919 season he had directed the Fighting Irish to an unbeaten season. In the course of his coaching career at Notre Dame, the team would enjoy five such unbeaten campaigns.

It was Rockne's various innovations that propelled Noter Dame's success during this period. Rockne introduced the box formation and the technique known as influence blocking, the coordinated line blocking schemes where the offence uses a variety of stratagems to maneuver the defensive players into a particular position on the field, as opposed to simply attempting to overpower the defense with strength. In this fashion, Rockne helped to make football a much more exciting game for its spectators, as his strategies emphasized deception and speed. Rockne also instituted what came to be called the Notre Dame shift, also known as the precision backfield move, where the running backs would adjust their positions in a synchronized fashion prior to the snap of the ball in an effort to confuse the defense.

The most enduring of the Rockne innovations may be platoon football, a technique later perfected by coaches such as Paul Brown and a standard procedure in football at every level today. Rockne was the first coach to organize groups of players, or platoons, into specific formations in an attempt to wear down the opposing team.

The innovations implemented by Rockne were so popular with spectators and so effective in neutralizing Notre Dame's opponents that other prominent college football coaches banded together in an attempt to limit some of these strategies by having them declared illegal, without success.

In the course of his tenure at Notre Dame, Rockne proved to be as skilled at the promotion of his team and program as he was a football tactician. By the time of Rockne's death in 1931, Notre Dame was the most recognizable and the most popular football team in the United States. Rockne was known by the nickname 'Rock', and he possessed the ability to turn a colorful and effective phrase when ever he was interviewed by the media. Rockne was held in considerable affection by the sports writing fraternity, who generally celebrated his coaching abilities in favorable articles in newspapers and magazines across America.

Rockne was, in many respects, both the coach and the equivalent of the modern sports information director at Notre Dame, as he promoted star players to ultimately promote his team. Rockne was one of the first coaches to cultivate and publicize star players as he did with George Gipp, an outstanding all purpose running back. During the 1924 season, the first in which Notre Dame finished with a national championship title, Rockne relied heavily on a quartet of players that he had trumpeted to the national media as the Four Horsemen of Notre Dame: Harry Stuhldreher, Don Miller, James Crowley, and Elmer Layden. This nickname has endured as one of the most evocative in the history of American college sports.

The most intense rivalry enjoyed by any of Rockne's teams was that with the United States Military Academy, the Army football team. It was during the half time of a game against Army that Rockne delivered one of the most famous of half time speeches, where he is reputed to have urged the Notre Dame team to go out and, "Win one for the Gipper," a reference to the then deceased former Notre Dame star and captain. This phrase was made famous through a 1940 film that starred future American President Ronald Reagan as George Gipp.

Rockne took on the duties of athletic director as well as his coaching duties in 1925. One of his major projects in this role was to direct the construction of a large on campus football stadium. In 1930, Rockne's final season as the Notre Dame coach, the Fighting Irish captured their third national championship under Rockne.

Rockne was a multi-dimensional personality and he was one of the most celebrated Americans of his time. Rockne wrote a regular newspaper column and authored two books during his Notre Dame career. By 1931 he had also begun a second career as a motivational speaker under contract with the Studebaker Corporation, a South Bend auto maker, to deliver inspirational speeches to its sales force. Rockne capitalized on his football fame in the launch of his own automobile company in 1931. Rockne was on his way to Los Angeles to discuss a movie project when the plane carrying him crashed in a Kansas wheat field on March 31, 1931, an event that President Herbert Hoover described as a national loss.

Rockne's enduring legacy is cemented by the fact that his winning percentage as a coach, .881, remains the best ever record among major college programs. Rockne was inducted into the National Football Foundation Hall of Fame in 1951. His statute stands in front of the College Football Hall of Fame.

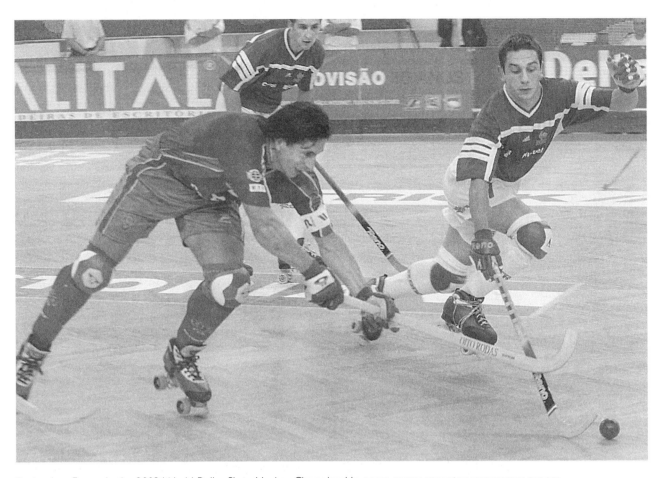

Portugal vs. France in the 2003 World Roller-Skate-Hockey Championship. **JOAO ABREU MIRANDA/AFP/GETTY IMAGES**

**SEE ALSO** Football (American); National Collegiate Athletic Association (NCAA); Sports Coaching.

# Roller hockey

Roller hockey has a long tradition as sport with a cult following in North America and in the various parts of Europe where ice hockey has long been established. Today the game, with two distinct variants, is far closer to the mainstream, with an international championship in each of its formats contested by both men and women, and national governing bodies for roller hockey established in over 20 countries.

Roller hockey was first played using the four-wheeled roller skates invented by James Plimpton (1828–1911) in New York in 1863, a successor to roller skate inventors whose work dated from the mid-1700s. Plimpton's invention lead to the development of the "quad" or "box" skate, with two wheels forward, capable of making a pivot, and two wheels on the rear of the skate.

The first application of the roller skate in another sport was that of roller polo, a game played in the eastern United States in the 1870s, when ice hockey was in its infancy. A game similar to modern roller hockey began in England in the early 1900s, and it was played internationally both before and after World War II. It was this form of roller hockey that was contested as a demonstration sport at the 1992 Barcelona Summer Olympic Games. It is variously known as rink hockey, hardball hockey, quad hockey, or international-style ball hockey. It has specialized rules and tactics.

With the development of the inline skate technology in the late 1980s, which permitted a skater to travel faster than was possible with the traditional quad skates, roller hockey evolved in a new direction. This variant of roller hockey, also known as inline hockey, has spawned leagues across North America and Europe that acted to create both high level competitions as well as those with a recreational sports focus. The Inline International Hockey Federation (IIHF) convened a world championship in 2005 that attracted 16 countries, including nations not associated with ice hockey success, such as Namibia and Taiwan.

The traditional roller hockey game played with the quad roller skate traced elements of its lineage to the sport of field hockey. The players use a stick, referred to as a "cane," that is similar in construction and design to that of a field hockey stick, with the object being to drive a hard rubber ball into the opposing goal. There are four players and the goaltender per team on the playing surface at any given time. The playing surface, which is enclosed by a barrier, may be of variable sizes but tends to be approximately 145 ft long (40 m).

Inline roller hockey is played on a surface similar in dimensions to a standard ice hockey rink, approximately 200 ft (60 m) by 100 ft (30 m). Given the characteristics of the inline skate, which has similar performance capabilities to that of an ice skate, the tactics and the dynamics of inline roller hockey are very similar to those of ice hockey. As with the traditional roller hockey version, inline hockey is played with four players a side, plus a goaltender; the players use conventional ice hockey sticks and the game is played with a ball or a puck, depending on the region where the sport is played.

Both versions of roller hockey require well-developed skating skills, with a premium placed on speed, agility on the skates, and an ability to change directions rapidly. Body checking of the type permitted in ice hockey is illegal in both forms of roller hockey, although the angling of an opposing player away from the ball or puck often leads to significant incidental physical contact.

The physical training necessary to succeed in either variant of roller hockey is similar in many respects to ice hockey strength and training exercises. Roller hockey is a sport contested in short bursts of activity, which places demands on the anaerobic energy systems. The ability to accelerate and turn quickly requires both explosive muscle power as well as the development of available fast-twitch muscle fibers. Interval training, where the athlete must work to a maximum level and then recovers, is essential to this sport, as is a measure of aerobic fitness, to provide the player with a base against which recovery can be made.

Both forms of roller hockey are played on a recreational level in North America, with inline hockey the more likely type of unstructured, or "pick up," game. Like ball hockey, the casual form of hockey played without skates in all ice hockey nations, roller hockey can be played wherever there is a hard, smooth surface.

SEE ALSO Ice hockey; Recreational sports; Roller skates.

# Roller skates

It is likely that the first roller skate was invented in the mid-1700s. The modern roller skate, a device with four wheels, two attached to the forefoot capable of making a pivot, and two wheels attached to the rear, was introduced in 1863 by American James Plimpton (1828–1911). The subsequent development of wheels that rolled easily, using internal ball bearings, greatly enhanced the performance of the roller skate. This design would become known as the "quad" skate, to differentiate it from the later and very popular inline skate.

Dedicated roller skating rinks became popular places of recreation in the 1930s, reflecting a corresponding public interest in various musical genres such as disco into the 1980s. Roller hockey, a game played on an enclosed surface with skaters who used a stick to direct a ball into a goal, also acquired a measure of international status. In the 1950s, roller derby, a sport that blended roller skating and physical, often contrived, contact, gained a solid fan base through the medium of television in North America.

The skateboard was created through the attachment of a wooden platform to roller skate wheels. Skateboarding is a hugely popular recreational activity, especially among young males, throughout the world. Skateboarding is also a competitive sport, with its athletes performing often extremely risky jumps, half pipe maneuvers, and other tricks; competitive skateboarding is often referred to as an extreme sport.

The advent of the inline skate changed roller skating, both in terms of the competitive sporting opportunities it afforded the participant, as well as the recreational opportunities it made available. The inline skate was first developed in the 1980s as a possible off-season training aid for ice hockey players. The skate was constructed in a fashion similar to that of the hockey skate, with four or five wheels aligned in a row, each constructed of a friction-educed plastic compound. An inline skater could travel much faster that a quad skater and users found that the inline design permitted a skater to cross rougher surfaces, such as pockmarked asphalt roads or sidewalks with relative ease. The American company, Rollerblade, Inc., became the industry leader by the mid-1990s, to the point where the company name became synonymous with the skating activity.

Inline skates became standard equipment in several sports, including inline hockey, which is a game played where similar tactics and strategies to those of ice hockey are employed, as the inline skate has similar turning, stopping, and acceleration

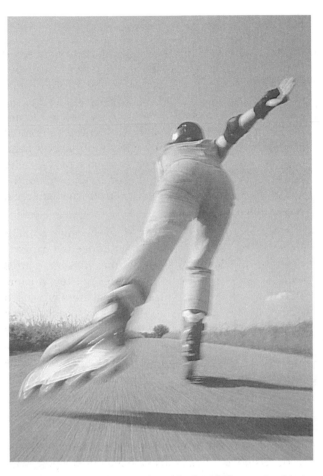

The inline skate was first developed in the 1980s as a possible off-season training aid for ice hockey players. © H. SPICHTINGER/ ZEFA/CORBIS

characteristics to those of the ice hockey skate. Another sport is speed skating, where the inline competitor races on an oval similar to that of the ice skaters, using identical race tactics. Distance races, conducted on courses such as those used by distance runners, ranging from 2-mi (5 km) routes to the marathon (26.2 miles, or 42.2 km). Skaters in these races use the same techniques concerning drafting, the formation of the skating pack, breaks and teamwork as are employed in cycling road races.

For fitness and recreational purposes, inline skating became a means of transport, using urban cycling paths, and as a summer training aid for cross-country skiers, particularly those athletes who employ the skating method of cross-country racing. The inline wheels are attached to a modified ski, and the athlete can replicate the skiing motion with poles and leg action on a road or other hard surface.

Roller skating in all forms can be an aerobic or an anaerobic exercise, depending on the application.

Roller skating requires efficient function of all of the muscle groups that form the leg structure; the gluteal (buttocks), groin, and abdomen are also important to the skating function as the skater must continually maintain balance. The ideal skating posture is similar to the stance often described as an athletic stance, or crouch with the body's center of gravity lowered through the bending of the legs, and the arms positioned for balance and the head erect.

Roller skating is also a sport that places emphasis on a flexible and limber body. Stretching exercises that involve the entire body will assist the athlete in develop the requisite form to achieve speed and to maintain balance through cornering, turning, and any changes of direction.

The most common forms of injury due to roller skating are the form of abrasions known as road rash, caused when the skater slides along the road surface or ground after a fall, and the variety of muscle pulls and strains that may occur through either overexertion or a lack of flexibility in a muscle group.

**SEE ALSO** Abrasions, cuts, lacerations; Endurance exercise; Recreational sports; Road rash; Roller hockey.

# Rowing

Rowing is one of the oldest forms of water transportation known to man. Rowing is the act of propelling a boat through the use of oars, long, bladed levers that are directed against the water for movement. Rowing evolved from the even more ancient methods of canoeing and kayaking, where the water craft was powered by a single person, using a single instrument, the paddle. Over time, ancient peoples, including the Egyptians, developed techniques where one person could use two paddles attached to the gunwales (sides) of the boat by a device later known as an oarlock, or two persons could each use a paddle working in synchronized fashion on opposite sides of a boat for propulsion.

Later cultures, particularly the Romans and the Viking Norsemen, advanced more sophisticated rowboats into an important part of their military campaigns. Rowing has been a means of support for fishermen and other water-related labor for more than 2,000 years. The rowboat remains a staple of transportation in many water-oriented communities today, for both commerce and as a pleasure craft.

Rowing as a sport competition first occurred along the Thames River in London. Rowboats had

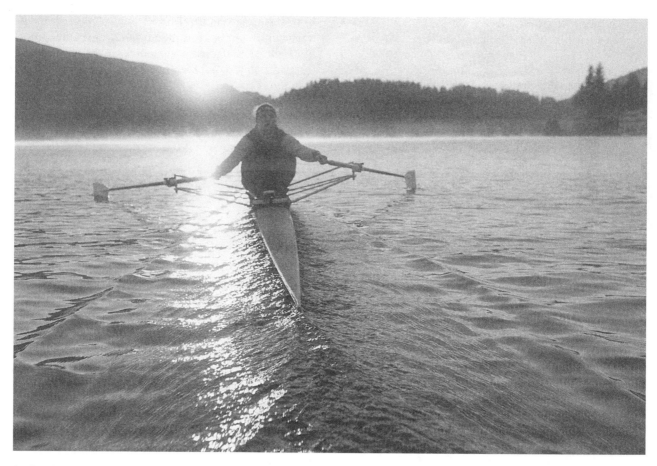

Sculling (rowing) in a single racing shell on the calm waters of Lake Union in Seattle, Washington. © JOEL W. ROGERS/CORBIS

been employed to ferry people and goods across the river as there were very few bridges constructed at that time. Competitions arose as to which oarsman was the fastest in crossing the river, out of which the first rowing race, the Doggett and Coach Badge Race, was held in 1716. The event was open to single competitors, conducted over a 5-mi (8 km) course along the Thames; this race remains an annual event.

Rowing as a competitive sport has a number of traditional events, including the Oxford University/ Cambridge University Boat Race (inaugurated in 1829), the numerous rivalries between American university teams, or crews, a biennial World Championship, and the pinnacle of competitive rowing, the Olympic Games.

With competition came technology and different competitive classes. Among the important developments in racing craft and oar design was the innovative rowing outrigger, first employed by Oxford in 1864. This device permitted the oars of the boat to be mounted farther from the gunwales, which made the boat more stable and permitted the hull of the

boat to become narrower and more hydrodynamic. Another innovation was the sliding seat. In 1870, the Yale University crew developed a seat that slid back and forth with the motion of the oarsmen; this device permits the crew to better use their leg power to drive their bodies and the oars through the water.

The traditional wooden boats gave way to increasingly lighter fiberglass and carbon fiber composite materials, making the boats faster and the oars more responsive.

The rowing classifications begin with the two different methods for the propulsion of the boat, sweep oar races where each rower powers one oar, and sculling, where each rower uses a pair of oars. In the sculling competitions supervised by the international rowing governing body, FISA, races are held in categories known as single scull (one rower), double sculls (two rowers), and quad sculls (four rowers). There are precise regulations as to the permitted dimensions of the boat, the oar specifications, and the material weight of the craft.

In the sweep oar categories, there are similar regulations regarding the boat equipment. Races are held with crews of two, four, and eight athletes. The sweep oar categories may also include a coxswain, or cox, the navigator of the craft who is also responsible for dictating and calling out to the crew of the desired stroke rate. In international competition, there are men's and women's divisions in each rowing category, as well as open weight and lightweight divisions. At an elite level, the ideal rower will possess a tall frame, to best extend the oar over the water, with a good strength-to-weight ratio, as the rower must propel his or her own mass most efficiently.

The standard international racing distance is 1.3 mi (2,000 m) in all racing divisions, with as many as eight boats racing in each heat. The competition is progressive, with the winner of a heat advancing to the next round, and the losers taking part in the *repechage*, a form of playoff among the unsuccessful heat competitors for a reentry into the main competition. Races are most often conducted on water that is protected to some degree from wind and wave action, to permit greater boat stability.

**SEE ALSO** Canoe/kayak; Endurance exercise; Exercise, intermittent; Rowing: Strength and training exercises.

# Rowing: Hydrodynamics

Hydrodynamics is the study of the characteristics and movement of an object in water; hydrodynamics is a branch of the physical science known as fluid dynamics. The hydrodynamics of a craft used in rowing is critical to both the speed of the boat as well as the efficiency with which it can be propelled. Rowing hydrodynamics involves an examination of two separate but related components: the movement of the hull in water and the movement of the oars through the water.

An important aspect in the assessment of the optimum movement of a boat hull through water is the determination of the *drag*, or the resistance exerted by either the oars or the hull of the boat during propulsion. Drag has three separate components that may be physically calculated: skin drag, or frictional resistance, the drag created between the hull and the water moving past it; foam drag, the turbulence created in the water as the hull passes through it; and wave drag, the loss of energy due to the creation of waves by the movement of the hull.

In determining the ideal hydrodynamics for a rowing shell, consideration must also be given to how the shape or contours of the hull will effect the resistance on the boat due to the air passing over it; the hull of the shell, the bodies of the rowers that extend above the hull, and the oars all are subjected to wind resistance. As a general design consideration, the hull of a racing boat accounts for 90% of the drag created against the boat, while the air resistance accounts for the balance.

The object of racing shell design is to achieve the greatest possible speed, while permitting the rowers to move with a measure of stability across the water. Speed is the product of the power generated to move the boat, less the resistance created by the boat. To generate greater speed, power is the variable; to double boat speed, the boat must receive eight times as much power. For these reasons, in a human-powered craft (such as a rowing shell), it is the resistance of the boat that is the focus of the boat design. As a general rule, a longer and slimmer boat will create less resistance in the water, as it creates less displacement (the shell will ride higher in the water), less turbulence, and less wake. Such designs are also less maneuverable, and subject to the design of the hull and the presence of a keel on the underside of the hull, the craft will be less stable. As hydrodynamics are determined with the optimal rowing techniques in mind, any variation from proper rowing form will have a dramatic impact on the performance characteristics of the boat. The rowing stroke has three distinct components—the drag, the catch, and the finish—and any variation that tends to create an up and down force on the hull will make it more resistant in the water. Smooth, level, and rhythmic strokes ensure that the power is applied evenly to the shell, making it move more efficiently.

The finish used on the hull surface is also a factor in the creation or elimination of excess drag. Hydrodynamics is often the subject of extensive testing with scale models operated in water tanks to simulate race course effects, and computer simulation to test both the hull materials and the finish to be applied in terms of the drag created.

The oars are subject to the same design considerations as the hull. A large flat-shaped oar might be a useful tool to move a large amount of water on each stroke, but the oar will create additional drag as it moves through the water, and it will create a lesser but significant amount of air resistance on each stroke when the rower drives the oar backward prior to the stroke. As a general rule, the blade surface area should be as large as the individual rower can manipulate.

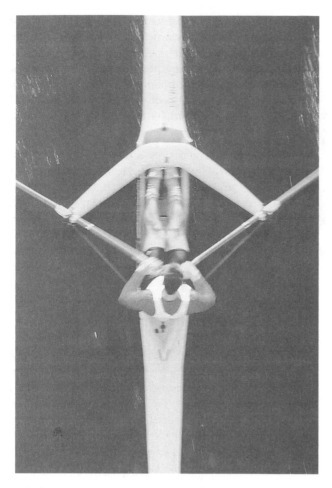

U.S. Olympic rower Jennifer Devine rows her single racing shell into the sunrise on the calm waters of Lake Whatcom in Bellingham, Washington. © JOEL W. ROGERS/CORBIS

Further physical considerations that stem from the material used in the construction of a racing shell that impact its hydrodynamics are the torque and flex of the hull. The stiffer the hull, the less the boat will tend to flex or bend on the delivery of each stroke; the bigger the boat, the larger the crew, the greater that these forces can be. Any deviation from the direction of the craft due to flex or torque will diminish its potential speed.

SEE ALSO Canoe/kayak: Hydrodynamics; Cricket: The physics of how the ball is bowled; Rowing; Soccer: Bending the ball; Water.

# Rowing strength and training exercises

Rowing is a demanding sport that requires a very high level of overall fitness from its participants.

Whether the athlete rows alone as a single sculler, or as a part of an eight-person crew, an effective rowing stroke is a well-balanced combination of technique, power, and endurance.

The sometimes contradictory physical demands of strength and endurance result from the repetitive nature of the basic rowing stroke. The rower is positioned on a sliding seat, with the feet of the athlete affixed to the frame of the racing shell through straps. The slide back and forth by the rower is accomplished through the push generated on each stroke by the rower's legs, and a pull back to the starting position that results from the actions of the oars and the resistance of the stroke in the water. A much as 60% of the power generated in a rowing stroke is developed in the legs and core (trunk) of the body.

An ideal rower will be tall and powerful, so as to both obtain the best leverage on the oar as it extends through the rowing stroke. A typical male Olympic rower in the men's eight will be over 6 ft 3 in tall (1.8 m) and weigh over 230 lb (105 kg). Height usually will provide the rower with a more optimum strength-to-weight ratio; the lighter the boat crew, the faster the boat will go provided the amount of power remains constant. The speed of the boat is the product of the available power, less the resistance to the boat as it moves through the water; the heavier the craft, including its occupants, the generally greater the degree of resistance against the water.

While rowing may present to the uninitiated as a relatively simple contest of human muscle power versus water, the mechanics of the rowing stroke are highly technical, especially when considered as part of a larger rowing crew that must move with complete synchronicity. Sole training and group training must be coordinated to achieve this end. The specific parts of the rowing stroke can be exercised on the water; one example is the use of a bungee cord or similar device to slow the progress of the oar and make the effort of rowing more difficult. Many rowers use interval training principles while on the water to develop both strength as well as recovery.

Rowing exercises must be broadly based to achieve these various performance goals. The development of technical rowing skills will be done primarily upon the water. A solo sculler or a crew can practice such aspects of a competition as the start, changes in cadence, and general unified strokes. Crews will sometimes use a large indoor swimming pool as a simulator, with the boat tethered, as a practice facility. Rowers can also use a stationary training device known as an ergometric rowing machine to simulate the resistance encountered in the rowing motion; these machines have the advantage of having a variable resistance.

The training that is nonspecific to the rowing stroke must be specific to the enhancement of the balance of power and endurance. The amount of the total training volume that a rower should devote to weight training is the subject of debate. In some countries, the national rowing program directs its athletes to engage in a hard weight workout two times per week; in others, the weight training may constitute up to one-third of the total training volume. There is no question that strength training cannot be left to the natural consequences of rowing participation, if the athlete is to improve on the water.

The power aspect of the power/endurance continuum can be developed through a focused total-body weight training program, one that combines free weights, exercise machines, plyometrics exercises, and leg training exercises such as squats, which mimic the drive of the legs forward and backward during the rowing stroke.

Endurance training will focus on cardiovascular fitness, which includes the various aspects of the body's ability to both row at a high speed, which is a function of the rower's stroke rate, as well as the rower's recovery from high intensity effort. One important component for the rower is the ability to use oxygen at the highest possible level, the $VO_2max$ of the athlete. In addition to rowing, running, both over distances as well as through interval sprints, and cycling are cross training devices that will aid the rower in this respect.

As rowing places significant and often explosive stresses on a number of large muscle groups, often while the athlete is in a seated position, stretching and flexibility exercises are essential to the maintenance of balance throughout these muscle groups.

**SEE ALSO** Canoe/kayak; Cross training; Exercise, intermittent; Rowing; Stretching and flexibility.

# Rugby

Rugby is the only major sport in the world named not for the nature of its primary element, but for the place where the game is reputed to have been invented. In 1823, near the English town of Rugby, the version of the soccer game then being played at Rugby School was varied to permit a player to handle the ball and carry it toward the opponent's goal. The sport quickly evolved to include the tackling of any ball-carrying opponents. The rules of rugby were not entirely formalized until approximately 1845, and by 1871, an association known as the Rugby Football Union was created and the rules of the sport were codified.

Rugby, or a game very similar to it, was first exported to North America by the British soldiers of the Quebec military garrison in the 1860s. Through games played against McGill University of Montreal, rugby became popular with the universities of the northeastern United States. The American form of rugby evolved once more into the sport now known as American football. Rugby, cricket, cross-country running, and soccer (in its organized form) represent four great English sports exports of the late 1800s.

It is said that the essential difference between soccer and rugby may be stated as a credo, that "soccer is a gentleman's game played by toughs, and rugby is a tough's game, played by gentlemen." Rugby permits and encourages significant physical contact, and one of the noteworthy features of the sport is that unlike American football and its specialized play, every player on the rugby field must have a basic command of all physical aspects of the sport: running, tackling, passing, kicking, and carrying the ball.

The basic rules of rugby are that the game is most commonly played with 15 players to a side; the game of seven per side employs the same rules of play regarding scoring and physical contact, with necessary modifications. The game is composed of two 40-minute halves. The rugby field (pitch) is 110 yd (100 m) from goal to goal, and a maximum of 75 yd (68 m) wide; the area behind the goal is a maximum of 24 yd deep (20 m). Due to the nature of the sport and the fact that the players wear very little protective equipment, natural grass surfaces are preferred.

The rugby ball is a rounded oblong shape, approximately 12 in (between 280 cm and 300 cm) long and 26 in (620 cm) in circumference; the chief objects of the game are to either advance the ball across the opponent's goal line for a "try," worth four points, or to kick the ball through the uprights of the opponent's goal for either a penalty, worth three points, or a drop goal, also worth three points. When a team scores a try, they may kick for a conversion worth two points. The shape of a rugby ball makes it conducive to the dropkick.

The 15 players play positions that are divided into two general groups, determined by their respective roles on the field. There are eight forwards, who are responsible for much of the effort to gain territorial advantage on the field, and seven backs, who tend to be the chief ball handlers and kickers. The player responsible for much of the coordination of the rugby team's attack is the "scrum half"; the fastest player on a rugby team is often the wing, who plays on the outside of the team formation.

The players are permitted to advance the ball towards the opposing goal line by running with the ball, kicking the ball, and passing the ball, so long as their teammate is behind them, as no player can be ahead of a teammate with the ball, the concept known as being onside. When the referee determines that a minor violation of the rules has occurred, the teams will form a "scrum," where the eight forwards on each team, known as the "pack," lock onto each other and attempt to obtain control of the ball that is placed into the scrum by one of the scrum halfbacks. The line of scrummage, the imaginary boundary between the two scrums, became the well-known expression in the line play in American football that is similar to the formation of the two rugby scrums.

When the ball goes out of bounds, the ball is returned to the field of play through a formation known as a "line out," where the forwards from each team form a line facing the in-bounding player, who throws the ball down the line, where the forwards attempt to either catch the ball or tip it to one of the teammates.

Although a rough and often fiercely physical game, rugby has strict rules regarding tackling. A player may tackle another player only when he has possession of the ball, and blocking or other types of physical interference are illegal. The tackle must not be delivered to the head or otherwise be done with a clothesline or spearing mechanism. Tripping, holding, or otherwise striking another player beyond the scope of a proper tackle will usually result in a penalty at the spot of the infraction. More serious breaches of the rule, such as kicking or punching an opponent, will commonly result in the offender's ejection. If ejected, a player may not be replaced for the balance of the game.

As with other English sport exports, rugby first flourished in the countries of the former British Empire. In addition to American football, Australian Rules Football is also a derivative of rugby. Rugby has been played for a considerable period in professional leagues centered in England, France, Australia, New Zealand, and South Africa. Rugby League, in contrast to the international game that is sometime referred to

Rugby Union, is a form of professional rugby popular in Great Britain, with 13 players per side and a modified scoring system for tries, penalties, and convert kicks.

Rugby first became prominent as an international sport through elite regional championships. The first of these was the Four Nations Cup, which began as an annual competition in 1882 between England, Scotland, Ireland, and Wales. France joined the group in 1910, and the current Six Nations Cup championship includes Italy. Rugby is played professionally in various parts of Europe, South America, and Australasia. Most of the world's competitive players tend to belong to rugby club teams, affiliated with a university or an adult volunteer-based amateur organization.

The Tri Nations Cup became an annual fixture between the rugby powers of Australia, New Zealand, and South Africa in 1996. In addition to these formal regional championships, the concept of the rugby tour is a sporting endeavor not replicated in other major sports. In a rugby tour, one of the acknowledged powerhouses of international rugby will play a series of games, often including strong local teams as well as the national team of the host country. The 2004 tour of Australia and New Zealand by the British Lions, an aggregation of some of the top English and British Isles players, is typical of the high level rugby played by touring national teams assembled by the international rugby powers.

As with many other championships, the World Cup of rugby has become the premier contest in the sport. Rugby is played officially in over 100 countries, and the World Cup, inaugurated in 1987 as a quadrennial event, is fiercely contested. In addition to the traditional powers of the sport whose roots extend to England, countries such as Argentina, Italy, Fiji, the United States, and Western Samoa all are usually ranked among the top 15 rugby nations. The World Cup and all aspects of international competition are governed by the International Rugby Board (IRB), founded in 1886. The IRB has vigorously promoted women's rugby, played according to the same rules as the men's game. Women's rugby has enjoyed significant growth throughout the traditional rugby world, also making inroads in North America, where rugby has been primarily a club sport as opposed to a league-structured competition.

Seven-a-side rugby is also contested as a separate World championship event. Seven a side places a greater emphasis on speed and ball handling than does the 15-a-side game, as the two sports are played on identically sized surfaces. The Hong Kong Sevens

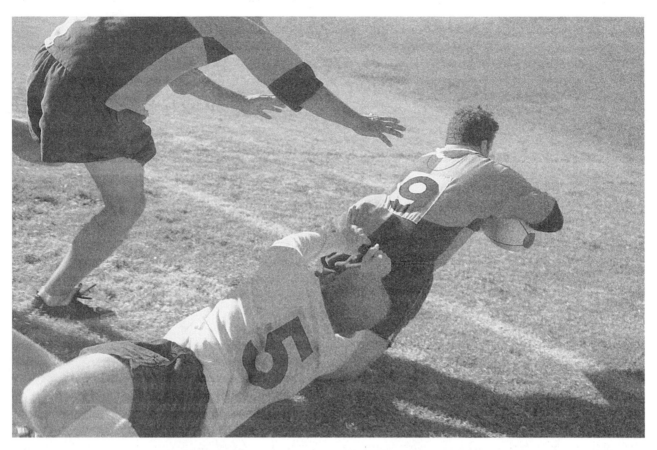

Rugby player scoring a try. © ROYALTY-FREE/CORBIS

is a longstanding and prestigious championship in seven-a-side rugby. Many players, particularly the smaller backs, play both versions of rugby.

The two general classes of players needed for rugby, forwards and backs, tend to encourage two distinct physical specimens to pursue the sport. The backs, who must perform the bulk of the ball handling and offensive thrusts, tend to be smaller and more compact in build. A back must possess sufficient muscle mass and strength to absorb the physical contact, with speed and agility. Forwards must possess the size to be assertive in scrum play, and yet be able to run up and down the field. Sports science analyses of elite rugby competitions suggests that a member of a forward pack will run over 3,000 yd (2,700 m) in an 80-minute contest, in addition to the expenditure of energy necessary to push in the scrum and tackle opponents.

The physical and hard-hitting nature of rugby is a sport paradox, in that the injury rate in contrast to sports such as American football and ice hockey is relatively low. Rugby produces a significant number of minor injuries, such as abrasions, cuts, bruising, and a variety of soft tissue injuries; the nature of scrum play often causes external injuries to the ears of the forwards (long-time forwards often exhibit the lumps of the surface of the ears similar to a boxer's "cauliflower ear") and broken noses are not uncommon. Significant physical damage such as a fractured leg or seriously damaged knee joints is relatively rare. The strict limits as to how an opponent may be tackled, coupled with the defined rules for scrum play, contribute to this relative degree of safety for the participants, as does the fact that, unlike American football and ice hockey, rugby does not permit protective gear that can be used as a offensive weapon.

**SEE ALSO** Cross training; Football (American); International federations; Rubgy: Strength training and exercises; Soccer.

# Rugby: The mechanics of the dropkick

The rugby dropkick is a technique that may be employed at any time on any part of the field by a player seeking to either score or to create an advantageous field position for the team. The dropkick is most effective as an offensive weapon when employed to attempt a drop goal, a kick that results in the ball traveling through the goalposts for three points.

There are no rules limiting who on the rugby field may attempt a drop goal. Typically, as the backs tend to handle the ball more often in the course of a game, they will be most proficient in this technique. Teams will often create offensive sets where they can put the ball in the hands of their best dropkicker to attempt a drop goal at an appropriate time. The dropkick is distinct from placekicking—when the ball is placed in a stationary position and the kicker runs up to kick it. Generally placekicks occur during conversions taken after a try or a penalty.

The mechanics of the dropkick begin with an understanding of the ball and its dynamics as it travels through the air. A rugby ball is oblong shaped, approximately 12 in (300 cm) long and 25 in (620 cm) in circumference, constructed of leather or a similar synthetic composite, with four separate panels and a stitched seam. The rugby ball is distinct from the round soccer ball and the less oblong, narrower American football. When kicked correctly, the rugby ball will spin on its axis in an aerodynamic spiral, and it is capable of being sent over 60 yd (52 m) by a skilled dropkicker.

The primary object of a dropkick is to strike the ball with the kicking foot the instant after the ball has been dropped to the playing surface. The progression made by the kicker to deliver an effective dropkick begins with the kicker holding the ball with two hands, positioned on either side of the ball, with the seam of the ball away from the kicker's body, toward the intended target. If the kicker is moving with the ball prior to the intended kick, the player will come to a stop, even for a brief period of time, to ensure that the mechanics of the kick can be executed from a stable body position. The ball ideally will be angled away from the kicker at an approximate 45° position, with the kicker's arms extended from the body. The kicker will seek to swing the kicking foot through the ball; for this reason, the kicker will first firmly plant the non-kicking foot into the playing surface, so as to maintain maximum stability on impact. As the kicking foot will usually follow a slightly sweeping motion, as opposed to a straight-on approach, the body of the kicker may be leaning at a slight angle away from perpendicular to the surface just before impact.

The ball is dropped to the ground, with care that the angle at which it was held by the kicker is

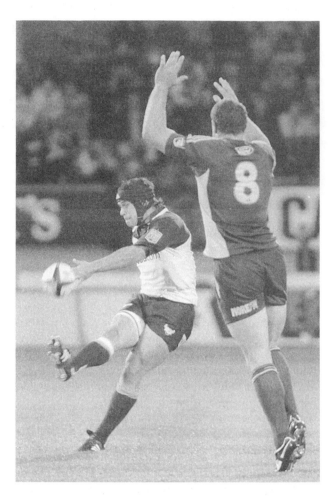

Rugby player attempting a drop goal. PHOTO BY ROSS LAND/ GETTY IMAGES.

preserved in its downward flight. The kicker will try to ensure that the point of the oblong makes contact with the surface, and not any greater portion of the ball. The kicker will then endeavor to strike the ball with the kicking foot the instant after the point of the ball has struck the ground. At this moment, the kicker's foot will be positioned in a downward (planter flexion) position to permit the length of the foot from the approximate point of the big toe joint through the instep to make contact with the ball. To achieve the desired height, trajectory, and distance on the dropkick, the kicking foot and leg will be in a smooth, powerful motion to generate a follow-through; the kicker's arms are generally positioned away from the body, once the ball is dropped, to provide balance.

Unlike the American football placekicker, the dropkicker will often resolve to attempt a drop goal in the open field due to an advantageous game circumstance. The kicker must develop a kicking rhythm that can be employed almost instantaneously.

The dropkick remains a legal tactic in American football, a reminder of the rugby roots of that sport. In 2006, quarterback Doug Flutie successfully executed a football dropkick for the first time in over 60 years, from a distance of 20 yd (17 m). Flutie's feat attracted significant media attention in North America. However, such a dropkick is entirely routine in rugby.

SEE ALSO Football (American); Rugby; Soccer: Bending the ball.

# Rugby strength training and exercises

As a multidimensional sport that places a variety of physical demands on the athletes, rugby training must be comprehensive in its scope. Every player on the field must possess a basic level of ability in the five major physical components of the of rugby: running, tackling, ball carrying, passing, and kicking. The various rugby-specific techniques needed to advance the abilities of the player cannot exist without these fundamentals.

Each of these fundamental skills must be developed in relation to the position played by the athlete. Rugby has 15 players per team (often referred to as a side), of whom eight are "forwards," who play in the more physical "pack" that scrums the ball. The forwards are primarily responsible for creating a territorial advantage for the team on the field. The remaining seven players are the "backs," who are aligned behind the forwards, starting with the scrum half who handles the ball most frequently, fanning out to the wing.

As a general rule, the forwards are the largest and strongest rugby players, and the backs are the most adept in ball handling, kicking, and running. While no successful rugby player can be a one-dimensional player, responsible for a limited series of physical tasks, the strength training and exercises devised for rugby athletes must balance the overall skills required by all players with those that are position-specific.

The strength training applicable to all rugby players will require overall muscular explosiveness, both in delivering a tackle, as well as in developing the acceleration necessary to sprint effectively. Players also need muscular endurance both to compete throughout an 80-minute game and to effectively recover from that exertion. Besides coordination and agility, musculoskeletal flexibility is important for the players. The better the range of motion the athletes can develop in the joints, the more responsive and the less likely they are to sustain a serious joint injury. For flexibility, conventional free weight training and dedicated stretching and flexibility exercises are most useful. Another critical component for players is muscular balance, particularly between the quadriceps and the hamstrings, which are subjected to both the stresses of running as well as the forces of tackling. A balance of the respective strengths of the quadriceps to the hamstrings in the approximate ratio of 3:2 is the goal.

The specific training needs of the forwards begin with their considerable size. At an international level, a forward may run over 3,000 yd (2,700 m) in the course of a contest. It is not uncommon for an elite forward to weight over 240 lb (109 kg); the larger the athlete, the more difficult the player will be to either tackle or to push in the opposing scrum. Comprehensive rugby forward training is an application of the principles of developing an ideal strength-to-weight ratio. Endurance training that is less stressful on the athlete's legs and joints is cycling or swimming. For the large player interval running achieves the dual effect of both running training and building the speed and explosiveness necessary on the field.

The forwards must possess overall muscular strength; much of the physical efforts they expend during a game are in the scrum, where significant energy is delivered through the drive of the athletes' legs to move the scrum forward. Leg training, such as squats, is provided by a scrum machine—a device constructed on a weighted sled—and replicates the forces experienced in the scrum. The scrum machine employs the same training principles as the American football blocking sled; it is a useful strength trainer because the athlete may derive the benefits of resistance and the opportunity to practice particular physical techniques used in scrum play.

The success of a rugby back will blend focused strength training, particularly in developing both speed and running power, with the muscular strength to combat tackles delivered by fast-moving or much larger players. Running training must emphasize the explosive nature of rugby, with both straight ahead and lateral movement. Plyometrics training and interval running assist in this development. Agility training may be incorporated into basic running movements through zig zag drills, where the athlete follows a predetermined pattern on a field or playing surface. Intervals that require the player to move backward, to simulate the fielding of a rugby kick (retro running), also build strength, reaction, and leg muscle balance.

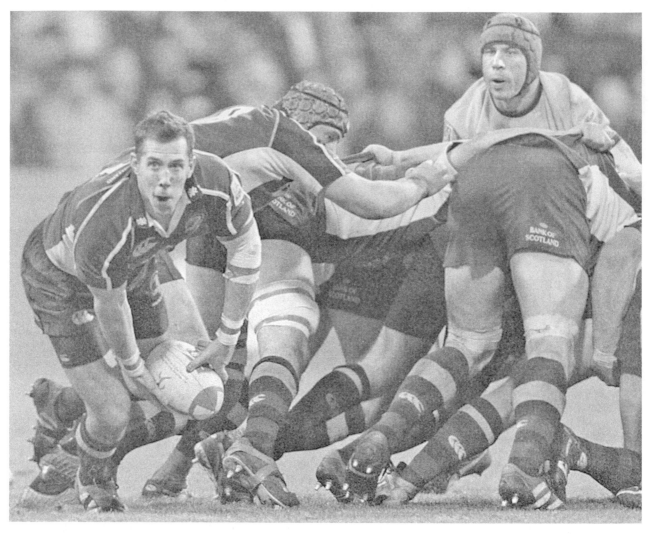

The strength training applicable to all rugby players will require overall muscular explosiveness. MARTIN BUREAU/AFP/GETTY IMAGES.

The backs must also possess an appropriate strength to weight ratio, for reasons counter to those of the forwards. A rugby back may run upward of 5,000 yards (4,500 m) in a game, much of the distance covered at a significant speed. The back must be light enough to move quickly, yet strong enough to sustain the multitude of blows encountered during an 80-minute game.

SEE ALSO Cross training; Exercise, intermittent; Free weights; Muscle mass and strength; Stretching and flexibility.

## Runner's stitch

Runner's stitch is the one condition that almost certainly befalls every runner at some time in either training or competitive circumstances. Known as a side stitch, or by the technical term exercise-related transient abdominal pain, runner's stitch is a painful but entirely transient and correctable physical problem. There are many explanations tendered through sports science as to its cause.

Runner's stitch is a painful cramping or stabbing sensation that is experienced by a runner during the course of the activity. The pain usually is felt most sharply under the rib cage, in the vicinity of the diaphragm and upper abdomen. In some cases, the pain will also seem to radiate to the runner's shoulder. Sometimes, the stitch will either slow the runner or immobilize him or her for a brief period while he or she endeavors to recover from the effects of the stitch. Although precise data on the point has never been gathered, there is strong anecdotal evidence in the running community that suggests that runner's stitch is more common among inexperienced or novice runners than among veteran athletes.

While the stitch manifests itself as a cramp, the accepted possible causes of the condition are wide ranging. It could occur due to impaired blood flow, or ischemia, to the abdomen and diaphragm during exercise. Another condition is the irritation of the muscle walls of the abdomen through the repetitive movements of running (the nerve structure from the abdomen ultimately radiates to the shoulders, accounting for the sensation sometimes felt there with the onset of a stitch. Stress placed on the connective tissues that support the diaphragm through movement occurs when the athlete has been breathing quickly, introducing short or shallow breaths into the lungs, and the diaphragm muscles may become stressed. In a related fashion, it is also believed that running will particularly affect the ligaments that hold the liver in place relative to the diaphragm (the liver is positioned immediately below the diaphragm), the repetitive bouncing motion created by the running stride creates undue tension on these ligaments that may create a source of stitch pain. Another possible cause of runner's stitch is cramping or muscle spasm directly within the muscles of the diaphragm.

In addition to the causes that have been identified as the potential reasons for a runner's stitch, cold weather running is often cited as an aggravator of this condition, as is the consumption of food within one hour of a race or workout.

A runner's stitch can often be remedied during the course of the run. The most effective approach is to stretch the diaphragm structure, which may be accomplished in a number of ways. The first effective diaphragm stretch is alter the breathing pattern; short, shallow breaths place a different stress on the diaphragm than do deep regular breaths. Often, a period of slower speed running or walking while taking very pronounced deep breaths will correct a stitch.

Another effective treatment is the application of manual pressure to the affected area. While the runner slows to a walk, he or she can firmly grasp the location of the stitch below the rib cage, pressing hard into the abdomen. While pressing against the muscles, the runner may then bend at the waist briefly to generate further pressure on the stitch location. The combined effect of the manual pressure with that of the bending of the runner's body often provides an immediate remedy that will permit the runner to resume the pace without recurrence of the stitch.

Biomechanical studies reveal that most runners instinctively coordinate their breathing with the rhythm of their foot strike. When the runner makes a deliberate effort to ensure that the inhalation and exhalation of breath are coordinated with their footwork, the diaphragm will then move in a more synchronized fashion with the body and be less likely to bounce as the runner moves, thus reducing any additional stress on it or the connective tissues that support it.

As with any other type of muscle difficulty, the overall strength of the abdominal muscles may contribute to the formation of a runner's stitch; improved overall fitness is the best prevention for runner's stitch. The runner's stretching program should include exercises directed to the lumbar (low back) and abdominal muscles, which ultimately support the efforts of the diaphragm.

SEE ALSO Cramps; Exercise and fluid replacement; Hydration strategy in distance running; Muscle cramps; Sodium (salt) intake for athletes; Water.

# Running: Cross country

While humans have run on natural trails since the dawn of time, cross-country running began as a competitive sport in England in the early 1800s. With competition centered around both running clubs, known as "harriers," as well as universities, the sport was exported to the United States in the 1870s, where it quickly became a university competition. The National Collegiate Athletic Association (NCAA) has convened national cross-country running championships since 1938. The International Amateur Athletics Federation (IAAF) has organized the world cross-country championships since 1967. Cross-country running is not an Olympic event, although a 3-mi (5-km) cross-country run is the last of the five events in the Olympic modern pentathlon.

Unlike other forms of running, cross country lends itself to team as well as individual competition. In the team format, points are awarded for the position achieved by each team member in the overall race standings. In IAAF competition, there are no standardized world records or course lengths, given the variability of terrain and conditions from course to course. An IAAF championship race course for men must be a minimum of 7.5 mi (12 km) in length; the women's race course must be a minimum of 3.1 mi (5 km).

The significant difference between cross-country running and the running that takes place on the road or the track is the variability of both weather and footing. For this reason, the training for cross-country running events is quite specialized. Many runners will compete in cross-country, road racing, and track events, but it is a rare and exceedingly talented runner who can win on a national or international basis in all three disciplines.

To effectively deal with the combination of terrain and elements, cross-country runners tend to develop a shorter stride than they might employ in a road or track event. By having the heel of the lead foot strike the ground closer to the body, the runner sacrifices stride length for greater stability and balance. The physics of the cross-country running's surface, and the corresponding effect on stride, also differ from those of the road and the track. A harder running surface will produce greater elasticity in the return of energy from the ground into the runner's legs; the softer, off-road trails where cross-country running takes place are less elastic, requiring the athlete to use more energy to cover the same distances. In addition to being more inefficient, in terms of the relationship between the energy expended by the runner and the distance traveled, cross-country running requires greater thigh muscle action and a resulting greater overall effort from the abdominal muscles and the lumbar (lower back) to support the leg action.

Unlike the stride cadence into which a road or track runner will quickly settle to assist in the delivery of an efficient and uniform stride, the cross-country runner must continually adjust the stride length to the terrain and weather conditions. The precise planting of the foot of the cross-country runner is often variable throughout the race. For these reasons, cross-country running is the most difficult of the running sports. Cross-country runners tend to be more versatile and adaptive athletes as a result.

Cross-country running training reflects the diversity of the conditions that an athlete might encounter. As a sport that primarily requires endurance, training that tends to strengthen the cardiovascular system will form a large part of the weekly training volume, particularly those exercises that enhance the body's capacity to process oxygen, the indicator known as $VO_2max$. To address the variability of the terrain, cross-country runners also devote significant time to hill training and interval repeat running. Cross-country running does not place significant emphasis on resistance training in the form of free weights, but some weight training is often relied on as a way of ensuring overall muscular balance and stability.

Stretching and flexibility exercises are an important component of all running training programs. Such exercises assist the cross-country runner in developing optimal range of motion, especially in the hip and leg joints, which assists the athlete in countering the effects of uneven terrain. Stretching also assists the cross-country runner in both warm up and cool down periods when the weather is cold and the muscles more prone to becoming tight. Runners often suffer injuries that are caused by weather and the running surface.

Cross-country running has tactical considerations that differ from other forms of racing. Most cross-country courses require a mass start for all competitors, which often lead directly into a narrow trail where passing a lead runner is difficult. To counter these circumstances, many successful cross-country competitors are front runners, athletes who can get to an early lead and hold their advantage for the entire race.

**SEE ALSO** Cold weather exercise; Exercise, intermittent; Running injuries; Stretching and flexibility.

# Running hurdles

From sprint races through the marathon and beyond, running is one the most elemental and instinctive of human movements. The musculoskeletal structure has evolved to permit power and efficiency in the body as it runs forward or backward. Running as fast as is possible, at any distance, is a demanding athletic goal.

Running the hurdles is the most difficult and the most technically challenging form of running because it involves both the athletic ability to generate muscle power and the science of integrating the speed of maximum forward movement with the efficient grace necessary to clear the hurdles. The elite hurdler has evolved in the past 100 years from a pure sprinter to an accomplished technician.

Hurdling is an ancient sport that was given prominence through its inclusion in the first modern Olympics in 1896; the rules on the competition are simple. Portable barriers are erected at predetermined locations on the track; the runner who reaches the finish line first after clearing the hurdles is the victor. Each runner must remain entirely within his or her own assigned lane of the track, and any interference with

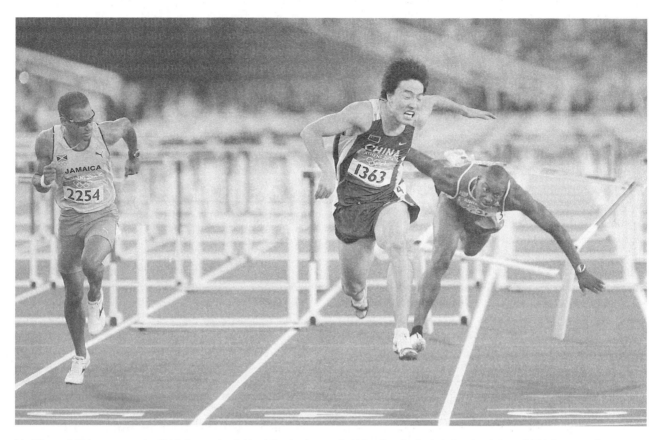

Liu Xiang of China crosses the finish line as he finished first in the men's 110-m hurdle final during the Athens 2004 Summer Olympic Games. **PHOTO BY STUART HANNAGAN/GETTY IMAGES**

the efforts of another competitor will result in disqualification. A runner is not obligated to successfully jump over every one of the hurdles, and it is common for one or more hurdles to be struck by the athlete during the course of a race; the athlete must not deliberately knock down a hurdle or he or she will be disqualified.

In outdoor hurdles races, a variety of distances may be contested; the most common are the 110 m, 200 m, and 400 m distances for men, while women race the 100 m and 400 m hurdles. Sixty meters is the most common indoor distance. In the sprint hurdles (races 200 m and under), the barrier is 42 in (1.2 m) high for men, and 33 in (0.8 m) for women; for the 400 m distance, the respective hurdle heights are 36 in (0.9 m) and 30 in (0.75 m). It is a testament to the difficulty of the hurdles that both the men's decathlon and the women's heptathlon include the hurdles as a component in competition; each is universally regarded as determinative of the title "world's greatest athlete."

All hurdles races begin with a traditional sprint start from the starting blocks. The same techniques employed by a conventional sprinter are those used by the hurdler, each emphasizing an explosive drive with the legs pushed against the fixed starting blocks, with the hips positioned above the hurdler's shoulders in the starting crouch.

Explosive power and reaction to the starter's pistol are of primary importance to the athlete. Hurdlers develop the physical abilities to achieve a strong start by the use of plyometrics exercises, repeat start training (where the starts are practiced in an interval fashion), and similar combinations of power and speed. The hurdler has other considerations that must be built into start training. In the sprint hurdles, the hurdler must plan from the position in the blocks how to run the first hurdle, fixed 15 yd (13.7 m) away, at full speed. In the 400 m hurdles, the first barrier is positioned 49.5 yd (45 m) from the starting blocks.

Hurdlers coordinate their start by determining which leg will be the first leg over the first barrier; the first leg is defined as the lead leg, and the second leg the trail leg. Through practice, the hurdler will know precisely how many strides he or she will take to travel from the starting blocks to the first hurdle; the hurdler will start with the lead leg positioned furthest back in the blocks to ensure the necessary pattern of strides culminating with the predetermined lead leg first over the first hurdle.

To achieve maximum running efficiency, the typical hurdler will take three strides between each sprint hurdle; as a general rule, given that all hurdlers at an elite level have excellent sprinting speed, the more efficient the runner and the fewer strides between hurdles, the more likely the success of the athlete.

The 400-m hurdles is generally regarded as one of the most difficult of races, as it combines the demands of the longest of the sprints with the necessary hurdling skill. The hurdles are spaced farther apart in the 400 m event than in the shorter distances, but the principles of efficiency and economy of stride remain the same. An elite international male hurdler will train to take between 13 and 15 strides between each of the 400 m hurdles; arguably, the greatest of these athletes, Edwin Moses of the United States, two- time Olympic champion who won over 100 consecutive international 400 m hurdles events between 1976 and 1987, raced taking 12 strides between the hurdles.

Hurdlers describe successful racing to require "attacking" the hurdles. The attack is the conversion of sprinting speed into fluid movement over the barrier; too high over the hurdle, and precious time is lost, and too low an approach to the barrier will result in contact with the hurdle and a disruption of the athlete's rhythm.

Hurdlers spend significant portions of their training at work on the individual components of the event. The start requires total body strength, including free weight training, squats, lunges, plyometrics exercises, and the enhancement of explosive speed. Flexibility, to both uncoil from the starting blocks as well as the movement of the body over each hurdle, necessitates stretching and flexibility exercises to promote joint health and the recovery from high intensity exercise. Additionally, the hurdler should perform knee lifts to be able to produce the lift necessary to take the lead leg consistently over the bar, with the trail leg smoothly clearing behind. Plyometrics exercises and bounding drills assist the hurdler in this aspect of the event, as it is the fast-twitch fibers of the leg muscles that are relied upon. Finally, the hurdler must practice take off and landing at each hurdle. The movement should be smooth and incorporated into each stride, with no bounce or deviation.

**SEE ALSO** Exercise, high intensity; Hurdles; Muscle fibers: Fast and slow twitch; Plyometrics; Stretching and flexibility.

# Running injuries

Running is a sport that, due to its diverse nature, presents a significant risk of injury to an athlete. The typical injuries encountered by a 100-m sprint specialist, where the focus of the athlete is the development of explosive power, may differ from those of the cross-country specialist or the marathoner. The sprinter, with a greater preponderance of fast-twitch fibers and likely greater muscular development, will undertake training regimes involving resistance training or other cross training that will likely differ significantly from those of the distance runner, thus exposing each group to different injury risks.

All running disciplines have injuries that result from the presence of one or more common factors. In almost every case of a running injury, one or more of these factors is present as a primary cause or as a contributor to the injury. Overtraining is the increase of training intensity or training volume, which often includes a sudden increase in the use of a particular training technique, such as interval running or hill training. Another contributor to injury is the nature of the training surface; as a very general proposition, hard artificial surfaces contribute to running injuries more often than do softer or natural surfaces. A switch to an unfamiliar surface may also contribute.

Important to preventing injury to the athlete is the quality of the running shoes used, either in terms of the condition of the shoes or with respect to the suitability of the footwear relative to the size and the physical characteristics of the athlete. Approximately 80% of all runners' feet strike the ground with "pronation," where the ankle and foot roll inward on impact; the remaining 20% of runners exhibit "supination," where the foot and ankle move outward. The shoe worn by the athlete must be one designed to accommodate the appropriate motion, or the athlete risks an unhealthy distribution of forces from the foot into the rest of the body on impact.

Structural misalignment, which directs unequal forces into a particular joint or bone, can cause a significant number of injuries. The most common misalignment is unequal leg length. Also, injuries can result from musculoskeletal imbalance, particularly between opposed muscle groups such as the quadriceps and the hamstrings. This imbalance is typically created through poor stretching and flexibility training.

In sprint running, including the hurdles events, the focus of the athlete in both the training that takes place on the track as well resistance training, is the development of explosive power, which the runner seeks to harness as speed. The tremendous forces

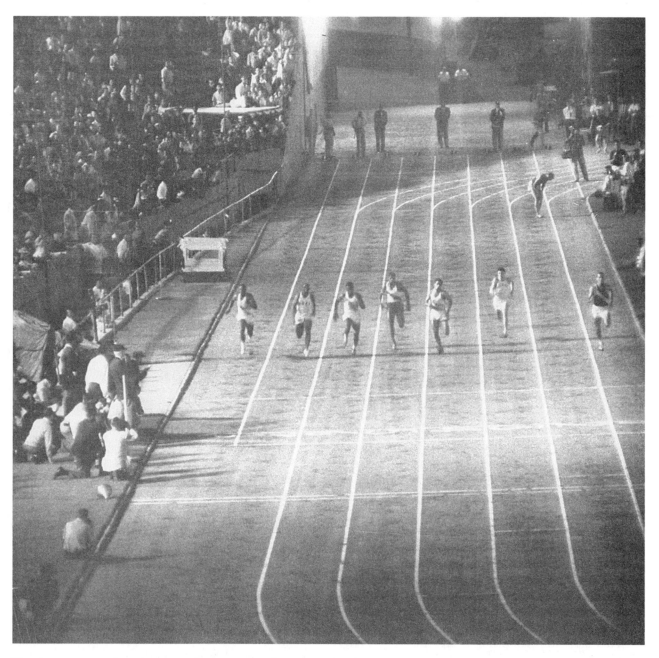

The diverse nature of running events (sprints and hurdles, to marathons) can put runners at a high risk for injuries. **PHOTO BY RALPH CRANE/TIME LIFE PICTURES/GETTY IMAGES**

generated by a sprinter out of the starting blocks place significant stress upon the knee joint, the hamstrings, and the quadriceps. From the crouched position of the start, where the hamstrings hold the knee in the flexed position, the quadriceps will extend the knee explosively at the start and drive the legs forward. It is a well-accepted principle of biomechanics that the ideal proportion in the relative strength of the quadriceps to the hamstring will be approximately 3:2. When this ratio is not observed

(generally the hamstring will be weaker of the two structures), the risk of a serious hamstring pull or tear is significant.

Other possible impacts on the sprinter that arise due to the power of the start are injuries to the Achilles tendon. Repeated movements from the starting blocks when the athlete has a structural imbalance due to muscle power or inflexibility will often irritate the tendon fibers, causing the painful condition of tendonitis, or may, in a worst case, rupture the tendon. The muscles of the lower leg, the gastrocnemius and soleus, are also at risk due to the movement delivered at the instant of the push off from the blocks, but in most cases the Achilles tendon bears the greater brunt of stress that may be magnified through a muscular imbalance. The groin muscles also have exposure to similar injury due to the function that they perform in sprint starts, the stabilizing of the body as it bursts forward.

Middle distance runners who train and compete primarily on hard surfaces as opposed to the newer cushioned track surfaces often develop plantar fasciitis, the connective tissue injury often diagnosed in conjunction with the formation of heel spurs on the bone of the affected foot. Research has determined that this condition is often a function of the hard training surface, inadequate attention to footwear (often lightweight racing shoes with less than optimal support through the arch of the foot, the location of the plantar tissue), and poor foot-specific stretching practices.

The popularity of distance running and the marathon that began in the later 1970s has directed corresponding attention to the specific injuries caused in distance running. Repetitive strain injuries, to all aspects of the musculoskeletal structure of the hips, legs, ankles, and feet of runners, are the most common running injuries. All five of the noted common causes of running injuries play a role in the formation of distance runner repetitive strain injuries. Of particular significance to distance runners are the issues of structural imbalance and stretching and flexibility training. What may present as a minor physical problem for the runner who accumulates a total weekly training mileage of 20 miles (35 km) will almost certainly become a full-blown and potentially chronic issue when the training reaches 50 miles (80 km).

The best way to avoid a significant running injury is to develop a comprehensive training plan. Planning requires preparation, which leads to a comprehensive assessment of physical needs. The identification of structural problems to be addressed by footwear selection, possible orthotic use to correct any imbalance, and the devotion to stretching and flexibility as a prevenatative measure are the most important parts of the runner's planning/injury prevention process.

**SEE ALSO** Achilles tendonitis; Common foot injuries; Groin pulls and strains; Iliotibial(IT) band friction; Knee injuries; Lower leg injuries; Osteoarthritis; Thigh and upper leg injuries.

# Running: Marathon

There is no more storied event in the modern Olympics than the marathon, a symbol of both ancient Greece and the heroism of Phillipides, the fabled messenger returning to Athens from battle. The ability of a runner to conquer both the marathon distance as well as the environmental conditions that often accompany such events has an appeal that transcends sport.

It was fitting that another Greek, Spiridon Louis (1873-1940), won the first modern Olympic marathon competition in 1896. His time of 2 hours 50 minutes was achieved on a 24-mile course (40 km); the modern standard distance of 26.2 miles (42.2 km) was established at the London Olympics of 1908, where the race course was lengthened to accommodate the wishes of the reigning monarch, King Edward VII (1841-1910), who wished to view the finish of the race from the balcony of his Windsor Castle home.

Paralleling the interest generated by the first modern Olympic competition, the inaugural Boston Marathon was run in 1897. Arguably the world's most famous road race, the expression "qualifying for Boston" has been a part of the distance-running lexicon for decades. The Boston Marathon is both an elite running championship, as well as a performance goal for the serious recreational runner.

Both the Boston Marathon and the Olympics have crowned and created running legends. Emil Zátopek (1922-2000) won the at the Helsinki Olympics marathon in 1952, only a few days after capturing the 5,000-m and 10,000-m championships; Abebe Bikila (1932-1973) won the 1960 Rome Olympic race running barefoot, and then repeated as champion in 1964 at Tokyo; Bill Rogers won the Boston Marathon four times between 1975 and 1980, and along with countryman and 1972 Olympic champion Frank Shorter, Rogers became an American running icon.

Marathon running has never been far from the public consciousness, given the attention paid to the Olympics and the Boston Marathon, even where recreational marathon participation was low in comparison to other sports. Consequently, information concerning equipment and training methods was not widely circulated beyond the hardcore running community. The first great running boom in North America in the late 1970s brought the marathon and its associated training systems into the mainstream.

Running generally, and marathon running particularly, has experienced a remarkable growth due to a

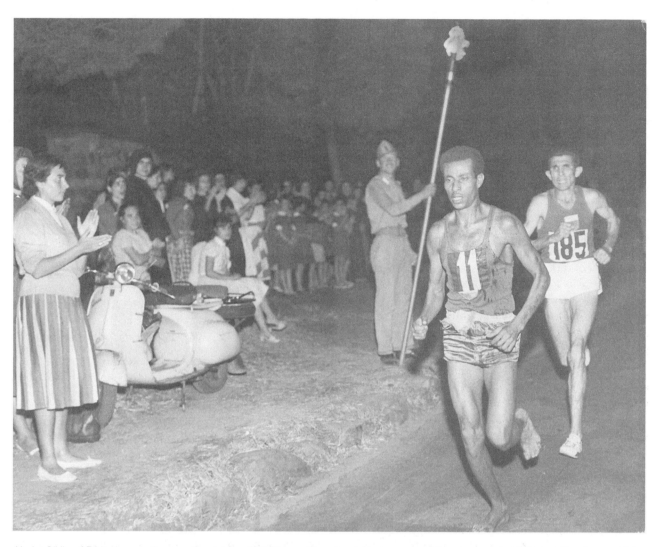

Abebe Bikila of Ethiopia won the marathon at the 1960 Rome Olympics, achieving a new Olympic record at 2 hours, 15 minutes, 16 seconds. **PHOTO BY CENTRAL PRESS/GETTY IMAGES.**

number of factors, the chief of which were a general increase in societal interest in personal fitness, the increased popularity of running among women, much improved running shoe technology and designs, including the waffle sole pioneered by Bill Bowerman, all joined with the social aspects of organized races. Training for and completing a marathon became a recognized athletic achievement, one that had a certain cachet for the recreational athlete.

The advent of the professional runner and prize money races also contributed to the marathon boom. London, New York, Rotterdam, Chicago, and numerous other major cities sought to attract large fields to their races by offering significant prizes to the elite racers, while creating an "event" atmosphere, designed to induce the recreational runner to attend.

The worldwide marathon boom is reflected in the data regarding the best times achieved in the marathon by men and women. From a best of 2 hours 50 minutes in 1910, the men's world record in 2005 had fallen to 2 hours 4 minutes. From 1967, when Kathryn Switzer became the first woman to participate in the previously male-only Boston Marathon, the best female marathon times have steadily fallen as participation levels have risen. The 2 hours 48 minutes standard set in 1979 has been reduced to the 2005 world record of 2 hours 15 minutes.

One of the attractions of the marathon is that, with training, almost anyone can physically complete the distance. Unlike team sports, the recreational runner and the elite racer are physically competing in an identical race; only the competitive result is different. Each is exposed to the same physical and mental stresses over the marathon distance, and each must approach their respective regimes in a similar fashion. Overuse injuries, brought on by excessive training or improper attention to rest and recovery, are the cause of the greatest number of physical problems for each group.

Training methods aside, the ability to run a marathon in a world-class time will be determined to a large degree by body type and related physiological factors such as oxygen uptake. Variables such as strength to weight ratio, stride length, individual biomechanics, and body fat percentage all factor into marathoning success. Sport scientific research conducted over the past 20 years confirms that the ideal male marathoner will typically be 5 ft 8 in (1.70 m) to 6 ft (1.80 m) tall, with weights between 120 lb (55 kg) to 145 lb (66 kg). For women, the ideal build will range between 5 ft 2 in (1.6 m) and 5 ft 10 in (1.75 m) in height, with weights between 90 lb (41 kg) and 125 lbs (56 kg). These optimum builds are ones that are significantly smaller and slighter than those of the typical North American or European male or female; the Olympic and world championship dominance of African marathoners in recent years, particularly those runners from Kenya and Ethiopia, is confirmation of the importance of size and physique in this demanding sport.

**SEE ALSO** Hydration strategy in distance running; Resistance exercise training; Running shoes; Running strength training and exercises.

# Running: Middle distance events

Middle distance races are not the subject of a hard and fast definition. Until approximately 30 years ago, the middle distances were thought to be all track races of between 400 m and the mile. Today, most observers regard a middle distance runner as one who competes in the races that range between 800 m and 5,000 m.

The middle distance runner is an athletic hybrid. These runners must possess excellent aerobic capacity, coupled with the power to drive forward for a finishing kick that may be as long as 300 m to 400 m, the point where almost all middle distance races are decided. The middle distances also require the greatest degree of tactical sense and intelligence in the runner, as the decisions that must be made concerning concepts such as front running, pack position, or the timing of an accelerating burst will all be determinative. The absolutely fastest or strongest runner does not always win a middle distance race.

While the men's 100-m Olympic championship is the most glamorous running event in the world, and the Boston Marathon is likely the best-known race, the one-mile race has a fabled history. The pursuit of the four-minute barrier in the mile by Roger Bannister of England, challenged by John Landy of Australia and Wes Santee of the United States, captured international sporting attention through the early 1950s, as did the later battles of Sebastian Coe and Steve Ovett in the late 1970s. American world record holder Jim Ryun and John Walker of New Zealand were two of the most famous international athletes when at the peak of their respective careers. It is a measure of the regard for the one-mile race distance that when the International Amateur Athletic Federation (IAAF) determined in 1976 that all of its records would be maintained in metric measure only, the mile was exempted.

The middle distances place physiological emphasis on a number of factors. The distribution between fast-twitch and slow-twitch muscle fibers in an elite middle distance runner is usually close to a 50% pattern, in keeping with the hybrid qualities of these athletes. To utilize this balance, most middle distance training programs combine aerobic and anaerobic training, with the anaerobic aspect often-intense speed training. In the 1980s, the successful middle distance runners of Africa, often athletes from the Rift Valley region, with an altitude of approximately 7,000 ft (2,200 m), pioneered a middle distance training program. In the program, the runners would warm up by running at a relaxed pace (7 minutes per mile) for approximately 4 mi (6.4 km). They would then run 40 400-m circuits of the track; each 400 m would be run in less than 60 seconds, with no more than one minute rest permitted between the 400 m intervals. Then the athletes would conclude the workout with another 4-mi run similar to that that began the session.

The focus of the African workout, which is extreme for any runner except those who are highly trained, is the mutual development of anaerobic strength (through the short recovery period), with the aerobic training that is supported by the significant volume of running (10 mi/16 km of high intensity track running, with 8 mi/12.8 km of easier unstructured running).

Sprint racing has no particular tactics to be employed; the runners go all out for as long as they can maintain speed. Marathon runners (as well as triathlon and Ironman participants) must employ tactics, but the nature of the event permits such race planning to be made over a relatively long period of time; instantaneous decisions are rare in such races.

Middle distance races are often decided by tactical decisions. In the 800-m race, the runners begin in lanes and they are allowed to get to the inside of the track oval, and thus run the shortest distance possible, after 100 m. The 1 mi/1,500 m begins with all runners behind a gently arcing start line. The runner must make a number of important decisions, each based primarily on the runner's physical attributes. A front running middle distance competitor is one who often tries to wear down the rest of the field with a strong early pace. Racers who possess a well-developed finishing kick will often wait in the pack of runners and attempt to push to the lead over the last 200 m to 300 m. Many athletes will feint a move out of the pack to test the resolve of the other racers. As with any sport that engages a high level of tactical consideration, the successful middle distance runner must spend considerable time developing a resilience and hypercompetitive attitude.

In middle distance races, each lap time is called out to the runners to orient their pace. In some middle distance events, particularly the mile (or the 1,500 m), race promoters may sometimes employ the services of a runner known as a "rabbit," often an accomplished 800-m runner who can take the runners into the second half of the mile at the highest possible pace. Rabbits have a long history in elite races.

**SEE ALSO** Muscle fibers: Fast and slow twitch; Running strength training and exercises; Sport performance.

# Running physics

Running, a sporting event and aerobic exercise, is the series of rapid leg movements—coordinated with arm motions—through long strides while on foot. To be considered an act of running, both feet must be held off the ground at regularly spaced brief intervals. Running is considered the fastest means for a human to move while on foot. Organized running events are part of the sport called track and field—those events performed on a running track. Such running events include the 100-, 200-, 800-, 1,500-, and 5,000-m runs. Longer running events include marathon races that are often run as a distance of 26.2 mi (42.2 km) and in other events as distances of 50 mi (80 km) or longer.

The runner's objective is to travel a given distance in a certain amount of time. When competing in a race, that amount of time becomes the least amount of time possible. In any case, to maximize the efficiency of running, the application of physical concepts is helpful. For instance, the speed of a runner is determined by the distance traveled with each stride (stride length) and the number of strides taken in a given amount of time (stride frequency, sometimes also called cadence). Stride length times stride frequency equals speed. For instance, five ft (1.5 m) per stride times three strides per second equals a speed of 15 ft (4.5 m) per second. To increase one's speed, a runner must simply increase one parameter without causing the other parameter to be reduced by a (more) comparable amount. For instance, to increase the stride frequency to four strides per second by reducing the stride length to 4 ft (1.2 m) per stride would result in a speed of 16 ft (4.8 m) per second—a good tradeoff between stride length and stride frequency.

The length of each stride taken by a runner is considered the sum of three separate distances. The takeoff distance is the horizontal distance that the body's center of mass (CoM) is ahead of the toe of the front (leading) foot at the instant the rear (trailing) foot leaves the ground. The flight distance is the horizontal distance that the body's CoM travels while the runner is in the air. The landing distance is the horizontal distance that the toe of the leading foot is ahead of the CoM at the instant the runner lands. These distances can also be further broken down to speed of release, height of release, angle of release, and air resistance.

The frequency of each stride involves the time of the stride, which can be further broken down to time on the ground and time in the air. During running, each foot contacts the ground for only a brief amount of time. At that moment, an impulsive force powers the body along a parabolic trajectory until the opposite foot touches the ground. At the instant that the foot leaves the ground, the vertical (upward) component of velocity for the body's CoM should be equal to its horizontal (forward) velocity in order to produce maximum range before the opposite foot hits the ground. Energy is depleted in raising the body's CoM for each stride. This energy is not recovered when the CoM is lowered again. The more that the up and down movement is minimized, the smaller amount of energy will be expended in motion that is not used to move forward. Up and down movement can be minimized by leaning the body forward while running. Such movement adds more horizontal component to the energy usage and, thus, contributes to a faster running speed with less energy expended.

In order to further minimize expenditure of wasted energy, both the arms and legs should be bent as much as possible. Hands and arms are swung from the shoulders and feet and legs are swung from the hips, similar to the swinging of a pendulum (from fingertip to shoulders and toe to hip). This arrangement is based on the principle of conservation of mechanical energy. As a result, the speed of a runner is directly related to the height of swinging objects (such as the length of arms and legs). If the arms and legs are bent while running, such positioning moves the CoM upward, which translates to a faster pace without increasing the amount of energy expended. This application of physics is the reason why runners run with their arms bent at the elbows, while holding their hands close to their waists, and why knees are bent as much as possible and shins are positioned parallel to the ground whenever the legs are swung forward.

**SEE ALSO** Running hurdles; Running strength training and exercises; Running: Marathon; Running: Sprinting.

# Running shoes

Running shoes are the single most important piece of equipment in both track and distance running. A well-constructed shoe, that balances protection of the athlete from undue physical stress with lightweight construction and responsiveness, will assist runners in the achievement of their ultimate goal: to run as fast as possible.

An effective running shoe must combine the features of shock absorbency, motion control when the foot strikes the ground, flexibility and responsiveness, and a measure of durability. Running shoe science began a remarkable progression that included the work of Adi Dassler (1900–1978) of Germany, the founder of Adidas, and the later creations of Bill Bowerman (1911–1999), the American track coach who developed the Nike "waffle" outsole in the early 1970s.

Each component of the modern running shoe has a specific function. The outsole is the outer tread of the shoe; it is usually made from a carbon rubber compound and provides traction for the runner. The midsole is the part of the shoe construction that provides both cushioning and stability to the runner. The midsole will appear to be made of a foam material, usually ethylene vinyl acetate (EVA), an extremely lightweight material, or polyurethane. It is common for running shoes to have a post implanted in the

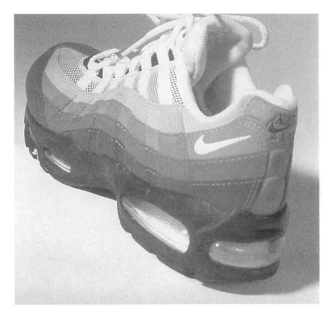

The Nike Air Max running shoe. PHOTO BY JAMES KEYSER/TIME LIFE PICTURES/GETTY IMAGES

midsole to provide further stability. Running shoes often have different densities of materials in the midsole construction, with the medial part of the midsole (inner) composed of a harder EVA, and the lateral (outer) side made of a softer material. This design is intended to counter the effects of "pronation," the inward movement of the foot on the contact with the running surface; 80% of runners tend to pronate. The midsole may also include a liquid or semi-gel, air, or specialized plastic compound to further absorb shock. Most distance runners will generate forces that are approximately three times their body weight on impact with each foot strike.

The upper is the part of the running shoe that encases the foot. It is padded and it is usually a synthetic material and typically washable. The heel counter is a hard, cup-shaped device set against the heel of the runner to promote stability and to limit the movements of the heel on impact (both laterally and vertically).

Many modern running shoes are built to accommodate a foot orthotic, used to correct the structural imbalances that are a primary cause of running injuries.

With each stride, the runner delivers a force through the shoe into the ground, as with classic Newtonian physics, every such action produces an equal and opposite reaction, with forces of impact directed into the foot. The more efficiently such forces may be distributed through shoe construction, the more responsive the shoe to the next stride and the less likely the musculoskeletal structure will be to unduly absorb these forces. The construction of the quintessential perfect running shoe is a marriage of the contrasting features of cushioning and responsiveness.

SEE ALSO Basketball shoes; Foot: Anatomy and physiology; Lower leg injuries; Plantar fasciitis; Running injuries.

# Running: Sprinting

Sprinting includes all races where there is no variation in the effort or the output of the athlete: the common phrase "all-out sprint" is a redundancy—the sprint is the maximum running effort. Race distances may be as short as 60 m for indoor competition; the 400-m race is generally regarded as the longest of the sprints.

While technique is important to the success of a sprinter, muscle strength and the ability to generate power are the overriding considerations. Beginning with the thrust of the runner out of the starting blocks, the entire body of the sprinter will be used to achieve maximum speed—the legs are the primary source of muscle power, with the arm motion an important thrust and counterbalance to the leg action. This desire to generate power means that all elite-level sprinters tend to possess a well-developed, muscular physique. Sprinters also invariably possess a greater number of fast-twitch muscle fibers as opposed to slow-twitch fibers; fast-twitch fibers are those where the neuron, the component of the nervous system that regulates an individual group of muscle fibers within a muscle structure, are "firing," or directing the fibers to move 10 times more quickly than those in the adjacent fibers.

The strength of the runner has a secondary consideration once the runner has left the starting blocks. The start is virtually instant acceleration, which continues for approximately 30 m to 40 m. After 60 m, the runner cannot accelerate any further and success in the race is then determined by how long the runner can maintain top speed, attempting to defeat the forces of deceleration acting on the body. The runner must continue to fully extend their stride without over-striding; the optimum placing of the feet with each stride is at a point in relation to the runner's body where the center of gravity of the runner remains exactly midway between the runner's feet. A shortened stride to endeavor to drive the legs harder and generate greater power will be counter-effective, due to the loss of distance covered by the shorter

stride. There is no perfect stride length, as the height and build of the runner will be the determining factor; but as a general proposition, a taller, powerful runner will tend to be more efficient in the sprints than a shorter, powerful runner.

The essential tactic in sprinting is to go as fast as one can for as long as one can. There are some important sprinting techniques, all of which are applications of the principles of physics, which will often determine sprint success. The first and most important technique is the development of a fluid, yet explosive start. Runners begin from a starting block, positioned to permit the runner to place both feet against a fixed mechanism and generate maximum force. Optimum effect is achieved where the runner's strongest leg is placed in the front block, with the hips raised above the level of the shoulders, for maximum thrust effect. The runner must also react to the starting gun; the starting blocks at elite levels are actually coordinated to the starter; in IAAF competitions, where the runner leaves the blocks less than 0.1 seconds after the gun, the runner is deemed to have committed a false start. Sprinters combine physical and mental training in their start techniques by replicating the start conditions and honing their concentration skills to block out all sounds but that of the starter giving instructions and sounding the gun.

The speed of a sprinter is a function of stride length as opposed to stride frequency; every sprinter will determine the appropriate relationship between those two factors, depending on the size of the runner. Stride frequency, also described as stride turnover, is the cadence that the runner can establish once top speed after the start is established. Runners who over-stride sacrifice the distance achieved with each stride for running efficiency.

The shoes worn by a sprinter are designed to assist in the maintenance of the balance between power and efficiency. A sprinter will wear spikes with a spike pattern on the forefoot only. Most sprinters do not run exclusively on the forefoot, but land on the side of the foot and roll forward to the forefoot for a powerful push off with each stride. Spikes on the rear of the shoe sole would create additional adhesion with the track surface and potentially slow the runner.

The runners' ability in the 200-m and 400-m sprints to run smoothly and effectively through the turns on the track are essential to success. In the 200-m race, the runners must start, proceed through what is the final turn of the 400-m oval, and then finish along a straight. "Running the bend" is the technique for 200-m racing; it is essentially a means in which

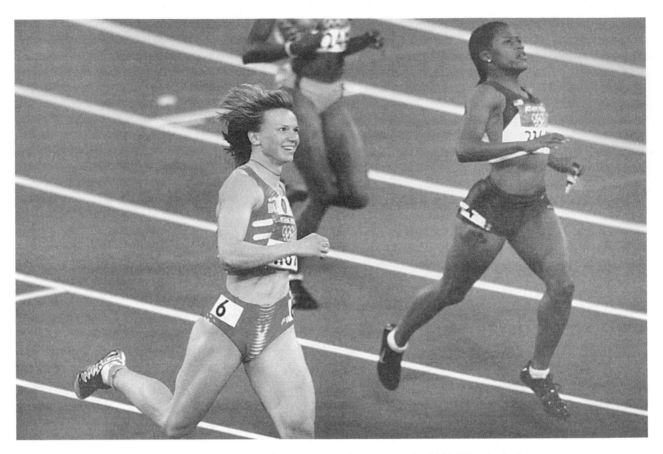

Yuliya Nesterenko of Belarus (left) runs to take the gold medal in the 100-m dash at the 2004 Olympics in Athens.
© S. CARMONA/CORBIS

the runner maintains maximum speed into the turn, with the track then acting much as a slingshot to propel the runner through the bend into the remaining straight. As the runner enters the bend, the runner will drop the shoulder closest to the inside of the oval slightly, to counter the effect of the centrifugal acceleration acting on the body. Four hundred meter racing has similar considerations as 200-m running with respect to running through the turns.

Sprints are often decided by fractions of seconds; lunging for the finish line is inefficient, compared to a thrust with the torso and head that is performed in rhythm with the cadence of the running stride.

**SEE ALSO** Plyometrics; Running strength training and exercises; Stretching and flexibility.

# Running strength training and exercises

Running strength training and exercises were regarded as an oxymoron as recently as 50 years ago. The relationship between running success and overall physical strength was poorly understood; it was believed that intense running workouts, conducted using varying speeds and surfaces, was the key to better performance. A prominent example of this approach is the career of Roger Bannister, the English runner who was the first athlete to break the 4-minute mile barrier; Bannister perfected interval and tempo run training, and he never participated in resistance or free weight training of any kind.

Modern sports science has confirmed the significant benefits of strength training in running, across all running disciplines. Sprinters require the development of maximum explosive power to drive themselves from the starting blocks, and the strength to maintain their speed through to the finish. They will look to resistance training that facilitates the development of overall muscular strength. The arms and the shoulders of a sprinter are essential to maintaining the counterbalance to the thrust of the legs on each stride as the athlete powers through to the finish. A hurdler has similar strength requirements to those of a sprinter in relation to an effective start, with the additional need for a powerful, yet fluid knee

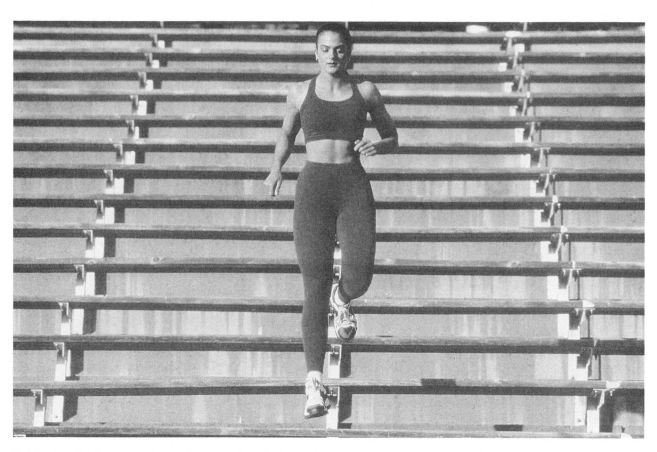

Training including intense running workouts, conducted using varying speeds and surfaces, aids in the development of the athlete's strength and endurance. © ML SINIBALDI/CORBIS

lift and thrust necessary to efficiently clear the barriers. The technical training for hurdles races will also combine the exercises that will enhance speed with the coordination of developing the precision of taking the same number of strides between each hurdle every time.

Middle distance runners, whose events may range in length from the 800 m to the 5,000 m distances, require strength balanced with aerobic endurance. For these athletes, the relationship between strength and weight is an important factor. Middle distances runners will employ training exercises that strike a balance between the fast-twitch muscle fiber speed capabilities and the slow-witch endurance component of these events.

The strength training undertaken by a marathoner is the converse to the approach of the sprinter; muscular power is subordinate to stride efficiency, oxygen uptake ($VO_2$max), and cardiovascular power, but muscle strength in the core muscles of the body will enhance the marathoner's form and the ability to have an effective countering mechanism to the operation of the legs. In every physical endeavor, the human body operates best when it is in balance. Strength training will achieve balance for the marathoner.

Strength training must also be assessed in terms of how the runner will be approaching the competitive season. All sports training, to be effective, should be "periodised." The athletic season, typically assessed with reference to the entire calendar year, is subdivided into the competitive season, the preseason, and the postseason, or off-season. Each of these periods may be further defined to take into account any factor that might impact on the quality or extent of training or competition. A period of travel, or academic or employment obligations are such factors. Within each period, the athlete sets training or competitive objectives. As a general proposition, strength training for running will be more important in the off-season and preseason than during the competitive season, but importance will be balanced against all other physical requirements.

The strength exercises useful to the sprinters and the hurdlers will be emphasized during the buildup and preseason; given the importance of strength to success, most athletes in these disciplines will continue with a modified degree of strength training throughout the year. These athletes will generally embark on strenuous free weight and resistance machine programs that engage the upper and lower body. Traditional routines such as bench press, curls, squats, leg press, and various extension exercises are useful. Sprint athletes also use resistance training in the form of stationary starts pulling a weighted object or employing the drag of a small parachute. These exercises have the additional advantage of simulating an aspect of competition while providing strength development.

All sprint athletes benefit from plyometrics exercises to assist with the development of explosive power in the start blocks. Hurdlers obtain a specific benefit from bounding plyometrics training to provide greater knee lift in clearing the hurdle and landing efficiently.

World-class 800 m and 1500 m races are run at lap times that average between 50 seconds and 60 seconds. The strength to generate a powerful kick over the final 200 m to 300 m is essential to success. These runners cannot be as bulky as a sprinter and expect to move a larger mass efficiently around the track. Middle distance runners seek to balance speed with efficiency through intense interval training, to replicate the kick distance, with high repetition/low weight resistance training; the middle distance runner requires excellent core strength (torso, gluteal, and abdominal muscles) to provide musculoskeletal balance.

Distance runners also benefit from whole body weight training at reduced work volumes. The stronger that the body may be constructed as an integrated unit, the less likely the chance that a muscle injury due to muscle imbalance will occur.

For all runners, strength training must be accompanied by flexibility and stretching exercises. Running, due to its precise and repetitive nature, creates a naturally inflexible muscle environment. Ideally, the runner should stretch before and after all runs; the same routines should be completed before and after all strength training.

SEE ALSO Cross training; Free weights; Resistance exercise training; Stretching and flexibility.

# Ruptured tendons SEE Tendinitis and ruptured tendons

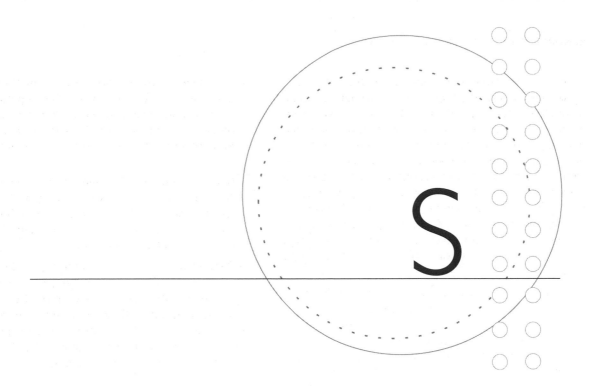

# Sailing

Sails translates the movement of wind into thrust that propels the boat. Sailing has a place in human civilization that likely extends as far back in time as man has possessed the ability to make crafts that could float on water. Sailing has a shorter history as a competitive sport, but it has been one of the most popular and intensely contested of sporting activities throughout the world. People have engaged in the organized racing of sailboats, crafts that range in size from dinghies (small open boats with one sail), to very large, multi-masted ocean going vessels for over 200 years.

Modern competitive sailing is governed by the International Sailing Federation (ISF), whose predecessor organization was founded in 1907. The chief purpose in the formation of the ISF was to bring standardization to the rules of international sailing. Today sailing is a vibrant Olympic sport; there are 11 different Olympic sailing events. In the international arena, the ISF sanctions racing in 81 different categories of sailboats, the largest of which are the multi these boats may be over 60 ft (18 m) in length. Sailing is one international sport where the racing activity on the club and regional levels throughout the world attracts greater interest than Olympic competition.

The best known of the international sailing races, the America's Cup, has been contested since 1851. The racing boats are classed as America's Cup class yachts and adhere to a complicated mathematical formula that considers boat length, beam (width), sail area, hull depth, keel size and dimensions, and other physical characteristics of the boat. Sailors, the sailor's home club, and syndicates that are formed in support of a particular boat, commence an America's Cup competition through the issuance of a formal challenge to race the Cup holder, known as the defender. The technology involved in the design and construction of these crafts is so sophisticated that challenges are mounted and races staged for the Cup in several year intervals.

The beauty and the enduring appeal of the sport of sailing springs from the fact that the principles of sailing are universal, applicable from the smallest of open sail boats, to the most sophisticated America's Cup challenger. The propulsion of a sail boat is achieved through the effect of the wind and combined function of the sails, the hull, and the keel (or centerboard). The techniques employed by a sailor to sail the boat in a particular direction are determined by the force and the direction of the wind.

The function of the sail in powering a boat is simple when the wind is directly behind the sailboat and the intended direction of travel is the same as the wind direction. The sail is positioned to permit the wind to strike it at angle perpendicular to the line of the sail. In this position the wind pushes the sail, and consequently the boat. It is for this reason that when the boat and the wind are moving in the same direction, the boat can never travel faster than the wind. Enlarged billowing sails called spinnakers, provide maximum surface area to catch the following winds.

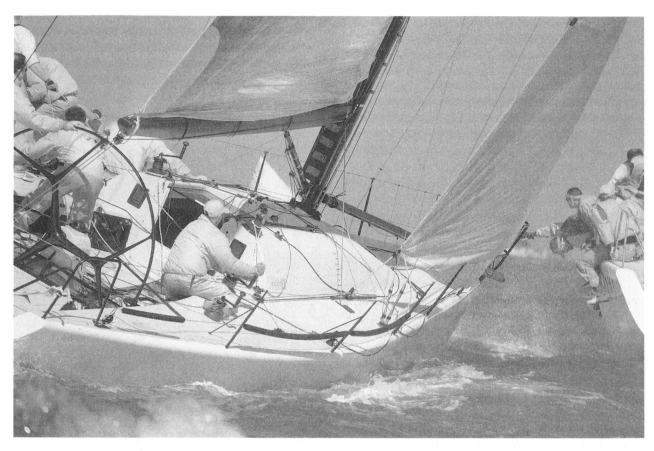

Key West Race Week. © SHARON GREEN/CORBIS

When the wind is moving in a direction that is angled to the direction of the boat, the sail no longer functions simply as a surface against which the force of the wind acts. The sail on a boat, with a curvature similar to an aircraft wing, now has the same relationship to the wind as does an aircraft wing to the air flowing both over and under it. As the wind strikes the leading edge of the surface of a sail at an angle, the airflow separates. The faster moving air naturally creates a pocket of lower air pressure in contrast to the higher air pressure formed on the opposite side of the sail that is in contact with the slower airstream. The sail, and, consequently, the boat will move into the region of lower air pressure.

Sails are airfoils in accord with Bernoulli's equation, which states that static pressure plus dynamic pressure equals total pressure. The sails are designed to maximize lift and minimize drag. The upper surface of a typical airfoil has a curvature greater than that of the lower surface. This extra curvature is known as camber. The straight line, joining the front tip or the leading edge of the airfoil to the rear tip or the trailing edge, is known as the chord line. The

angle of attack is the angle that the chord line forms with the direction of the air stream.

The stagnation point is the point at which the stream of air moving toward the wing divides into two streams, one flowing above and the other flowing below the wing. Air flows faster above a wing with greater camber since the same amount of air has to flow through a narrower space. According to Bernoulli's principle, the faster flowing air exerts less pressure on the top surface, so that the pressure on the lower surface is higher, and there is a net upward force on the wing, creating lift. A sail is a wing oriented along the axis defined by the mast of the boat and so lift becomes a horizontal driving force, a form of thrust, to propel a boat through the water. The camber of a sail is varied by devices that slightly alter the shape of the sail.

A sailboat can be sailed into the wind (upwind) to within approximately 30° of a direct upwind position. So long as the wind direction permits the creation of the two pressure regions on the sail, the wind will power forward movement. Any attempt to sail closer to the direction of the wind causes turbulence and a loss of air contact with the sail surface. Lift, and hence the driving force of the sail, is lost.

The hull of the boat is the physical outer structure that is in contact with the water. The front or nose of the hull is the bow; the rear is the stern. Attached to the hull in the approximate center of the boat is the keel, a larger structure that extends from the hull into the water. The general function of the keel is to provide stability to the boat. The specific purpose of the keel in relation to the function of the sails is to resist any lateral forces created by the wind as it pushes against the sails. If the sailboat did not have a keel, when the wind struck the sails from an angle the boat would be pushed both forward and laterally. The keel operates to convert the lateral forces of the wind into forward motion.

Tacking is the most common steering technique used in sailing. Tacking is the maneuver employed when the destination of the sailboat is in an upwind direction. The sailboat is steered in a series of angular courses forming a zigzag pattern across the water into the wind, to maximize the wind power available. Tacking requires the sailor to use the rudder to change direction, while making a simultaneous shift in the position of the sail to capture the maximum available wind. The boat moves into the wind by taking turns to the left and right of the wind to maintain a proper angle of attack for the sail. The tacking results in net forward motion into the wind with the movement to the left and right of the desired direction of travel offset by the opposing tacks.

The hull of the sailboat and its characteristics are also subject to intense scientific testing as the basis for the hull designs used in racing craft. The performance of a hull in water is a branch of the science known as hydrodynamics. Computer technology permits a significant level of design testing to be done by way of computer simulation, where an infinite manner of variables, including different sail configurations, weight, wind, lake or ocean current, and material design may be examined and tested at a relatively low cost.

SEE ALSO Computer simulations as a training tool; Sailing and steering a sailboat; Windsurfing.

# Sailing physics

Sailing is the control of a vessel moving across a body of water that uses wind power for propulsion. The physics of sailing has many subtleties, and the act of successfully sailing a boat is a combination of art, scientific principles, and the experience of the sailor. Those subtleties will be grounded in three distinct aspects of sailing—the function of the sails, the shape and the configuration of the hull, and the function of the keel.

The sails are the most distinctive physical feature of any wind-powered vessel. The sail is designed to act as a foil, with similar physical properties to those of an aircraft wing. As wind moves across the surface of a sail, the air moves at a higher speed where the wind strikes the surface. The faster moving air produces lower pressure upon the sail than does the slower moving air on the opposite side of the sail. It is a rule of physics, referred to as the Bernoulli principle, that the vessel will move into the area of lower air pressure, in the same fashion that an aircraft wing, angled upwards, will lift when air is directed against it.

If the wind striking a sail is coming from directly behind a sailboat, the boat will travel in the same direction as the wind and at the same speed as the wind. The boat cannot travel faster than the wind speed because the sails block the path of the wind, an act that decelerates the wind. When the wind is striking the sails at an angle toward the direction of travel of the boat, the power of the wind is directed into forward motion through the stabilizing effect of the keel. The keel is the device attached to the hull that extends below the water surface and provides both ballast as well as a counterforce to the wind. The wind force that strikes the sails at an angle to the path of the boat does not take the boat in a lateral direction, because the keel counters all such direction through the creation of opposite pressures in the water.

The function of a sail as a foil means that a boat can be steered upwind (into the wind), so long as the boat is not headed directly into the wind. The degree to which a boat can be sailed upwind varies with the construction of the boat and the type of sails. As a general rule, sails will not act as a wind foil if the wind direction is less than 30° from the centerline of the boat, with the bow first.

Applying these principles, the sailboat is sailed upwind using a combination of the rudder and wind direction to traverse a zigzag path across the water, a technique known as tacking.

Sails on boats large and small are generally controlled by one or more pulleys. A pulley is a type of lever, that may both change the direction of a force applied, or when used in combination, the pulleys may multiply the forces applied to it. The rope found in a common pulley is the lever, and the grooved wheel in which the rope rests is the device used to change the forces.

When a single pulley is employed to move a sail, the amount of force required to move the mass of the sail is unchanged. The pulley makes the action of applying the force easier, as the direction from which the force is applied is adjustable to the convenience of the user. Normally, the more pulleys used to move a sail, the less force required.

As a general rule (although different physical considerations apply to vessels such as windsurfers), the larger the sailboat, the faster it will be able to travel. Where boats are designed to displace water, as in the case of a keel boat, the length of the boat is an important component in determining the physics of the maximum boat speed. The maximum boat speed is referred to as hull speed, calculated using the formula 1.34 multiplied by the square root of the length of the waterline (in feet). The waterline is the location of the hull where the boat rests on the surface. The result provides a maximum hull speed in knots, the measure of speed in nautical miles per hour. (A nautical mile is 1.15 miles, the distance described by 1 minute of 1 degree of longitude.)

As an example, the hull speed of a sailboat with a hull that is 25 ft long at the waterline would be calculated as $1.34 \times 5$, or 6.7 knots.

The boat cannot travel faster than the wave created by the bow of the boat as it moves through the water. Windsurfers are not subject to these considerations because they do not displace water like a keelboat does, but are intended to plane on top of the water. Windsurfers do not push water aside, as does a large keel boat, but skips along the water in the fashion of a stone that is thrown to bounce across the surface of the water.

SEE ALSO Sailing; Sailing and steering a sailboat; Windsurfing.

# Sailing and steering a sailboat

Sailing is the movement of a boat powered by wind across a body of water. The science of steering a sailboat is the application of a series of physical principles that underlie the fundamental relationship between wind speed and direction, the size and shape of the boat, and the characteristics of moving water.

The wind forces acting upon a sail are often compared to the effect of wind upon the wing of an aircraft. A boat may be thought of as possessing two wings, one above the water (the sail), and one below the water (the keel). As wind strikes the sail, the sail acts as a foil, causing the air current striking the sail to move at different speeds on each side of the sail. The side of the sail exposed to slower moving air is subject to greater air pressure, creating lift. Lift is a force that acts perpendicular to the direction of the force created by the air, as lift causes the boat to move in the direction of the higher speed air, which results in lower air pressure on the sail. This effect above water is counterbalanced by the water forces acting upon the keel, the portion of the boat that extends below the waterline to provide both ballast (counterweight) to the boat and to prevent the boat from moving sideways.

The steering of the boat is performed through the combined action of the positioning of the sail, using the sheet (the rope or ropes that control the sail position), and the rudder, an airfoil shaped board attached by a hinge to the stern (rear) of the boat where it immersed in the water. The rudder is controlled by the helmsman (the sailor responsible for steering the boat) through a tiller extension, a mechanism that permits the turning of the rudder by either a steering wheel or on a smaller sailboat, by direct linkage to the rudder called a tiller.

The steering of the sailboat, as a part of the setting and the maintenance of a particular course across the water involves four fundamental sailing manouvers—tacking, jibing, heading up, and bearing away. The combined effects of the sail and the keel mean that the boat may be steered in any direction except directly into the wind. The fastest and most nimble racing vessels can only sail as close to the wind direction by as much as approximately 35% into the wind.

The rudder and the tiller operate as a large lever. A turn is accomplished by pushing the rudder through the water. To turn the boat to the right, the tiller must be pushed to the right; a left turn requires a push to the left. The foil design of the rudder creates a pressure differential that steers the stern of the boat into the low-pressure zone. The bow swings to the opposite direction.

Tacking (also known as "coming about") is a steering concept that recognizes that the boat cannot sail directly into the wind. Tacking to achieve a change in direction is distinct from the "tack" (the direction that a boat may travel). Tacking is the maneuvering of the boat in an upwind direction (against the wind), creating a zigzag motion across the direction of the wind, without ever proceeding directly into the wind, where the sails would be ineffective. The bow of the boat is at all times facing the direction of the wind when the boat is tacked. As the wind moves in a direction across the boat into the sails that is perpendicular to the boat's direction of travel, the boat is not pushed in the direction of the wind due to the drag force exerted by the keel. The drag force acts to negate the wind effect, and as the keel is aligned with the hull of the boat, the boat is directed forward and not sideways. A sailboat will often perform a number of tacking movements to achieve a desired steering result across a body of water. At each tack, the sails are brought from one side of the boat to the other, through the movement of the boom, the pivoting hardware to which the sails are attached, mounted perpendicular to the mast to redirect the force of the wind; the rudder is correspondingly adjusted. In many tacks, depending upon the wind speed, the size and construction of the boat, or the condition of the water, the boat may heel, the crew of the boat will have to move from one side of the boat to the other to stabilize the boat against the forces of the wind during the tacking process.

Jibing (also spelled in various authorities as gybing and gibing) is a steering technique that is similar to tacking, except that jibing is performed when the boat is being steered in the same direction as the wind, with the stern at all times facing the wind. Jibing is often a more dynamic steering movement than a tack, because the sails remain full of wind throughout the maneuver. A boat moving on a downwind path is able to navigate more directly to an intended destination; variations in course direction a downwind course are achieved through jibing. As with a tack, the crew will usually move to the side of the boat opposite the sails to maintain the balance of the boat (a movement that recalls the old expression "maintaining an even keel").

Heading up the boat means to steer the boat closer to the direction of the wind. To achieve this result, the sails must be brought closer to the centerline of the craft; if boat is too close to a position directly opposed to the wind direction, the sails will flutter, or luff, without power and the boat will not move. Heading up the boat is the preliminary aspect of tacking. Bearing away the boat is to direct the boat to permit the wind to come from the stern; jibing is the steering technique that will follow an effort to bear away.

**SEE ALSO** Sailing; Sailing physics; Windsurfing.

# Ulrich Salchow

8/7/1877–4/19/1969
SWEDISH
FIGURE SKATER

Ulrich Salchow was a notable contributor to the sport of figure skating. His name has been preserved in modern times through the skating jump that bears his name, the Salchow, a standard maneuver that forms part of the repertoire of every competitive figure skater.

Salchow won a total of 10 world championships in his long skating career; he was runner-up on three other occasions. Salchow also captured the gold medal for figure skating in the 1908 Summer Olympics (figure skating was then a summer competition as the first Winter Olympics was not held until 1924). After his retirement from the competitive arena, Salchow was a key figure in the rise of the International Skating Union (ISU), acting as the president of the ISU from 1925–1937. Salchow is one of the most successful athletes in the history of Sweden.

The Salchow jump was first performed by Ulrich Salchow in 1909. It represented a remarkable athletic technique for the time, as it requires the skater to take off into the jump from the back inside edge of one skate, landing on the back inside edge of the opposite skate. The skater uses the free leg (the leg not involved in the take off into the jump) in a wide, sweeping motion, to provide the rotation to carry the skater's body through the air. If the skater is able to generate both sufficient lift and a powerful free leg rotation, he or she can execute a multiple number of rotations in the air prior to landing on the opposite foot. The various jumps are therefore classed as a single, double, or triple Salchow, depending upon how many rotations are performed. A quadruple Salchow has been successfully completed on only a very few occasions in competition.

The Salchow is one of the first jumps that an aspiring figure skater learns to perform, in part because the footwork necessary to execute the Salchow takes the skater naturally into other defined skating maneuvers. The judging in figure skating is based in part on purely subjective considerations, and in part on international standards for jumps such as the Salchow. Despite efforts by skaters to use the Salchow as a two-footed take-off jump, the ISU has remained true to the original Salchow, and skaters are carefully scrutinized in competition to ensure that the Salchow is performed with a one-footed takeoff, regardless of how many rotations that the skater seeks to include before landing.

**SEE ALSO** Figure skating, ice; Motor Control; Visualization in sport.

# Salt

Salt is one of the best-known and most important substances ingested by the human body. Essential systems regarding the hydration of the body, the maintenance of the acid/base balance essential to human survival, and production of muscular energy cannot occur without the consumption of dietary salt and its regulated presence in every cell.

Salt, often described as table salt given its widespread use as a condiment, is the chemical compound created by the union of two elements, sodium, a metal, and chlorine. Their product, sodium chloride, is expressed as the chemical formula $NaCl$. While in popular speech salt is commonly used in an interchangeable fashion in description of sodium's characteristics, sodium represents only 40% of the composition of table salt by weight. Salt is a mineral, a substance that is mined underground in various parts of the world; salt is also easily extracted from seawater. The term salt is used to describe both the sodium chloride compound as well as the more generic class of metals that are capable of replacing an existing hydrogen atom in an acid. Potassium, calcium, and magnesium are classified as salts in this respect.

Salt is the most common flavoring added to food in the world. Salt has been used as a food preservative for thousands of years, and it is today employed, either in its common form or in a similar chemistry such as monosodium glutamate (MSG), in thousands of food preparation processes. Sodium nitrate, a preservative, and sodium bicarbonate, used in food preparation, are also common sources of sodium in compounds similar to salt. Salt that is sold commercially as a flavoring or condiment is usually distributed with iodine added; iodine is an essential element to human function that assists in the prevention of various thyroid gland conditions, including goiter, a pronounced enlargement of the gland which can restrict its operation, leading to an impairment of the regulation of the body's entire metabolic function.

Throughout the industrialized world, salt is consumed through food in amounts far in excess of the body's actual requirements for either sodium or chlorine. In the United States, the recommended daily allowance (RDA) of sodium for an adult is between 1,100 to 3,300 mg per day; the average American adult consumes between 4,000 and 5,000 mg of sodium. Many foods have salt or sodium in their composition, including all milk products, green vegetables such as celery, root vegetables such as beets, and others. Salt is commonly added to meats and all manner of prepackaged or processed food products. Paradoxically, no matter what amount of salt is ingested by the body through regular diet, additional salt is essential to athletic performance, and most sports drinks and other nutritional supplements will have salt or simple sodium added.

Sodium and chlorine play distinct roles in effective human function. Each element is absorbed into the body through the digestive processes of the small intestine, where the elements are broken into their single elemental forms. The key processes to which sodium is directed from the point of absorption into the body include water (fluid) balance within the body; acid/base balance in the body, known as the pH level; the specific relationship between sodium and the element potassium creates what is often referred to as a potassium/sodium "pump," a fluid pressure system essential to the generation of energy within each cell; and a related role in the effective transmission of impulses through out the central nervous and peripheral nervous systems.

The most common negative impact of excessive salt consumption is the generation of excessive levels of sodium within the body. Excess sodium is a negative impact on the rather delicate fluid balance levels within the body, the most direct effect of which is hypertension, or high blood pressure. Hypertension is a critical factor in reduced cardiovascular health, including significantly increased risk of stroke and other forms of system failure.

Conversely, an overly restricted dietary salt consumption can lead to the relatively common condition experienced by endurance athletes, hyponatremia, a disruption of the sodium balance that interferes with the body's ability to regulate fluid levels under the stresses imposed by endurance sport.

Chlorine is not given any where near the critical scrutiny of that afforded excess sodium consumption. Chlorine comprises only 0.15% of the body weight of an adult person, and it is stored by the body almost entirely within the intracellular fluids. Chlorine is also important to the body's ability to regulate the acid/base balance. Chlorine is important to the body's ability to absorb potassium, as well as being a part of the function performed by the blood in transporting waste carbon dioxide from the tissues to the lungs to be exhaled. Chlorine is essential to the digestive process, in that chlorine joins with hydrogen to form hydrogen chloride, the major component of stomach bile.

Unlike sodium, excess chlorine is not believed to present any significant problems to overall body function.

**SEE ALSO** Diet; Hydration; Minerals; Sodium (salt) intake for athletes.

# Salt intake SEE Sodium (salt) intake for athletes

# Salt tablets

In the modern era where sport technology has played such an important role in the training programs formulated for both elite competitors and recreational athletes seeking a personal best, sophisticated sports drinks and gel products abound in the nutritional supplement market. The simple salt tablet is a decidedly "old school" athletic supplement.

Salt in its natural mineral form is one of the oldest known diet supplements. The effect on the function of the body of one of salt's constituent elements, sodium, has been well understood for at least two centuries. Formed into salt tablets, salt was used by laborers in warm, heavy industrial environments of North America in the late 1800s; it was also provided to soldiers by a number of national armies during World War II to assist combatants in dealing with dehydration in hot jungle and desert environments. For more than 50 years, salt tablets have been a staple in North American preseason football training camps, which are often held in the heat of July and August.

Unlike some of the modern-age training supplements that are marketed with little scientific backing for the claims advanced as to effectiveness, there is no scientific question concerning the benefits of salt, and particularly sodium, for athletes involved in warm weather sports.

Sodium is directly related to the body's ability to perform. Sodium is of primary importance in its role as a regulator of how much fluid is present in the body at any time, both in terms of volume, which ultimately will impact on the blood volume available to the cardiovascular system for all of its processes

associated with human performance, as well as sodium's role in relation to the maintenance of the acid/base (pH) balance throughout the body. Muscle energy is developed through a complex series of processes in the individual cells, a portion of which is tied to the "pump" mechanism established through the proper balance between potassium and sodium in the intracellular fluids that support each cell. A sodium deficit can have a catastrophic effect on one or all of these human systems. The condition known as hyponatremia is the ultimate result of a sodium deficit, in which the body's sodium imbalance is so severe that even when dehydrated, the body will not absorb available water from the stomach through the small intestine because the sodium level has triggered the body to take no more water without sodium being available.

Sodium is lost to the body during exercise through perspiration and urine excretion. Sodium can only be replaced through dietary sources or supplements; the body has no independent mechanism to warehouse sodium.

In warm weather exercise, the amount of sodium that an athlete may lose through perspiration is varied. Athletes who are acclimatized to warm environmental conditions of high temperatures and humidity will generally lose less sodium per volume of perspiration than those who are not so accustomed to the conditions. A typical adult will lose sodium at a rate ranging between 100 mg and 700 mg per liter, and the athlete will lose between 1.0 l to 2.5 l of fluid to perspiration per hour, subject to variables such as intensity and body type. Most commercial sport drink products contain sodium, but the typical quantity ranges between 50 mg and 170 mg of sodium per 8 oz (250 ml) bottle, meaning that the consumption of sport drinks, while a benefit, in terms of fluid replacement, is not necessarily a solution to sodium deficit. To achieve sodium replacement through the sports drink, the formulation might taste more like seawater than a sports drink. Five hundred milligram-sized salt tablets, which are chemically 40% sodium and thus provide approximately 200 mg of sodium to the athlete, might assist the athlete in counteracting a sodium deficit.

Salt tablets present problems for athletes if taken orally to correct sodium deficiencies. In their raw form, salt tablets are often difficult to digest, causing gastric irritation, with accompanying nausea and diarrhea a common side effect. The stomach has difficulty in the immediate digestion of salt tablets, meaning that the benefit of the sodium is delayed; sports drinks, and their nutrients, are far easier for the body to absorb. Swallowed alone, without significant fluid to accompany the salt tablet, the sodium will act to further accelerate the dehydration of the body.

In endurance races, such as triathlons, the Ironman, marathon, and ultra-marathon running, and ultra cycling events, salt tablets have been successfully employed as a supplement to the sports drink supplements. Salt tablets, taken either with sports drinks (that have their own sodium component) or fruit drinks that naturally contain potassium, serve to increase the sodium levels in a form that is far easier to digest and therefore be of more immediate use to the fluid level and acid/base balance of the body.

Salt tablets, even when consumed with a volume of sports drink, should be tested; the athlete can ingest the tablets during training to determine how the athlete's body will react after they are consumed.

SEE ALSO Hyponatremia; Salt; Sodium (salt) intake for athletes; Sodium and sodium deficits.

## Scottish Highland Games competition

The Scottish Highland games, part cultural festival and part athletic competition, are the modern-day embodiment of the war games and contests that were held in ancient Scotland. Highland Games are at least as old as the ancient Olympic Games of Greece.

In the modern variant, Highland Games are held all over the world; Scottish music, particularly bagpipes, is a common feature. In the modern Highland Games, women and men compete in separate athletic divisions. The athletic competitions are generally divided into light athletics, including highland dancing, sprint races, and jumping events, and heavy athletics, a series of demanding strength events that, to the sports world, are the essential Highland Games competitions. Unlike the ancient Highland Games, where membership in a Highland clan was a precondition to competition, the modern competitions are open to anyone who can match the set qualification standards.

The heavy events at a typical Highland Games competition will include the "caber toss," officially known as turning the caber. A caber is a long, tapered wooden pole with a shape similar to that of a ship's mast or a telephone pole and a weight between 100 and 180 pounds (45–82 kg). The caber is placed upright, then picked up at the smaller end by the competitor;

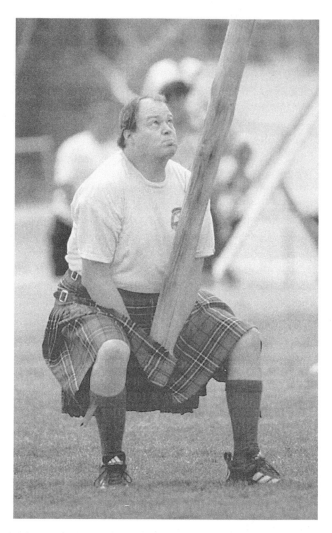

Highland Games athlete in the "caber toss." BOB BIRD/GETTY IMAGES

the thrown caber must pass through the vertical (90 degrees from the ground) to be considered "turned." A valid throw will fall away from the competitor within a 180-degree semi-circle, and the closer to a straight line from the competitor the end of the caber is turned when it lands, the more successful the toss. Another heavy event is the stone put, an event similar to the shotput, in that the stone, weighing 22 lb (10 kg) is thrown from behind a line for the furthest distance. The hammer throw, another event similar to the Olympic competition, is a competition in which a hammer is attached to a line and thrown, with the athlete using the principles of centrifugal force to assist in generating speed. The weight toss is an event in which a 56-lb (25.4 kg) weight is thrown for the furthest distance. Finally there is sheaf tossing, whereby a heavy sheaf of grain, encased in a burlap type sack, is thrown using a pitchfork.

These seemingly rustic events are exceedingly demanding. The ideal Scottish Highland Games heavy athlete will be powerful; the throwing of heavy weights often is facilitated by a relatively low center of gravity. Leg strength, particularly the development of required muscular power needed for the explosive force to deliver thrust in all five of the heavy events, is essential to success.

Highland Games circuits have developed in the past 20 years, in Scotland and across North America, mirroring the increasing popularity of the heavy events. World championships have been held in Scotland, as have world master's Highland Games (for those over 40 years of age). A number of successful heavy athletes have also competed in other strength competitions, most notably the "World's Strongest Man" events made popular through the television media.

**SEE ALSO** Hammer throw; Short, high intensity exercise; Shotput.

## Sex testing

Sex testing, also known as gender verification testing, was employed in various types of athletic competition as a means of ensuring that all of the female competitors in a particular sport were in fact, biologically women.

There is a significant chorological gap between the first documented case of gender subterfuge in international sport and a scientific response. At the 1936 Olympics in Berlin, Herman Ratjen competed in the women's high jump competition under the first name of Dora. Ratjen finished fourth. Ratjen concealed his masculine identity by, among other measures, binding his genitals. Ratjen's subterfuge was not confirmed until 1955, when he stated that he had been forced to compete as a female by the Nazis.

In the early 1960s, there were suspicions that a number of Eastern Bloc athletes who competed as females may have been men. Other than physical examination, there existed at that time only primitive scientific technology to confirm gender. In 1966, the first gender verification testing was performed at the European Track and Field championships. The testing procedure was simple; female athletes were required to either undress before a panel of medical doctors, or otherwise be examined manually.

In 1968, the International Olympic Committee (IOC) introduced an element of science to the sex

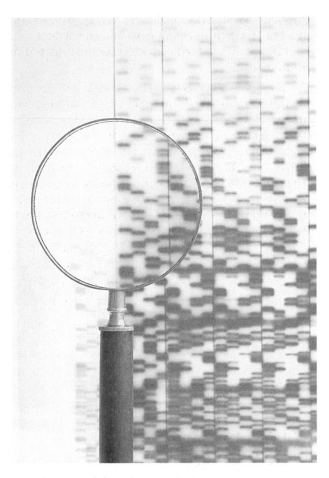

Examining a karyotype. © ROYALTY-FREE/CORBIS

testing process. Female athletes at the Olympics that year were required to provide a buccal swab (a cellular sample form the inside of the cheek) that was analyzed to confirm the presence of a sex chromatin (a portion of the nucleus of the cell that could be identified as female).

By the time of the 1992 Olympics, the IOC employed DNA testing that accurately identified the presence of the Y chromosome present in the genetic material contained in the cell of all females. Even with scientifically verifiable testing procedures, it was accepted in the scientific community that a very small number of females possessed a genetic structure that might provide a result that suggested that the female was a male. Such athletes might be disqualified from participation even though they were actually women.

The International Amateur Athletics Federation eliminated sex testing in 1992 as being of no value in the present day. The IOC followed suit in 1999. The only female athlete ever permitted to compete at the Olympics without submitting to sex testing was

Britain's Princess Anne, daughter of Queen Elizabeth, who competed in the equestrian events.

SEE ALSO Gender in sports: Female athletes; International Olympic Committee (IOC); Sports psychology.

# Sexual and reproductive disorders

Sexual disorders are those conditions, both physiological and psychological, that affect the sexual function, desire, or performance of any person, male or female. Reproductive disorders are related to sexual disorders, in the sense that the function of the same general bodily systems may be affected. Reproductive disorders are those that interfere with or limit the ability of persons to produce the cellular material required to conceive a fertilized ovum (egg) within the female reproductive system, or otherwise permit the natural development of the ovum to fetus and ultimately birth as a child.

Public discussion and awareness regarding both sexual disorders and reproductive disorders is a relatively recent phenomenon. Throughout most of human history, such circumstances were considered to be private issues, discussed only between adult partners, if at all. The level of understanding among typical adults as to the function of their reproductive systems and the related sexual organs did not extend to how sexual disorders were caused or how such conditions might be treated or prevented. The limited public information concerning such matters was generally restricted to physical conclusions—a male might experience "impotence," a woman was often said to be "frigid". Married couples who were not able to conceive were not generally able to access any scientific resources to treat the underlying cause of such conditions.

An example of the greater public willingness to discuss matters pertaining to sexual dysfunction is the widespread success of the erectile dysfunction medications Viagra, Cialis and their pharmaceutical competitors. These medications are marketed in a fashion that both promote a general knowledge of the medical condition that underlies the sexual disorder, as well and the resulting benefit to the user.

Sexual disorders can take one of many forms for both men and women; a number of causes are applicable to both sexes. The sexual organs in both men and women are controlled to a significant degree by the body's endocrine system, whose major glands, the thyroid, pituitary, and adrenal glands, influence and coordinate the production of estrogen and testosterone, the female and male sex hormones. Where the production of these chemicals is reduced within the body, due to injury or disease, sexual function will invariably decline.

Reproductive disorders may affect any part of the glands, organs, or external genitals. Such disorders may impact the course of reproduction from conception (the fertilization of the female ovum with male sperm in the fallopian tubes, the portion of the female reproductive system leading to the uterus). In addition to the sexual dysfunctions that would prevent fertilization of the ovum, a number of conditions will potentially prevent reproduction. Sexually transmitted diseases (STDs) are a common cause of infertility. STDs are a broad class of infectious diseases, which includes infectious diseases such as gonorrhea and acquired immune deficiency syndrome, AIDS.

The consumption of a number of varieties of both prescription and non-prescription drugs can significantly affect sexual function. SSRI (selective serotonin reuptake inhibitors), a class of anti-depressant drug of which the brand names Zoloft and Prozac taking the medication. Alcohol, a central nervous system depressant, reduces sexual drive in the same fashion. The long term usage of both SSRIs and alcohol have been demonstrated to inhibit sexual drive in both men and women.

In the athletic community, various types of anabolic steroids have been established as having both pronounced physiological and physiological effects on the user that detract from sexual performance. One of the most studied side effects of anabolic steroids is the physical effect of the primary male sexual organs, the penis and the testicles, and the secondary sexual organs, the male breasts. The consumption of anabolic steroids will often cause the testes, the glands located in the male scrotum which produce testosterone, to shrink. There exists a clear correlation between anabolic steroid usage and diminished sexual function, while promoting uneven moods and breast development.

Androgen insensitivity syndrome (AIS) is a genetic condition that affects the development of male testicles and external genitalia. This condition is genetic in origin, caused by the presence of a mixture of male and female chromosomes within the body. In it most common manifestation, a baby may be born with a sufficient quantity of male chromosomes that a require a verification test (sex test) to confirm that the subject is male, even where the subject is female in appearance. In the complete form female triad is often observed among athletes in sports where body image and physical appearance form a part of the competitive basis of the sport; gymnastics and figure skating are two such examples. The individual medical conditions that constitute the triad are osteoporosis (reduced bone density), eating disorders (where the subject seeks to improve their self image and to lose weight through either binging and purging or reducing calorie consumption to unsafe levels), and ammorhea, the loss or disruption of the menstrual cycle. Ammorhea in particular can contribute to reproductive health difficulties for women, as the long term disruption of regular menstruation cycles may be difficult to reestablish.

**SEE ALSO** Health; Hormones; Musculoskeletal injuries.

# Craig Sharp

7/5/1930–
BRITISH
SPORTS SCIENTIST, DOCTOR OF VETERINARY
MEDICINE, DISTANCE RUNNER

Craig Sharp is hailed within the international sports science community as the founder of sports science in Great Britain. In 1971, Sharp commenced his academic work in the field as a Professor of Physical Education at the University of Birmingham, the only British institution to then offer what is now referred to as a sports science degree. In the following years, Sharp established a reputation as a respected academic who was skilled in taking sports science theory and developing useful practical applications. Sharp founded the Birmingham Human Motor Performance Laboratory in 1973, an innovative step in the advance of the study of high-performance athletes. Sharp later co-founded the British Olympic Medical Center in 1987, an institution which functions as a support facility to the British Olympic program.

Through the efforts of Sharp and others in Great Britain, sports science is now a recognized and well-regarded course of academic study, with numerous universities offering undergraduate, masters, and doctoral programs.

In his many published articles on sports science, Sharp has emphasized several recurring themes. He has long advocated the expansion of the sports science knowledge base to make knowledge more broadly available to both athletes and coaches. Sharp is a believer in the ongoing physical testing of athletes, using methods such as detailed treadmill and

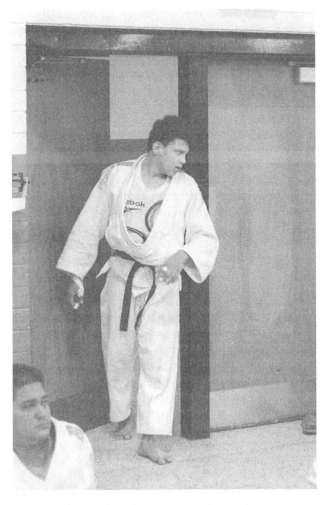

Brazilian judo competitor, Edinanci Silva, at the 2000 Olympics. Silva suffers from androgen insensitivity syndrome (AIS). ANTONIO SCORZA/AFP/GETTY IMAGES

of AIS, the child will be born with testes that are subsequently removed through surgery.

At the 1992 Summer Olympics, five female athletes tested as male from a total of over 2,400 people. At the 1996 Games, eight women tested as males due to AIS. It is to be noted that persons with AIS, a genetic condition, are distinct from transgendered persons, whose decision to undergo gender altering surgery is usually rooted in the presence of a psychological condition, a gender identification disorder. Renee Richards, the transgendered tennis player who was the first such athlete to compete in the United States Open in 1977, is the best known example of a transgendered person participating in a sport in their new gender.

Among female athletes, the medical community recognizes a set of physical and psychological conditions that are referred to as the female triad. The other physiological research as a tool to improve performance.

A noteworthy feature concerning the contribution of Sharp to the development of sports science is his remarkably diverse background and personal range of interests. Sharp was a capable distance runner as a young man, at one time holding the record for the fastest run to the peak of Mount Kilimanjaro in Africa. He was also a professional squash player. Sharp is likely the only prominent sports scientist to have begun his professional career as a doctor of veterinary medicine, a profession that he pursued with some distinction for 14 years. Sharp is also an authority on Scottish poetry.

SEE ALSO Sports medicine education.

# Shoes SEE Athletic shoes

# Shoes, running SEE Running shoes

# Shooting

Shooting, also known as sport shooting has been a competitive sport in a variety of forms since the mid-1800s. Competitions that involved pursuits such big game hunting, target shooting, and the hunting of a wide variety of birds were all contested in various parts of the world. The first prominent organization created to advance the interest of serious sport shooters and marksmen was the National Rifle Association, formed in the United States in 1871.

Throughout its history as a competitive sport, shooting has encompassed many different types of firearms. "Gun" is a term used interchangeably with firearm. At its most basic, a firearm is any barreled device capable of discharging a projectile. By the time of the first modern Olympics in 1896, competitive shooting was conducted in separate divisions for three types of firearms; rifles, pistols, and shotguns. A rifle is a long barreled firearm that has spiral grooves machined along the interior of the barrel; the spiral grooves, or rifling, create a rotary motion when the bullet is fired. The spin imparted to the bullet by the rifling tends to produce a more accurate shot. A rifle is typically discharged from the shoulder position of the shooter. A pistol is small firearm designed to be held and discharged from a single hand of the shooter. Both pistols and rifles may be powered by the force of conventional gunpowder contained in the cartridge that contains the bullet to be fired. The explosive force of the gunpowder is initiated when the trigger on the firearm is pulled by the shooter. Other types of both pistols and rifles are powered by systems that employ either compressed air mechanisms or pressurized gases.

A shotgun has a long barrel, one typically shorter and thicker than that of a rifle. The inside of the shotgun barrel is smooth, as the projectiles discharged are not a single object, as with a rifle bullet, but are numerous tiny projectiles, referred to as "shot". Shotguns are not as accurate as either rifles or pistols, but are an effective device in covering a wider area with the discharged ammunition.

The International Sport Shooting Federation, ISSF, is the governing body for shooting competitions through out the world. There are 17 different categories of shooting recognized at the Olympic games, seven open to women and 10 restricted to male competitors. Until 1996, a number of shooting categories at the Olympics were designated as mixed events, open to competitors of either gender. In addition to the various types of rifle and pistol shooting where the marksman attempts to shoot at a distant target, there are two general classes of moving target competitions involving trap and skeet. The trap is a device that propels specially constructed clay targets into the air at a specified distance from the shooter. In Olympic competition, the shooter must attempt to shoot 125 of the targets, from a total of five different shooting positions. In the event called double trap, two clay targets are released simultaneously at differing angles, requiring the shooter to make successive shots on the targets.

Skeet is also an event involving shot guns. The shooters assume a series of positions during the competitions, attempting to strike the targets, sometime referred to as "clay pigeons" after they are propelled into the air.

Shooting also is an important element of a winter sports discipline, the biathlon, where the competitors complete a series of laps on a cross country ski course, with intervals in which the athletes are required to shoot at set targets with a rifle from both prone and standing positions. The combination of endurance, strength, and precise marksmanship, accomplished while the athlete attempts to steady their body from the rigors of skiing, make the biathlon one of the most difficult Winter Olympic sports.

As with many sports where muscle power is not a prerequisite, shooting appears deceptively simple.

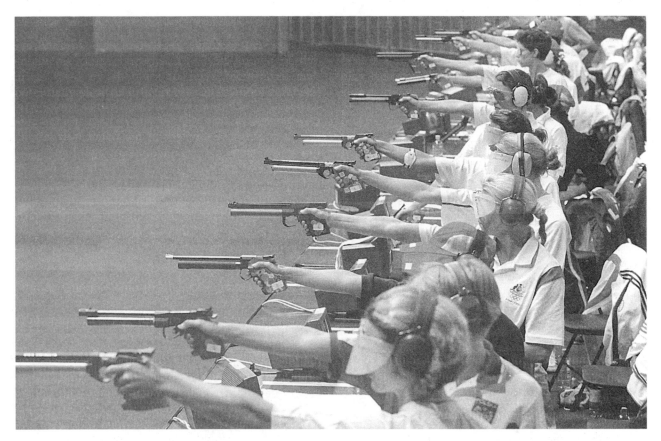

Female athletes shooting air pistols as part of 2000 Olympic Games (pentathlon). © JACQUES LANGEVIN/SYGMA/CORBIS

The ability to steady hand and mind to deliver a sequence of shots requires well-developed powers of concentration and emotional control. Elite shooters spend considerable training time developing skills in visualization, where they direct their mental powers to the entire sequence of a successful shot, as an aid in coordinating their physical and mental efforts.

The greater the level of physical fitness possessed by a competitive shooter, the more likely they are to achieve competitive success. Many shooters attempt to fire at a target between heartbeats, when the body is at its most stable. The more fit the athlete, generally, the lower the heart rate. A lower heart rate will provide the shooter with a greater window within which to deliver the shot. The breathing exercises that are often performed by shooters during competition to relax the body have a more pronounced effect on a body that has both a fit cardiovascular and cardiorespiratory system.

Shooting has known its share of performance enhancing drug concerns. The best known of the drugs used by shooters to relax themselves and potentially slow their heart rate are alcohol and beta blockers, both banned substances on the World Anti-Doping Agency (WADA) Prohibited List. Beta blockers are drugs used to treat a number of cardiovascular conditions; they have the effect of slowing heart rate and reducing blood pressure, an advantage in shooting.

**SEE ALSO** Motor Control; Skiing, Nordic (cross-country skiing); Visualization in sport.

# Short, high intensity exercise

Short, high intensity exercise can take many forms, but it has certain constants—the exercise will be purely anaerobic in its nature (usually activities or individual segments of a longer exercise of fewer than 90 seconds duration), and it will require the athlete to perform at between 75% and 85% of the maximum physical capability.

Short, high intensity exercise can be the component of a longer and otherwise aerobic program; running high speed intervals in the middle of a longer slower run is a common example. Common short, high intensity exercise will include sprinting, weight-lifting, and the traditional field athletics such as the shotput, hammer throw, high jump, and discus. In each case, there is a very large expenditure of energy within the short time period. The intense effort required of the athlete is also highly focused toward the athletic goal, with very little extraneous effort. For this reason, short, high intensity exercise activities tend to be ones where technique, economy of movement, and execution are as important as the energy that the body is able to generate to complete the physical actions involved.

Short, high intensity exercise has a number of physiological attractions to the recreational athlete who is interested in fitness and weight loss, as these activities tend to require the body to expend a greater number of calories than medium or low intensity pursuits. The average adult person who runs three miles at a rate of eight minutes per mile will expect to expend approximately 300 calories; the same person who runs the same distance over the same terrain at a pace of 6.5 minutes per mile will expect to expend 350 calories. There is also a greater benefit derived by the athlete after the workout is concluded; high intensity exercise provides a greater boost to the metabolic rate for up to 24 hours after the activity is completed, where the corresponding low or medium intensity exercise creates a negligible difference in metabolic rate. For short, high intensity exercise that is added as a component to an ongoing fitness program, the athlete can expect overall body fat to be reduced by between 3% to 5% over a six-month period, assuming that there are no other variables.

The other crucial benefits of short, high intensity training are the improvement of the person's $VO_2max$, the measure of the ability to process oxygen, and a generally greater strength built throughout the musculoskeletal system. The resistance inherent in short, high intensity exercise that is directed to the body will both build muscular strength and prevent bone density reduction.

Most short, high intensity exercises place significant emphasis on explosive movement at some point in the activity. Success in these disciplines will ultimately involve the specific training of the fast-twitch fibers in the target muscle groups. Plyometrics is the type of training engaged to enhance fast-twitch muscle response and to generally develop an explosive ability that may be sustained throughout the duration of the exercise.

The relative brevity of the exercise requires the athlete to pay even greater attention to the warm up/cool down cycle. A warm up will permit both the musculoskeletal system and the cardiovascular system to be brought to the operational status necessary to work at the body's maximum rate; stretching and flexibility components to the warm up that address the muscle groups to be used at high intensity tend to reduce injury by as much as 50%. Cool down serves to gently reduce the body's heart and respiration rates, while keeping the muscles loose.

Short, high intensity exercise is sometimes viewed as a weight loss panacea by persons with poor fitness who wish to lose weight. Such persons are at significantly greater risk of injury as short, high intensity exercise, by its nature, places demands on the body to which an unfit person will be unaccustomed. Unless the person possesses excellent fitness, short, high intensity exercises or training must be approached incrementally.

SEE ALSO Exercise, high intensity; Exercise, intermittent; Plyometrics; Running: Sprinting; Variable resistance exercise.

# Shot put

Unlike most of the traditional Olympic athletic events that were first contested at the modern Games in 1896, the shot put most likely owes its lineage to the Scottish Highland games competition, the stone put. The shot put is contested in both men's and women's categories at the Summer Olympics as well as the biennial World Track and Field championships.

As with all other field events, the shot put is a deceptively simple sport. The competitor is required to throw a 16 lb (7.2 kg) steel ball, using a prescribed method where the ball is held in one hand, in a position under the competitor's chin. From a 7 ft (2.2 m) circle, within which the athlete must remain during the throw, the ball is thrown in a thrusting motion; the ball must land within a sector of the field whose apex begins at the throwing circle. In Olympic competition, each shot putter is given six throws, with the best effort counting as the athlete's score.

The shot put is primarily a strength event, but the technique used to generate the efficient and powerful movement of the athlete in the throwing circle will usually determine success. Two different techniques are employed by shot putters to deliver the shot. The first is known as the glide technique, where the thrower moves across the throwing circle quickly to develop speed, and with one fluid motion throws the shot, twisting the body at the point of the delivery to

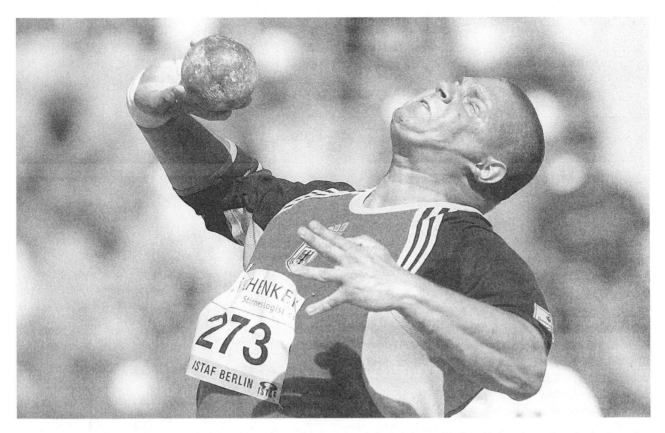

The combination of the athlete's speed as they move across the throwing circle and the angle of projection determines the horizontal motion of the shot after it is release. **PHOTO BY FRIEDEMANN VOGEL/BONGARTS/GETTY IMAGES.**

ensure not to end up outside the throwing circle and fault, which will void the throw. The second technique is described as the spin, where the thrower begins the movement with the back to the target area. The athlete then takes a quick step and turns the hip as quickly as possible to generate maximum velocity in the throwing circle. The thrower then transfers the weight as forcefully as possible to the foot closest to the edge of the circle, thrusting the throwing arm to release the shot while the body is moving forward.

The angle at which the shot is delivered is also crucial. Unlike objects such as a discus or a javelin, which must be thrown with the aerodynamics of their intended flight considered, the shot put angle of projection will be the ideal combination of the speed of the shot as obtained from the movement of the thrower across the circle, and that will defeat the effect of gravity the longest.

It is the combination of the speed of the athletes as they move across the throwing circle and the angle of projection that will determine the horizontal motion of the shot after it is released. The vertical effects on the shot are determined by the force of gravity on the ball, which is a constant. The flight of the shot is always a parabola, due to the influence of the force of gravity on the horizontal speed of the shot.

Other than specialized track spikes, which give the throwers additional stability as they move through the throwing circle and then plant their feet to deliver the throw, and the chalk, which is permitted to improve the athletes' grip on the steel ball, the shot putters are not permitted to use any other aid or equipment to deliver the throw.

A successful shot putter will possess a very strong and well-developed upper body, powerful legs with which to drive across the throwing circle, and a measure of agility necessary to execute this maneuver in a confined 7 ft (2.1 m) circle. It is a testament to the difficulty of the shot put that it is one of the 10 events that form the ultimate track and field athletic challenge, the decathlon.

While there is significant differences in the technical approaches to each discipline, the training that is required to develop a shot put athlete is similar to that employed by a hammer throw specialist or a discus thrower. Intensive weight training that emphasizes the chest and the shoulders of the athlete will be stressed.

Leg exercises such as squats, lunges, leg presses, and other forms of exercise to heighten the explosive ability of the thrower's legs to deliver upward thrust at the time of the release of the shot are crucial to success.

As with many Olympic athletics events, the limelight is on these competitors only once every four years. Shot putters and other field competitors toil in anonymity in other regional or collegiate competitions. It is noteworthy that in this strength event, unlike other Olympic competitions, the world records for men and women have not fallen since 1990 and 1987, respectively. This stagnation in record progress tends to coincide with the greater ability of the sport scientists to detect anabolic steroid use.

**SEE ALSO** Decathlon; Hammer throw; Plyometrics; Short, high intensity exercise.

# Shot put: Throw mechanics

The shot put is a track and field event that involves throwing a heavy metal ball called a shot as far as possible using only one arm in a pushing motion, what is called putting. The shot put athlete (or shot-putter) needs strength, but must also be quick and coordinated in order to create momentum and maximum force during the throwing motion. The shot-putter begins at the back of a marked circle that is 7 ft (2.1 m) in diameter. The shot-putter faces away from the throwing direction while positioning the shot against the shoulder and under the chin. In two quick steps, the shot-putter turns, moves quickly to the front of the circle while launching the shot by thrusting the arm forward.

The throw mechanics of the shot put involve primarily four factors. Projection speed (v) is measured from the point the shot-putter releases the shot; projection angle (θ) is the angle between the horizontal and the initial shot direction, range (R) is the horizontal distance from the release of the shot to where it lands; and height difference (h) is the distance from the ground to the vertical release point.

The projection speed (v) is the most important of these factors. It is determined by the magnitude and direction of the forces applied to the shot and by the distance over which these forces act.

The optimum projection angle (θ) for achieving maximum horizontal range (R) depends on the size, strength, and throwing technique of each particular athlete. The optimum projection angle usually ranges from 26 to 38°. The projection speed (v) and the launch height

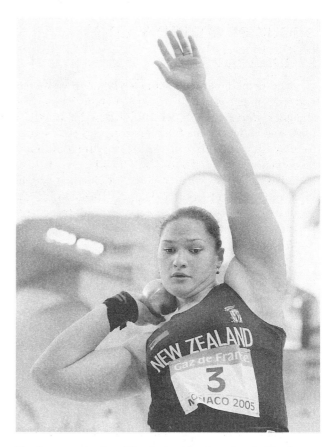

The throw mechanics of the shot put involve primarily four factors: projection speed, projection angle, range, and height difference. **PHOTO BY IAN WALTON/GETTY IMAGES.**

(h) are dependent on the projection angle. Experiments have shown that the projection speed generated by an athlete steadily decreases with increasing projection angle. The decrease in projection speed with the increase in projection angle is the result of two factors.

As the projection angle increases, the shot-putter must expend a greater effort to overcome the weight of the shot, and so less effort is available to accelerate the shot (or produce the projection speed). The muscular and skeletal systems of the human body is better able to exert forces in the horizontal direction than in the vertical direction.

In the end, the release height of the shot put is determined by the athlete's body position at the moment of release. If all other factors are equal, the athlete who attains a position in which the throwing arm, trunk, and legs are fully extended at the instant of release will achieve greater distances than the athlete who is in a less-desirable position.

**SEE ALSO** Shotput; Skeletal muscle.

# Shoulder anatomy and physiology

The omni-directional shoulder is the most mobile and the most versatile of the human joints. The shoulder, in conjunction with the elbow joint and the ulnar and radial bones of the forearm, may be operated to create a powerful lever to perform lifting or prying movements. The ability of the shoulder to rotate is essential to all throwing, catching, or shooting actions in a multitude of sports. The construction of the shoulder permits the arm to be rotated 360° from every position relative to its connection to the shoulder.

The inherent flexibility and the range of motion present in the shoulder is due to the unique structure of the joint. Virtually every joint in the body brings two or more bones into close, one-on-one contact. The musculoskeletal framework of the shoulder mechanism relies to a much greater degree on the connective tissues of the shoulder, as opposed to its bones, to provide the joint with its strength as well as its ability to absorb significant force. The shoulder has the greatest risk of soft tissue injury of any of the joints that propel human limbs.

The skeletal components of the shoulder include humerus, the long bone of the upper arm that is a part of the elbow and the shoulder joints; the scapula, or the shoulder blade, positioned on the posterior (rear) of the shoulder on the upper back; the clavicle, or the collarbone, aligned between the neck and the outer limit of the shoulder; and the sternum, or breastbone, which is not a primary bone in the formation or function of the shoulder joint. The sternum is a bone that supports the opposing end of the clavicle from the shoulder.

Each of the shoulder bones has articular cartilage covering the head of the bone that comes into contact with another bone, reducing the degree of friction created by two bones moving against one another. Articular cartilage also provides a measure of cushioning between the bones. Osteoarthritis is a common form of disease in the shoulder region among athletes who, through the wear and tear of repetitive motions such as throwing, sustain a gradual thinning or wearing away of the articular cartilage.

Shoulder movement and any corresponding injuries are commonly described with reference to the shoulder joint, as if the structure had a single means of flexion, extension, and rotation. The shoulder comprises four separate joints, each an integrated device that is capable of a degree of independent movement.

The glenohumoral joint is the largest and the most prominent of the joints that contribute to shoulder movement. It is this part of the shoulder that is most commonly described as the shoulder joint. The glenohumoral structure is created by the meeting of the head of the humerus and the portion of the scapula known as the glenoid. These two bones create a "ball and socket" mechanism, which permits the shoulder to rotate freely. The flexibility of the glenohumoral joint is the result of its own intricate ligament structure as well as the position of the rotator cuff relative to the glenohumoral structure. The joint is powered in part through its connection to the biceps tendon, which provides the linkage to the biceps muscle. The remainder of the joint's movement is directed through the muscles and tendons of the rotator cuff. The entire glenohumoral joint is enclosed in a loose membrane capsule that contains a small quantity of synovial fluid that also assists in the movement of the joint.

The acromioclavicular (AC) joint is formed between the clavicle and the region of the scapula known as the acromion. It is the AC joint that is subject to injury when a shoulder is said to become "separated," which refers to the clavicle becoming detached within the AC joint.

The sternoclavicular joint is created at the junction between the sternum and the clavicle, at the base of the neck.

The scapulothoracic articulation is not a joint in the technical sense of two or more bones in conjunction; this structure is a muscle and tendon mechanism that permits the scapula to slide without obstruction along the upper back as the arm is raised or extended during the movements of the shoulder.

The rotator cuff is the most important soft tissue structure in the shoulder. The rotator cuff is essential to any action in relation to the throwing or catching of objects in sport. The rotator cuff, positioned on the top of the glenohumoral joint, provides the muscle power to assist the shoulder in movement, permitting circular motion. The rotator cuff also limits the joint from being overextended when the arm is extended upward. Of the four muscles and tendons that form the rotator cuff, the supraspinatus muscle and its tendon, which extends from the rotator cuff to the top of the humerus, are the most frequently injured of the rotator cuff tissues. Baseball pitchers, athletes who often sustain an injury described generally as a rotator cuff tear, most often sustain a specific injury to the supraspinatus tendon.

The next most important of the soft tissue features of the shoulder are the two bursa, located at the highest part of the shoulder. The bursa, which are

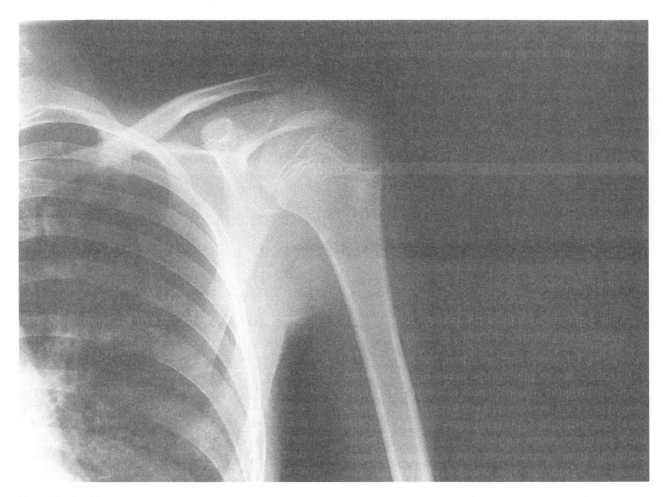

X-ray of a shoulder. © MAXINE HALL/CORBIS

small, fluid-filled sacs constructed of fibrous material, provide cushioning to the joint; the bursa work particularly to protect the rotator cuff from excessive contact with the acromion, a bony extension of the scapula. Overuse of the shoulder, most often through repetitive throwing, will often irritate the bursa fibers, creating an often chronic condition known as bursitis.

**SEE ALSO** Back anatomy and physiology; Bone, ligaments, tendons; Musculoskeletal injuries; Shoulder injuries.

## Shoulder injuries

The shoulder joint is exposed to as broad a range of forces as is any other joint in the body. Every sport requires the full function of the shoulder, whether to throw an object, strike an opponent or a target, the propulsion of the athlete, or to provide balance in movement. No matter how extensively an athlete works to protect and to strengthen the shoulder and its supporting structure, the joint is constantly exposed to a variety of sports injury.

The shoulder joint is both powerful, flexible, and fragile, as there is less bone-on-bone contact within the shoulder joint than other joints of the body, such as the hinges created at the knee or the ankle. Less bone means a correspondingly greater reliance on the muscle and the connective tissue to support the stresses of joint movement, and a greater risk of soft tissue injury. The skeletal components of the shoulder are the humerus, the long bone of the upper arm, the scapula (shoulder blade), and the clavicle (collarbone). In a technical sense, the sternum (breastbone) is also a shoulder bone as it supports the end of the clavicle that is opposite to the shoulder. Each of these bones is covered at the end with articular cartilage, with reduces the friction that otherwise results from movements where bones make contact against one another within the joint.

The shoulder is commonly referenced as if it were a single entity; the shoulder structure is in fact four distinct joints, each an integrated unit that functions within the shoulder. The four joints include the glenohumoral joint, which is the largest of the shoulder joints and is the most exposed to injury; it is the "ball and socket" created between the head of the humerus and the portion of the scapula known as the glenoid; the acromioclavicular (AC) joint, formed between the meeting of the clavicle and the portion of the scapula called the acromion; the sternoclavicular joint, created where the opposite end of the clavicle is secured to the sternum, providing the shoulder with stability; and the scapulothoracic articulation, a structure that is often classified as a joint, when it is more accurately described as a muscle and tendon configuration that permits the scapula to slide along the back as the shoulder is raised and lowered.

Each of the individual shoulder joints has its own supporting network of ligaments. The entire shoulder is encased in various muscles and tendon groups to power the variety of movements of which the shoulder is capable. One of the most important of the connective tissues is the rotator cuff, an assembly of four muscles and tendons positioned on top of the shoulder, under a portion of the scapula, that serves to both permit the arm to be raised and used in a powerful fashion, as well as hold the shoulder joint in place. The joint capsule that surrounds the glenohumoral (ball and socket) joint is also commonly examined in cases of shoulder injury. A further soft tissue component of the shoulder structure is the bursa, located between the glenohumoral joint and the rotator cuff. The bursa is a gel-filled fibrous cushioning device that absorbs some of the forces directed into the shoulder.

Shoulder injuries are most often caused by one of three general mechanisms. The first is overhead motion, during which the hand and forearm are extended through shoulder movement to a point furthest away from the body, the point where the shoulder is at its most vulnerable to overload. The second cause is that of repetitive movement, which places a strain on the shoulder structure. The repetitive strain injuries may be in the form of tendonitis, bursitis, rotator cuff injury, or over the longer term, osteoarthritis. The third class of injury is that caused by a blow absorbed by the joint, caused through a fall or by trauma. These injuries may take the form of a fracture to one or more of the bones of the shoulder, or soft tissue damage such as a joint dislocation.

Rotator cuff injuries are very common in sports. Baseball pitchers may have the highest incidence of occurrence, but all sports where the shoulder and arm are moved forcefully and repetitively create an environment for an entire range of shoulder cuff problems. American football quarterbacks, swimmers, golfers, and volleyball players commonly experience these injuries.

A rotator cuff injury will most often be the result of a wearing against the surface of the rotator cuff structure, creating a tear to the rotator cuff tendon. The same repetitive movement can create a pinching between the cuff and the overlying scapula bone of the shoulder joint. The injury may reveal itself as either a sudden onset of significant pain and reduced shoulder movement, or a more gradual decline in apparent joint function. The inability of a pitcher to throw as hard as previously, or a loss of power in a volleyball player's spike are the type of diminution caused by a damaged rotator cuff.

A rotator cuff injury may also present as an impingement of the shoulder motion. In such cases, often in repetitive movements such as throwing, swimming, or the motion to deliver a tennis serve, the acromion region of the scapula repeatedly rubs against the surface of the rotator cuff. Impingements, while a less serious form of rotator cuff injury than a tear of one of the four soft tissue components, represent a significant problem for an athlete because impingements are a present limitation in the athlete's range of motion in the joint, and also tend to become progressively worse.

Rotator cuff injuries are revealed through the use of x rays (often by way of an arthrogram, the injection of a dye into the joint for a better x-ray image), or through magnetic resonance imaging (MRI). Physiotherapy, with a particular emphasis on the preventative strengthening of the surrounding shoulder muscle structures, is the preferred remedy in over 90% of rotator cuff injuries. Stretching and flexibility exercises are essential to maintain an optimal range of motion in the recovering joint. Nonsteroidal anti-inflammatory drugs (NSAIDs) have also been proven as effective in the management of shoulder pain arising from both the rotator cuff injury as well as the discomfort experienced in rehabilitation. In more extreme cases, especially where there has been a degree of tearing to the rotator cuff, corticosteroid injections are used to manage the inflammation. Rotator cuff surgery is decidedly a last resort, as it is invasive and depending on the extent of the rotator cuff tear, surgery is successful in only 80% of all cases.

A separated shoulder is a common injury that results from physical contact to the shoulder region.

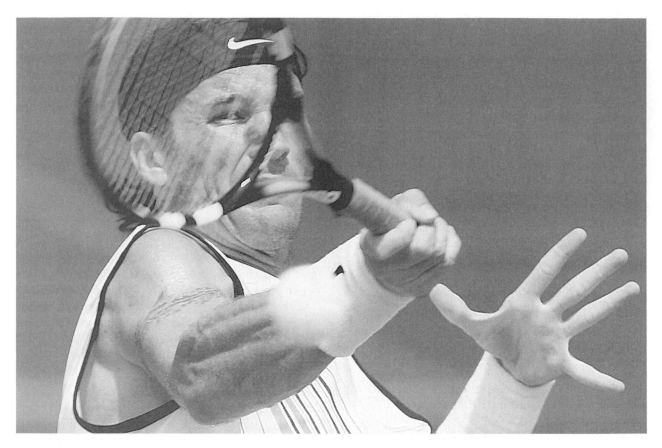

Mid-way through this match, Carlos Moya (returning the shot) ended the match due to an injury to his right shoulder. NICOLAS ASFOURI/AFP/GETTY IMAGES

The injury is actually sustained to the AC joint on the top of the shoulder, where the force of a blow, often a fall on the shoulder, causes a tearing of the ligaments that joint the clavicle and the scapula. The injury is immediately noticeable to an athlete, as there is significant pain and a bump forms at the site of the injury. The degree by which the bones are separated at the AC junction dictates the severity of the injury. Most separated shoulders heal with rest, the frequent application of ice in the first 48–78 hours after the event, and the use of a sling to permit the arm to be rested.

A dislocated shoulder is the coming apart of any of the joints of the shoulder, but is most common in the ball and socket joint. In contact sports such as American football, rugby, or ice hockey, the shoulder, as the body's most mobile joint, can be struck from almost any angle with great force. In competitions such as downhill skiing and gymnastics, an athlete can fall awkwardly with significant force and dislocate the joint. The force of dislocation may cause the humerus bone to become detached from the joint capsule in which it is held;

the surrounding ligaments or tendons may also be torn on impact. The rehabilitation for such injuries is similar to that of the separated shoulder, with a likelihood that the progress will be slower as the injury is usually more serious.

A fractured clavicle (collarbone) is the most common type of fracture to any of the bones of the shoulder joints. Usually the result of a hard fall, a fracture will result in the immediate impairment of the athlete's ability to use the arm. There is most often a noticeable sharp lump under the skin in the immediate vicinity of the break. Subject to related damage such as a ruptured blood vessel or nerve damage, the clavicle will heal cleanly within six to eight weeks of the injury.

In cases where the shoulder has been subjected to the progressive wearing away of the articular cartilage of the shoulder bones, the resulting osteoarthritis may require joint replacement surgery. This procedure is most common as a result of osteoarthritis in the glenohumoral joint. An artificial socket is the remedy, permitting the humerus bone to move against a synthetic surface.

SEE ALSO Baseball injuries; Musculoskeletal injuries; Shoulder anatomy and physiology; Tendinitis and ruptured tendons.

# William A. Shroyer

1888–1944
AMERICAN
INVENTOR, BASEBALL PLAYER

In the early days of American baseball, prior to 1890, the rules regarding the length, width, and configuration of a baseball bat were yet to be standardized. It was a common practice for players to manufacture their own wooden bats. Because bats broke, or became rough, with use rather frequently, players had to switch to a new, homemade bat. The replacement bat would often create a different "feel" in the hands of the batter, creating a period of adjustment for the player with the new bat.

The first technological advance in the manufacture of baseball bats occurred in 1884, when John Hillerich (1867-1946), an aspiring professional player who was also employed in his father's wood working factory, manufactured a bat from white ash, a very strong and durable wood, for a player on the local Louisville, Kentucky professional team. The new bat was found to be very well made, and soon the "Louisville Slugger" became a highly prized piece of baseball equipment. The Louisville Slugger is the world's best known baseball bat, designated the official bat of Major League Baseball.

The Louisville Slugger, and the various models of bats that followed it were functional and effective. The market for baseball bats and all other type of baseball equipment expanded in the twentieth century throughout America. Wooden bats remained prone to breakage and splintering no matter how well the bat was made. The "sweet spot" on wooden bats, the point in the barrel of the bat where the ability to strike the ball was most consistent, varied in both location and size on a wooden bat. It was in this era that a former baseball player turned inventor in Dayton, Ohio, William Shroyer, developed his ideas regarding a long lasting, economical and perhaps indestructible bat, the metal bat.

By way of patent number 1,499,128, as filed with the United States Patent and Trademark Office in June, 1924, Shroyer filed detailed diagrams and a description of the proposed metal bat design. Shroyer described the purpose of his design as one that would provide the lightness, springiness, and resiliency of the current wood construction. Shroyer sought to avoid the wood splitting and splintering that commonly occurred with wood. Shroyer also set out in his patent diagrams a threaded aperture in the head of the bat, a device that provided a place for the insertion of additional weight in the bat barrel if desired by a batsman.

It is evident from the patent office records that Shroyer had directed considerable care to his invention. It is equally apparent that Shroyer never commercially marketed his all-metal bat, and there is little evidence to suggest that he was ever able to manufacture a model beyond that of a prototype. No example of the Shroyer bat exists today; its inventor and patent holder died in relative obscurity.

The Shroyer metal bat patent is significant in the history of sport science for its prescience. The first aluminum baseball bat sold as a mass marketed item was produced by the Worth Sports Company in 1970. From that point, large baseball equipment companies such as Easton established significant markets for their aluminum bats in the softball, lob ball, and collegiate baseball markets.

Major league baseball banned the aluminum bat from competition almost from the moment it was available. Aluminum possesses a significantly higher coefficient of restitution than does wood, resulting in a correspondingly greater ability in the aluminum bat to return the energy of a pitched ball to the ball with the swing of the bat, causing the ball to travel further on a hit. Aluminum bats would render most professional baseball parks as home run derbies. Studies conducted by both the National Collegiate Athletic Association (NCAA) and private research groups confirm that an aluminum bat will send a baseball a minimum of 10% farther when hit with equal force by a wooden bat.

SEE ALSO Baseball.

# Sida cordifolia

Sida cordifolia, more commonly known as the mallow plant, is a small, green, seed-bearing plant that has been prized for over 5,000 years for its medicinal properties. Sida cordifolia is widely used in the Indian alternative medicine philosophy called Ayurveda, "the science of life." Ayurveda is a series of concepts that are rooted in the Hindu religion, with principles that are believed to be even older than those of the traditional Chinese medicines. Ayurveda remains a prominent part of modern Indian medicine, with designated schools that instruct students in applications of Ayurveda healing techniques. Ayurveda advocates a whole mind/whole body approach regarding the treatment of physical ailments; yoga and meditation are also components of the holistic philosophy that is Ayurveda.

Sida cordifolia is not of the same botanical family as the well-known medicinal herbs ephedra or the North American variant Mormon tea, but Sida cordifolia shares a common medicinal component with each: the alkaloids (plant-based substances) that include ephedrine, pseudoephedrine, and vasicinone.

Sida cordifolia and ephedra have a similar amounts of ephedrine present within their structures. While all parts of the Sida cordifolia plant have ephedrine present in them, the seeds of the plant possess the greatest percentage of the stimulant. Ephedrine is a well-known stimulant, which when consumed in any form, will tend to have an immediate effect on a number of the processes of the body. The most pronounced of these effects is an increased heart rate, and a corresponding increase in blood pressure.

Ephedrine has been used for many years and in many forms as a stimulant for athletes to assist with concentration and to reduce fatigue. It is also prized as a catalyst to facilitate weight loss (often described in various applications as "fat burning"). Ephedrine, like every other stimulant, will increase the body's metabolic rate. Persons who are engaged in significant weight training or other muscular strength and development activities often consume dietary supplements that contain varying proportions of Sida cordifolia to obtain the effect created by its ephedrine properties, caffeine (often present through the natural plant root guarana), and either willow bark or aspirin, each valued for the anti-inflammatory qualities of its chief ingredient, salicylic acid. These training products are known to strength athletes as the "ECA stack." This particular type of formulation is designed to provide the athlete with the stimulation of the ephedrine and caffeine, coupled with the analgesic effect of the aspirin, desirable for those who train hard and with great frequency.

Sida cordifolia was first determined to possess ephedrine in 1930, and for this reason it was subsequently recommended in India by physicians as a heart stimulant. In Ayurveda practices, Sida cordifolia had three common applications: Mashabaladi Kvatha, where the plant seeds were mixed with other ingredients to relieve muscular pain; Balataila, a process for the treatment of nervous system complaints, stomach problems, and as a cardiac tonic; and the crushed leaves of the plant as an astringent for the treatment and dressing of wounds or skin injuries.

Sida cordifolia has another alkaloid present within its structure that also has a pronounced effect on the body. Vasicinone, a substance formed from carbon, hydrogen, nitrogen, and oxygen, is expressed as the chemical equation $C_{11}H_{12}N_2O$. Vasicinone is an effective bronchodilator, tending to assist the body in the opening of restricted breathing passages.

Ephedrine poses risks to the body based on its chemical structure. The increase in heart rate and blood pressure creates an increased risk of heart attack. There are no formulations in which ephedrine is contained that reduce those risks. Ephedrine, coupled with the ingestion of a companion stimulant such as caffeine, can serve to accelerate the effects of ephedrine. All stimulants create a risk of both dependency for the user, and a danger that the user will feel compelled to increase the amounts consumed, risking toxicity.

The legal restrictions on the use of Sida cordifolia are not entirely clear in North America. Ephedrine, the subject of considerable debate in international sport as to its impact as a stimulant, given its broad availability and popular use in various cold and decongestant remedies, remains a prohibited substance in any competition that is subject to the control of the World Anti-Doping Agency (WADA), where the concentration of ephedrine found in the system of an athlete exceeds 10 mcg per milliliter of urine when tested. In the United States and a number of other Western world countries, the ephedra plant and its herbal products have previously been the subject of bans by regulatory agencies; Sida cordifolia (and other ephedra containing herbs such as bitter orange) are not similarly restricted.

**SEE ALSO** Dietary supplements; Ephedra; Herbs; Mormon tea; Stimulants.

# Skateboarding

The sport of skateboarding has undergone significant changes since it was introduced in the United States in the early 1950s. Originally a land based offshoot of surfing, the original skateboards were wooden boards attached to roller skates. Skateboarding at that time was an activity primarily carried out on streets and sidewalks.

Skateboarding is today a multi-dimensional sport that includes persons who ride their boards in the 1970s was significant innovation. Urethane permitted the rider to obtain greater traction on a paved surface, and the wheels ran much more smoothly, making the skateboard safer to operate.

Many skateboard tricks have acquired their own name. the most notable is the "ollie," regarded as the foundation to the majority of jump maneuvers performed in skateboarding. The ollie is executed by the rider applying a sudden force to the rear of the skateboard, and moving their feet forward to counteract the rear force, and sequence that propels the board into the air. Another common skateboard technique is "grinding," where the bottom of the board is made to slide along a hard surface. There are many examples recorded in the media where a skateboarder has sustained a spectacular fall when endeavoring to grind their board along a handrail or similar structure.

Skateboarding has significant safety concerns, particularly when the rider attempts a jump from a ramp, or any other stunt that takes the rider above the ground. Helmets, knee pads, wrist protection (to prevent injury to the hands and wrists in a fall), and elbow protection are common.

World Cup Skateboarding is the organization that sanctions professional skateboard events through out the world.

**SEE ALSO** Extreme sports; Snowboarding; Wakeboarding; Youth Sports Injuries.

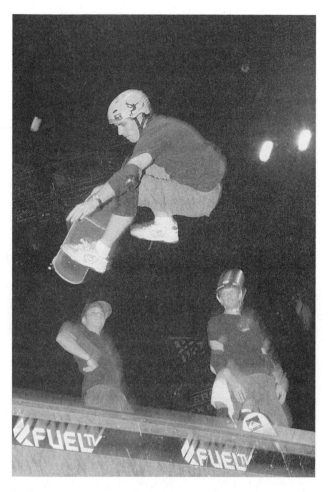

Professional skateboarder Andy Macdonald performs a trick above the half pipe while professional skateboarder Tony Hawk (R) looks on. **PHOTO BY MAT SZWAJKOS/GETTY IMAGES.**

public areas as well as the boarders who use specialized skateboard parks equipped with ramps and half pipes in which they can perform elaborate and often dangerous stunts. Skateboarding has a close connection to street fashion of young people and it has encouraged an easygoing attitude toward participation, in contrast to other more traditional sports. Skateboarding is a world wide sport, most actively pursued by youths and young adults.

Skateboarding has received a significant boost in its world wide popularity due to the combined effect of its inclusion in the X Games, the profile of professional skateboarders such as American Tony Hawk, and various videogames that have served to promote skateboarding and the extreme sports nature of the stunts that can be executed.

From the flat plywood board attached to a set of roller skate wheels that constituted the first skateboards, the invention of the first urethane wheels in

# Skates, roller SEE Roller skates

# Skating, figure SEE Figure skating

# Skating leaps and throws SEE Figure skating dynamics of leaps and throws

# Skeletal muscle

The skeletal muscles are those tissues that are attached to the bones of the body beneath the skin. As the muscles on examination appear to be constructed of varying lengths of strips, due to the manner in which the muscle fibers are situated, these muscles are also known as striated muscle.

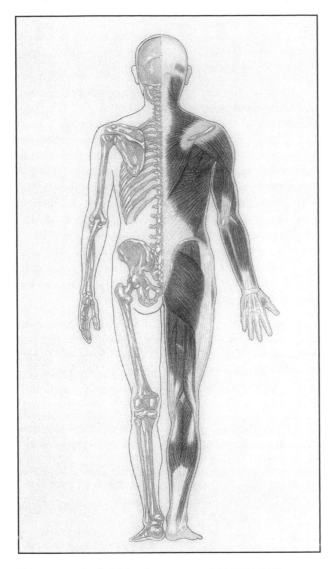

Human musculo-skeletal system. CARLYN IVERSON/PHOTO RESEARCHERS, INC.

Skeletal muscle is a distinct type of specialized muscles found within the body. Cardiac muscle (heart muscle) is used only to power the contractions of the heart. Cardiac muscles are controlled through the function of the autonomic nervous system, the aspect of human function regulated by the hypothalamus region of the brain. Smooth muscles are located within every hollow organ in the body, with the exception of the heart. Smooth muscles are also controlled involuntarily, performing such functions as the pushing of blood within the arteries of the cardiovascular system and the movements of ingested foods within the digestive system.

All skeletal muscles are positioned relative to the bone in a similar fashion no matter where in the body they may be positioned, irrespective of the muscle function. The prime place of attachment between a skeletal muscle and the adjacent bone is the point of origin for the muscle. The muscle will taper at its opposite end into a more slender connective tissue, the muscle tendon, to the connection with the bone, the point of insertion. Imbalances between the strength of the skeletal muscle, the laxity or otherwise in the tendon, and the connection to the bone surface are common causes of muscle injury in athletes.

Skeletal muscle can only exert its desired force on the skeleton to produce movement when the muscle is contracted. Almost all joints in the body are comprised of muscles that operate in pairs: one muscle acts as an extensor, to extend or straighten the joint, and the other muscle in the pair acts as a flexor, to facilitate the bending of the joint. The biceps and triceps muscles of the upper arm are an extensor/flexor pair for the elbow joint, as are the quadriceps (extensor) and the hamstrings (flexor) in the movements of the knee.

The muscle fibers that are the substance of each muscle are of similar construction throughout all skeletal muscles. The fibers are generally long, slender cylinders that extend from the point of origin to the tendon that connects at the point of insertion. The fibers are bundled, in quantities ranging from a few fibers to several hundred. The contraction of each muscle fiber bundle is controlled through the nerve impulses directed into the fiber bundle by a neuron, a type of electrical relay that is connected to the larger nervous system. The speed with which the neurons communicate impulses to the muscle fiber group determine whether the fibers will be a fast-twitch fiber (useful in sports that require, power, strength, and reaction time), or a slow-twitch fiber (best suited to endurance sports). In fine motor control muscles, such as the eyelid, the neuron may only control a group of 10 muscle fibers or fewer. In a large muscle such as the quadriceps or the gastrocnemius, each neuron may be connected to as many as 2,000 fibers. The fibers are made up of myofibrils, filaments that run the length of the muscle fiber.

The operation of the nervous system and its relation to the skeletal muscular system is sometimes referred to as the neuromuscular system. When nerve impulses are communicated to the muscle, a complex series of electrochemical reactions convert the impulse into a muscle contraction. Central to the reaction is the balance between sodium and potassium in the muscle membrane fluid. Sodium floods the membrane at the time the impulse is registered, replaced by potassium to return the membrane to a rest state. The reactions occur very quickly, and a muscle can be restored to its rest position after the activity generated by an impulse in approximately one millisecond.

Muscle fibers require resistance to grow stronger; an inactive muscle cannot ever become stronger. The act of applying resistance to the muscle, such as is achieved through weight training, is not itself an immediately strengthening act; the muscle repairs itself during rest between resistance training sessions. As the body rests, the muscle fibers attract cells known as myoblasts, which fuse with the existing fiber, causing the muscle fibers to become denser and stronger. Muscle size is not limitless, and the fibers will not attract unlimited numbers of myoblasts for repair, due to the presence of myostatin in the muscle cells. Myostatin is the hormone produced by the body that regulates muscle size, a natural limit on how large muscles can grow.

The actual muscle contraction generate within the muscle is fueled by the chemical reaction that occurs involving the compound adenosine triphosphate (ATP), which participates in a series of energy-producing reactions that involve creatine phosphate, present in the muscle cell, and gylcogen, transported to the cell through the blood as glucose.

SEE ALSO Bone, ligaments, tendons; Muscle fibers: Fast and slow twitch; Musculoskeletal injuries; Skeletal muscle function and energy metabolism.

## Skeletal muscle function and energy metabolism

Skeletal muscles are the mechanism for powering human movement. While individual muscles are typically regarded as distinct organic structures, the skeletal muscles are the largest organ grouping in the body (the skin is the largest contiguous organ). Virtually all joints are moved by pairs of muscles working in contrasting but complimentary ways, one set providing the extension of the joint (extensors), the opposing, or antagonist, set countering with flexion, or bending capability.

All muscles are composed of specialized muscle fibers. While the fibers are made up of the similar kinds of cells, fluids, blood vessels, and nervous system components, muscle fibers have certain key physical distinctions that create two distinct kinds of fibers, fast-twitch (type II fibers) and slow-twitch

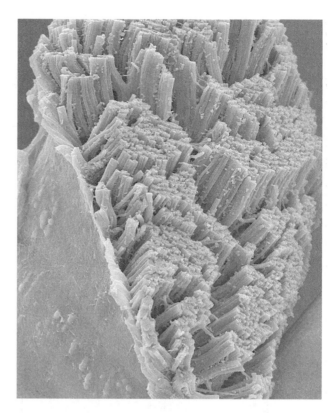

Skeletal muscle fiber (magnified 220 times). © VISUALS UNLIMITED/CORBIS

(type I fibers). Some fibers exhibit characteristics that place them between the two broad types, but closer to the fast-twitch variety; these fibers are often classed as the type IIa group.

The fast-twitch and slow-twitch fibers are distributed throughout the muscles of the body. The percentage distribution is determined genetically and it is unique to every human being. There is considerable scientific authority for the proposition that, through specific training such as intense endurance training, the composition of muscle fibers in an athlete's legs can be altered, converting fast-twitch fibers for use as slow-twitch fibers to better support the endurance activity.

Whether a muscle fiber functions as a fast-twitch or slow-twitch fiber is subject to a number of physical and neurological factors. Slow-twitch fibers are governed by slow conduction neurons, the relay switch of the nervous system that governs a group of muscle fibers ranging in size from as few as 10 to as many as 2,000 fibers. Fast-twitch fibers are governed by fast-acting neurons, which are capable of transmitting or firing the nerve impulses that command movements by the muscle 10 times more frequently than the slow-twitch neurons will fire.

The energy metabolism characteristics of each type of fiber also contribute to the function of each type. Fast-twitch fibers store glycogen within the cells of the muscle fiber. Glycogen, the storage form of the carbohydrate product glucose, is then utilized at the muscle in the cycle of electrochemical reactions that produce adenosine triphosphate (ATP), the source of energy within the muscle. To utilize this store of energy, a process known as glycogenosis occurs within the cell, where glycogen is converted to a compound, glucose-1-phosphate, which then participates in the energy production cycle within the cell involving creatine phosphate and ATP. The muscles store glycogen in quantities that total approximately 1% of the muscle mass, a reserve that is quickly depleted through intense exercise; the muscles can only produce ATP through glycogenosis for an approximate maximum of 90 seconds. As the ability of the fast-twitch cells to produce ATP and energy is limited, the fast-twitch cells quickly become fatigued. Examples of this energy metabolism frequently occur in sports such as sprinting. Races such as the 400 m and 800 m events are often described as the toughest of the running distances, because optimum performance is demanded of the body as it is running out of the energy stores capable of being generated in its fast-twitch fibers.

Slow-twitch fibers require glycogen, broken into its constituent glucose, before energy can be produced in its cells. The requisite glycogen is transported to the cells through the circulatory network that ends in the capillaries that service the cells of each muscle fiber. Because the energy production process in slow-twitch fibers is much slower, it can be sustained for much longer periods, and the slow-twitch fibers do not fatigue as readily as the fast-twitch fibers.

The mitochondria is the portion of the muscle cell where the energy production occurs. The mitochondria in the anaerobic fast-twitch fibers are significantly larger than that of the slow-twitch aerobic fibers. It is within the mitochondrial membrane that, depending on the energy sources available, either fatty acids are reduced for energy production, or glucose is ultimately converted to lactate as a part of the ATP energy cycle.

The skeletal muscles also perform important roles relative to the body's energy system while the body is fasting or otherwise not ingesting foods to be converted into useful energy sources. The skeletal muscles release amino acids during periods of fasting, particularly alanine and glutamine. These acids work in the bloodstream to maintain the body's blood glucose levels, stimulating the conversion of glycogen stored in the liver into glucose.

**SEE ALSO** Glycogen level in muscles; Muscle fibers: Fast and slow twitch; Muscle glycogen recovery; Skeletal muscle.

# Ski area avalanche control

An avalanche is the most destructive and dangerous event that can occur in a ski area. The torrent of snow that obliterates everything in its path is the ultimate natural disaster in a mountain region. The famed St. Bernard dogs of the Swiss Alps acquired their legendary reputation from the rescue of travelers caught in snow falls and avalanches. Death from exposure, injuries, or suffocation are a common fate for a skier caught in an avalanche.

Avalanches have a measure of predictability in that they can only occur on certain types of mountain terrain. An avalanche will rarely occur on a slope that is angled at less than 30°; these events similarly almost never occur on slopes greater than 45°, as it difficult for snow to accumulate in sufficient volumes on a steeper angle to precipitate a descent. As avalanches typically occur year after year in the same places, the force of the avalanche creates a well-defined path on a mountainside. New avalanche sites are often inadvertently created through the removal of forest cover for development or road construction.

A large volume of snow on a mountain side is not the sole cause of an avalanche. The type of snow, the layers of snow that may be created by a series of snowfalls, and the degree of adhesion between each layer of snow are all factors. Avalanches will take one of two forms: movement that involves loose snow, the less serious type of avalanche, and those that are known as a slab advance, created when various layers of the season's snowfall adhere and create a single wall of snow moving down a slope. The slab advance avalanche is the most destructive form, commonly extending over hundreds of feet/meters in width.

An avalanche can move along the terrain in three distinct fashions. The snow can move through the air, as occurs when the avalanche moves over a cliff or rock outcropping. Avalanches most often move along the ground; in some circumstances, the movement may be a combination of ground and air.

An avalanche may be triggered by natural and artificial, or external, means; avalanches are often

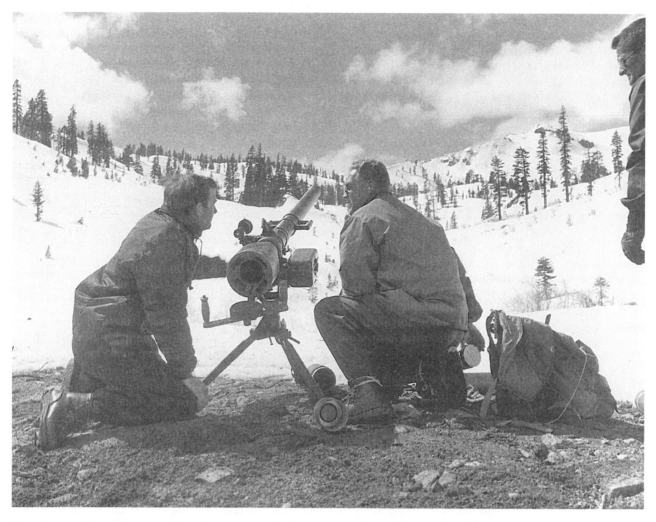

Men shoot recoilless rifles at snow formations to control avalanches at the 1960 Winter Olympic Games at Squaw Valley. One of the men works for the Forest Service as an avalanche control expert. © CORBIS

triggered intentionally for control purposes. The most common natural precipitating event is the fall of new snow on an already unstable snow mass. Skiers moving across or in the vicinity of an area of unstable snow are the most frequent cause of an inadvertent avalanche.

To control the ski area from the consequences of an avalanche, the first preventative step is to ensure that avalanche forecasting can be performed with some measure of precision. The forecast will include daily examinations of the current snow cover, including its type and its apparent density as well as meteorological forecasts.

Avalanche control has two essential components: the modification of the terrain where the avalanche is expected to occur prior to the ski season, and physically redirecting the snow once it has fallen and accumulated in a potentially dangerous fashion.

Terrain modification may entail a number of physical changes to the avalanche area. These steps are taken after the terrain has been carefully assessed and the most common avalanche pathways have been mapped. A common modification is the erection of snow sheds in the vicinity of road ways, buildings, or other structures that potentially fall in the path of an avalanche. A snow shed is commonly constructed of concrete, to withstand the force of thousands of pounds of advancing snow. The shed is not designed to stop the avalanche so much as to deflect the advancing snow away from the protected structure or feature.

Steps may also be taken to alter the physical terrain through earthmoving or the placement of barriers to divert the path of a future avalanche. A mountainside will often be divided into segments for the purpose of avalanche control, to prevent one avalanche from triggering companion slides on adjacent ski areas. Lightweight but strong metal fencing is often placed high on a mountainside to prevent the formation of the snow slabs that cause the most avalanche damage.

Once the snow has fallen and begins to accumulate in a manner that may precipitate an avalanche, the danger may be controlled by a number of artificial means. Through avalanche forecasting, the fracture zone, the place on the snow surface where the slab is most likely to break off from the existing snow cover, is capable of being identified. Explosives can be placed in the fracture line to trigger an artificial and more manageable event; mortar shells are sometimes fired from a distance into the fracture line to reduce the risk associated with a person physically skiing to the desired area for this purpose. A technique known as ski-cutting is also employed, where ski patrollers, working in pairs, use their skis to ski along the area of the fracture line and cause a limited and predictable avalanche.

**SEE ALSO** Cold-related illnesses and emergencies; Exposure injuries; Ski conditions; Skiing, Alpine; Skiing, Nordic (cross-country skiing).

# Ski conditions

Ski conditions are defined as the amount and the state of the snow for the purpose of skiing. For this reason, the expressions ski conditions and snow conditions are often used interchangeably. An assessment of the applicable ski conditions is an important, sometimes primary consideration in both Alpine skiing and Nordic (cross-country) skiing as to how the athlete will approach the tactical decisions required for a particular course. In the third of the skiing disciplines, freestyle skiing, ski conditions are less important to the performance of the athlete because the freestyle skier competes on a manicured snow surface on a generally much shorter race course.

The condition of the snow will dictate how the skis will perform on the snow surface. The altitude at which the skier is performing, the temperature of the snow, and the effect of sunlight and wind will all play a role in how the snow surface will react to the forces directed against it. Snow conditions often vary dramatically from the top of the mountain to the bottom in Alpine skiing; on a 12-mi (20 km) Nordic course, temperatures may change by as much as 20°F (8°C)

from the beginning of the event to the end, causing the snow to physically change as the race progresses.

How snow falls will determine how it initially forms on the ground. Snow is classified into various types. Powder refers to the softest form of snow, and usually accumulates in a dense, packed formation, and when untracked, powder is a surface on which Alpine skiers find that they can execute turns, control their downhill speed, and generally hold their edges with greater ease. When powder has been skied on, it is described as "tracked out," where the surface has various lumps and ruts that reduce some of the cushioning.

When the snow has been subjected to a freeze and thaw cycle over a period of time, the snow surface may often have a crust of ice form on top, which also becomes more granular in its texture. The same freeze and thaw temperature cycle in reverse can produce an opposite result, slush, where the snow becomes wetter and heavier and makes skiing movement more difficult. The most challenging snow condition faced by both Alpine and Nordic skiers is ice, created where a soft or wet surface freezes; icy ski conditions are not 100% solid water, but are sufficiently hard to create an extremely slick ski terrain.

Ski conditions will dictate the type of ski wax applied to the equipment of both Nordic and Alpine skiers, although the purpose of the wax is specific to each ski discipline. Ski waxes tend to be one of two general types: glide wax and kick wax. Wax for skis has a dual purpose, the primary of which is to create an optimum sliding surface between the snow and the ski. The secondary purpose behind the application of wax is to protect the surface of the ski from damage caused by the contact between the ski and the icy ruts and imperfections of the course.

Glide waxes, in an almost infinite variety of formulations, are used by both Alpine and Nordic skiers. Most skis are subjected to some form of factory prewaxing; the skis will be subjected to very high-end waxing treatments in preparation for all training and competition runs. A number of glide waxes are applied through a heat process to create a better adhesion between the ski and the wax. The glide wax is generally composed of a mixture of either hydrocarbon (oil) byproducts, or a fluorocarbon base. Glide waxes function by creating a microscopically thin cushion of water between the ski and the surface as the skier races over the snow, which reduces the amount of friction between the ski and the surface.

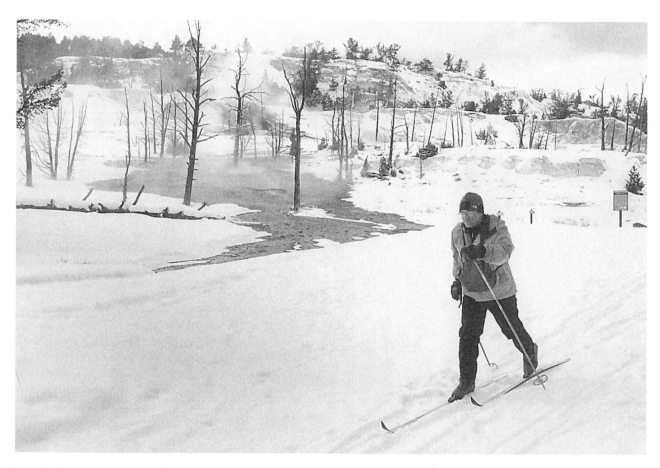

Knowing the current ski conditions enables skiers (downhill and cross-country) how to prepare for and approach the tactical decisions required for a particular course. **AP PHOTO/THE LIVINGSTON ENTERPRISE, ERIK PETERSEN**

Kick wax is a substance used exclusively by Nordic skiers to create a more effective skiing motion. The longer and thinner cross-country ski has two distinct areas that are often treated with different kinds of wax; how extensively the two types of wax are applied depends on whether the skier will be skiing in the classic style, where the skier moves the skis forward in alternating strides, or the modern skating style. Kick wax is applied to the ski surface under the boot bindings to make the ski move easily over the snow. On cold or very firm surfaces, the wax will be a hard wax, which permits a degree of grip onto the icy surface necessary to permit the skier to get the traction necessary to kick forward with every stride. When the snow is soft or wet, the wax substance will be a softer "klister" wax, which permits the skier to glide more efficiently in the heavier snow. In elite-level Nordic racing, the ski technician is a very valuable member of a ski team. The technician will often be required to change the waxes a number of times during an event to counter the changes in weather or snow conditions.

**SEE ALSO** Skiing, Alpine; Skiing, freestyle; Skiing, Nordic (cross-country skiing).

## Skiing, Alpine

Alpine skiing includes all forms of the sport that involve skiing in mountain settings; the Alpine classification is derived from the Alps mountains of south central Europe where this form of skiing originated. Alpine skiing today is a popular recreational activity in any mountainous area of the world where there is snow. The competitive forms of Alpine skiing are especially popular in North America, in the Rocky Mountains and the ski areas of the northeastern United States, and throughout many European countries. Alpine skiing has a worldwide following through the annual World Cup ski circuit. The Alpine events at the quadrennial Winter Olympics are among the most popular of that competition.

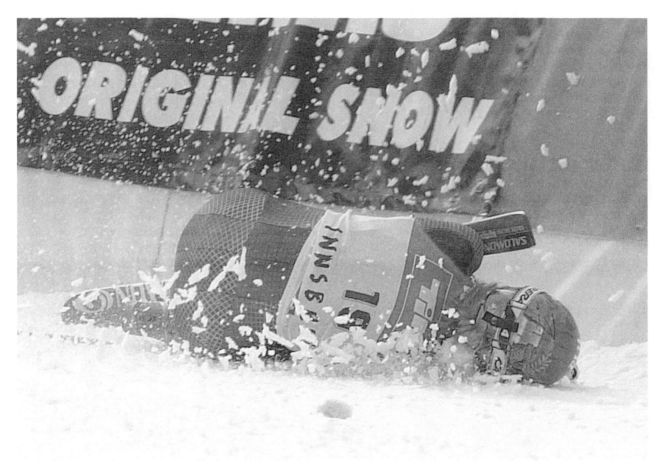

Due to the speed of the event, injuries in the downhill are often catastrophic in nature; concussion and serious knee injuries are common.
AP PHOTO/RUDI BLAHA

Competitive Alpine skiing is divided into a number of distinct pursuits, each of which has its own technical, equipment, and training requirements. There are few subjective aspects to any of the Alpine events—subject to the skier successfully negotiating preset gates placed on the course, the fastest competitor down the mountain will win the race.

Alpine skiing comprises five separate events; many elite racers will compete in all of them. Alpine skiing is contested in both men's and women's categories. The downhill, like the 100-m sprints in track and field, is the most glamorous of the Alpine events. Dominated for decades by European skiers such as Jean Claude Killy of France and Franz Klammer of Austria, Canadian downhillers such as Ken Read and Steve Podborski, and American Picabo Street made the downhill a more international competition. An event that typifies courage, the downhill requires an intense adherence to technical form to both maximize speed (usually in excess of 60 mi/100 km per hour) and to keep the skier on the course.

Due to the speed of the event, injuries in the downhill are often catastrophic in nature; concussion and serious knee injuries are common if the skier falls. The downhillers must be adept at three separate components of ski movement: starts, getting a strong push from the start gate at the top of the hill to obtain the highest speed as quickly as possible; turning, often on icy surfaces at high speeds as the skier takes an optimal line down the course; and gliding, where the skier creates an aerodynamic body position, known as a "tuck" to maintain speed and balance through the flatter sections of the course. The downhill racers often must land from jumps on the course, a technique that requires skiers to relax their body to absorb the force of the high-speed landing, while maintaining an efficient position and not compromising speed.

The super giant slalom, known as the "super g," is an Alpine skiing event that is a combination of the speed of the downhill and the more technical requirements of balance and negotiating gates that are essential to the shorter slalom events. This race, like the downhill, will consist of one run down the mountain.

The giant slalom is a race course where the skier must negotiate a series of gates that require the skier to maintain speed, while in a low position to cut through the gates with a minimum of wasted effort. A missed gate is a disqualification. The race will be composed of two runs, with the skier's total time the basis of the score.

The slalom is the shortest of the Alpine courses and the most technically demanding. The gates are placed closer to one another, and the skier must execute high-speed turns back and forth through each gate. Slalom skis are shorter than those used in super g and the downhill, to improve the maneuverability of the skier through the gates. Skiers are allowed to make contact with the gates so long at they do not avoid the gate: slalom skiers often use their shins and forearms to power through the obstacle with the minimum distance traveled, and they wear significant padding along the shins and forearms, as well as a full-face masked helmet to permit the skier to pass close to the gate without being injured by the contact.

All Alpine ski events are relatively short in duration. For this reason, all Alpine disciplines have certain common training features. As with many elite disciplines, especially those where the competitive season is dictated by environmental conditions such as cold and snow fall, Alpine skiers have a well-defined training calendar of preseason and post-season training. Alpine skiers must have a strong upper body to generate drive with their poles and to counter the very powerful forces of the skis. Downhill racers will encounter significant g forces, the force of acceleration due to gravity, as they descend the course and execute turns; physical strength is required to adequately counter this effect. The leg movements made at high speed on the course require considerable explosive muscular ability, developed by various types of plyometrics exercises. The recovery time of alpine skiers is promoted through an aerobic exercise component.

The ability of the skier to absorb the often extreme forces of the jumps and bounces created on an alpine course mandates intense attention to flexibility exercises. Stiff or otherwise unresponsive joints, particularly in the ankles, knees, and pelvis, will mean more force being directed into the body and detracting from the desired forward and efficient motion of the skier.

**SEE ALSO** Cold-related illnesses and emergencies; Plyometrics; Range of motion; Ski conditions; Skiing, Nordic (cross-country skiing).

# Skiing, freestyle

It is a paradox of the world of winter sports that freestyle skiing, the most seemingly unstructured of the skiing disciplines, is judged almost entirely on a subjective basis. However, the Alpine and Nordic events, much more restricted in terms of technique and approach, are assessed by the most objective of measures: the clock.

Freestyle skiing can trace its roots in the rebellion against the established structure of Alpine skiing in the 1960s. There arose a movement among skiers, particularly in North America, to have a competitive ski environment that permitted far greater freedom of expression among its athletes. Freestyle skiing first grew in a cult fashion in the northeastern United States' mountains and the resorts of Quebec. The Canadian Freestyle Skiing Association was the first governing body in the nascent sport, formed in 1974. The International Olympic Committee (IOC) had been resistant to the inclusion of freestyle skiing in the Winter Olympics; the IOC expressed reservations that the sport was too dangerous. Nevertheless, the first Olympic freestyle competition was held in 1992, for both men and women, with the number of events available within the sport growing with each Olympics. Over 30 countries now have national governing bodies in freestyle skiing.

Freestyle skiing has two general types of competition, and athletes tend to specialize in one area only. Moguls competition is a series of events where the competitor descends a steep hill that has a pitch of as much as 30° and has been artificially groomed with an asymmetrical series of bumps of unequal dimensions. The snow surface for the course is packed to make the skis move with as little friction as possible. As the skiers move down the hill, they are required to execute a series of jumps, twists, and other acrobatic maneuvers. Each maneuver is scored in terms of its degree of difficulty and complexity, as well as the speed with which the jump was executed. The total time taken to cover the entire course is also a factor in the mogul scoring system.

Dual moguls events are conducted in the same fashion as single moguls, with two competitors descending side by side on the hill. Given the nature of the scoring for the jumps and other maneuvers, the first freestyler to descend the hill is not necessarily the winner of the event.

The second freestyle ski discipline is that of aerial freestyle, or aerials. Aerial events require the skier to descend a steep hill and leap from a ramp to perform a predetermined maneuver. The skier is

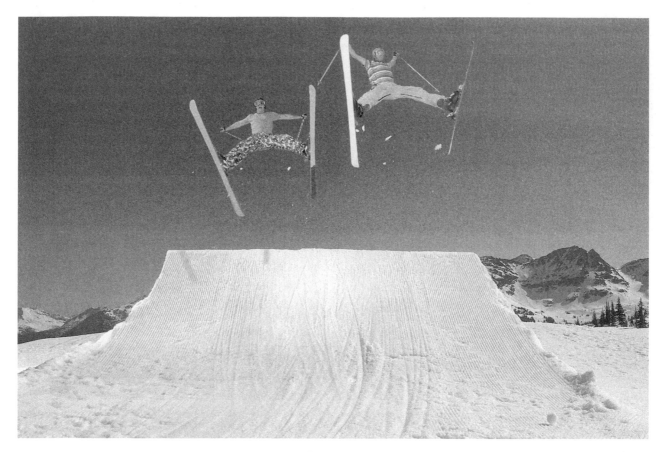

Freestyle ski jumping. © RANDY FARIS/CORBIS

judged by the level of difficulty of the jump, the technical execution of the jump, the quality of the landing, and artistic factors. Aerial freestylers are generally heralded as the glamour athletes in the freestyle world, as they will perform their routines in the air having left the ramp at speeds approaching 60 mph (100 km/h), with twisting body movements that may take them 50 ft (15 m) above the ground. The aerialist is required to land on a steep hill without losing balance.

Freestyle skiers do not require a high level of classic skiing ability. An ideal mogul skier will possess excellent balance, leg and core strength to successfully negotiate the moguls, and an extremely well-developed sense of body control, to complete jumps and land on the uneven mogul surface in rapid fire succession. Aerial skiers must possess similar physical attributes as those in moguls, with an additional emphasis on extremely well-developed flexibility.

The training required of a freestyle skier differs dramatically from that in which either Nordic or Alpine competitors will engage. Both forms of free-

style skiing are high intensity sports, the moguls typically lasting as long as 90 seconds, and the aerial event approximately 20 seconds. The development of the athlete's anaerobic energy systems is crucial.

The range of motion required in the joints of a freestyle skier is profound. The ability to both generate the power necessary to jump explosively, coupled with making a soft landing to permit the skier to move on to the next element is essential. All freestyle skiers engage in significant stretching and flexibility training.

Freestyle skiing is a sport where simulation is an essential training aid. An athlete can practice the various aerial maneuvers contemplated in both moguls and aerials on a trampoline; the trampoline represents a very safe and cost-effective way for an athlete to work on the performance components in a warm indoor environment. In a number of countries, summer freestyle ski training sites have been constructed, using an artificial snow surface on the jumping hill, with the skier landing in a pond of water. As with the trampoline training, the athlete may practice intensively with a reduced risk of injury.

SEE ALSO Exercise, high intensity; Ski conditions; Skiing, Alpine; Skiing, Nordic (cross-country skiing); Plyometrics.

# Skiing, Nordic (cross-country skiing)

Modern Nordic skiing traces its roots to the ancient forms of transportation employed by Scandinavian people to travel across their snow-covered landscapes. Nordic skiing evolved into a series of distinct competitive disciplines in the late 1800s. Cross-country skiing is at the heart of Nordic competition; in both international and the Olympic Winter Games, the Nordic events also include the biathlon (skiing and rifle target shooting), ski jumping, and the Nordic combined event (cross-country skiing and ski jumping). Nordic skiing is administered through the international governing body for all skiing disciplines, the International Ski Federation (FIS).

At its essence, cross-country skiing requires long, narrow skis with bindings that permit considerable flexibility in the movement of the foot, lightweight boots, ski poles, and clothing appropriate to the conditions; cross-country skiing can take place in conditions where the air temperature is above freezing, to those where the effect of wind chill may approach −40°F (−40°C). The skis are designed to support the weight of the skier over their greater length, creating efficiency in movement through less resistance against the surface of the snow. The skis are not fixed boards, but each is constructed with a degree of flex, which permits the skier to push with the foot and receive energy from the ski in return; unlike a flat solid surface, the ski has a significant coefficient of restitution, a physical measure as to how much energy is returned by an object from an applied force. Modern cross-country skis are made of lightweight, composite carbon fiber and fiber glass materials for this reason.

Ski conditions will vary tremendously from day to day, and occasionally from hour to hour, on a Nordic ski course, as temperatures and sunlight striking the snow fluctuate. Snow will generally be either a hard, icy surface or a softer, wetter compilation sometimes tending to slush. Specialized waxes are applied to the running surface of the skis to provide more efficient movement across the surface as well as providing the skiers with the ability to obtain a degree of traction against the surface as they stride forward.

Glide wax is often applied to the ski by way of a heat process to create maximum adhesion between the ski surface and the wax. Where the wax is applied to the surface of the ski and in what quantity it is applied are dictated by the ski conditions and the style of the skiing to be done, either classic technique or skating. Glide waxes are formulated to reduce the friction between the ski and the snow surface. Kick waxes are applied to provide the skier with grip against the snow surface. In classic ski technique, the skier strides forward with the skis moving parallel to one another. The skier strides with a kick motion, and the kick wax permits the ski to adhere to the surface long enough to create resistance, which in turn allows the skier to generate force to produce propulsion along the surface. In extremely icy conditions, a very thick wax called "klister" will be applied to the skis. Elite skiers and cross-country ski teams will have ski technicians, whose sole responsibility is to maintain the proper type of waxes for the prevailing conditions.

Classic skiing represents the original means of cross-country skiing. The skier moves with the ski propelled in parallel; the binding permits the heel of the boot to be raised with each stride. Classic skiing is sometimes referred to as "kick and glide," with the kicking motion of each foot complimented by the skier's double pole technique, with the poles being pushed into the surface with each stride for extra forward movement and for balance.

The modern form of cross country technique is the skating style. Skating skiers employ shorter skis and poles, and a motion where the skis, each positioned at approximately 30° of angle from the direction of travel, are pushed into the snow surface in a skating motion, with the poles driven into the surface in coordination. Skating permits the skier to go faster than in the classic discipline; most elite racers will compete in both types of events and, in international competition, there are races where the skier must use both techniques, with ski and equipment changes at a midway point.

The biathlon requires the skier to complete a prescribed number of laps on a course with target shooting required between laps. There is a considerable physiological and mental challenge posed in this sport, as the skier, whose heart rate may exceed 170 beats per minute while skiing, must, through coordinated deep breathing, reduce the heart rate to permit accuracy in shooting at a target positioned 55 yd (50 m) distant.

Ski jumping embraces an entirely different set of physical considerations. The athletes launch from a ramp that descends from the hill; the take-off

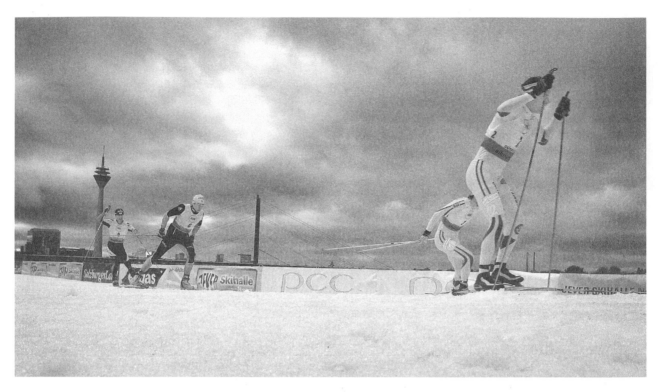

Men skiing on the cross-country ski run during the first stage of the 2005 Nordic Skiing World Cup, in the western town of Düsseldorf, Germany. VOLKER HARTMANN/AFP/GETTY IMAGES

speed for an elite jumper will exceed 55 mph (90 km/h). The skiers then extend as far over the ski tips, positioned in a "V" formation. This aerodynamic body position maximizes the skiers' degree of lift in the air; depending on the hill and the wind conditions, an elite jumper may travel as far as 135 yd (120 m) in the air.

Cross-country skiing engages a number of important physiological considerations for the competitive racer. Fitness is crucial since cross-country skiing is a very demanding sport, requiring primarily well-developed endurance capabilities, including oxygen uptake, VO$_2$max, to service the significant energy demands of movement. Strength-to-weight ratio is also important. Cross-country skiers are often relatively tall, to obtain a longer, more efficient stride and to secure optimal leverage with the ski poles. Cross-country skiers must possess excellent overall muscular strength, with a measure of explosive sprint capability to sprint at the end of the races.

Hydration is an important consideration as cross-country skiers will build up significant heat production and corresponding perspiration loss through the demands of the sport even in very cold temperatures. Also, acclimatization to cold and difficult conditions is essential.

Nordic cross-country ski competitions have a variety of events, from relay races to shorter sprint distances 5 km and 10 km, to the longest World Cup and Olympic event, 20 km. The courses are often designed to include significant uphill and downhill segments. Most elite cross-country skiers will compete in both classic and skating disciplines. Norway has won the most championships of any country in cross-country skiing, with Finland, Sweden, Russia, Germany, and Italy all recognized world powers in both men's and women's racing.

While cross-country skiing is at one level an elemental battle between skier and snowy course, there have been a number of doping incidents in international championships. Blood doping is the artificial enhancement of the athlete's erythrocyte (red blood cell) levels to create a greater ability to transport oxygen within the blood stream. Common techniques involve either the administration of a synthetic version of the hormone erythropoietin (EPO), which governs red blood cell production within the body, or through the intravenous transfusion of another person's enriched blood. Blood doping was the cause of a disqualification of members of the Finnish Nordic team at the 2002 Winter Olympics. In 2006 at the Turin Olympics, Russian skier Olga Pyleva was stripped of her silver medal in cross country when the banned stimulant carphedon was detected in her system.

SEE ALSO Blood doping; Ski conditions; Skiing, Alpine; Skiing, freestyle.

## Skiing, water SEE Water skiing

## Skin injuries SEE Abrasions, cuts, lacerations

## Skin and muscle blood flow during exercise

The skin is the body's largest organ, accounting for approximately 15% of the body mass of the average adult. The skeletal muscles are the largest collection of common structures, totaling 40% of the body mass. The skin and the skeletal muscles are each significantly affected by blood flow during exercise.

The skin is composed of two defined parts, the epidermis and the dermis. The epidermis is the outer covering of the body, acting as both a shield against foreign objects that might enter the various bodily systems, as well as insulation and support for the internal organs and tissues. The dermis is located below the epidermis, and contains the capillaries, the blood vessels that provide the tissue with its necessary nutrients, the subcutaneous glands that release oils and perspiration from the skin, and the roots for human hair. During exercise, the dermis is immediately affected by changes in blood flow.

Skeletal muscles are the source of power for all skeletal movement by the body through their contraction, which is stimulated through a complex interplay of nerve impulses. Skeletal muscles also assist in the support of the entire bodily structure. The individual muscles are each composed of a series of fibers, arranged into bundles of various sizes. The muscle fibers contain cells where the energy-to-power movement is produced. These cells are supplied with oxygen and nutrients, such as glucose or fatty acids, through the capillaries that extend directly into the muscle. The blood also removes the waste products that occur through energy production in the muscle cells. Each muscle fiber is encircled with three or four capillaries. When the body is performing with efficiency, oxygen and nutrients are carried to the

muscle cells by the blood at the same rate with which waste carbon dioxide and other metabolites are removed.

An increase in blood flow is described as active hyperemia. The effect of exercise on the flow of blood within the body is progressive. To accommodate the demands for oxygen, the heart will begin to beat faster and to pump more powerfully. An increased heart rate will stimulate increased blood pressure within the cardiovascular system as well as increased blood volume to counter the demands of exercise. Depending on external factors such as temperature and other environmental conditions, the thermoregulatory system of the body will seek to achieve a balance between the maintenance of the body's core temperature and the release of perspiration to cool the body. These functions cause blood to be directed toward the surface of the skin. The warm blood from the internal areas is cooled through this exchange; perspiration causes a reduction in blood volume over time unless the fluids are replaced. In warm weather conditions, as much as 30% of the cardiac output goes to direct the flow of blood to the skin for cooling; the evaporation of perspiration will act to reduce body temperature. The control of the capillaries that expand and contract in the process of increasing and decreasing blood flow to the skin is determined through the nerve structures connected to the autonomic nervous system, the specialized regulation by the brain of a number of essential body functions.

In cold conditions [when the body is exposed to temperatures that fall below 40°F (4°C), the autonomic nervous system will seek to maintain the warmth of the vital internal organs, and blood will correspondingly be directed away from the extremities and the skin surface to the internal organs. In such circumstances, the skin temperature will fall and the skin, both the epidermis and the underlying dermis, becomes vulnerable to freezing, leading to the injury known as frostbite.

When the body is at rest, approximately 20% of the cardiac output is directed to the maintenance of blood flow to the skeletal muscles. The rate of skeletal muscle blood flow in the body's resting state is 3 ml/minute per 100 mg of muscle mass. Very shortly after the start of exercise, the blood flow rate to the muscle will increase by as much as 20 times the resting rate. In sports such as swimming, cross-country skiing, or running, where the entire body and almost all skeletal muscles are working in some capacity, the cardiac output directed to the skeletal muscles approaches 80%. There is a rough correlation between blood flow increases and the increase in the amount of oxygen consumed during exercise.

The increased blood flow is directed through a cardiovascular device known as the skeletal muscle pump. The veins that direct the spent arterial blood back to the heart and lungs are constructed with a one-directional valve that promotes venous return, permitting the body to recycle and recharge the blood more quickly.

SEE ALSO Blood volume; Cardiovascular system; Cold weather exercise; Muscle cramps.

## Sky diving

Sky diving is the sport form of parachuting, an activity defined as the controlled descent of a person to the surface of the earth from an aircraft, using a parachute to control the rate of descent. Sky diving is often grouped with sports such as bungee jumping and para-gliding, activities which are often described as the aerial extreme sports.

The history of parachute jumping pre-dates the modern concept of extreme sport by several hundred years. Leonardo da Vinci (1452-1519), the noted Renaissance inventor and artist, designed a parachute intended for use in the rescue of persons from burning buildings. A number of French balloonists experimented with parachutes from heights of over 2,000 ft (600 m) beginning in the late 1780s.

With the advent of powered aircraft in the early part of the twentieth century, parachuting became a important component of military troop deployment, tactics, and aircrew safety. The paratrooper is a specialized soldier used in a wide number of combat roles in present day military operations.

The first sport parachuting competition was held in Yugoslavia in 1951. Sky diving, like most extreme sports, places a far greater emphasis upon the personal experiences of the participant, as they seek to achieve a personal goal, rather than focusing on the attainment of a competitive objective. Sky divers have established a number of records that are a testament to human endurance. The most notable example is that of the parachute jump from the greatest height ever recorded. In 1960 Col. Joseph Kittinger of the United States Air Force traveled 102,800 ft (31,000 m), a fall that lasted approximately 4.8 minutes, in which Kittinger reached

speeds approaching 700 mph (1,100 km/h) over a desert in New Mexico.

Sky diving requires primary importance to be placed upon the safety of every participant. In the United States, a prospective skydiver must be a minimum of 18 years of age (16 years of age if they have the permission of a parent or guardian to make a jump). The subject must also obtain a certificate of physical fitness from a physician, and all sky divers must complete a training program known in most jurisdictions as a first jump course. The first jump will generally take one of two training formats, a tandem free fall jump, or an instant opening/static line jump. In a tandem free fall jump, the student and instructor jump together from the aircraft at an altitude of approximately 10,000 ft (3,000 m), attached to the same parachute system. The two persons enter free fall (where they are pulled without restriction towards the earth by the force of gravity) for approximately 30–50 seconds, when the parachute is activated. In a instant opening jump, the student jumps and the parachute opens immediately upon the student exiting the aircraft.

A significant aspect of sky diving is the execution of group parachute jumps, where the participants seek to create different shaped formations in the air as they fall. The group formation divers wear skin-tight jump suits to reduce the effect of drag on their bodies as they fall through the air. During the period prior to the activation of their parachutes by the sky divers, the formation moves in a group free fall. Drag is the force created upon any body moving through the air; skydivers will also reduce the effect of drag in the creation and maintenance of the shape of the desired formation during descent, by altering the profile of their bodies as they descend. These sky divers will reach speeds of approximately 100 mph (190 km/h) prior to the deployment of their parachutes.

At several locations through out the world, wind tunnels are utilized by sky divers to simulate the conditions experienced by a skydiver as they descend in free fall.

Sky divers often describe their sport with any number of adjectives that convey the excitement of the rush towards the earth's surface; exhilarating and breath-taking are two that are commonly employed. The determination of the physical fitness of the participants centers on the healthy function of the subject's cardiovascular and cardiorespiratory systems. The risks associated with sky diving are

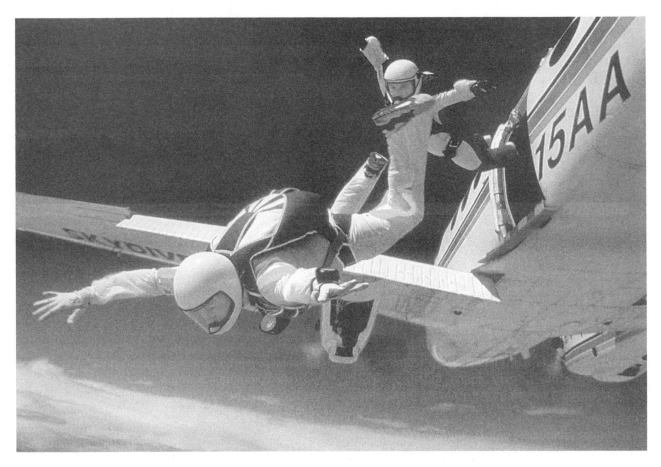

Two men skydiving. © DAVID MADISON/ZEFA/CORBIS

more often identified with substandard safety practices both in flight and at the drop zone, such as the proximity of trees or power lines to the descending sky diver. In the United States, there are approximately 15 sky diving fatalities for every one million jumps annually.

An important physical skill learned by sky divers is the absorption of the forces generated on landing. A favored technique is the entering into a sideways roll immediately upon impact, with the hands and arms kept close the sky diver's torso. This technique is known as the parachute roll; if the landing forces are not absorbed effectively, the skydiver risks serious injury to the feet and lower legs. If the skydiver is overweight, the risk of forces at impact causing injury are magnified accordingly.

**SEE ALSO** Balance training and proprioception; Environmental conditions and training; Motor control.

# Slam dunk SEE Basketball: Slam dunk

# Slapshot SEE Ice hockey: Slapshot velocity and hockey stick technology

# Sleep

Sleep is as essential to health as air, food, and water. Human performance, in everyday life and in sports, will depend on the quality and the regularity of sleep. From a technical perspective, sleep may be defined as the natural state of rest where the person sustains a partial or complete loss of consciousness. The body during sleep is less responsive to external stimuli, and the brain activity is altered during sleep, where the brain sometimes engages in dreams.

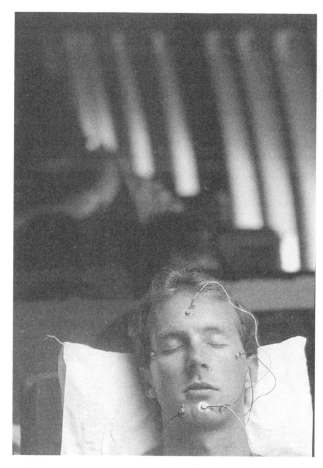

Stanford University student being monitored for heart rate and temperature during a flight from California to Tokyo as part of a study on jet lag. © LOUIE PSIHOYOS/CORBIS

The primary purposes of sleep are to rest the body, to permit the repair of musculoskeletal tissues, and for the body to generally recover from the stresses imposed on it during the waking hours. The amount of sleep that an individual requires will vary from person to person; as a general proposition, an adolescent will requires over nine hours of sleep per day, a consequence of their body's growth. An adult typically requires between seven and nine hours of sleep per night. Persons who are active in sports will generally require a greater quality, if not quantity, of sleep each night.

The effectiveness and the duration of sleep is governed by two distinct factors. Sleep/wake homeostasis is balance that the body strives to maintain between its wakefulness and sleep as a restorative process. When the body has been subjected to a very demanding period of activity, it will seek to have the sleep period be one of corresponding quality and duration to achieve homeostasis (balance).

The second factor governing sleep patterns is the circadian biological clock, sometimes referred to as the body's circadian rhythms. The circadian biological clock tells the body when it is most alert and when it is required to sleep. These rhythms are governed by the hypothalamus, the region of the brain that governs a diverse group of functions, including body temperature, hormonal release, and how the body responds to light and darkness. Most adults experience their most powerful desire to sleep between 2:00 a.m. and 4:00 a.m., with a lesser rhythm present between 1:00 p.m. 3:00 p.m. daily.

Circadian rhythms are not constant; external factors such as prior sleep quality and jet lag will disrupt the rhythms. The desire to nap during the course of a given day is tied in part to the presence of the rhythms; the afternoon *siesta* that is a part of the culture of many warm-weather countries is consistent with these natural rhythms.

Sleep can be disrupted by a multitude of conditions, some of which are a consequence of physical illness or disease, others more transient and often environmental in nature. Snoring, which disrupts the quality of sleep for both the snorer and any sleep partner, can be caused by a number of physical factors; overweight persons tend to snore more frequently. Medications, particularly those that have a steroid in their formulation, may disrupt sleep. Caffeine consumption (or other stimulants) artificially counters the effects of fatigue, the body's natural signal to rest. Alcohol is a central nervous system depressant, creating an artificial desire to sleep and a disruption of the body's cycle.

Jet lag is the well-known expression for the effect on the circadian biological clock caused by travel to different global time zones. Jet lag can be particularly disruptive to the achievement of peak athletic performance. The athlete's body, which may be accustomed to afternoon or evening performance times, is essentially tricked by the imposition of a lengthy time difference. Jet lag generally affects athletes who are competing in a time zone more than four hours apart from their home time zone.

Restless leg syndrome is a nervous system condition where the legs move spasmodically through sleep, affecting sleep quality. Another condition, sleep apnea, is a breathing disorder that creates temporary obstructions of breath as the sleeper inhales and exhales. In a rare worst-case scenario, sleep apnea could lead to a cardiopulmonary disruption; sleep apnea contributes to poor quality sleep. Nocturia is a need to urinate at night; a number of kidney disorders and medication side effects will disrupt the sleep of persons in this fashion.

Sleep inertia is a condition that may arise in persons who enjoy a full night's sleep. In some persons, sleep inertia can create a state where the person suffers from an impairment of the cognitive abilities that may last as long as two hours upon awakening. The portion of the brain responsible for the formulation of plans and the solving of problems, the prefrontal cortex, does not reach an active level at the same speed as other parts of the brain. Caffeine, through coffee, is the typical manner in which people counter the effects of sleep inertia.

SEE ALSO Exhaustion; Fatigue; Fitness; Health; Sleep deprivation and sports performance.

# Sleep deprivation and sports performance

All humans are biologically programmed to require sleep, as essential as air, food, and water. The demands of sports training and competition make good, regular, and restful sleep even more important. No athlete can ever realize his or her true sport potential unless their sleep is as vigorously pursued as all other aspects of the athletic life.

Sleep deprivation is not one or two nights of inadequate rest. Sleep deprivation is also referred to as a cumulative sleep debt, the product of ingrained sleep habits. Adolescents who normally require over nine hours of sleep per night to accommodate the growth processes ongoing in their bodies will often desire even more sleep if they are participating in sports. Athletic adults of all ages require more sleep than the general requirement for inactive persons of between seven and nine hours of sleep per night.

The physical effects of sleep deprivation have been the subject of considerable scientific study, particularly as the condition might affect shift workers, or doctors and nurses working very long shifts in an environment when an error due to fatigue might have fatal consequences. As a general rule, when a person has remained awake for periods of 24 hours, the ability to perform relatively basic mathematic problem solving and memory skills will diminish by over 20%. Another comparison is the condition of a sleep-deprived person and someone whose motor skills are significantly impaired by the consumption of alcohol; sleep deprivation is similar to a blood alcohol level reading that will support the criminal offense of

impaired operation of a motor vehicle in most countries of the world.

The physiological effects of sleep deprivation on athletic performance are profound. They include an impairment of the athlete's motor function. The inability of the athlete to control all aspects of muscular movement will result almost invariably in substandard sports performance. Examples include races such as the hurdles, which depends on the fluid combination of power and the striding over each hurdle, or sports where the athlete must coordinate a series of movements in rapid succession, a drive to the basket in basketball or the pole vault. As a consequence, the risk of injury to the sleep-deprived athlete is significantly greater than normal.

Another effect is an impairment of the athlete's visual reaction time. In sports where the athlete must react to an object, such as a hockey goaltender or a cricket batsman, this impairment will mean the difference between success and failure. Until 2005, major league baseball turned a blind eye to the widespread use by its players of stimulants such as amphetamines. These drugs were a preferred method through which players could combat the sleep deprivation and fatigue caused by back-to-back games and extensive travel, that would otherwise impair reaction time.

Sleep deprivation also causes delays in an athlete's auditory reaction, such as the reaction to a starter's pistol or a teammate calling out information during a game. There is general impairment of an athlete's tactical and decision-making capabilities. As for aerobic performance and endurance, the storage, conversion and metabolism of glucose as an energy source are decreased through sleep deprivation. It is estimated that glucose metabolism will deteriorate in a period of seven to 10 days of limited sleep by as much as 30% to 40%. In addition to the limitations that sleep deprivation will impose on physical performance, this condition will impair the ability of the body to properly store the glycogen necessary to provide the body with reserves to use during vigorous training or competition.

The psychological effects of sleep deprivation on an athlete are as profound as its impacts on the body. A sleep-deprived athlete will often believe he or she is even more fatigued than they actually demonstrate, with all of the usual symptoms of fatigue exaggerated in the mind of the athlete. Absence of sleep will also trigger the endocrine system to produce greater levels of cortisol, the hormone sometime referred to as the stress hormone, an adverse effect on mood. With cortisol, and the other physiological consequences of sleep deprivation, the athlete will often feel irritable and short-tempered.

Overtraining is a well-known athletic condition where an athlete overreaches in the training objectives for a period of time, either through excessive training volume, intensity, or both. If an athlete is deprived of proper sleep, the overtraining syndrome may occur on a much smaller work volume or intensity, because the body's lack of proper sleep reduces the maximum that it can safely endure.

When sleep deprivation has affected an athlete, the remedy is not so simple as one or two good sleeps, although such a development is a start. The athlete must incorporate sleep in properly defined measures into the training program as with any other training component. In typical cases, sleep deprivation can be completely addressed within a few weeks of proper attention.

SEE ALSO Exhaustion; Fatigue; Motor control; Sleep.

# Slow pitch SEE Softball: Slow pitch vs. the fast pitch

# Smilax

Smilax is the name given to a number of different varieties of climbing vines that grow throughout South America, the Caribbean, and parts of North America. The variant known as *Smilax medica* produces a root that is widely reputed as a highly effective herbal medicine. Smilax is also known as sarsaparilla, which is distinct from the well-known flavoring for root beer; the smilax root is essentially tasteless if consumed in its natural form.

Among the indigenous peoples of South America, smilax was employed in the treatment of headaches, and as a counter to general physical weakness, sexual impotence, joint pain, and skin diseases such as dermatitis. Smilax was later regarded as a powerful blood purifier by European explorers who had contact with native medicines; smilax was particularly renowned as a cure for syphilis. Modern scientific research with respect to smilax have confirmed the presence of saponin, a type of plant steroid, which is believed to be theoretically capable of synthesis by the body into either testosterone or estrogen, the male and female sex hormones. Saponin is also found in the tribulus herb, which is also touted as a strength

supplement by various factions of the weight training and body building community.

Smilax also contains various flavanoids, which are phytochemicals with antioxidant properties, substances that protect the body from the actions of free radicals. These radicals are commonly oxygen molecules ($O_2$) that have one or more pairs of electrons absent from their structure, making them chemically unstable. The radicals seek to obtain their absent electrons from otherwise stable cells, rendering that cell unstable and in turn forcing it to "steal" necessary electrons from a neighboring cell, a process that will touch off a chain reaction in a larger group of cells, resulting in permanent damage to the cell structure. Antioxidants act as scavengers among the free radicals they encounter. Through the donation of their own electrons, the antioxidants render the radical neutral.

Smilax became known as a dietary supplement on the basis of the erroneous belief that it would be converted into testosterone within the body. Smilax is marketed extensively in the strength training and bodybuilding community on this premise. There is currently no scientific evidence in support of the theory of testosterone or estrogen conversion; smilax has no known side effects associated with its use.

SEE ALSO Chinese ginseng; Dietary supplements; Ephedra; Herbs.

# Snowboarding

Snowboarding is a winter sport in which a person glides, turns, and jumps on snow using a board that is reminiscent of a surfboard. Unlike a surfer, the snowboarder remains attached to the board by wearing special boots that are secured to the board via bindings.

Snowboarding has its roots in the 1960s, when a popular winter toy called the "Snurfer" was invented. Essentially a very wide, short ski with an attached rope handle, the Snurfer enabled the rider to balance and ride downhill. One of the early users of the Snurfer was Jake Burton. His refinements of the Snurfer produced today's version of the snowboard. Burton snowboards remain one of the sport's most popular brands.

In the early 1980s, snowboarding had appeared, but was still a fringe pastime. By the middle of the decade, the sport exploded in popularity.

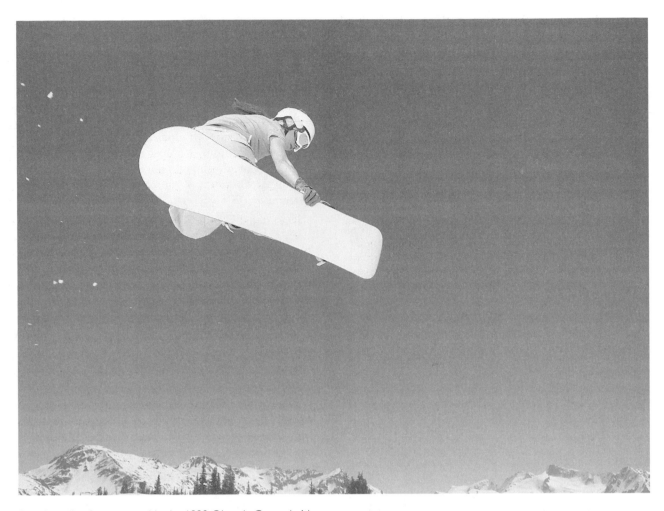

Snowboarding first appeared in the 1998 Olympic Games in Nagano. © MIKE POWELL/CORBIS

There are a variety of snowboard styles. The typical recreational snowboarder moves down the hill in a series of S-shaped curves, alternately shifting his or her body weight forward and backward to carve through the snow using the edges of the board. This type of snowboarding is known as alpine snowboarding.

Many snowboarders will also incorporate jumps into their run. Most snowboarding facilities have a terrain park, an installation that houses snow mounds that are used as jumps and various types of rails that the snowboarders can ride up on and attempt to maintain their balance as they traverse. A terrain park is similar to a skateboard facility, where the rails and jumps allow for various jumps, spins, and other maneuvers. The latter include a 360° spin performed while sliding along the snow, a spin done while airborne, and grabbing the raised tail of the snowboard while airborne. This more adventurous snowboarding is called freestyle.

Still other snowboarders called freeriders will forgo the prepared terrain of a resort for the natural challenge of snowboarding down unprepared slopes. Snowboarding through glades of trees and through deep powder snow adds to the challenge of freeriding, which is usually the domain of accomplished snowboarders.

Competitive snowboarding events now include high-speed runs down the mountain, similar to downhill or giant slalom races in skiing, as well as events where the aim is to successfully accomplish as many jumps, spins, and flips as possible while negotiating a "half-pipe"—a bowl-shaped run with steep-walled sides. Snowboarders can also race down a prepared course as a group with the object of not only completing the course in the quickest time, but also avoiding collisions with fellow competitors. All these forms of snowboarding are now Olympic medal sports.

As with skis, the design of snowboard equipment reflects their intended use. A freestyle snowboard tends to be shorter, wider, and more flexible along its length than other boards, to make maneuvers easier to do. The board is symmetrical, with both ends being the same. Either end can be the leading end.

An alpine snowboard is meant to proceed in a certain orientation, similar to a ski. The board is not symmetrical in design; the tail is narrower than the tip. Still, the board can be ridden with the tail pointed downhill (a position referred to in the jargon of the sport as "Fakie").

Those snowboarders who crave a high-speed run will tend to use a narrower snowboard. These so-called race boards look much like a very wide ski. Their narrower design allows the rider to quickly shift weight from one edge to the other, which is essential to maintain control when moving quickly down the hill.

The placement of the feet can differ also. Free-style snowboarders often opt to position both feet parallel to each other and perpendicular to the long axis of the board, to permit either end of the board to initiate a turn. In contrast, alpine snowboarders will tend to use one foot preferentially as the leading foot, angling that foot with the toes pointed slightly toward the front of the snowboard to provide more stability and control. Alpine snowboarders typically wear boots that are stiffer than other snowboard boots, also to provide increased stability.

Snowboard boots are fixed to the board by means of bindings. There are two binding designs. Both have a back plate that extends upward to provide support to the back of the foot and lower leg. In one design called the strap binding, the boots are physically strapped in after being positioned in the binding. This binding provides a very stable support. Strap bindings differ in rigidity and height of the back plate, depending on their use. For example, the increased control provided by a higher back plate is desirable for higher speed turns.

The second binding design automatically secures the boot in place as the snowboarder steps down. While eliminating the need to manually strap in the boots, the step-in binding does not provide as much stability and control of the snowboard.

Another recommended piece of snowboard equipment is a helmet. Indeed, many resorts no longer permit snowboarders access to the hill unless they wear a helmet. Optional equipment includes padding on the knees, wrists, hips, and gluteus.

**SEE ALSO** Snowboarding injuries.

# Snowboarding injuries

The sport of snowboarding can be traced to the invention of a device known as a snurfer, created in the United States in the 1960s. By the 1990s, the snowboarding was the fastest growing winter sport in North America. With the growth in snowboard popularity, there was a parallel rise in the incidence of snowboard injuries. Most snowboard injuries are caused by mechanisms unique to the characteristics of the snowboard and the corresponding movement of the user (often referred to as a "boarder").

As many people who take up snowboarding are attracted to its apparently freewheeling and less structured style, there has been traditionally less attention paid to both snowboard instruction and the use of safety equipment. Snowboarding also has a decidedly acrobatic element; many ski resorts have constructed specially designed half pipes and similar layouts to permit snowboarders to practice aerial maneuvers.

Snowboarding has been a popular Winter Olympics sport since its introduction in 1998, with a variety of individual disciplines contested in men's and women's categories. Events such as the half pipe competition are scored subjectively; the giant slalom and snowboarder cross are races where the winner is the athlete with the fastest time to complete the course.

Contemporary snowboards are usually constructed from a fiberglass or composite material board that has two defined edges. The board surface has a measure of flexibility in its construction, and the board is accordingly capable of absorbing a degree of the forces directed into it. Unlike a conventional Alpine ski binding, the snowboard bindings do not release to permit the boarder's foot to become detached from the board during a run. The boots worn by the boarder are one of three styles–hard, soft, and hybrid. The soft boot is the most common style worn by recreational snowboarders, as it permits the boarder a measure of flexibility in their ankles as they maneuver the board. Hard boots are favored for performance and elite racing; the hybrid includes characteristics of both hard and soft boots.

The most common snowboard injury are those sustained to the wrist and surrounding bone structure. As the bindings of the snowboard do not permit the feet of the boarder to be released if the boarder loses their balance during a run, many boarders instinctively react by thrusting out their hand and arm as they fall, causing a significant force to be directed into the wrist. It is this mechanism that causes almost all of

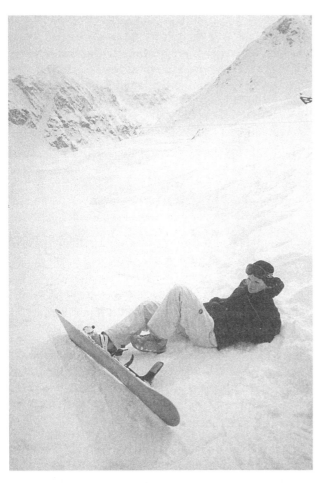

In the 1990s, snowboarding was the fastest growing winter sport in North America—along with that came a growing incidence of snowboarding injuries. © JONNY LE FORTUNE/ZEFA/CORBIS

the wrist injuries that occur in snowboarding. The typical damage sustained to the wrist in a fall ranges from a sprain of the ligaments that connect the ulnar and the radius bones of the forearm at the wrist joint, to a single or multiple fracture of one of the many small bones of the wrist joint. One bone that is particularly vulnerable to fracture in this fashion is the scaphoid bone, located in the wrist immediately below the thumb joint. Scaphoid injuries are sometimes not discernable from x ray; due to its structure, if the scaphoid is fractured there will be a disruption of the blood supply to the bone, with the potential result of necrosis, or bone death.

It is the same type of fall with an outstretched arm and resulting impact that is the cause of the second most common type of snowboard injury, those occurring in the shoulder joints. The largest of the shoulder joints, the scapulohumeral joint [the structure created by the meeting of the humerus

(upper arm) and the scapula (shoulder blade)], may become dislocated. This injury arises when the force of the impact directed into the boarder's outstretched arm radiates into the shoulder. The boarder may also sustain a separation of the clavicle (collarbone) and the acromion, the bony segment located at the top of the scapula, a circumstance known as an AC joint injury, or separated shoulder.

Ankle and lower leg injuries are relatively common in snowboarding; the nature of the injury will depend to a large degree upon the type of boot worn. Boarders who favor soft boots will sustain ankle injuries, usually sprains of the ligament sets that connect the talus (ankle bone) to the tibia, fibula (the bones of the lower leg), or calcaneus (heel bone). Fractures of the ankle are not common in snowboarding unless the boarder strikes another object while riding. When the boarder wears hard boots, the twisting forces sustained by the ankle joint that can cause an ankle injury to the soft boot boarder are directed by the hard boot into the boarder's knee, exposing the boarder to knee ligament injury. In most cases, the knee is not a prime injury target; unlike Alpine skiing, there is little independent twisting motion in the knee as the board is propelled; the boarder's entire body tends to twist in unison with the board as it moves across the snow.

Spinal injuries are not common in snowboarding beyond the bruising of the buttocks due to hard falls. In extreme cases, snowboarders have sustained compression fracture injuries to the spine, where the forces of falling have been directed into the lumbar (low back) vertebrae with sufficient force to fracture the vertebrae.

Head injuries most commonly occur when a snowboarder strikes another object, such as a tree or natural obstruction, or where the boarder fails to properly execute an aerial maneuver and lands on their head. Helmets, which are not always worn by recreational boarders, reduce much of the risk of serious head injury.

In addition to the different types of boots, a number of different kinds of specialized snowboard safety equipment have been devised in recent years. Wrist protectors, fashioned as a support and guard for each hand, protect snowboarders from wrist and shoulder injuries in the event of a fall. Along with the use of wrist protection, snowboarders are encouraged to use the "parachute roll" where the boarder learns to fall with their hands and arms close to the body, to reduce the degree of force directed into the wrist and shoulder.

As important as the safety equipment is the level of physical fitness of the boarder. Snowboarding, with its absence of many of the formal rules and conventions of other sports, possesses one common element with other sports with respect to injury prevention—fitness, particularly as developed through strength and flexibility. Fitness is the best protection a boarder has in avoiding injury.

**SEE ALSO** Musculoskeletal injuries; Ski conditions; Skiing, Alpine; Wrist injuries.

# Sir Garfield St. Aubrun Sobers

7/28/1936–
BARBADIAN (BAJAN)
CRICKET PLAYER

Garfield Sobers is one of the great players in the history of cricket. An all rounder, Sobers was an able batsman, bowler, and fielder who could adapt his style of play to any circumstance. Sobers was the lynch-pin of the West Indies international teams from 1952 to 1974.

As a batsman, Sobers was renowned as an aggressive player who was not afraid to play an attacking game. In cricket, batsman are usually classified as those that produce runs and those that bat defensively, working to protect the wicket while their batting partner produces runs. Sobers often positioned himself at the very edge of the batsman's crease when awaiting the ball, standing as close to the bowler as is legally permitted. Sobers batting technique was so well developed that the shortened distance between himself and a very fast bowler did not impair his ability to stroke a fast bowled ball.

A common tactic in cricket bowling is to begin a match with the team's fast bowlers, (the pace bowlers) and follow their speed with the changes of paces and unpredictable ball movement that is in the arsenal of the spin bowlers. Sobers was the rare cricket batsman who could hit fast bowling and spin bowling with equal ability.

Sobers prowess as a batsman is reflected in the cricket record books. In 1960 versus Pakistan, Sobers scored a record 365 runs not out (meaning that Sobers was not out when the last run of the game had been scored). This record was not broken for 24 years. Sobers was known primarily as a powerful batsman, with the dexterity generated by supple wrists to use a flick type stroke to control the direction in which the ball was hit with considerable precision.

In cricket, each batsman faces a bowler for the segment of the match known as an over, an interval in which six balls are bowled at the same wicket, after which the bowler delivers the balls at the opposite wicket to the other batsman. Sobers was the first man to hit all six balls in an over beyond the boundary of the playing field, scoring six for each ball, the maximum score available in a single hit.

Sobers was also regarded as one of the finest athletes ever to play cricket, possessed of excellent reflexes and speed in the field when ever he was called upon to make a play on a batted ball.

Sobers reputation was strongest as a batsman, but he also had a significant reputation as a bowler. Sobers, who was left handed, was generally regarded as a medium to fast bowler, with mastery over a number of different deliveries. Sobers best type of ball was the bowling referred to as a 'chinaman,' a variation of the googly. The googly is a deceptive ball, as opposed to one that is intended to overpower a batsman. It is thrown by a right handed bowler in a manner that upon striking the pitch, the ball appears as if it will make a leg break (a break in the direction away from a right handed batsman); the googly instead breaks in towards the body of the batsman (an off break).

A chinaman (the term is a reference to the first player ever to thrown this type of ball) is the same type of ball as a googly, except it is thrown by a left handed bowler. The ball is thrown with the fingers of the bowler placed across the single seam of a cricket ball to impart the desired spin. The chinaman is thrown with a medium velocity (approximately 70 mph (110 km/h), in contrast to the fast bowling speeds of over 100 mph (160 km/h). It is similar in its movement to that of a screw ball in baseball.

Sobers, as an all rounder, made contributions to his teams in every respect. While playing for South Australia as a professional, Sobers once batted over 1000 runs and took 50 wickets as a bowler in two seasons, a double that has never been achieved on one occasion by any other player in the elite Australian league. He was the captain of the West Indies cricket sides for 16 years during his career. He was a cricketer who seemed to inspire awe tinged with immense respect, as Sobers was regarded as a consummate sportsman. On number of occasions during his career, Sobers called himself out on a play where the umpire had not made such a signal, as Sobers knew that he had made a play that the umpire could not have observed.

Sobers status in the cricket world was the basis for his knighthood by Queen Elizabeth in 1975. Sobers was declared a National Hero by the country of Barbados in 1998.

SEE ALSO Cricket; Cricket batting; Cricket: The physics of how the ball is bowled.

# Soccer

To its worldwide following of fans who number in the hundreds of millions, soccer is "the beautiful game." Soccer is the world's most popular sport, the only game is played at an elite competitive level in every country on Earth.

A large measure of soccer's appeal is its simplicity. Played on a large field, with 11 players per side, the object of soccer is straightforward: to direct the ball with either the feet or one's head into the opponent's goal. The rules of the game are equally direct, establishing in the single referee the absolute and final authority for matters on the field. While physical size and speed are useful attributes in a soccer player, another aspect of the popularity of soccer is that anyone can play the game, and while age may diminish a player's speed or ball-handling skills, soccer can be a competitive pursuit at any age.

Soccer has likely been played in one form or another in many cultures over the centuries, as the act of kicking an object is a natural one. Soccer as an organized sport began in England in the mid-1800s, both as a school competition and among workingmen for recreation. The Football Association, the world's oldest governing body for soccer, was formed in England in 1872. The Laws of the Game, as propagated by the Football Association, have remained the rules bedrock on which soccer has enjoyed its worldwide development. The first international play took place among the countries of the British Isles, and by 1900, the game was being played widely throughout Europe.

Soccer enjoys the tradition built in many very prestigious professional leagues, particularly in Europe; the European soccer governing body, UEFA, is a very influential organization in its own right, with over 50 member countries and their national soccer associations. All of the interest in international soccer reaches a crescendo in the glamorous and intense, often super-heated environment created through the quadrennial World Cup, and the over two years of qualifying play downs that precede the selection of the 32-team field. The international game, both at the World Cup as well as in any regional championships such as the European Cup or African Cup, is ultimately conducted in accordance with the rules of the Federation Internationale de Football Associations (FIFA). The governing body of international soccer rivals the International Olympic Committee (IOC) for the claim to being the most powerful sports governing body in the world.

The field on which soccer is played is as simply configured as the game itself. The field, or pitch as it is called in Europe, is a rectangular shape; in international play, the field must measure a minimum of 110 yd to 120 yd in length (100–110 m), with a minimum width of 64 yds to a maximum of 75 yd (70–82 m). Each of the outside boundaries is patrolled by a linesman, who determines whether the ball has gone out of play. These officials also advise the referee as to whether a particular play is offside. The goal is also rectangular, 24 ft wide by 8 ft high (7.3 m by 2.4 m). An 18 yd (16.5 m) penalty area is marked in another rectangle on the field adjacent to the goal; for fouls committed by a defensive player within this area, a penalty kick is awarded and the ball placed for a single penalty shot from a mark 12 yd (11 m) from the goal.

By FIFA rule, international soccer has been played on natural turf surfaces only. Earlier generation artificial surfaces tended to cause the ball to bounce more than was desirable; the plastic turf also posed the significant risk of abrasions to players who slid to make a tackle or goalkeepers making a save. FIFA have authorized the testing of the softer, newer generation artificial surfaces, with a view to integrating these surfaces into FIFA competitions, as FIFA recognizes that natural turf cannot be properly maintained in some climates.

Soccer, like rugby and basketball, is a sport where the successful player must have command of a broad athletic skill set, irrespective of the position played. The player must have a base level of endurance that will permit the athlete to run for a full 90-minute game, with often intense bursts of running and other physical activity interspersed within that period. The goalkeeper is often a tall and very agile athlete, with well-developed hand-eye coordination and the ability to anticipate offensive strategy. The defenders are often the largest players on the field; they must be able to run with the position's speedy forwards, to clear the ball from the defensive zone with either a "header" or a clearing kick, as well as being able to make a strong and accurate pass while under opposing player pressure.

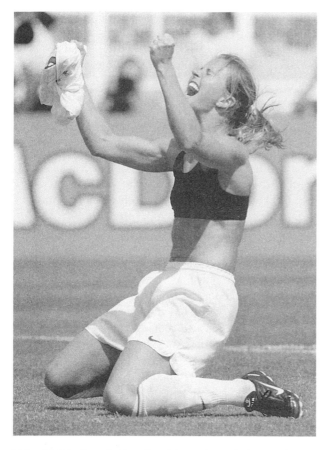

U.S. midfielder Brandi Chastain celebrates her winning penalty kick to defeat China at the 1999 Women's World Cup soccer final. © REUTERS/CORBIS

The midfielder must possess the best all-round skills on a soccer team, capable of breaking up offensive sorties by the opponent, as well as moving forward to join the attack against the opposing goal. The forwards, often given the designation "the striker," have a primary responsibility to carry the attack to the opponent, seeking to create opportunities to score goals. Unlike rugby and American football, the sports that have their origins in soccer, soccer games are typically low scoring. A striker who can convert the relatively few chances to score is a valuable soccer commodity.

One of the great attractions of soccer is that no matter how sublimely talented a player may be, teams are only successful when they are working in unison. Team concepts such as the spacing of the players and the determination with which they move the ball into an attacking position as a team will usually trump an outstanding individual player who attempts to monopolize the ball.

Soccer is a sport where the individual technical components can be broken down into discrete parts for training and improvement. Those basic areas are dribbling, in which the control of the ball by the individual player is a precondition to success in a dynamic 11-player team concept. Dribbling a soccer ball is all of the techniques used to control the ball when it is at the feet of a player, both while the player is stationary and when the player is moving with the ball. Soccer demands that a skilled player be able to make a multitude of different passes, all of which are dictated by the circumstances with which the player is faced. Soccer passes range from delicate touches of the ball that merely change its direction to a teammate, to huge 60 yd (55 m) kicks to reach a teammate attempting to outrun the opposing defense. Receiving a pass can be required in a similar variety of circumstances from almost any place on the field; the key aspect to receiving a pass is the control of the ball with the feet, legs, torso, or head.

Shooting the soccer ball is elevated to an art form in a game where scoring chances are relatively few. Kicks directed at the goal are rarely taken from a stationary position; offensive players are often on the move, and they are required to make instantaneous decisions concerning both the direction and the speed of the intended kick. The header is an essential skill for every player on a soccer field. Heading the ball is used to clear the ball away from a player's own goal to control and to maintain possession of the ball through the midfield, and to direct the ball, often in remarkable feats of agility and coordination, into the opposing goal. When the ball is kicked out of bounds by a player, the opposing team is permitted to throw the ball onto the field of play. The throw must be made with both feet on the ground and an overhead motion.

The corner kick is when the ball is kicked out of bounds behind the goal line by the defensive team, and the attacking team is awarded a corner kick, taken from the corner of the field and directed into the goal area to create an offensive chance for the attackers, either as a header or a kick. The corner kick is usually struck by the player to create spin on the ball, causing the ball to bend. All high-level teams attempt to run a set play from a corner kick, often with an offensive player running into the goal area as the ball is delivered by the kicker.

The penalty kick is an important feature of soccer, both as an award for a foul committed in the goal area during the game, and as the tie-breaking device at the end of regulation play. Soccer was the first major sport to provide for a series of penalty shots

SOCCER: BENDING THE BALL

as its tie breaker, as opposed to the continued play of the game until a sudden death goal was scored (Olympic ice hockey now has a penalty shot tie breaker).

Like basketball, soccer is nominally a non-contact game as well as an extremely physical sport. "Marking" is the well-known European term for the actions of a defender to keep an opposing forward for either getting free to take a pass or to deliver a shot if the forward received the ball. The closer the action comes to the goal, the more prominent the battles for physical position between forwards and defense. In international soccer, the referee often will not call an obvious foul if there was no advantage gained to the player in question.

Speed and anticipation are essential to both control the defensive end of the field and to make attacks on the opponent.

Technical skill will usually take a team a great way toward success. The pinnacles of the game are reached by teams that play with a particular and well-defined style. Brazil has dominated World Cup play since the 1950s with a quick, highly entertaining brand of soccer, while countries such as France and Germany have been successful with a more measured and deliberate approach. Decisions regarding the style of play to be employed are often a combination of philosophy and athleticism.

While the world market for soccer is immense and continually growing, North America represented in many ways an unassailable fortress against which soccer could not secure a foothold. The North American Soccer League flourished in a few cities in the early 1970s, when the league secured the star power of one of the game's legendary players, the Brazilian Pelé. Soccer could never penetrate the professional sports consciousness on the North American continent, and the interest in professional soccer appeared to fade. A vibrant youth soccer movement that began in the 1980s, coupled with both the success of the American women's national team and the securing of a place in the 2006 World Cup by the American men's team, have created a positive image for the sport. In Canada, youth soccer registrations now outnumber those for ice hockey, the national game.

**SEE ALSO** FIFA: World Cup Soccer; Musculoskeletal injuries; Soccer injuries; Soccer: (U.S.) Strength and training exercises.

# Soccer: Bending the ball

"Bend it like Beckham" is both an offbeat title to a feature motion picture, as well as a universal catchphrase recognizing the superlative skills possessed by David Beckham, the English national captain, and soccer icon. Using both his innate feel for the ball and through the application the principles of physics as they relate to objects traveling through the air, David Beckham has demonstrated throughout his career an unsurpassed ability to kick a soccer ball around a wall of free kick defenders, charting an elliptical route to the goal.

David Beckham is not the only noteworthy practitioner of the bending art in soccer—Roberto Carlos of Brazil and the legendary Pelé were equally adept at driving the ball from seemingly impossible angles on free kicks for a score. Bending the ball is a technique practiced by all soccer players who seek to develop comprehensive ball skills.

The "bend" is soccer jargon for the curve of the ball as it travels through the air on a free kick. Like the curve ball thrown by a baseball pitcher, or a volleyball when served, the spinning soccer ball when kicked tends to deflect the air moving past it, and the air responds by deflecting the ball on its path.

This physical principle is referred to as the Magnus force. When the ball is spinning after being kicked, the air through which the ball travels tends to follow a longer path around one side of the ball than the other, as the air is dragged along by the turning surface of the ball. The air following this longer path will bend more sharply, which results in a significant drop in air pressure on that side of the ball. The ball will then be pushed toward its low-pressure side, causing deflection.

A further physical consideration in understanding the bend of the soccer ball in flight is the wake deflection force. As a moving ball will leave a turbulent wake of air behind it, the spin of the ball will deflect the wake to one side. This deflection will shift the air stream flowing around the ball; the air stream will in turn push back on the ball. The Magnus and wake deflection forces operate in the same direction, contributing to the remarkable curvature on free kicks from players such as Beckham.

In a relatively low scoring game like soccer, the ability to take advantage of every offensive opportunity is critical to success. The "bending" power of a

WORLD of SPORTS SCIENCE

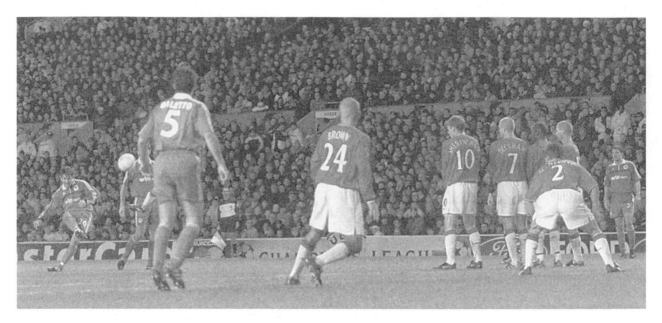

Player (L) bends the ball around the Manchester United wall to score. GERRY PENNY/AFP/GETTY IMAGES

skilled player has the effect of extending a teams effective scoring range.

SEE ALSO Baseball curve ball.

# Soccer goalie geometry

The geometry of the soccer goalkeeper, or goalie, position can be summarized by the expression "playing the angles." Other than possessing the ability to catch a ball struck toward the net, as well as being sufficiently agile to dive to block or cover shots, a goalie's understanding of the angles at which balls will be directed at the goal will usually decide goaltending success or failure. The goalkeeper, the last line of defense on the soccer field, is responsible for the protection of a goal that is 24 ft wide and 8 ft high (7.3 m and 2.3 m). As a basic geometric proposition, the closer the goalie can get to the shooter, the less net area the shooter has available as a target.

The understanding of goalie geometry is not restricted to the horizontal angles of a shot toward the goal. The goalie must also appreciate the vertical geometry of the flight of the ball, an understanding of the fact that the ball can be directed along a horizontal and a vertical axis. When the goalie may cut down a shooter's angle by moving closer to the shooter, the goalie may then become vulnerable to a shot lofted above the goalie, known as a "chip."

There are three specialized situations in which goaltender angle play is of particular importance: the corner kick, the free kick, and the breakaway.

A corner kick arises on a number of occasions in the course of a soccer game, where the ball is kicked or directed past the goal line by a defender. The corner kick is an offensive set piece, with the offensive players moving in a coordinated attack as soon as the ball is struck. The goalie must be positioned at the place in the goal crease where he/she can move most efficiently to block either a kick, a volley, or a header that will be attempted on the corner kick.

A free kick is awarded on a defensive foul that occurs outside of the penalty area. A defending team will usually set up a wall of five or six defenders; the offensive player will either attempt to bend the ball with a spinning kick around the wall for a direct shot on goal, or fake the direct kick and pass to a teammate who has a better shooting angle on the goal, avoiding the wall. The goalie's optimum position will depend on the angle between the ball placement and the goal; commonly, the goalie takes up a position where he/she can see around the wall, without entirely eliminating his/her ability to move laterally along the goal line to respond to the kick.

A breakaway is the greatest challenge faced by a soccer goalie. If the goalkeeper is positioned at the goal line waiting for the shooter to make a move, the shooter will control the angle and be able to move to his/her most desired position to take a shot. If the goalie rushes at the shooter to cut down the angle,

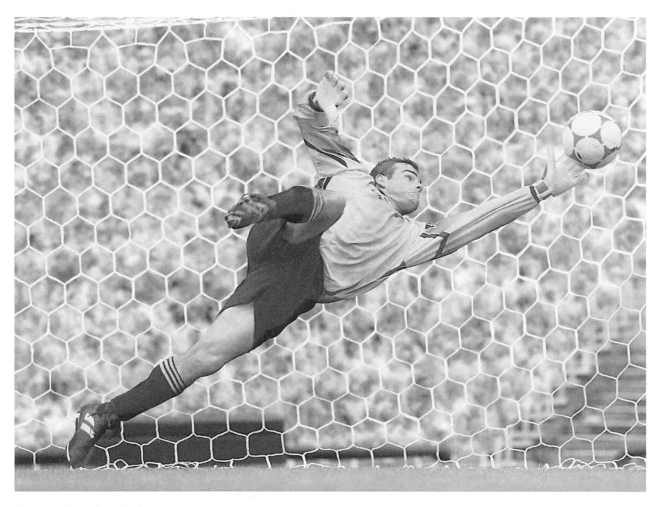

Soccer goalie trying to block a goal. © ROYALTY-FREE/CORBIS

the shooter may elect to "chip" the ball over the onrushing goalie's head. A goalie must take a position that reduces the shooter's angle without entirely compromising the goalie's ability to stop a lofted shot.

SEE ALSO Basketball shot dynamics; Soccer; Soccer: Bending the ball.

## Soccer injuries

As a dynamic, high speed game where physical contact occurs both incidentally and deliberately, soccer creates many circumstances where injury may result. Most soccer injuries are relatively minor in terms of the degree of disability created; more serious injuries often result through the execution of a hard sliding tackle or other sudden physical collisions between players. Data from researchers

regarding soccer injuries indicates that there are over 150,000 soccer injuries reported annually in the United States, among a playing population of over three million athletes; approximately 45% of these injuries occur in players under the age of 15 years.

As would be expected in a sport that centers on kicking a ball, injuries to the lower legs are the most common injuries in soccer. Ankle sprains are another common occurrence, often created by either an awkward plant of one of the feet while running or changing direction, or by stepping on another player's foot, causing the ankle to twist forcefully. Most soccer players wear a cleat that is low cut to permit greater maneuverability, and this footwear is not naturally supportive of the ankle.

The Achilles tendon is vulnerable to two kinds of injury. Given the explosive movement required of a soccer player, the Achilles must instantly respond to the impulses of musculoskeletal movement. If the Achilles tendon is imbalanced in terms

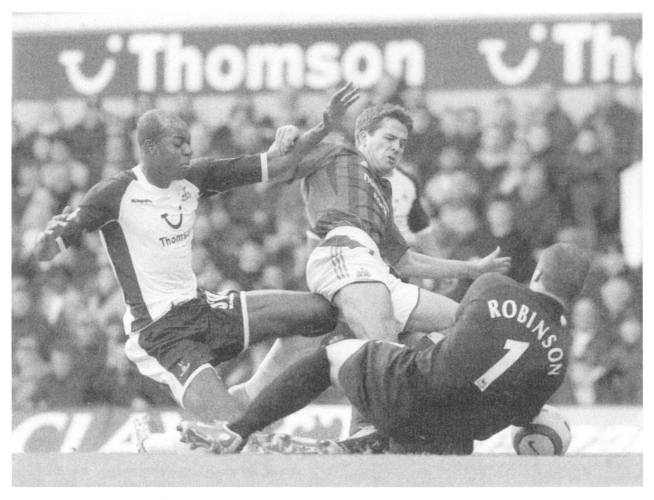

Injuries to the lower legs, ankles, and feet are the most common injuries in soccer. © LINDSEY PARNABY/EPA/CORBIS

of either its strength relative to the connected muscles of the calf, or if the tendon is not sufficiently flexible, the fibers of the tendon can become overstretched or subjected to micro tears. The second type of injury to the Achilles results from the tendon being kicked from behind by an opposing player. The resulting trauma can significantly damage the tendon fibers.

Soccer players are subjected to numerous varieties of accidental kicks from an opponent in the course of play. Most of these kicks result only in contusions, as the players wear relatively durable shin guards. More serious injuries to the lower leg may occur as a result of a defender's sliding tackle, where the defender slides forcefully along the turf to strip the ball from an opponent. If the tackle is not executed cleanly, the offensive player's leg may be caught and twisted, the mechanics necessary for either a significant ankle sprain or a fracture of the tibia/fibula bones in the lower shin.

The knee can also be injured by a sliding tackle, if the offensive player's leg is planted on impact and the knee joint is forced laterally (sideways); this type of collision prevents any of the force of impact being directed and absorbed anywhere but the knee joint. In such circumstances, the anterior cruciate ligament (ACL), a large connective tissue between the femur and the tibia in the knee joint, is at the greatest risk of injury. Other knee injuries occur in the same fashion as ankle injuries, where the leg is planted forcefully on an uneven surface, and the ultimate stress radiates directly into the knee.

Thigh injuries in soccer are typically one of two types. The first are contusions, as the thigh is exposed to all manner of physical contact in the course of a game. The second type of injuries are those common to all other running sports, muscle strains and pulls caused by repetitive and often explosive acceleration. Soccer players who have an imbalance in the function of the hamstring, which provides flexion to the knee, and that of the quadriceps, which gives the knee its ability to extend, will often experience injuries to these muscle and tendon groups.

Groin injuries are often the bane of the high-level soccer player. The structure of muscles, tendons, and ligaments in the upper thighs and the lower abdomen is complex; these tissues are also vulnerable to injury in soccer due to the almost constant lateral and stop and start movements that place stress on them. The abdominal injury that has attracted attention throughout the sports world that is popularly called a sports hernia is, in fact, a tear of the groin inguinal hernia, first identified among English professional soccer players in 1980. Such injuries require surgical repair.

Other than contusions, injuries to the upper body in soccer are less common. The collisions in the sport will occasionally cause a shoulder separation, which is damage to the acrimoclavical (AC) joint, the connection between the shoulder blade and the collarbone. Soccer goalies are more exposed to shoulder injury as a result of diving across the crease to make saves and striking the goal post.

Head injuries may occasionally arise due to collisions with opponents—concussion and damage to the player's teeth are the greatest risk. Many players wear mouth guards to protect their teeth, which has the additional benefit of reducing the effect of concussions by keeping the tempomandibular joint (TMJ) from being driven upward into the skull. Since the mid-1990s, there has been controversy in the international sports science community as to whether the repeated heading of a soccer ball will cause damage to the brain or to the muscles and structure of the neck. Various studies initiated by soccer nations have not yet resolved this question.

**SEE ALSO** Ankle sprains; Groin pulls and strains; Lower leg injuries; Musculoskeletal injuries; Soccer.

## Soccer tackling mechanics

In soccer, a tackle is a defensive maneuver where the defender endeavors to take the ball from the opponent's possession. Unlike the tackling that is at the heart of American football and rugby, a legal soccer tackle must be executed so that any physical contact is incidental to the play on the ball.

A tackle may take various forms, with each technique known by different names in different parts of the world. A block tackle is the most basic form of

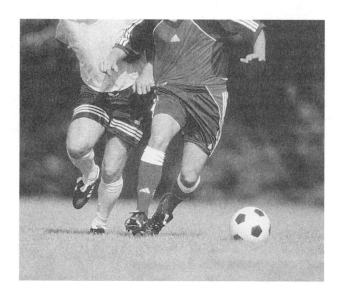

Soccer players tackling. © H. SPICHTINGER/ZEFA/CORBIS

upright tackle. The defensive player approaches the opponent from a front-on position, and while maintaining a low, crouched stance to ensure stability, the defender plants one foot and drives the other low, seeking to strike the ball with the inside of the foot and then secure it from the opposition player. A shoulder charge is a more aggressive challenge brought by the defender, where the defender will make shoulder-to-shoulder contact with the offensive player in the effort to take the ball. The player is not allowed to use the shoulder to knock over or push aside the offensive player, but contact incidental to the challenge is permitted.

The slide tackle is the most dramatic and the most dangerous form of tackle permitted in soccer. By rule, the defensive player is permitted to slide along the playing surface to attempt to take the ball from the offensive player. A sliding tackle will generally be both ineffective and dangerous if the offensive player has the ball in their feet. The sliding tackle is best employed when the offensive player is running with the ball out in front of the body. When executed correctly, the defender begins the approach in a crouched position, beginning the slide with one leg extended. The defender slides across the path of the offensive player to make contact with the ball, knocking it from the possession of the offensive player; there is often quite significant incidental contact with the offensive player being knocked down after the ball has been contacted by the tackler.

When performed in a careless or reckless manner, the sliding tackle has a significant potential for injury to the player being tackled, as the offensive player's knees and lower legs are exposed to the sliding force. The defender will be penalized if the sliding tackle is attempted from an angle where the offensive player cannot see the defender; the defender is subject to ejection from the game if the tackle is made from behind or if, in the opinion of the referee, there was no legitimate attempt to play the ball.

**SEE ALSO** Soccer; Soccer injuries; Soccer (U.S.) Strength and training exercises.

# Soccer (U.S.) strength and training exercises

The simplicity of soccer disguises the intense physical requirements to succeed in the sport. Simply playing soccer by the hour will make a player better, but it is the focused and specialized training, directed at every segment of the player's necessary skill set, that will take a good player to the next level of ability and accomplishment.

Soccer training is intended to build the individual skills of the athlete, while creating a bridge to team tactics and coordinated play. All soccer players will participate in strength and training that enhances some physical aspects of the sport; the degree with which any one or more of these discrete abilities is emphasized will depend on the individual player and the position played. The physical aspects of the game include speed, including acceleration and explosiveness; agility and balance; body control, particularly in jumping and heading the ball; leg strength; and endurance.

The development of each of these physical capabilities must be incorporated into the training required to build the individual technical components of play. Those technical areas are dribbling the ball; passing the ball and receiving a pass, using the feet, legs, torso, or head to control the ball as may be necessary; shooting the ball; heading the ball; inbounds thrown in; corner kicks; the penalty kick; and defensive marking and tackling techniques.

The speed required for soccer can be developed as with all other running sports. Interval running is used for this purpose, especially that which incorporates an agility component. Intervals that simulate game conditions, such as those that replicate the explosive bursts of between 10 yd and 60 yd (10 m and 55 m) to run to a ball, or the acceleration required to run down an opponent are examples.

Interval training is a primary means for the soccer player to stimulate fast-twitch muscle fibers. Interval repeats simulate game conditions, where the player may be required to accelerate quickly many times in a 90-minute match.

Endurance training is the backbone to the physical capabilities required in soccer. As with sports such as boxing, rugby, or basketball, where the primary means of gaining an advantage in competition will be through the shorter, anaerobic bursts of muscle energy, strong aerobic capacity assists the player in making a speedier recovery between the intervals, which in a game setting may be from 10 seconds to 30 seconds in duration.

Muscle mass alone is not a highly prized physical attribute in the soccer player, unless the athlete is able to move efficiently. Soccer does require a measure of physical strength to assist the player in maintaining a position obtained on the field. There is a significant amount of physical contact between opponents, some of it inadvertent such as two players contesting a ball in the air. Other physical contact is either reckless or deliberate, such as the hard sliding tackle by a defender. Weight training that emphasizes strength, but not the development of mass, is valued. High repetition/low-to-medium resistance training achieves this end.

To develop the leg strength necessary for jumping and driving the ball powerfully, a variety of exercises are employed. Plyometrics programs, emphasizing explosive jumps, are directed to the ability of the player to go as high as possible to head a ball. Weight training that is leg-specific, including leg presses, leg squats, and lunges, build the quadriceps, the muscle group that extend the knee joint to deliver a kick.

Calisthenics and other flexibility training assist the athlete in developing an optimal range of motion in all joints. The greater the degree of flexibility, the more agile the player and the better the player will be equipped to move responsively. Due to the repeated lateral movements required of soccer players during games, these athletes are especially vulnerable to groin strains and pulls. Soccer strengthening and flexibility exercises will stress this region of the body, in conjunction with the neighboring abductors, which assist in the lifting and powering of the thigh, and the abdominal muscles.

For competitive players who compete either regionally or internationally, acclimatization to both heat and altitude may be incorporated into a player or team training schedule. Soccer is played throughout

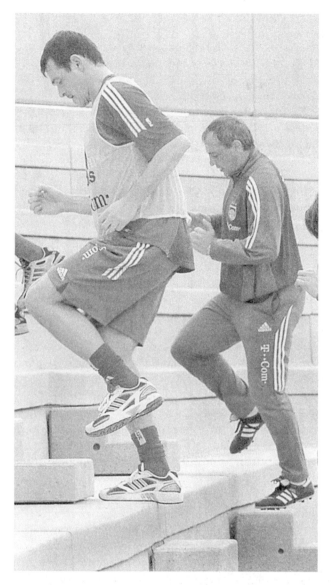

Soccer player performing step-climbing strengthening exercises during training camp. **AP PHOTO/AZIZ SHAH**

areas of the world that experience intense heat and humidity; there are many stadiums that host international matches located at altitudes greater than 5,000 ft (1,500 m), an environment that tends to tax the aerobic capacity of the player through the reduced amount of oxygen available in the air. In ideal circumstances, soccer teams playing at altitude will arrive a minimum of seven days prior to the competition to permit the athletes to acclimatize, a process that begins with the body's increased production of the hormone erythropoietin (EPO). EPO will trigger the production of a greater number of erythrocytes, the red blood cells that transport oxygen. The greater amount of red blood cells available to the player

during high altitude competition, the more efficient the player's cardiovascular system.

**SEE ALSO** Exercise, intermittent; Motor control; Plyometrics; Soccer; Soccer injuries; Stretching and flexibility.

# Sodium (salt) intake for athletes

Every person in the Western world consumes more than sufficient quantities of salt through their diet to satisfy their bodily needs for sodium, one of the two elements that form salt; 90% of all dietary salt consumed is excreted through the urine as excess. In the pre-industrialized world, the reliance on whole, non-processed foods created a natural balance in the body between sodium and potassium, present in most fruits and vegetables. Salt is one of the most important substances consumed by athletes, as salt is crucial to the proper function of a number of bodily systems, all of which are essential to athletic performance. Salt is composed of the elements sodium and chlorine, with sodium comprising 40% of the total weight of salt. Sodium is chemically classified as a metal of the type known as an electrolyte, capable of carrying and transmitting an electrical charge.

Sodium is essential in many bodily processes, including the maintenance of optimal fluid levels within the body; sodium levels are the key determination of how much water will be retained within the body and how much water will be excreted as urine. Sodium is a substance that is very soluble in water and virtually all sodium ingested into the body will be absorbed through the small intestine. The hormone aldosterone, which is produced in the adrenal gland, is the chemical that regulates sodium levels.

Sodium also maintains the acid/base level within the body, usually expressed as the pH balance. Additionally, it helps in the relaying of nerve impulses into the skeletal muscles, through a mechanism known as the sodium/potassium pump, where sodium and potassium act in concert to maintain the electrochemical balance within the muscle cells that permits the impulse to reach the muscle fiber.

Sodium is depleted in exercise through a number of mechanisms within the body. Approximately 85% of the sodium in the body is contained within the bloodstream. Sodium levels are constantly influenced by the generation of perspiration and urination. A healthy person requires a maximum of 3,000 mg of sodium per day to maintain proper sodium/fluid balance. The body does not possess an organic facility in which sodium can be stored and accessed at a later time. In vigorous exercise, or in warm weather conditions, an athlete may lose more than 1,000 mg of sodium per day. The primary cause of sodium loss is through perspiration and resultant fluid loss. When sodium and fluids are depleted together, a chain reaction is triggered. The sodium in the bloodstream that is necessary to maintain the body's balance will be depleted as fluids are lost, which creates a reduced blood volume. Lower blood volumes will result in lowered blood pressure in the cardiovascular system, which generally will reduce the ability of the system to function at an optimal level. A common physiological result of this sodium loss progression is muscle cramps, particularly in the lower leg and calf muscles.

When an athlete replenishes the fluids lost through perspiration with water only, producing an unequal replacement of water versus sodium, the desired sodium balance, or osmolarity, present when the body is in homeostasis (balance) is correspondingly reduced. This condition is known as hyponatremia, or water intoxication. This conditions renders the athlete extremely fatigued, uncoordinated, and at risk of significant further dehydration, as the water ingested into the body will flood the cells, and it will not be absorbed into the bloodstream to boost blood volume, as the body will involuntarily seek to maintain as high a sodium level in the body's fluids as possible. This condition also causes poor carbohydrate metabolism, which reduces the ability of the body to generate musculoskeletal energy.

The opposite state experienced by athletes who consume too much sodium relative to their fluid levels is hypernatremia, created when the body senses that the ratio of sodium to fluid is too high. The body releases the anti-diuretic hormone, ADH (vasopressin), to chemically trigger a shutdown in the production of urine, in an effort to keep the level of fluid higher in relation to the increased sodium level.

The body excretes excess sodium through the urine processed by the kidneys. Excess sodium to the extent of causing toxicity in the body is rare among athletes. The greater risk of excess sodium is the creation of either transient high blood pressure or hypertension, an indefinite condition that places undue stress on the function of the entire cardiovascular system.

The sodium levels necessary for an athlete to perform are maintained entirely through diet; it is during and immediately after competition that additional sodium is beneficial. Almost all conventional sport drinks do not possess sufficient amounts of sodium to assist in the replacement required by an athlete in warm or physically taxing conditions; to achieve total sodium replacement the drink would have to have the composition and the taste of seawater. As an athlete should ideally consume sufficient fluids to replace all perspiration lost, the amount of sodium contained in that lost fluid must be replaced as well. Salt tablets are often used to bolster sodium levels because they contain a far greater concentration of sodium than does any sports drink. Athletes who compete in ultra-marathons or Ironman competitions, events that take place over many hours, sometimes employ low-tech strategies in the consumption of additional sodium. Eating salty pretzels is a favorite among some members of the ultra-marathon community to increase sodium consumption during an event or lengthy training session.

**SEE ALSO** Diet; Hyponatremia; Renal function; Salt; Sodium and sodium deficits.

# Sodium and sodium deficits

Sodium is an essential component to many aspects of human performance. Sodium is readily available to the body through the consumption and digestion of the salt, the mineral composed of sodium and chloride. Salt is expressed as the chemical equation $NaCl$, of which sodium is 40% of the composition.

The usual concern regarding sodium and its impact on health is the consumption of excess sodium, given the dietary practices prevalent throughout many parts of the world. Most commercially prepared foods have salt or a similar sodium compound in their formulation. Elevated levels of sodium place significant stresses on the body's fluid and blood volume balance. Sodium is the major underlying cause of transient high blood pressure and chronic hypertension present in a significant proportion of the adult population of most Western countries. As the body does not store water-soluble sodium for lengthy periods, the sodium must be disposed of and excreted through the production of urine in the renal system. The kidneys are placed under additional stress to process and excrete the additional sodium.

Sodium's properties as an electrolyte (a substance capable of carrying an electric charge) make it invaluable to the ability of the body to transmit nerve impulses to its muscles; sodium and potassium operate in a form of chemical partnership at the cellular level to facilitate the transmissions. The level of sodium within the bloodstream, which is the body's measure in the regulation of fluid levels, is maintained at a constant proportion of water versus sodium. The sodium level is maintained by the regulation provided to the body by the autonomic nervous system, an involuntary control mechanism centered in the hypothalamus region of the brain.

For an inactive person, a sodium deficit is not likely to be noticed immediately; for an athlete, any significant deficit in sodium levels will have an embedded and pronounced and negative impact on the body's performance both in muscle function and with respect to the ability of the athlete to maintain a healthy fluid level.

A deficit is a pronounced reduction in the optimal amount of a substance within the body, a gap between ideal and actual that is not capable of compensation by any other process. A sodium deficit, which often occurs in a gradual and cumulative fashion as a training session or a competition progresses, will most profoundly impact various aspects of athletic performance, including insufficient or incomplete rehydration, which occurs when sodium levels are below optimum. The body will not absorb all of the required water to bring fluid levels to the desired level, because the body will not absorb water into the bloodstream to create a ratio of sodium to fluid that is much below the recommended operating range. This incomplete rehydration will have its greater impact on performance the day following the creation of the sodium deficit, as the fluid level to support activity the next day will be inadequate, which often leads to dehydration at a far earlier point than would otherwise be expected.

Muscle cramps tend to occur in the larger working muscles of the body, particularly in the gastrocnemius and soleus (calf) muscles, and the quadriceps. Muscle cramps are a direct result of reduced sodium levels, as the nerve impulses that direct the muscles to function during sport are not transmitted to the muscle. The transmission of the impulse is facilitated through the sodium/potassium pump, an electrochemical reaction involving the electrolytes sodium and potassium, which alternate in an ebb and flow through the cells of the muscle, a part of the electrical current that carries the impulse to its intended cellular target. When sodium is deficient, the pump is not in balance and the transmission of the impulse cannot be completed. The end result for the athlete is a painful, often disabling muscle cramp. Unless sodium is absorbed into the body,

proportionate to additional fluid as the body loses sodium through perspiration, cramping will persist.

The condition of hyponatremia is the most serious of the consequences of sodium deficit. When sodium levels become reduced through the perspiration created through athletic activity, the body may block the absorption of any additional fluids to preserve the existing sodium balance. Water may remain in the stomach, or, if it is passed through the small intestine, the water is stored in the cells of the body. Known as water intoxication, hyponatremia can quickly lead to significant neurological dysfunction, including drowsiness, a lack of coordination, and ultimately to unconsciousness. The solution to the sodium deficit is often an intravenous injection of a hypertonic saline solution with 3% sodium chloride, administered in regular intervals over a 24- to 48-hour period. Poorly treated, hyponatremia is fatal.

SEE ALSO Hydration; Hyponatremia; Minerals; Salt; Sodium (salt) intake for athletes.

# Softball

Softball, a variant of baseball, was invented as an indoor recreation in Chicago in 1887 by newspaper reporter George Hancock. In the period prior to 1900, the game began to be played outdoors, using a larger ball than employed in baseball, and on a smaller playing field. Variously known throughout the American Midwest and Canada as "kitten ball" and "pumpkin ball," the name softball was formally adopted in 1926. Women had participated in organized softball since the early 1900s.

The United States has been the dominant force in softball since the game's invention. The National Softball Association became the governing body in the United States for the sport, an organization that led to the standardization of the rules of the sport (which had varied significantly from region to region) in 1933. Softball began to slowly develop an international constituency following the end of World War II, which spurred the formation of the world governing body for softball, the International Softball Federation. The first world championships were convened for both men and women in 1966.

While men's softball continued to be played in various countries around the world, softball became more closely associated with female competition. The National Collegiate Athletic Association (NCAA) sponsored its first-ever American intercollegiate women's national softball championship in 1982; over

600 institutions now participate in one of three competitive divisions. Softball has the distinction, along with the sport of field hockey, of being one of only two sports exclusively reserved for female competition in the NCAA.

The culmination of the progress of women's softball as a world sport occurred with the designation of softball for inclusion as a full medal sport at the 1996 Olympic Summer Games in Atlanta; softball was also contested in the 2000 and 2004 Summer Olympics. However, in 2006, the International Olympic Committee (IOC) voted to discontinue both softball and men's baseball as Olympic competitions after the 2008 Olympics in Beijing. The IOC decision was a curious one, given the stated goal of the IOC to ensure that in time, the Olympics would have an equal number of men's and women's competitions.

Softball, as regulated by the National Softball Association, developed two distinct variants: fast-pitch softball and slow-pitch softball, a game sometimes described as simply slow-pitch or lob-ball. The chief distinction between the two games is with respect to the speed with which the pitcher is permitted to deliver the ball to the batter, and the corresponding response of the defensive team to the batted ball. Slow-pitch is an extremely popular game in North America, played by men, women, and in coed formats, in both recreational and competitive leagues.

The rules of fast-pitch softball create a game that is similar to baseball in terms of the number of players, the shape of the field, equipment, and the general strategies to be employed both offensively and defensively. The game is played with nine players in the field, including four infielders, three outfielders, a pitcher, and a catcher. Each team is permitted to bat until they make three outs. When each team has been to bat for three outs each, an inning is concluded. There are seven innings in a softball game.

Softball is played on a field popularly known as a diamond, given its shape; the field may not be any longer than 225 ft (68 m) from home plate to the outfield fences. The field is divided into an infield, which is defined by the positioning of four bases, and the outfield, the area between the infield and the outfield fences. The infield is comprised of four bases, commencing at home plate. The bases are 60 ft apart (18 m).

The pitcher delivers the ball toward home plate from a pitcher's plate (often referred to as "the pitching rubber"), which is 43 ft (13 m) from home plate. The pitch must be delivered in an underhanded motion, known as a "windmill" motion. The pitcher's rear foot must remain in contact with the pitcher's plate throughout the delivery. Women's softball does not permit a hop or jump in the pitching motion, while men's softball permits a hop movement, which permits the pitcher to deliver the ball with greater velocity.

All players wear cleated shoes and uniforms; all defensive players use a fielding glove designed for the particular position played. The catcher wears equipment for safety, including shin guards, a chest protector, helmet and face mask, and heavily padded glove. Players may be substituted, but once a player is replaced in the course of the game they are not permitted to return to play.

The ball, at 12 in (30 cm) circumference, must have a coefficient of restitution (COR) of a maximum 0.47. This characteristic comes into clearer focus when contrasted with the legal COR for a baseball, which by rule must be between 0.514 and 0.578. The lower the COR of any material, the less energy is returned to any object coming into contact with it. The lower COR of a softball is an important distinguishing factor in the distances traveled by it when compared to a baseball when struck with a bat.

The bat has regulated dimensions of length, weight, and circumference; the most important aspect of a softball bat is its construction, which typically is aluminum or a composite metal material.

Unlike baseball, where a base runner is permitted to lead off from the base in preparation for either attempting to steal the next base or to secure a advantage if the ball is put into play, the softball base runner may not leave the base until the ball is struck by the batter.

The general offensive and defensive strategies employed in softball are similar to those used in baseball. Offensively, the team attempts to advance its players around the bases to score runs by hitting, running the bases, and advancing their base runners through devices such as when a batter "sacrifices" an out to permit a teammate to gain an extra base. Another strategy is drawing a walk, the one-on-one battle with a pitcher where the pitcher throws four balls before he or she is able to either throw three strikes over the plate or otherwise induce the batter to hit the ball until he or she is out. It is the differing role of the pitcher in each sport that defines the strategic differences.

In both baseball and softball, a talented pitcher is the key to team success. In softball, that importance is magnified by a number of factors. The pitching

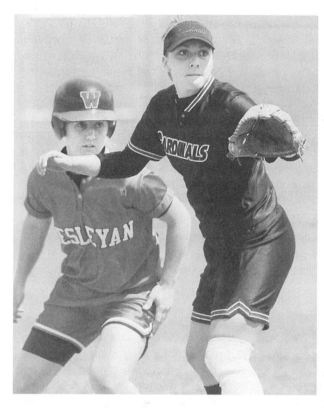

Female softball player waiting for a throw. AP PHOTO/PARKERS-BURG NEWS & SENTINEL, JEFF BAUGHAN

mechanism permitted in softball places a lesser amount of stress on the pitcher's shoulder and elbow than does the overhand mechanism of the baseball pitcher, who is the most player most injured in baseball. Softball pitching and its fluid, natural rotation of the shoulder, coupled with a forward stride, permit the softball pitcher to pitch with less risk of either injury or fatigue, while maintaining pitch velocity.

In baseball, it is common for modern pitchers to be relieved after six or seven innings of the standard nine inning game, with the pitcher resting for three days following the game. In softball, a dominant pitcher can often pitch with less rest. In the 1970s, the softball world's most dominant pitcher, Canada's Pete Landers, regularly pitched complete games in both ends of a doubleheader (two games played consecutively in a single day).

Pitching dominance and a less lively ball place a premium on what is sometimes referred to as "small ball." Batters seek to get the ball in play, where the fielder must make a throw and the batter hopes to cover the 60-ft (18 m) distance to first base in advance of the throw. With the same number of players on a surface that is at least 35% smaller than in baseball, coupled with the greater ability of the pitcher to dominate the hitter due to the reduced distance between the two opponents, the ability to hit the ball to a vacant area on the field is correspondingly reduced.

The game of slow-pitch is also governed in the United States by the National Softball Association, but the game has taken a developmental path that is strikingly different than that of its fast-pitch cousin. Slow-pitch has a tremendous recreational appeal due to the fundamental distinction as to the role of the pitcher: in slow-pitch, the unstated premise of the game is that the ball will be put into play by every batter. Given the greater emphasis on offense in slow-pitch, the game provides for 10 players, with an additional outfielder. The other equipment used by the players is similar to that of fast-pitch. At the elite levels of slow-pitch, the bases may be set 65 ft or 70 ft (20–21 m) apart.

**SEE ALSO** Baseball; Exercise, intermittent; Motor control; Softball: Slow pitch vs. the fast pitch.

# Softball: Bat speed and hitting

Within softball, the bat is generally made out of hardwood, metal (aluminum), or composite materials (polymer arrangement usually of glass, carbon, and Kevlar fibers). International regulations dictate that a softball bat be no more than 34 in (86 cm) in length, 38 oz (1 kg) in weight, and 2.25 in (6 cm) in diameter. Bat speed is defined as how fast a bat moves through its arc when a softball batter swings it. It is generally determined at the bat's center-of-mass. The softball varies in size depending on the type of softball play. The International Softball Federation generally permits a ball to have a circumference of 11 in (28 cm) or 12 in (30 cm).

When swinging a bat at a softball thrown from the pitcher—either delivered at maximum speed with a flat arc, as in fast-pitch softball, or at slower speeds with an steeper arc, as in slow-pitch softball—the batter will either miss the ball or hit it. Hitting a softball is defined as striking a ball with a bat so that the ball lands in fair territory (either in the infield or the outfield) within a softball playing field.

In preparation for swinging a bat with a particular speed and hitting a softball, the batter will stand facing the pitcher inside a batter's box—either on the first-base side box for a left-handed hitting batter or on the third-base side box for a right-handed hitting batter. The bat is held with both hands near the handle-end while positioned over the shoulder and away from the pitcher. The batter hits the ball by

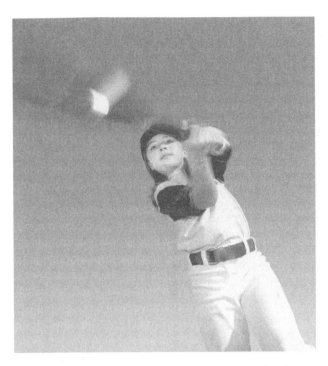

When swinging, rotational (angular) mechanics rather than linear (straight-line) mechanics are primarily involved. © ROYALTY-FREE/CORBIS

stepping forward with the front foot while making a swinging motion with the bat.

When a ball it hit by the batter within fair territory, it is designated as different terms depending on the result. A batted ball that is hit high in the air is generally called a fly ball. However, when a fly ball is hit at an angle greater than 45° (based on the angle between the horizontal ground and the ball's initial angle-of-flight), then it is considered a pop fly. A batted ball is called a line drive if it is hit into the infield at a height above the ground where an infielder could possibly catch it. However, a batted ball that hits the ground within the infield is considered a ground ball.

When swinging a bat to hit a softball, rotational (angular) mechanics rather than linear (straight-line) mechanics are primarily involved. Although the effects of gravity, airflow drag, and other minor considerations occur during swinging and hitting, there are two major forces acting on the bat to create bat speed. Angular momentum is the transfer of the body's rotational momentum to the bat that occurs when the hands are quickly swung in a circular arc. Angular momentum is generally defined as the cross-product of the position of an object and the linear momentum of the object.

Torque is the other major force and is the application of a rotational force at the bat's handle by the combined efforts of the hands, arms, and shoulders. Torque is generally defined as the force applied to an object multiplied by the distance from the axis of rotation to the point on which the force is acting.

When the path of the hands makes a circular arc as the batter's body rotates during the bat swing, the body's angular momentum is transferred to the bat in the form of accelerated motion (acceleration). This transference of momentum is generated as the arms swing the hands in a circular arc and as the barrel-end of the bat swings around the hands.

Torque is the result of two forces being applied to an object from opposite directions so that the object is forced to rotate about a point. Torque is applied to the barrel-end of the bat in the swing by the pushing and pulling actions of the forearms and hands.

To maximize bat speed, the softball batter must apply torque throughout the swing and maintain the hands in a circular path. In order to accomplish these actions most effectively, the upper body (shoulders, arms, and hands) should rotate around a fixed axis (the spine). For a well-hit bat, the collision occurs over a period of about one-thousandth of a second. The effect of this brief collision—that of the ball reversing direction—is brought on entirely because of the bat swing. The bat applies force to the ball, which compresses it, and the ball then exerts force on the bat upon regaining its original contours. The recoil action from this exerted force drives the ball quickly away from the bat. However, the recoil force is less than the compressive force because some of the collision energy is absorbed by frictional forces. In essence, a softball travels farther if it is struck by a bat that is swung faster.

**SEE ALSO** Baseball bat speed; Baseball bats: Sweet spots and tampering; Softball; Softball: Slow pitch vs. the fast pitch.

# Softball: Slow pitch vs. the fast pitch

From its invention in 1887 as an indoor game, softball grew rapidly in the United States and Canada through the early part of the twentieth century. Fast-pitch softball had its rules codified in 1933, and the game acquired an international following, precipitating the formation of the International Softball

Federation (ISF) in 1952. By the time of the 1996 Summer Olympics, when women's softball made its debut as an official Olympic competition, the ISF had approximately 90 member nations.

Slow-pitch softball, also known as "lob ball," also grew in popularity across the United States beginning in the early 1950s. The manner in which the ball is delivered by the pitcher is the key distinguishing feature between the two types of softball. Where the fast-pitch game depends on a powerful pitcher who can deliver the ball with either great velocity or with deceptive ball movement, slow-pitch encourages the batter to hit the ball, put the ball in play, and force the defensive team to make strong fielding plays to generate outs, as opposed to strikeouts by the pitcher.

There is a third variant of softball, modified pitch softball, that has a more limited following. Played with nine players in the field, the ball must be delivered by the pitcher underhanded in a prescribed manner, similar to slow-pitch.

In slow-pitch, the pitcher must deliver the ball underhanded, with a minimum arc of 6 ft (1.8 m) and a maximum arc of 12 ft (3.6 m). The umpire has the discretion to rule a pitch as illegal due to insufficient or excessive arc. Most pitchers attempt to deliver the ball in such a fashion that the ball is dropping in an arc that is as close to perpendicular to the ground as possible. The closer to perpendicular the path of the ball, the more the hitter will be inclined to swing at the ball with an uppercut, as opposed to a level swing. When the player swings with an uppercut stroke, the player tends to use only the arms and the shoulder muscles, limiting the power and the speed with which the bat will strike the ball. An uppercut stroke is also less likely to make maximum contact between the bat and the ball surface.

When the ball is delivered with a flatter arc, a capable hitter will swing with a more level stroke, striding forward from the plate, driving the ball with both arms and shoulders, as well as the torque generated by the twist of the batter's torso, hips, and legs. A poorly thrown slow-pitch ball will often be delivered for a homerun. Prodigious homerun hitters in slow-pitch softball take advantage of two physical principles inherent in the batter's stroke: the fact that an aluminum bat can be swung faster, thus generating greater bat force upon the ball, and the "trampoline effect," which is the physical reaction of the ball when it makes contact with the aluminum bat barrel.

Slow-pitch softball and fast-pitch softball are played on fields with similar dimensions. In addition

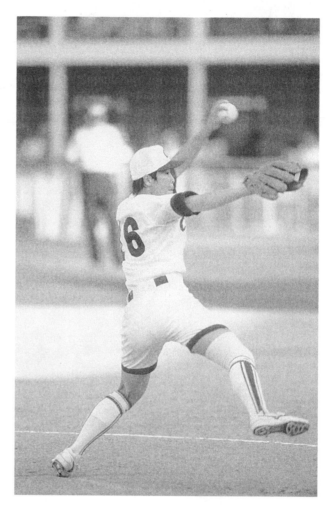

Slow-pitch softball is very popular in recreational leagues throughout North America. © WALLY MCNAMEE/CORBIS

to the methods of pitching the ball, there are other rules that have a significant impact on how the two games are played. Fast-pitch is played with nine players in the field, including the pitcher and the catcher; slow-pitch is played with 10 players, with the additional player almost always positioned in the outfield, either in a relatively fixed location or as a rover. The additional player in slow-pitch is intended to counter to some degree the additional hitting and offense that is invariably a part of the slow-pitch game.

Fast-pitch softball is played with virtually all of the rules of traditional baseball and therefore employs very similar strategies. A strategy common to both games is the use of the bunt, the deliberately restricted swing and contact with a pitch by the batter to place the ball in the infield to either permit the batter to reach first base or to advance a teammate as a "sacrifice." The bunt is not permitted in slow-pitch; it is umpire's discretion as to rule a poorly hit ball that rolls a short distance in front of home plate as intentionally played.

Another tactical limitation placed upon slow-pitch is the prohibition against base stealing, a strategy available in both fast-pitch and baseball. The rationale for this limit is the fact that the offensive team has better opportunities to advance a runner through the batter.

The most striking difference between fast-pitch and slow-pitch softball may demographical. Through the removal of the high-speed offering from the pitcher to the batter, slow-pitch by definition is both a safer and an easier game to play. It is very popular in recreational leagues throughout North America for this reason; it is one the few sports that enjoys significant popularity as a mixed gender sport, both recreationally and competitively. Slow-pitch is also well suited to age group competition.

SEE ALSO Baseball; Exercise, intermittent; Softball; Stretching and flexibility.

# Annika Sorenstam

10/9/1970–
SWEDISH
PROFESSIONAL GOLFER

Annika Sorenstam is one of the most accomplished golfers, male or female, in the history of the sport. Sorenstam's career has been one of ceaseless achievement on both the Ladies Professional Golf Association (LPGA) tour and on a broader international level.

Sorenstam was born into a family with pronounced athletic interests. After taking up golf at age 12, she joined the Swedish junior national program at age 14. Sorenstam ascended to the Swedish national team at age 17, in 1987.

Sorenstam was one of the first foreign born players recruited to National Collegiate Athletic Association (NCAA) women's golf when she accepted a golf scholarship to the University of Arizona in 1990. Arizona had produced a number of highly successful professional players, the most noteworthy being Masters champion Phil Mickleson. Sorenstam won the NCAA women's title in 1991.

After the 1992 college season Sorenstam left Arizona to become a professional golfer. Sorenstam joined the LPGA Tour in 1993, and by the end of the 1994 season she had finished in the top ten at LPGA events five times. Sorenstam earned her first victory on the LPGA tour in 1995, at the U.S. Women's Open, a victory that touched off a remarkable run of success. By the end of the 1996 LPGA season Sorenstam had won four more tournaments, as well as capturing the LPGA Player of the Year award.

Notwithstanding the challenges mounted in individual tournaments from notable players such as Kerrie Webb and Lori Kane, Sorenstam continued to be the player all other LPGA players aspired to match. Sorenstam was never a competitor to be perceived as resting upon her hard earned playing laurels, and she forged a reputation as one of the hardest practicing players in golf, male or female.

Sorenstam's hard work in practice paid off in both the 2001 and the 2002 LPGA seasons, as she became a breathtakingly consistent golfing machine. In 2001 Sorenstam reclaimed the Vare Trophy, awarded to the player on the LPGA tour with the lowest scoring average, with a 69.42 scoring average, only one one-hundredth of a point below Webb's record breaking 1999 average, and then in 2002 Sorenstam shattered the record with a 68.70. Sorenstam hit the green from the fairway 80% of the time that season, making her the most accurate golfer, male or female, in the world.

Sorenstam remained committed to a total fitness and strength training regimen notwithstanding her success. In 2001, armed with her new strength and her consistency, Sorenstam shot the best single round of golf ever by a woman on the LPGA Tour. At the Standard Register Ping tournament in 2001, Sorenstam shot a 59, something that only six male golfers have done in the history of the sport.

In the 2002 year, Sorenstam tied another long-standing LPGA record by winning 13 tournaments in a single season, matching the standard set by LPGA Hall of Fame player Mickey Wright. Sorenstam's achievement was all the more impressive because she compiled her 13 wins in only 25 LPGA tournaments, where Wright played in 33 events in setting the record in 1963.

The process for admission into the LPGA Hall of Fame is unique in professional sport. Unlike those sports where Hall of Fame status is first advanced by a nomination and followed by a subsequent vote by a committee tasked to determine the eligibility of the prospective member, the LPGA adopted a points system as a more objective standard for Hall of Fame inclusion. LPGA major wins are worth a set number of points towards the Hall of Fame total, as are lesser amounts for regular LPGA tour event wins. In addition to points accumulated on the LPGA tour, the player must have won at least one Vare award, and have played on the LPGA tour for at least 10 years. Sorenstam became the earliest inductee into the LPGA Hall of Fame in 2003, as she accumulated her 49th tour victory and easily surpassed the requisite point total for Hall of Fame admission.

From the commercial perspective of women's professional golf, Sorenstam's career winnings of over 18 million dollars as of the commencement of the 2006 season was the record for the most money ever won on the LPGA tour.

An enduring question in competitive women's golf is that of the comparison between the elite women's players, such as Sorenstam, and the best of the men's PGA tour. At 5 ft 6 in (1.7 m) tall, Sorenstam is much smaller than most male players, and there is little question that her average driving distance off the tee of approximately 260 yd (200 m) pales in comparison to that of many capable male amateur players, let alone a elite level PGA touring professional. In 2003, in an event designed for a television audience, Sorenstam competed against leading male professionals Fred Couples, Phil Mickleson, and Mark O'Meara in an event called the Skins Game.

Sorenstam's most controversial participation in a men's golf tournament occurred in May, 2003, when she was invited to play through the device of a sponsor's exemption in the PGA Colonial tournament at Fort Worth, Texas. Sorenstam's entry attracted some stinging commentary from a number of male professionals, most notably that of elite player Vijay Singh, who was so aggravated by the Sorenstam entry into the tournament that he declared that he would not play if he were paired with Sorenstam during the event. At the Colonial, Sorenstam became the first woman since Hall of Famer Babe Zaharias in 1945 to play in a men's event. Although she failed to make the cut, Sorenstam' creditable play against an elite male field placed her at the 96th position, out of 111 golfers.

Sorenstam has another distinction on the LPGA circuit, as her sister Charlotte has toured for a number of seasons as very capable professional in her own right. Two sisters playing on the LPGA tour at the same time is a rarity.

In golf, given the influence of technological advances in both clubs and golf balls, it is difficult to compare the performance of players from one era to another. Sorenstam is demonstrably one of the greatest player in the history of women's golf.

SEE ALSO Golf; Golf swing dynamics.

# Albert Goodwill Spalding

12/2/1850–9/9/1915
AMERICAN
PROFESSIONAL BASEBALL PLAYER, SPORTING GOODS MANUFACTURER

Albert Goodwill (A.G.) Spalding used his fame, acquired as a stand-out pitcher for the Boston Red Stockings of the fledgling National League, to create the world's first sporting goods empire. The Spalding company pioneered the sale of baseballs, footballs, basketballs, and other newly developed sports equipment beginning in the late 1870s.

The A.G. Spalding Company was built by its namesake and founder beginning in 1878. Al Spalding had been a dominant pitcher with the Boston Red Stockings between 1871 and 1876. In those six seasons, Spalding led the league in victories each year. He was the first pitcher to win more than 200 games, playing in an era when relief pitchers were virtually unknown and a starting pitcher was expected to complete the games that he begun. Spalding finished his playing career with the Chicago White Stockings, later known as the Chicago White Sox, where he both pitched and played first base.

Spalding was such a skilled pitcher that he could have been elected to the Baseball Hall of Fame strictly on the strength of his playing career. Spalding was enshrined in the Hall as an executive and builder in 1939.

Spalding combined his growing sporting goods business with his work as the team president of the White Sox, a position that he held for ten years. Spalding's teams won three league championships during his presidency. In 1888, Spalding organized a world tour to promote the game of American baseball to other countries, with mixed success; the tour also served to promote the Spalding sporting goods line.

Baseballs were the most important product manufactured by the Spalding Company in its early years of operation. Baseball was a rapidly growing pastime throughout America, and baseballs were a commodity in great demand. Spalding, as White Sox president, had little difficulty in persuading the other National League teams to use the Spalding baseball as the league' official baseball. Spalding provided the balls at no cost to the league, and used the endorsement provided by the National League to nationally market his product. At that time, the National League was the only major league, as the American League was not operational until 1901.

Baseball players in the early 1870s did not wear gloves when playing in the field, nor did catchers wear masks or protective equipment. Baseball players were expected to be hard men who could play with a measure of pain, and gloves were seen as a sissified aspect of the sport that ought to be discouraged. The earliest documented use of a glove by any player was a catcher with the Cincinnati team, Doug Allison, in 1870. While playing first base for Chicago in 1877, Spalding designed for his own use a padded, but fingerless glove, that had the appearance and dimensions of a modern cyclist's glove. The Spalding glove proved to be very popular with catchers, as there were no specialty gloves designed for use at a particular position until after 1890.

In the early 1880s, Spalding began the manufacture of an all leather baseball shoe, constructed with steel cleats. He incorporated very soft and supple kangaroo leather into the uppers of the shoe to improve fit and performance; kangaroo leather was also used by ice hockey skate manufacturers in their early products for this reason.

In 1887, Spalding perceived that the new sport of American football was likely to expand, creating a further need for its own specially designed products. Spalding developed a leather football, with rawhide laces; his ball became a standard by which others were measured.

Spalding's success with his baseball product spurred other sports equipment manufacturing innovations. In 1894, at the request of James Naismith, the inventor of basketball, Spalding developed a distinct ball for use in the sport. Since the invention of basketball in 1891, Naismith had used a soccer ball for his basketball games. Spalding created a leather covered ball with a rubber bladder, designed to be both durable and with sufficient grip that it could be easily handled by the players.

In 1895, Spalding again designed and manufactured a ball for a newly developed American sport, volleyball. The first volleyball was of leather construction.

Spalding solidified his hold on sporting goods manufacture in this period through his publication of various official rule books and guides with respect to a number of sports. Baseball, as the game Spalding knew best, was the most documented.

By 1901, Spalding had established 14 sporting goods stores that sold his products exclusively; the bulk of the Spalding business was by way of mail order. Spalding extended his manufacturing processes to include any equipment required for any sport being played in America. After Spalding's death in 1915, his company continued to expand its merchandise base; golf clubs and related golf products became a Spalding mainstay. With the exception of soccer, the equipment produced today by Spalding are traditional American sports-basketball, football, volleyball, baseball, and softball.

**SEE ALSO** Baseball; Basketball; Football (American).

# Special Olympics

The Special Olympics Athlete's code is "Let me win. But if I cannot win, let me be brave in the attempt." Those words are perhaps the clearest expression of what the Special Olympics movement is about.

The Special Olympics concept was given its initial momentum in the early 1960s by American Eunice Kennedy Shriver, who wished to create opportunities for persons with intellectual disability in the wider world through their participation in organized sport. The first Special Olympic Games, modeled to a large degree on the format of the traditional Summer Olympics, was held in New York in 1968. Since that time, the Special Olympics have become both a winter and summer quadrennial sports festival open to participants worldwide. Other Special Olympics competitions are convened in a wide range of team and individual sports throughout the world on both a local and a regional basis.

It is a measure of the global interest in Special Olympics activities that the Special Olympics Law Enforcement Torch Run, first run in the United States in 1981, is now a fundraising event organized in 35 countries around the world.

It is the stated mission of the Special Olympics movement that its participants obtain the advantages of year-round sport training in Olympic-type sports, with an emphasis on fitness, participation, and friendship within a competitive atmosphere. The Special Olympics seeks to be a part of the life of persons with intellectual disabilities in assisting them to be as productive as possible in society at large. It is this point that distinguishes the Special Olympics from both the Paralympics and Olympics movements, where competition at the highest possible level is an overarching objective of the participating athletes. The Paralympics, competitions standard for the participation of persons with intellectual disability, are similar to those established by the Special Olympics; there is no formal overlap between the two organizations.

Special Olympics International (SOI) is the governing body of worldwide Special Olympics programs. SOI is composed of representatives of its various member nations, which in turn are composed of regional and state Special Olympics bodies.

The Special Olympics movement advances its mission through inclusivity. The intellectual disabilities of the Special Olympians render these athletes indistinguishable from 90% of the general population. Special Olympics competition is open to any athlete who is a minimum of eight years of age and who meets certain criteria, including the athlete has been identified by an appropriate professional or agency as a person with a mental disability, or the athlete has been similarly identified as a person with cognitive delay, often referred to as a "slow learner"; a slow learner is usually considered to be a person who is more than two years behind their peers in their educational progress. Another criterion is that the athlete has been determined to possess a significant learning disability or vocational problem. The Special Olympics movement uses adaptive skill areas, aspects of life such as social skills, self-care, and vocational abilities, to assess athlete eligibility.

Certain individuals who might otherwise qualify for admission to all Special Olympics programs are restricted in the extent of their participation for safety reasons. An example is certain athletes with the genetic disease, Down syndrome, which often imposes a companion condition, atlantoaxial instability, which renders the cervical vertebrae located immediately below the skull (vertebrae C-1) vulnerable to injury with physical contact.

The Special Olympics include a broad range of sports that are inspired by the Olympics format, with appropriate modification. The Winter Special Olympics has two events, snowshoeing and floor hockey, added to suit the requirements and the skill set of the athletes. The Special Olympics variety of floor hockey is also modified for broader participation, a six-player per side indoor game played with a pole and a felt disc with the center removed; the disc is advanced through its propulsion through the insertion of the pole into the disc center.

One Special Olympics sport that does not require significant modification form the standard Olympic format is power lifting. Special Olympic athletes lift weights in squat, bench press, and dead lift competitions.

Special Olympics equestrian competition preserves the Olympic format in that male and female athletes compete in the same events. Unified Sports

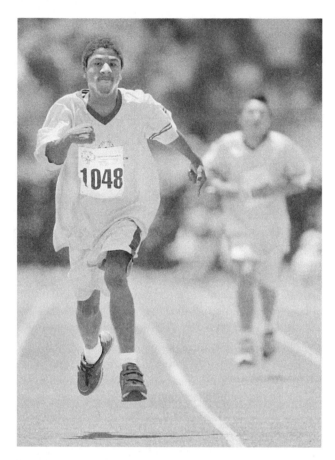

The 400-m run at the 35th Annual Summer Games of the Special Olympics. AP PHOTO/RIC FRANCIS

is a feature unique to the Special Olympics equestrian competition. Unified Sports pairs a Special Olympics athlete with an athlete who is not intellectually disabled, and these athletes compete on their mounts as a team in various relay and drills events.

Another feature of Special Olympics team events are the individual skills competitions. Examples are basketball dribbling and passing events, and floor hockey shooting contests. In most skills competitions, all of the members of the team are able to participate regardless of ability. In regional or state Special Olympics competitions, the skills competitions are used to seed teams into their appropriate level of play. The team sports such as basketball or floor hockey will generally provide for up to four competitive divisions. Basketball, a very popular Special Olympics sport, uses the same rules of play as would a regular competition at its highest ability level, with modifications to accommodate the level of intellectual disability in the remaining divisions. Such aspects of the Special Olympics are another component of the inclusivity that is desired in all aspects of the competition.

SEE ALSO International federations; International Olympic Committee (IOC); Paralympics; Sports coaching.

# Speedskating

Speedskating is a sport in which the object is to skate around an oval ice track for various, defined distances in as quick a time as possible. Athletes' times are often separated by only a few hundredths of a second. The course can be either a long course 400-m oval (the same dimensions and shape as is used in track and field competitions) or a short course of 200 or 250 m. The latter course can be accommodated on a conventional ice hockey surface.

The sport can be carried out on ice ovals that are located outdoors or indoors. For competitions such as the World Championships and the Winter Olympics, all speedskating events are held indoors, where the ice temperature can be precisely controlled and where wind is not an issue.

Long course speedskating has a lengthy competitive history. The first recorded event took place in Oslo, Norway, in 1863. The sport's governing body, The International Skating Union (ISU), was formed in the nineteenth century, and has been the organizer of world championships since 1893.

Short course (or short track) speedskating also has a long history. Originally conducted as a race with a mass start by a larger group of participants, this type of speedskating made its Olympic debut at the 1932 Lake Placid Olympics. The ISU officially adopted the short course version as a competitive sport in 1967; international competition began in 1976, and the first world championships were held in 1981. The event became a demonstration sport at the 1988 Calgary Olympics, where its combination of speed and ever-present danger of crashes immediately proved to be a crowd and broadcast favorite. By the next Olympics, short course speedskating had become a medal event.

The standard 400 m long course speedskating oval consists of two lanes. The turns at either end of the course have a diameter of 54–56 yd (50–52 m). Even though athletes race against the clock instead of one another, each race in a speedskating competition involves two skaters. Typically, the skater who begins the race in the inside lane wears

an arm band of a designated color, while the skater who begins in the outside lane wears a differently colored arm band. To ensure that each covers the same amount of distance each lap of the oval, the skaters must cross from their starting lane to the other lane at a defined point in the race (the first straightaway after the first turn).

Each skater is allowed one false start (when the skater begins the forward motion before the starting signal has been given). If the athlete incurs another false start in the same race, he or she is disqualified from the competition for that distance. Other reasons for disqualification include entering the adjacent lane other than in the designated crossover zone, not changing lanes, and interfering with the other skater during the lane change.

Long course speedskating distances most often include sprints of 500 and 1,000 m, where an explosive start and quickness throughout the race are paramount (elite athletes can exceed 37 mph/60 km/h), to longer distances (1,500, 5,000, and 10,000 m) where the ability to maintain form and a steady pace are keys to success. Women may also participate in a 3,000-m event. Typically, the sprint events are run as two races, with the time for each race tallied to produce the overall time. Pursuit races—where teams of skaters compete, each skater alternately assuming the lead for a time, in an effort to catch up to another team—can also be run, particularly in short course competitions. All races are run in the counterclockwise direction.

In both the long and (especially) short course competitions, falls can occur. When skaters fall, they can get up and continue the race, although the added time will almost certainly eliminate them from the medal podium. If a fall in a long course event disrupts the other competitor, the race can be appealed and run over again.

Speedskating is an aerodynamic event. Skaters wear tight-fitting lycra suits that include hoods to allow them to move as quickly and efficiently as possible through the air. The suits must follow the natural contours of the body. Many skaters wear goggles or glasses to prevent their eyes from watering during a race. Posture is also important. Racers adopt a hunched position to cut down on wind resistance and increase the power of the leg muscles applied to each stride and, in longer races, hold the inside arm behind the back and rhythmically swing the outside arm to make movement as efficient as possible. Swinging the arm also helps a skater maintain balance and direction through the turns.

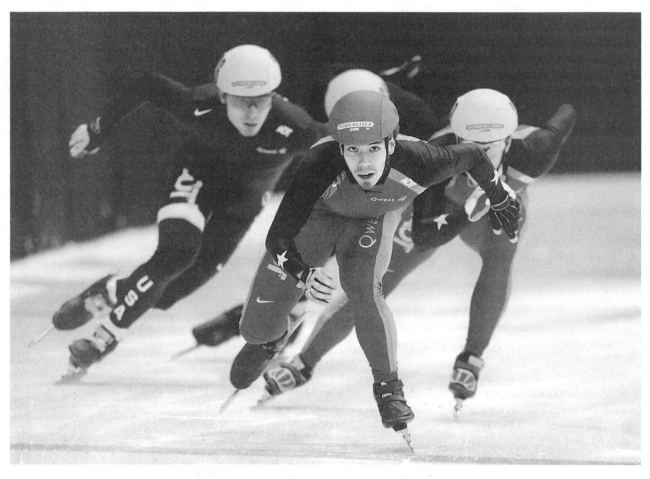

Competitors at the 1000-m final during the U.S. Short Track Speedskating Championships, 2005. **PHOTO BY MATTHEW STOCKMAN/ GETTY IMAGES.**

Another distinctive speedskating gear is the long-bladed skate. The 15–17 in (38–45 cm) blade is much longer than the boot, providing more surface to dig into the ice and power the athlete forward (the blade is sharpened to be flat to allow for a long gliding stride, in contrast to hockey skates, which have two edges on the underside of the blade to assist in rapid stopping and direction change). The blade length comes at a cost; turns need to be carefully executed so that a skate blade does not catch as one foot is crossed over the other.

Until the mid-1990s, the boot was designed with the blade fixed to the underside of the boot along its entire length. Then, a new design was introduced, in which the blade is fixed to the boot only near the toe. This hinged design allows the boot to flex forward while still maintaining the blade in contact with the ice. As the foot moves downward after a skating stroke, the blade snaps back into position. The distinctive sound had given the "clap skate" its name.

Both designs are available for use, depending on an athlete's preference. The clap skate is used by the majority of competitors in longer distance events, where the added assist from the blade becomes important during the tiring late stages of a race.

Elite speedskaters will have their skates custom built to the dimensions of their feet. Some skate barefoot, in an effort to maximize their control.

Speedskating was long dominated by European and Canadian athletes. However, the sport is now truly international, with elite competitors from around the globe attaining world-class performances. A noteworthy American performance occurred at the 1980 Lake Placid Olympics, when Eric Heiden won gold in all five of the men's events.

SEE ALSO Figure skating, ice.

# Spike, volleyball SEE Volleyball: Set and spike mechanisms

# Sport nutrition

Human nutrition and sport nutrition are closely related concepts. Nutrition is the process of nourishment of the human body through food, and whether in a non athletic, day-to-day existence, or for the purposes of high performance sport, proper nutrition has the same basic principles. Diet, as distinct from nutrition, is the composition of the various foods that are ingested into the body. Nutritional benefits may be derived from whole foods or through dietary supplements.

The difference between regular nutritional practices and those that pertain to sport is the fact that even the most minor departures from optimal nutritional practice can have a significant impact on sport performance; greater latitude in nutrition will not necessarily be noticed in circumstances where human performance is not measured.

The nutrients consumed through food are divided into two broad classifications: macronutrients and micronutrients. The macronutrients are carbohydrates, proteins, and fats. For the past 40 years, the generally accepted proportion of each of the macronutrients in a healthy diet was 60–65% carbohydrates, 12–15% proteins, and less than 30% fats. Sports-focused research has provided significant data about the ratio of carbohydrate, proteins, and fats for optimum macronutrient consumption for athletes. This research has confirmed that different sports will dictate different macronutrient consumption patterns for their participants.

Nutritional research has also been motivated by secondary factors in relation to sport performance. Nutritional guidelines are sometimes varied in consideration of health and fitness developments that indirectly impact on sports performance. The rapid rise in obesity rates in many countries, related in part of the equally dramatic rise in both juvenile and adult (type 2) diabetes, has spurred further examination of what constitutes optimal nutritional.

Carbohydrates are essential to athletic performance; athletes simply require more energy than do sedentary persons. A carbohydrate-restricted diet and effective athletic participation are incompatible concepts. Further, carbohydrates provide the energy for all brain and central nervous system activity. Carbohydrate consumption by athletes that is out of proportion to other macronutrients is also not necessarily a healthy choice. High-carbohydrate and low-fat diets, as are sometimes engaged in by endurance athletes such as marathon runners or by athletes seeking to remove the perceived weight gaining properties of dietary fat from their diet, will tend to reduce the production of high density lipoproteins, the so-called "good" cholestrol that negates the effect of the lower density, plaque-causing cholesterol that contributes to cardiovascular disease.

Dietary fats are crucial to athletic performance, as the fats, stored within the body as triglycerides and released into the bloodstream as the energy source, fatty acids, are also essential to the absorption of fat-soluble vitamins such as vitamin A and vitamin D. Without the proper absorption of vitamin D into the body, the companion absorption of the mineral calcium, essential to the formation and repair of bones, will be impaired. Proper sport nutrition requires a supply of fat in the athlete's diet; the adjustment of the precise quantity and quality of fats into the body is often essential. Dietary fats present in many diets are both saturated fats, the cause of the "bad" cholesterol, and the trans fats, created through the use of partially hydrogenated vegetable oils that make liquids solid. While a non-athletic person should limit consumption of these products, which have no nutritional value and which present well-established health risks, these fats in significant quantities will impair athletic cardiovascular performance.

Conversely, the fats can provide an athlete with a significant macronutritional benefit beyond the absorption of fat-soluble vitamins. Polyunsaturated fats are essential to the function of the body; there are two primary polyunsaturates, better known as omega-3 acid omega-6. In the formulation of a diet that addresses specific needs, the athlete should become familiar with food package labeling; in most countries in the Western world, and in regions such as Australasia, the identification of both the quantity and the quality of food ingredients such as trans fats and the relative percentages of other product components must be clearly marked.

Protein was long misunderstood in its application to sport performance, particularly in activities where musculoskeletal strength is crucial. Protein is the essential macronutrient in the building and repair of muscle and connective tissues, as well as essential to the formation of certain hormones and enzymes. The classic weight training programs encouraged the consumption of large amounts of dietary protein, such as animal meats, to contribute to muscle development. Modern sport research confirms that it is the type of proteins that consequently supply the correct essential amino acids that are as important as protein quantity. A healthy, non-athletic person will require a certain amount of daily consumption of protein to maintain muscle health; an athlete may consume only slightly more protein, even during intensive training, so long as the amino acid composition within the protein is correct.

Strictly speaking, fiber is not a macronutrient or a micronutrient, as it is not digested into the body; fiber tends to be present in both nutritional groups and it possesses significant sports nutritional benefits as a facilitator of the digestion and absorption of both types of nutrition sources. Dietary fiber has profound benefits in the proper and orderly digestion of foods and processing of waste products; regularity in both areas is essential to athletic performance. Dietary fiber is of particular benefit to the body in the maintenance of its blood glucose levels. Fiber that is not naturally occurring in a food product is described as functional fiber; studies confirm that while any fiber will assist in the digestive processes, dietary fiber is preferable.

The micronutrients are those components of diet that occur in smaller amounts than the broader carbohydrate, proteins, and fats that form the macronutrients. While no athlete will be able to compete at any significant sporting level if he or she does not consume proper proportions of the macronutrients, it is the effect of the micronutrients that often attract considerable sports science attention. It is the adjustment of micronutrient levels that may spell the difference between adequate and superb performance. Micronutrients include all vitamins, most minerals, and the class of substances known as the phytochemicals, or phytonutrients, which are present in many foods.

Vitamins are present in foods in one of two categories. Fat-soluble vitamins, which include vitamins A, D, and E, require the presence of fatty acids to be absorbed into the body. Fat-soluble vitamins are capable of being stored in the liver. Water-soluble vitamins, the most prominent of which are vitamin C and the vitamin B complex, are absorbed through the digestive process by the small intestine. Water-soluble vitamins cannot be stored within the body and each must be replenished through diet each day. Each vitamin is necessary to the function of one or more of the multitude of bodily systems.

A key example of vitamin absorption and athletic performance is that of the water-soluble vitamin B group. Different vitamins within the complex are essential to the regulation and function of carbohydrate absorption and the orderly storage of glycogen. Similarly, the presence of adequate levels of vitamin D is fundamental to the processes by which the bones are built, maintained, and repaired. Although the mineral calcium, along with phosphorous, is the prime construction material in bone cells, vitamin D must be present for the cell formation to occur. Both optimal glycogen storage and bone repair are fundamental to sport success.

Minerals, generally defined as substances that are produced from the Earth, are present in a wide variety of foods. Many minerals have a significant impact on general performance; many different mineral deficiencies are potentially catastrophic to effective athletic performance. There are over 20 minerals present in varying amounts in the body; key minerals are calcium, phosphorous, magnesium, and iron. A separate class of minerals with electrolytic properties includes sodium and potassium.

A sodium deficiency will create a chain reaction of increasingly serious problems in athletic performance. Sodium is essential to the maintenance of fluid levels and the acid/base balance within the body, as well as with respect to the transmission of nerve impulses into the muscles, in an electrochemical partnership with potassium. Calcium deficiencies will contribute to a loss of bone density and related structural problems, especially given the stresses of sport on the musculoskeletal system. Iron performs a number of important functions within the body, none more important than its presence within the hemoglobin of erythrocytes, the compartment of the red blood cells that transport oxygen.

The phytochemicals, like the fiber they are often contained within, have no caloric or energy value. Some common types of phytochemical actions and related food sources include antibacterial agents, the best known of which is allicin, the active ingredient of garlic that provides the vegetable with its characteristic strong odor. Allicin is a chemical that acts as an effective agent against bacteria entering the body. Antioxidants are found in a variety of plant sources. An antioxidant is a chemical that tends to seek out any molecules in the body that have an unpaired electron, known as free radicals, molecules that tend to form cancer-causing cells. Phytochemicals sources such as fruits, carrots, onions, and other vegetables are well-regarded antioxidants. Lycopene is a powerful antioxidant found in the skin of tomatoes that acts effectively in preserving the health of the cells in the cardiovascular system.

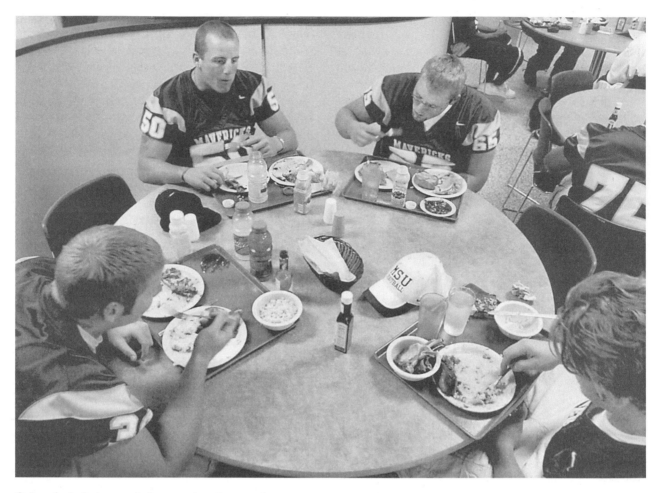

College football players enjoying a meal on the eve of a game. AP PHOTO/PAT CHRISTMAN, MANKATO FREE PRESS

Alkaloids have phytochemical actions as well. The most important alkaloid is caffeine, the world's most consumed stimulant, possessing a powerful effect on the central nervous system. Digoxin is found naturally in the foxglove plant, and is used as a medication in the treatment of heart failure, as it acts to regulate and to strengthen a failing heart rate.

Flavanoids are chemicals found in a number of fruits, such as cranberries, raspberries, grapes, and blueberries that often act as antioxidants. Flavanoids also work to inhibit the progress of low-density lipoproteins in the cardiovascular system, the form of cholesterol that causes plaque and contributes to the narrowing of arteries and the development of arteriosclerosis. Red wine has been long regarded as possessing flavanoids.

Beta-sitosterol is a substance found in peanuts, wheat germ, and various rice products; these chemicals tend to reduce cholesterol levels, especially in men with prostate problems.

While phytochemicals can be added to an existing diet by way of dietary supplements, these substances are best absorbed into the body through a balanced diet that contains significant fresh fruits and vegetables. Two food types that are often overlooked concerning phytochemical benefits are the consumption of dried fruits, which lose little of their phytochemical effect in this form, and the liberal use of herbs and spices with meals. Most dried herbs, such as basil, thyme, and oregano, are rich in various phytochemicals. The active ingredient in many types of red pepper, capsicum, is an effective antioxidant agent.

**SEE ALSO** Diet; Minerals; Nutrition; Phytochemicals; Sodium (salt) intake for athletes; Vitamin C; Vitamin E.

# Sport performance

Sport performance is the manner in which sport participation is measured. Sport performance is a complex mixture of biomechanical function, emotional factors, and training techniques. Performance in an athletic context has a popular connotation of representing the pursuit of excellence, where an athlete measures his or her performance as a progression toward excellence or achievement. There is an understanding in sport that athletes interested in performance tend to the competitive or elite level; athletes interested in simple participation, for broader purposes such as fitness or weight control, are most often recreational athletes who do not set specific performance goals.

On one level, the determination of sport performance in most sport disciplines is a simple matter. In those activities where the result is measurable and defined, such as a race, a jump, or an object to be thrown, the end result is quantifiable. In these sports, it is the quest for performance improvement that drives the analysis of the individual components of performance. When an athlete and the coach can isolate areas on which to focus in training, the ultimate result is likely to be improved.

Sport performance has four distinct aspects, each of which has a number of subcategories, some of which are rooted in physical certainty, others of which tend to the highly variable. The four areas include neuromuscular factors, the relationship between the nervous system and its dimensions and the musculoskeletal system; mental control and psychological factors; environmental conditions; and coaching and external support for the athlete.

The neuromuscular factors that impact sports performance are typically the most comprehensive and represent those aspects of performance that occupy the greatest degree of focus and preparation time. In many sports, no matter how devoted to training the athlete may be, if he or she is not physically equipped to compete, the performance will not improve.

The neuromuscular component of sports performance is subdivided into its own discrete elements. Each of these elements must be the subject of specific training approaches, including body type. Many sports lend themselves to a particular, generically predetermined physical frame or stature; American football linemen and rugby forwards must have a significant degree of physical size. Unless the athletes have a natural predisposition to having a large build, they cannot competitively succeed at these positions. Similarly, large-build athletes will not be successful distance runners or high jumpers as their genetics are essentially a disqualification from the serious pursuit of such sports; they will be limited, no matter what

passion they may possess for the sport, to more recreational participation in such pursuits. In many sports, such as gymnastics and basketball, athletes with desirable natural physical attributes are directed into these pursuits.

Another neuromuscular component is muscular strength, both in terms of muscle mass and muscle power. While body type will tend to significantly influence the ability of an athlete to develop muscle strength, training will permit strength development in all athletes; strength, whether in terms of discernable power or as a function of the core strength, the neatly counter-balanced relationship between the upper body and lower body musculoskeletal structures when in movement.

Endurance, which is the ability of the body to perform over time, is essential to success in all sports. In high-intensity sports of a short duration, such as sprinting and weightlifting, endurance is similar to a backbone to the activity, assisting in the speedy and efficient recovery from the stress of the event or training. In sports where endurance is a central aspect, such as distance running or cross-country skiing, maximal endurance, as reflected in the ability of the athlete to consume and process oxygen, expressed as the athlete's $VO_2max$, is of prime importance.

Flexibility is the counterpoint to muscular strength; the greater the range of motion present in the joints of an athlete, the greater the ability to move dynamically. An inflexible athlete is unlikely to ever achieve outstanding athletic performance. Inflexibility in human joints creates imbalance in the connective tissues and muscle structures, which will reduce the ability of the muscle to achieve maximum power, and will increase the risk of injury.

The ability of the body to respond to external stimuli in sport, such as the movement of an opponent or the starter's gun, requires the development of aspects of the athlete's motor control. These specific neuromuscular abilities include the feature of reaction time.

Agility, balance, and coordination are three interrelated concepts. These aspects of sport performance are also influenced by heredity and body type to a significant degree, but all can be enhanced through training. Most sports have specific drills developed to further each of these areas, such as the simple running drills where an athlete must run through a pattern laid out on the running surface. When the drills are run in reverse or in varying sequences, the drill is intensified. Each of these neuromuscular features of sport performance is less influenced by the strength of the musculoskeletal system, and more impacted by technique and repetition.

Speed is built by training that is focused on the development of the fast-twitch fibers of the skeletal muscles. The distribution of fast-twitch fibers through the muscles of the body is also regulated by genetics, but training can maximize the fast-twitch effect.

In many sports, the ability of the athlete to develop a rhythm to the performance will be crucial to success. Running, cross-country skiing, cycling, and speed skating are sports where the establishment of an effective rhythm or cadence will keep the athlete organized and physically efficient. The development of a rhythm is the imposition of a cadence on musculoskeletal activity.

Mental control and the related psychological factors in sport performance are intangibles that are reflected in the final result of an athlete's effort. In many respects, the mental elements of sport are the most difficult to master, as they usually require a high level of athletic experience and maturity to reach fruition. Examples abound in every sport of the supremely physically gifted athlete who is said to "choke" or "fold under pressure," because the athlete was not able to master emotions during competition. This development of athletic emotional control is capable of being examined from a number of perspectives, including intelligence, which is a valued commodity in an athlete. Logic and analytical power assists an athlete in any sport to dispassionately review where they must improve.

The ability of an athlete to self-motivate is essential to success, both in competition and training. Additionally, creativity is also an intangible that will separate the successful athletes from the merely talented. Creativity manifests itself in team games through clever or well-conceived tactics. In individual sports, creativity is often reflected through the athlete's approach to training routines.

Discipline is a factor in both practice and games. Undisciplined performance will inevitably lead to error; a failure to adhere to practice schedules by the athlete will usually result in substandard performance.

The level of alertness and mental acuity that the athlete brings to performance is a function of a number of combined factors, including physical fatigue or stresses unrelated to sport, such as personal circumstances, education, or employment pressures.

Environmental factors are rarely within the athlete's personal control; the ability of the athlete to adapt to unexpected environmental factors is often determinative of performance success. There are important environmental factors that can affect success. Playing conditions are the same for all competitors, be it the surface of an Alpine ski run, a sudden rainstorm soaking a rugby pitch, or unexpected heat in a distance race. An athlete seeking to maximize performance must not only exercise the mental control to avoid being upset by weather or the condition of a playing surface, the athlete must examine ways to make the conditions work in the positive.

Equipment will sometimes impact performance. A broken hockey stick or a baseball bat that fractures on impact in a tied baseball game can dramatically affect an outcome; deficient equipment can also take a psychological toll on an athlete. The 2006 Winter Olympics provided a remarkable example of an equipment failure becoming a motivating factor for an athlete, when Canadian cross-country skier Beckie Scott had a ski pole break during the women's relay, mentally deflating Scott and crippling her efforts. As Scott fell behind the pack, the Norwegian national director of cross-country skiing ran out to Scott and provided her with an extra pole. Scott raced ahead with renewed vigor; Canada ultimately won the silver medal.

Coaching and external support for the athlete is as important as any factor in sport performance. For young athletes, if there is not a parent or organized sport group providing direction and assistance to the aspiring competitor, success is unlikely. In certain disciplines, such as skiing or figure skating, when there are significant expenses with respect to securing practice time and specialized coaching, an athlete's opportunity to progress absent parental or other support is highly unlikely.

Coaching will impact sport performance, either positively or negatively, in two separate ways. Coaches provide the primary direction to an athlete in terms of training, tactics, nutrition, and sport technique. It is the coach who must keep current with respect to all advances in the sport. A lack of appropriate coaching direction in any of these aspects will prevent the athlete from achieving the best result. As importantly, a coach is one of the athlete's primary emotional support, due to the intensity and the immediacy of the relationship.

**SEE ALSO** Fitness; Health; Motivational techniques; Sport psychology; Visualization in sport.

# Sport psychology

Psychology is the study of the nature and function of the mind, with particular emphasis placed on the relationship between thought and physical action. Psychology has become increasingly important in sports, particularly with respect to the improvement and maintenance of athletic performance. Sport psychology is an aspect of sport training and preparation; this science is primarily directed at assisting individual athletes and teams maintain an optimal balance between mind and body, both in terms of the physical execution of the technical aspects of the sport and the related functions of emotion and mood. Many athletes who possess superior physical gifts are rarely able to seemingly combine athletic talent and mental control; sport psychology is directed at the building and reinforcement of that connection. Sport psychology is a separate but related study from sports medicine.

Formal psychological training is a combination of intense academic study and practical applications; sport psychology is an accepted subscript of the science. Sport psychologists typically are persons with an interest in and an understanding of the mechanics and the dynamics of both sport and sport coaching. At an elite competitive level, the athlete/coach/psychologist triangle is usually very tightly formed, particularly in support of athletes who compete in individual sports.

Sports psychology was not generally accepted as a formal science until the 1970s, when a body of knowledge began to develop concerning how athletes could be motivated to train harder and to maintain a peak emotional level prior to competition. Modern sport psychology is a multifaceted science, covering a broad and sometimes contradictory range of professional opinions about how to best stimulate the mind of the athlete to assist in the achievement of a desired result.

There is no single sports psychology approach. Team sports and the dynamics of group interaction are entirely different than the pursuits of individual competition. The nature of the sport itself will play a significant role in how the athlete may be assisted; certain sports, by their nature, are likely to attract certain types of personalities. A cross-country skier and the object of the sport are a polar opposite to the goals of a weightlifter or a boxer. While individuals in their sport may require varying psychological approaches, the science of sports psychology is founded on a number of constants. Sport psychology, as a support to the athlete, will invariably include work in three general areas: goal setting, imagery and simulation, and development of better powers of concentration.

Goal setting is a planning process that occurs as a part of an assessment of the overall needs and abilities of an athlete. Goals must ultimately be realistic; to set objectives that are unattainable for an athlete is to guarantee failure. Goal setting involves the determination of such issues as the athlete's ability to self-motivate and the personal measure of self-confidence. The sports psychologist, along with the athlete and the coaches, can play a role in the prioritizing of competitive events within the training year; effective coaches will create a schedule that is often referred to as periodization of training, when the year is divided into the constituent parts of competitive season, off-season and preseason. Sport psychology principles are of particular application in the athlete's development of a feedback loop, where the constant analysis, reevaluation, and refocusing of training and competitive direction, occurs regarding performance.

Imagery and simulation training and techniques form the second branch of sport psychology. Although commonly treated as a single entity, imagery and simulation are two distinct psychological approaches to sport training and preparation.

The physical training undertaken by any athlete requires the development of the athlete's brain and the pathways of the nervous system, particularly those of the peripheral system that extend to the musculoskeletal structure that is directed and powered to achieve movement. The more specific and focused the nerve impulses initiated by the brain in respect of the intended physical movements of the sport, the more effective the athlete will be in execution of the required movements of the sport.

Imagery is a psychological technique where the athlete is conditioned to prepare for sport through the use of the mind. Imagery includes the development of set thought patterns, composed of often abstract words or images that the athlete finds helpful in reinforcing the focus on the activity. Images are developed between the athlete and the psychologist to trigger certain types of emotions that the athlete may wish to harness at appropriate times. The common emotions that are tied to imagery are those that calm the athlete in a tense environment, ones that motivate the athlete to increase intensity where the athlete may be at a lower level of intensity than is desired, or images to heighten the ability to block out all extraneous activity or distraction.

The images may be personal to the athlete's experience, or they may be created to spur a particular reaction. Once taught, imagery is a self-motivational tool, portable in that the images and their keys are carried in the athlete's mind. An example is the use of the word "wind" and words associated with the performance and the nature of wind in relation to how a distance runner might imagine his or her own performance. The abstract wind is connected to the reality of what the athlete seeks to achieve.

Simulation is a mental training process that is a direct linkage between mental control and the sport. Simple simulations include the mental rehearsal of sport-specific techniques such as the mental review of all aspects of a foul shot in basketball, from the first approach to the foul line to the ball falling through the cylinder. An important component of effective simulation is the appreciation of all of the senses that the athlete would expect to engage at the time of the actual event being simulated. Using the basketball foul shot as an example, the player would be encouraged to think not only of the mechanics of the shot, but how the ball feels in the shooter's hand, the sensation of the player's shoes on the floor, and the sound made by the ball as it swishes through the mesh of the basket on a successful attempt. Simulation seeks to build the entire act and its surrounding physical circumstances in the mind, to better equip the athlete to deal with those related sensations during competition.

Simulation is the mental companion to the physical training involved in sports practice. The live drills used by teams to prepare for competition are the mirror to the mental training and psychological preparation of simulation. The overriding purpose of both imagery and simulation in sport is to assist in the development of confidence in the athlete.

The development of the athlete's powers of concentration is the third general component of sport psychology. In many respects, the maintenance of concentration powers is the most difficult mental effort extended by an athlete, as concentration is influenced by both physical circumstances such as fatigue or injury, as well as the mental aspects of competitive pressure and other distracting variables. Sports psychologists often seek to develop a number of specific attributes to mental performance as a general increase in the powers of concentration in an athlete. The first of these qualities is focus. In both training and competitive situations, an athlete must maintain a relentless attention on the matters at hand. Focus is applicable to both the mechanics of the sport, as well as the maintenance of the required intensity to perform at the desired level.

Mood is the next factor to be controlled in the enhancement of concentration powers. Sport psychology provides for an intensely individualized analysis when determining the ideal mood suitable for the best performance in any given athlete. As a general proposition, the psychologist will seek to assist the athlete in attaining the desired mood. Imagery is sometimes employed, as are external stimuli such as music.

The athlete's activation level is a concept closely related to the mood of the athlete, as every athlete has an emotional point where he or she is sufficiently mentally stimulated to possess the desire and the drive to perform, without being so excited by the prospect of competition that the athlete loses concentration regarding the execution of the required physical aspects of the sport. The phrase "to get psyched up" is a simple example of words that are used to take the athlete to the activation level. Another tool to maintain activation level in an athlete is positive self-talk, where the athlete is encouraged to talk silently for constant self-encouragement throughout an event.

Sports psychologists will also seek to equip the athlete with personal stress management tools; if an athlete succumbs to the stress of competition, he or she will not be able to succeed. The control of stressful factors by the athlete, especially when the athlete is able to direct some of the energy that is created by stress into positive performance, is among the goals of the psychologist.

Pressure is a more generalized emotional factor that is closely related to stress. Pressure is often driven by external circumstances, such as the expectations of a parent, a team, or a coach. It is a factor that tends to undermine the power of concentration. Pressure is often subtle and more diffuse than the stress that is associated with a specific event. Pressure may often be related to insecurity or a poor self-image on the part of the athlete. Sports psychologists often work with athletes to establish reasonable expectations to assist with the ability to deal with the variables of sport performance.

The overall maintenance of mental and emotional balance on the part of the athlete's mental outlook is a powerful weapon against overtraining. The science of psychology has long recognized two general classifications of personalities, labeled type A and type B. Type A persons are those who are intense, perfectionist, and demanding individuals;

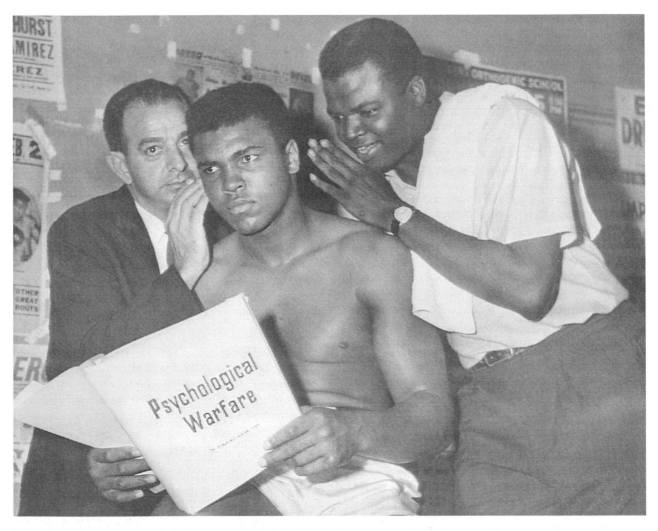

Muhammad Ali engaged psychological as well as physical skills in his fights. © BETTMANN/CORBIS

Type Bs are relaxed and easygoing people. Type A athletes are the most vulnerable to overtraining syndrome, as these persons will tend to push themselves past healthy physical and emotional limits in their pursuit of excellence.

**SEE ALSO** Motivational techniques; Sport performance; Sports coaching; Visualization in sport.

## Sports coaching

Sport coaching is as difficult and as demanding as any other aspect of sport. Good coaching and poor coaching often have impacts on the individual athlete or a team and can become magnified out of proportion to the coaching direction itself. The complete and well-trained sports coach is seemingly a multi-dimensional personality, possessing a wide range of technical, communication, and interpersonal skills.

There is no one source from which strong sports coaches are produced. Many successful coaches were sports players with average physical talents; others developed coaching skills through formal academic or sports institute education. All sports coaches must possess certain attributes, some in greater measures than others, to provide effective direction to their athletes or teams. An important attribute is a technical knowledge of the sport. A passion for the sport is a coaching asset on its own, but a love of the game standing in isolation is not a sufficient grounding for coaching effectiveness. While it may not be essential that the coach possess tactical genius (although the further one moves to elite competition, the more important tactics will be to a primary coaching consideration), the coach must have a thorough grounding in the fundamentals of the sport, or the coach will not be able to provide the necessary direction to the athletes in either training programs or competitive events. In North America, the knowledgeable technical coach is sometimes referred to as one who understands "the Xs and Os," a reference to the visual aids often used by coaches to diagram a play or a maneuver.

Other coaching skills include preparing physical training programs and practice planning. Technical sports knowledge permits the coach to plan how the athletes will best develop their skills for competition. A critical part of coaching is the establishment of realistic overall performance goals. To achieve such goals, the thorough coach develops training programs that build on the concept of the periodization of training. Through periodization, the coach will plan a training year that is divided into the general periods of preseason, competitive season, and off season, with each of these periods divided into sub-periods to take into account such events as a special competition or injury rehabilitation. The macro planning of the athletic season works in tandem with the micro planning that a coach will employ to prepare individual practice and training sessions. All training is directed toward a training objective, which in turn must be focused toward a distinct competitive or performance goal. A coach must have a solid understanding of performance and the function of the body in every respect, as the coach must appreciate the limits of human capabilities if training is to be maximized without exceeding athletic capabilities.

Mental and psychological training for the athletes is critical. The coach is the prime motivational support for both individual athletes and teams. It is the coach who sets the tone for the quality of training sessions. Coaches also lead the effort to motivate and to maintain the athlete's emotional control during competition.

A coach needs to impart tactical ability in competitive situations. Many coaches are very skilled at scouting an opponent and devising a strategy, commonly described as the development of a game plan. The execution of the game plan by a team often depends on the coach's ability to make tactical adjustments during the course of the competition. A coach must develop a resolute emotional control to minimize the influence of external competitive forces, such as officiating and crowd noise, to implement the game plan or to make such adjustments to the plan as circumstances may demand. An effective coach in a game situation will usually be able to detach to a certain degree from these influences without losing touch with the emotional state of the

team or individual athlete. Tactical success also requires the coach to remain current with every development and performance trend in the sport.

In an overarching way, the coach will be the primary personal support for the athlete in many cases. Coaching is, at its heart, a trust relationship between coach and athlete. At its best, the coach is a supremely influential figure for good in the life of the athlete, a sporting mentor with whom the athlete has a powerful emotional bond. The successful coach puts the interests of the athlete ahead of his or her own in every circumstance. In rarer cases, the often well-intentioned coach becomes a Svengali, a hypnotist who controls the athlete in every aspect of his or her life. Such coaches often lose sight of their primary duty to develop the skills of the athlete, rendering the athlete a part of the coach's personal agenda instead. Such situations are ultimately self-defeating for both athlete and coach.

SEE ALSO Computer simulations as a training tool; Motivational techniques; Sport performance; Sport psychology; Visualization in sport.

# Sports injuries

The treatment and management of sports injuries has become a multi-faceted and highly visible aspect of sports science. Sports medicine is a distinct area of professional study within the broader field of medical science because sports injuries frequently engage concepts not relevant to the treatment of any other type of physical injury.

An injury is defined as any form of harm or hurt sustained by the human body, no matter how it may have been caused. An injury may be precipitated through one's own actions, such as a sprained ankle sustained while playing basketball, or through the impact of an environmental force, such as heat or cold. Injuries may be accidental, they may be caused by the deliberate actions of a third party, or the harm may be self-inflicted. The body makes no physiological distinction between sport and non-sport injuries; the body responds to any damage sustained to a tissue, bone, organ, or system no matter how the injury was caused.

When employed as an adjective to describe a type of injury, the term sports is defined as any game, competition, exercise or training program that requires physical activity. At one time, sports injuries were deemed to be only those that occurred in the course of competition. Injuries sustained while the athlete is practicing are equally sports injuries.

Sports injuries are best understood as a part of a cycle or a continuum of physical activity. Sports injuries do not occur in a vacuum, where the injury leads in a progressive fashion to treatment and then recovery. Sports injuries occur against a complex backdrop that includes the athlete's level of ability, the athlete's experience in the sport, general health and fitness history, and the athlete's desire to return to the sport after recovery. The background factors will often dictate the approach taken by an athlete and medical personnel to treatment and rehabilitation.

Injuries are a fact of a sporting life. In most sports, it is not a question of if an athlete will ever sustain an injury, but rather when an injury will occur and to what degree of severity. Athletic injuries may result from participation in the sport itself, as with a boxer sustaining a concussion as a result of absorbing an opponent's punch to the head, or a basketball player sustaining a tear of her anterior cruciate ligament (ACL) in a knee. Alternatively, participation in a sport may reveal the existence of a pre-existing or underlying physical condition.

Examples of a sports injury acting as an agent that exposes a pre-existing physical condition include the presence of an unequal leg length in a runner; unequal leg length contributes to the unequal foot strike forces that commonly result in a stress fracture of the tibia. Other latent physiological conditions that are revealed by exercise include weaknesses in the cardiovascular system, such as an irregular heart beat.

There are a number of sports where the typical participant in the activity brings a particular mental outlook to the sport that carries with it a greater likelihood of injury. An example is the training approach adopted by many endurance athletes, such as marathoners and triathletes, one that is often expressed as "no pain, no gain." At its most basic articulation, this approach advances the proposition that if the athlete is not suffering to some considerable degree in workouts, the athlete will never achieve competitive success. Numerous studies have confirmed that such athletes fall victim with far greater frequency than any other to overuse and over-training injuries, such as stress fractures and serious joint damage. It is a significant challenge to dissuade an athlete with this fundamental training mindset from this approach with the intent of reducing their personal risk of injury.

In a similar way, the external mental pressures that may be directed towards an athlete often contribute to an over zealous approach to training that results in a sports injury. The parental pressure upon a young athlete to excel, or the similar pressure directed from coaches towards athletes may create a mindset that makes the likelihood of injury greater.

The chief distinction in the treatment of sports injuries as opposed to the injuries sustained in the general population is the extent and the purpose of the rehabilitative treatment directed to each. The medical profession, whether in general practice or in a sports specialty, has an over riding obligation to treat any debilitating physical condition. The imperative behind sports injury treatment is a combination of speed, a desire to return the athlete to action as quickly as possible, and to work towards the prevention of a similar injury in future. In professional sport, there is usually an additional factor, the often significant financial incentive for both a team and an individual athlete to make a speedy recovery.

An example of the speed that typically attaches to both the diagnosis and the commencement of treatment of a sports injury is found in the nature of the diagnostic tools employed by the treating medical personnel—x rays, magnetic resonance imaging (MRI) technology, and computer tomography (CAT) scans. Most professional sports teams and many collegiate programs, such as the elite Division I schools participating in National Collegiate Athletic Association (NCAA) competition in the United States have immediate access to these tools.

Arthroscopic surgery is the single most important development in sports injury treatment since 1980. The arthroscope is a small surgical device equipped with a camera that permits the surgeon to examine the interior of an injured joint through a small incision. Arthroscopic procedures revolutionized the treatment of injuries to the knee, elbow, and shoulder, as the surgeon was not required to perform an invasive procedure to achieve a modest surgical objective.

Many technological advances in arthroscopic techniques since 1980 have been driven by the desire to fully rehabilitate an athlete to their former athletic productivity and income generating potential. The now standard operation to repair the elbow ulnar cruciate ligament (UCL), often damaged as a result of the stresses inherent in baseball pitching, was first developed by Dr. Frank Jobe, a California sports medicine orthopedic specialist, in 1973. Many arthroscopic procedures used in shoulder and knee repair were initiated by American sports medicine expert James Andrews, commencing in the mid-1980s.

The frequency of sports injuries is often described in terms of an injury rate, a term that carries different meanings in different contexts. As an example, the National Football League has often had attributed to it a 100% injury rate, meaning that every player in the league is in injured at one time or another during a season. However, the expression of an injury rate in such broad terms is misleading if the data does not make reference to other factors, such as the severity of the injuries sustained, the days lost or games missed by an injured players, and in what context the injury occurred (preseason training camp, practice, games, or in the player's personal off season conditioning program).

In 2003, a comprehensive study into the incidence of sports injuries was undertaken in the United States entitled the SuperStudy of Sports. The study was directed to the establishment of clear definitions of sport injury. In addition to considerations of classifying severity of injury, the study sought to demarcate the boundary between sport and non-sport activities. As an example, a 15-year-old boy who falls from his skateboard and fractures his wrist has sustained a sports injury; his mother who accidentally trips over the same skateboard and falls in her driveway, breaking her wrist, has not sustained a sport injury.

The SuperStudy set out four general classifications of sport injury, where each class of injury is tied to the amount of time the athlete was required to spend away from the sport due to injury.

A Level I injury will not interrupt the athlete's participation in the sport or activity, and there is no subsequent problem resulting from the injury. Examples of Level I injuries include a soccer player with a bruised shoulder that does not affect his or her mobility. A Level II injury is one that requires the athlete to miss at least one training session or competitive event, but no more that 1 month of activity (practices or competitions).

A Level III injury can sideline the athlete for a minimum of 1 month of activity. A Level IV injury has the same definition as a Level III occurrence, except that the athlete was require dot obtain medical treatment at a hospital emergency room, undergo surgery or other medical intervention.

The European Community authorized a sports injury study that employed a similar methodology in 2004.

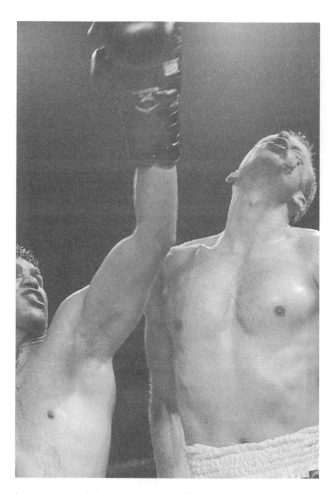

In most sports, it is not a question of if an athlete will ever sustain an injury, but rather when an injury will occur and to what degree of severity. © SHAWN FREDERICK/CORBIS

The rehabilitation undertaken to recover from a sports injury will often engage a number of allied professionals. To correct or protect an injured joint or structure, orthotics and other protective devices may be constructed to assist the athlete in achieving optimal physical function. The physical work required of the athlete to return to their pre-injury fitness often requires the athlete to learn a variety of stretching and flexibility exercises to rebuild or to improve an existing range of motion in a joint. This rehabilitation is often supervised by either a physiotherapist, an athletic trainer, or both.

In some cases, the most profound consequences of a sports injury are psychological. In many sports, the difference between success and failure is razor thin; if the athlete has lost consequence or acquired doubts as to their abilities to perform as a result of the injury sustained, the mental training will become as important as physical rehabilitation. This phenomenon is often observed in athletes who race in high speed or other inherently dangerous circumstances. Alpine skiing, particularly the down hill event, is one where if the athlete makes a complete physical recovery from an injury, but cannot mentally sustain the willingness to ski to the very edge of physical control, the skier is unlikely to regain their top racing form.

The ability of an athlete to psychologically recover from an injury is sometimes as demanding a process as the physical rehabilitation. There is an extensive body of academic material on this aspect of sports injury recovery alone. When one distills the various psychological approaches to this problem, the result is that the athlete must be encouraged to participate as they did before the injury, as opposed to participating in such a fashion that their goal is to avoid the circumstance that lead to their injury.

**SEE ALSO** Musculoskeletal injuries; Sport Performance; Sports Medical Conditions; Sports Medicine Education.

# Sports medical conditions

Medical conditions have a relationship to two related, but distinct, sport issues—the ability of an individual athlete to generally participate in sport, and the more refined pursuit of sporting excellence. Depending on the nature of the condition, medical circumstances will either influence or dictate sport outcomes.

The consideration of medical conditions that affect sport is not made in a uniform manner. Child and adolescent athletes are subject to different considerations than are adults, particularly with respect to the general musculoskeletal development of young persons, and with regard to growth plate considerations in particular. Conditions that are directly related to the aging process such as osteoarthritis and other physiological considerations will influence the relationship between medical conditions and sport participation for older persons.

The determination of what effect, if any, a medical condition may have on the performance of a prospective sport by an athlete will first require an assessment of the relative risk posed by participation to the athlete. The American Pediatrics Association developed a useful categorization formula in 1994 that is now widely employed in pre-participation sport assessments made by physicians. In this method, the risk of participation is examined with reference to the degree of physical contact in the activity. Sports are classified as contact or collision sports, limited/incidental contact sports, and non-contact sports.

Contact or collision sports include ice hockey, American football, rugby, and Alpine skiing (due to the risk of high speed falls or collisions with fixed objects on the ski hill). Limited or incidental contact sports include basketball, soccer, cycling (risk of falls), inline skating (risk of falls), baseball and softball (base runner collisions), and various athletics field events where contact is made with a landing area, such as the high jump. Sports that are of limited risk to the athlete when performed in isolation may present a more significant risk where there are repetitions required in training.

Non-contact sports include all running disciplines, volleyball, sailing, athletics field events such as the shotput, and archery.

In any circumstance where there is an issue as to the physical durability of the person proposing to participate in a particular sport, these classifications are useful. However, the degree of risk to a particular participant is not limited to the degree of physical contact created in the sport. An equally important consideration is the level of physical intensity with which the participant is expected to perform in the sport. Intensity can be weighed in most sports through the impact that participation imposes on the cardiovascular and cardiorespiratory systems and their related functions.

Intensity is a measure that itself has a number of different dimensions. Intensity has been defined as a combination of the dynamic demands on the cardiovascular system, or the volume of work imposed on it by a sport activity, and the static demands, the pressure placed on these systems. Intensity is also affected by the related factors of training levels and the emotional level of the competitive environment and those required of the athlete to compete. A sport that places the athlete at moderate risk of injury caused by physical contact, such as volleyball, places significant mental and emotional demands on the competitor when the venue is a state championship or an international tournament. Emotional considerations apart, high-intensity sports include running, rowing, cycling, cross-country skiing, and lacrosse. Moderate-intensity sports include volleyball, sailing, baseball, and cricket. Curling, golf, and archery are examples of low-intensity sports,

With the two different methods of defining the relationship between sport and a known medical condition, the athlete can be cross-referenced against two valid standards. Some common medical conditions have two means of comparison to explain how the impact of a medical condition can be assessed in a particular sport. Skeletal and structural conditions are often revealed through sport participation and not before. Factors such as uneven leg length, a congenital weakness in a bone formation or reduced bone density, the onset of osteoarthritis, and similar medical conditions are made apparent through sport when they were not necessarily apparent in daily life. The assessment of these conditions from a contact/collision perspective is very important; in some high-intensity sports, the stress of repetitive action may pose significant problems for the athlete. When the preexisting skeletal condition is known, sports posing physical risk should be avoided. In some cases, when the assessment reveals a structural imbalance, the athlete will be encouraged to obtain an orthotic or other corrective device.

Identified cardiovascular system problems will require an intense physical assessment as a part of the participation analysis. Potential cardiovascular conditions that have a significant impact on athletic participation include self-induced conditions such as hypertension and arteriosclerosis, usually precipitated by poor dietary practices, as well as congenital problems such as a heart murmur, heart arrhythmia, and various types of irregularities in the heart muscle wall. The true extent of these conditions is sometimes impossible to define; common tools to assist in the determination are stress tests involving heart monitors and related assessments.

Eating disorders such as anorexia nervosa and bulimia often occur among young female athletes in sports where there exists considerable pressure, both among peers and coaches, as well as that imposed by the nature of the sport itself to possess a particular body type. When such disorders are identified, the athlete should be removed from the competitive and training environment in which the disorder arose until the disorder has been entirely resolved. An eating disorder is well recognized in the medical community as a serious mental illness that requires thorough medical attention; sport participation should not be renewed until the athlete is well.

Diabetes is increasingly common in both adolescents and adults; in most circumstances, a diabetic condition can be properly controlled through diet. Many athletes have succeeded in high-intensity settings with a diabetic condition with proper monitoring and support.

Neurological conditions, such as a history of concussion caused by blows to the head or jaw, can produced cumulative effects; each successive blow to the head represents a progressively greater risk of permanent brain injury than the previous incident. The athlete must be assessed not only from the perspective of the general risks of the particular sport, but what level of risk within the sport remains for the particularly vulnerable athlete, if the maximum amount of protection were available.

In most cases, the safety of the athlete is of lesser consideration when a partial loss of vision will be primarily a performance issue. An example is American ice hockey player Bryan Berard, who lost all of the sight in one eye playing in a National Hockey League (NHL) game in 2000. Berard continued his career after satisfying league officials that he could perform at a professional level with one fully functional eye.

As a neurological condition, epileptic seizures will require a careful assessment of the seizure history of the athlete and the effect of available anti-seizure medication on different types of sport-imposed physical stress.

People who are either clinically obese or who are significantly overweight must proceed with a physical training program with considerable caution. The chief risks associated with sport in these circumstances are the additional stresses placed on the joints of the body, as well as the pressures created for the cardiovascular system.

People who have had a kidney removed must approach sports involving significant fluid losses and rehydration with caution; warm weather and endurance exercise require the kidneys to operate at maximum capacity in the maintenance of optimal sodium/fluid balance. On the other hand, damaged internal organs, such as a damaged kidney or an enlarged spleen, are almost always a condition that will exclude participation in sports that involve even a slight risk of physical contact. Further assessment must be made of the organ capacity in relation to its function relative to the demands of the relevant non-contact sport.

Existing skin disorders, such as herpes simplex I, are contagious. Sports where the athlete will have significant skin contact with apparatus or floor mats, such as gymnastics, or where there is significant skin-to-skin contact required in the sport, such as wrestling and boxing, should be those where participation is excluded until the skin condition is definitively cleared.

Asthma and related breathing conditions are among the most common of medical conditions that affect sports participation. The cause of asthma, which is an inflammation and a consequent narrowing of the bronchial passages and airways leading to the lungs, is both hereditary and environmental in nature. Certain types of people have a predisposition to asthma; other persons are susceptible to a condition known as sport-induced asthma. Almost all forms of asthma can be treated for the purpose of permitting an athlete to fully participate in any sport with appropriate and carefully monitored medical support. Other asthma conditions are those that the young athlete tends to outgrow. The most common medication used to treat asthmatic conditions are inhaled corticosteroids, which are generally taken on a daily basis. When the athlete feels the distress from the onset of an asthma attack during competition or training, a bronchodilator is employed, such as Albuterol, a beta$_2$ agonist (a chemical that mimics the effect of adrenaline and tends to work to open the affected passages).

SEE ALSO Eating disorders in athletes; Health; Psychological disorders; Sport psychology; Sports medicine education.

# Sports medicine education

Sports medicine is a relatively recent medical specialty. Until the 1980s, the team physician in a high-level sport program was often an orthopedic specialist with an interest in sport; there was no defined training or educational programs to support sport medical practices. The primary focus of the physician was reactive, as opposed to preventative, in nature. The diagnosis, treatment, and repair of injuries was the most important ongoing function in sport medicine.

The increasing sophistication with which athletes and their coaches approached training and competition was the impetus in the development of the sports medicine as a recognized discipline within the medical profession. Sports medicine education today embraces a wide range of sciences, each of which contributes to the healthy training, diagnostics, treatment, repair, and rehabilitation of athletes. A sports medicine practitioner will be a part of a coordinated treatment effort involving a number of allied experts.

Modern sports medicine is not directed simply to the treatment and repair of injuries; the ultimate goal with respect to an athletic injury is the promotion of healing, recovery, and a limitation-free, pain-free return to sport. Sports medicine education is directed toward all of these objectives.

Sports medicine is influenced by a number of forces, some of which are within the traditional realm of the physician, with others rooted in various applications of sport performance. Those forces include medicine, with particular emphasis on the orthopedic specialties, both surgical and non-surgical treatments, and physiatry, the rehabilitative and physical medicine specialty. Anther discrete medical specialty that is a part of sport medicine education is the subscript of orthopedics, joint reconstruction. Medical research, with which all sport medicine education must be closely allied, is an ongoing, dynamic field that is driven by the study of disciplines such as biomechanics and bone biology.

Other sports medicine application are podiatry, the medicine of the foot and its processes, and exercise science (kinesiology), the study of human movement. The effective treatment and management of sports injuries requires a solid grounding in the mechanics of the body.

A sports medicine expert may not physically direct a day-to-day course of athletic therapy; an understanding what the therapist can accomplish is fundamental to the prescription of treatments for the injury. However, how an athlete is coached is an important component to the understanding of the likely course of rehabilitation and recovery to be experienced by the athlete.

A large and important aspect of general nutrition, health promotion, and wellness is the counseling and direction of athletes concerning the use of dietary supplements, and the dangers of contaminated or otherwise illegal performance-enhancing substances.

Sports medicine education will embrace each of the sports science fields. No one specialist is likely to possess the skills and the training to act as the primary treatment professional in each component; many sports medical professionals act as coordinators of care programs that are directed to each aspect of the science. As with all sports science disciplines, the professional will have sufficient knowledge to know when to engage the input of another specialist.

Sports medicine education places a primary emphasis on the need to provide athletes with a physical assessment prior to their participation in a sport. This assessment will often be provided in conjunction with coaches or athletic therapists, if there are concerns regarding a preexisting injury or condition, or when the medical personnel are seeking to identify a congenital condition such as heart arrhythmia (irregular heart beat). In many sports, the sports medicine professional will be engaged to provide

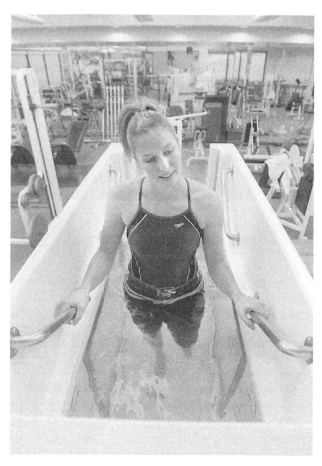

Noelle Pikus-Pace of the U.S. Olympic Skeleton Team, using the AquaCiser as part of her physical rehabilitation after a broken leg.
PHOTO BY EZRA SHAW/GETTY IMAGES

in-season assessments and testing of the athlete. In professional sport, when the athlete is often a party to a guaranteed contract and remunerated whether or not he or she is sufficiently healthy to play, the pre-season medical assessment, known in as the physical, is a mandatory clearance for the athlete to enter competition. Subsequent physicals will be conducted by a team's sports medicine personnel when an athlete proposes to return to competition from injury.

Given the demands of sports competition on the body, a significant component of sports medicine education will invariably be devoted to the diagnosis and testing of athletes in relation to injury. These processes often focus on the mechanics of movement, engaging the combined principles of both exercise science and medicine.

Orthopedic medicine, the science of the diagnosis and treatment of musculoskeletal injuries, is a central aspect of sports medicine. Developments concerning arthroscopic surgical techniques, increasingly sophisticated micro-surgery techniques that are a less invasive repair of joints such as the knee or elbow, are a rapidly developing specialty within orthopedic medicine. Since the year 2000, advances in the preservation of articular cartilage in the joints have included Cartrell cartilage implants and other procedures to rebuild cartilage and corresponding joint function.

Physiatry, the rehabilitative and physical medicine specialty is an important aspect of sport medicine education. Related to all rehabilitative efforts is the direction of all efforts that support the recovery of the athlete beyond the scope of traditional medical training—the creation of appropriate orthotics, and the utilization of alternative treatments such as physiotherapy and massage.

**SEE ALSO** Chiropractic medicine and sport; Sports medical conditions.

# Sports security and terrorism

Terrorism is the deliberate and systematic use of violence and intimidation in anywhere the actions are intended to achieve or to influence a political result. Terrorist acts have been perpetrated for as long as there have been political disputes. The term was first employed by British statesman Edmund Burke (1729–1797) to describe the actions of the Jacobins during the French Revolution in the late 1790s. Notable terrorist actions in recent history include those of the Irish Republican Army against Britain at various times throughout the twentieth century, the efforts of various terrorist groups that have been directed against the state of Israel since its founding in 1948, and the coordinated attacks upon various American targets made by Al-Qaeda agents on September 11, 2001, the events collectively known as the 9/11 attacks.

Sporting events, particularly those with global appeal, are an obvious terrorist target, as such attacks will attract the attention of the world to the particular terrorist cause. The capture and the subsequent murder of 11 Israeli Olympic team members at the 1972 Summer Olympics was such an act. Members of the Palestinian group "Black September" sought the release of 200 Palestinian prisoners held by Israel through these means. The deaths of the Israeli athletes is regarded the one of the most significant terrorist acts ever committed prior to the 9/11 attacks. A related issue that remains controversial was that made by International Olympic Committee president Avery Brundage with respect to the continuation of the Games in the wake of the Israeli team killings. Brundage directed that the Games would continued as scheduled, after a one day delay.

Prior to 1972, the Olympics had not previously been the target of any significant terrorist activity. The murder of the Israeli athletes at Munich altered the nature and extent of sports event security forever. At every Games held since the 1972 Olympics, security has been a significant and highly visible presence. In addition to on site protection, the police forces of the host nation seek and obtain information from other nations with respect to any possible terrorist risk that might manifest itself at the Olympics.

While terrorism on the level of the Munich killings has never been replicated at an international sporting event, a number of terrorist acts have been perpetrated with an indirect impact upon international sport. A notable example was the destruction of a Korean Airlines jet by a terrorist bomb in 1987. Subsequent investigation revealed that the perpetrators intended to disrupt the lead up to the 1988 Summer Olympics that was ultimately hosted by South Korea. In 1996, a bomb planted by a domestic terrorist was detonated in the Atlanta Games Olympic Park, with one person killed and over 100 injured. In 1997, the Olympic stadium in Stockholm was severely damaged by a terrorist bomb, planted by a group who were opposed to a Swedish bid for the 2004 Olympic Games that were ultimately awarded to Athens.

The 9/11 attacks served to further heighten security concerns, especially with respect to both the potential threat to American athletes competing abroad and the staging of events on American soil. Teams representing the United States in events as diverse as the Ryder Cup golf championship and international tennis tournaments have been the subject of close security protection for this reason.

At the 2002 Winter Olympics at Salt Lake City, the American organizers of the Games instituted two measures then unique to Games security. A 52 mile no-fly zone was imposed around the entire Games site, and sharpshooters were placed on various mountain top positions to protect specific competition venues.

The Maccabiah Games are often referred to as the "Jewish Olympics," a quadrennial sports festival that attracts Jewish athletes from around the world to Israel to compete in an Olympic styled format. The Maccabiah Games are held in Jerusalem, and the proximity of the Games to Israel's Arab neighbors, particularly the nearby Palestinian population, has been a point of significant friction since the Games were first held in 1950. Threats from various terrorist groups directed towards the Maccabiah Games and its competitors are common.

The Maccabiah Games attracts approximately 7,500 athletes and many thousands of visitors; at the seventeenthMaccabiah Games in 2005, over 2,000 Israeli soldiers were deployed at the competition venues, with larger numbers at the opening and closing ceremonies. All athletes were assigned a non-transferable identification card, with several built in security features, including encryption to prevent counterfeiting.

The World Cup of soccer is a 32 nation championship that is contested in a number of different stadiums in the host country. While international soccer has been plagued in recent years by "hooliganism," the excessive fan behavior made most notorious by the supporters of English soccer. FIFA, the world governing body of the sport has implemented security measures, including the deployment of police and private security forces *en masse* at every game, coupled with an extensive behind the scenes security work up, including the obtaining of lists of every known undesirable person who might attend the World Cup from any of the participating countries.

Prior to the 9/11 attacks, the level of security present at most North American sporting events was relatively modest, as the security concerns were chiefly directed to spectator behavior, such as the prevention of spectators from interfering with the event, or entering the stadium without a ticket. As an example of heightened concerns regarding terrorist activities, the organizers of the 2006 Major League Baseball All Star game held in Pittsburgh, utilized 100 trained bomb detection dogs as a part of an enhanced security program developed for the event.

**SEE ALSO** FIFA: World Cup Soccer; International Olympic Committee (IOC); Maccabiah Games.

# Sprains and strains

Sprains and strains are common soft tissue athletic injuries. These two terms are often used interchangeably, when in fact each is a distinct injury both in causation and effect.

A sprain is an injury to a ligament, the connective tissue that joins two bones together in a joint. The injury is the result of the ligament fibers being overstretched, often causing a micro-tear, as opposed to the severing or the rupture of the fibers. The overstretching is most often caused by a movement of one beyond the possible range of motion of the joint, either through a hyperextension (overextension), or by a twisting action. Hyper-extended and twisted knees are examples of knee sprains. Ligaments are composed of a type of collagen, which is formed from specific amino acids ingested in the body through dietary protein. Collagen is a naturally elastic substance found in various formations in all of the connective tissue within the body. Collagen provides the overstretched fibers that constitute a ligament sprain with the ability to heal through the action of the body's restorative processes; vitamin C is essential to ligament strength and elasticity.

A strain is an injury that occurs to a muscle or a connecting tendon. A muscle strain is an injury caused to the fibers of skeletal muscle; the other types of muscle, cardiac muscle and smooth organ muscles are not susceptible to strain because they are not controlled by voluntary nervous system impulse. Skeletal muscle is composed of long, thin, cylindrical fibers that are arranged in bundles; a strain is an overstretching or micro-tear of the fiber. Tendons are also formed from a type of collagen, although a tendon is generally a less elastic tissue than a ligament.

Sprains commonly result from a twisting motion in a joint that creates either overextension or overflexion of the supporting ligaments. A common example of this injury mechanism is a sprained knee caused by contact in sports such as soccer, American football, or rugby. These sprains result from circumstances where the athlete is moving in a forward direction, when the knee is twisted, either through physical contact with an opponent or through a sudden change of direction by the athlete, sometimes accompanied by irregularity or unevenness on the playing surface. The forces that directed the knee forward are suddenly directed laterally, creating torque (a force that causes rotation in the joint), causing the ligaments to stretch. The same mechanism, with a greater degree of force applied, will result in the more serious tear or rupture injury to the ligament.

Another common sprain is to the individual fingers or the wrist, due to an object such as a ball forcefully striking the body and bending the specific structure past its normal range of motion.

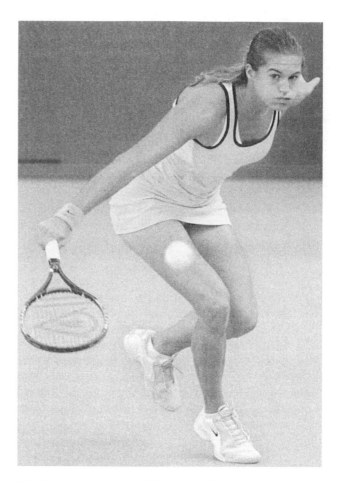

World number one Amelie Mauresmo of France returns a shot to Lindsay Davenport of the U.S. during 2004 match. Mauresmo later withdrew with a recurring left-thigh strain. OLIVER LANG/AFP/ GETTY IMAGES

A muscle strain, often referred to as a pull, is most often caused by either repetitive motion that overtaxes the muscle, or through an imbalance in a set of muscles. Almost all joints in the body operate through the function of a muscle pair: one muscle, the extensor providing the joint with the ability to extend or straighten, the other, the flexor, permitting the joint to bend. The knee, with the extensor quadriceps and the flexor hamstring is such a joint. A general ideal ratio of strength between the four muscles of the quadriceps and the hamstring is 3:2; muscle and tendon strains are common in both muscle groups when there is an imbalance, which creates additional stress on the weaker of the pair when the forces of motion are applied.

The groin, given its location within the body, is a set of tissues connecting to the abductor muscles of the upper thigh and the lower abdominals, is a common site for a strain injury, as imbalances between the groin and the muscle groups connected to the groin can lead to injury. Groin pulls are very common in sports requiring sudden lateral movement.

Ligament injuries are most often a result of the nature of the physical movement associated with a particular sport, and as such these injuries are not always preventable. Muscle strains are more often caused by a preexisting structural imbalance. A focused and whole body stretching and flexibility regime, where the muscle groups throughout the body are balanced with one another, is the most effective way to minimize muscle and tendon strains.

The overriding goal in the treatment of sprains and strains is the avoidance of a recurring injury. For both injuries, the application of the RICE (rest/ice/compression/elevation) treatment for the first 48 to 72 hours after the occurrence will reduce swelling in the injury and will facilitate healing. Most strains and sprains will not require any external support other than wrapping; crutches may sometimes be necessary when the athlete has sustained a significant strain of a knee or ankle ligament that is short of being torn or ruptured.

SEE ALSO Groin pulls and strains; Hamstring pull, tear, or strain; Musculoskeletal injuries; Quadriceps pulls and tears; Tendinitis and ruptured tendons.

# Sprinting SEE Running: Sprinting

# Spurs SEE Heel spurs

# Squash

Squash is a fast paced indoor court racquet sport whose evolution has been largely independent of any other sport, including racquetball, which bears some superficial similarities to squash. The central object of squash, which may be played in a singles or doubles format, is to play shots off the walled court with a racquet in such a fashion that the ball strikes the floor twice before the opponent can make a return.

Squash was first played in its modern form at Harrow, an English boy's school, in the years after 1850. Squash was descended from rackets, an outdoor walled game itself descended from early forms of tennis. Squash became a popular game at various English schools, and its appeal spread to North America and various parts of Europe in a short time. The

first international squash competition took place between teams from the United States and Canada in 1922. The governing body of international squash, the World Squash Federation, (WSF) has over 120 national organization in its current membership.

As squash is actively played in over 150 countries, the WSF has made a concerted effort to secure the inclusion of squash as an Olympic Sport, without success. Squash is a medal sport in both the Commonwealth Games and the Pan American Games. The Professional Squash Association sanctions a vibrant professional squash series for both male and female competitors, with events staged throughout the world.

The squash court is a four walled rectangle, divided into sections through the placement of dividing lines that govern the placement of shots. A singles court is approximately 32 ft long and 21 ft wide (9.75 m by 6.4 m); the front wall is 15 ft high (4.57 m). Service boxes are laid out of the floor of the court, the area from which a player must make their serve. A doubles squash court is approximately 50% longer and 20% wider than the singles court.

The front wall has three lines marked across it. Closest to the floor of the court is the tin; approximately half way up the wall is the service line, and near the top of the wall is positioned the out line. A legal serve must strike the area between the tin and the service line, and land in the opponent's half of the court behind the service boxes. Once a legal serve has been made, both players may drive shots that strike the front wall between the tine and the out line. Players may use any of the walls to make shots, so long as the shot does not strike the wall above the out line.

There are two scoring systems used in squash. In the first system, known as the English system, points are only scored on the player's service. A typical match is the best of five games, with each game determined by the first player to reach nine points. The alternate scoring system, used most frequently in professional squash, awards a point to the successful player in every rally, with a game won at 11 points.

The most important pieces of squash equipment are the racquet and the ball. The racquets used today are invariably light weight (some are as light as 4 oz (110 g), with a very strong construction. The racquets are made from composite materials such as carbon fiber and are usually 27 in (68 cm) long. The materials used in the construction of the racquet create a degree of flex in the racquet that permits the player to transfer a greater measure of muscular power through the racquet into the ball on a stroke.

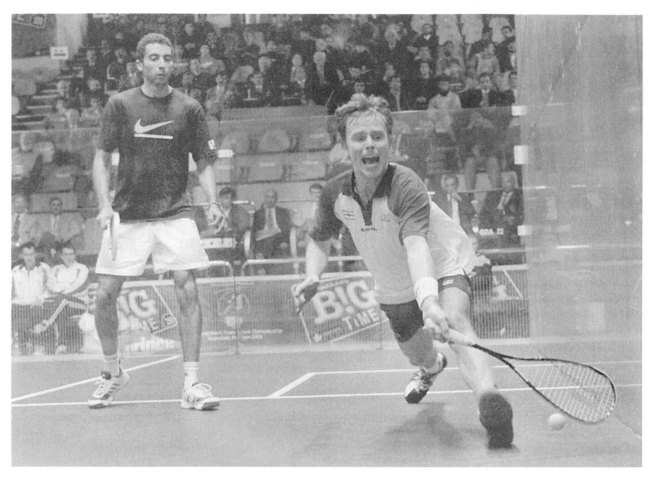

Men playing at squash championships (2005). FAROOQ NAEEM/AFP/GETTY IMAGES

There are five different kinds of squash balls approved for various types of competition by the WSF. As a general proposition, the more experienced the players, the less lively the ball used will be; conversely, inexperienced players who have difficulty returning shots will enjoy the game more if the ball is livelier and is capable of bouncing higher from the court surface. The speed and resilience of the balls sanctioned by the WSF are classified by the color of the ball, ranging from "blue" (fast) to "double yellow" (super slow). At the highest levels of squash competition, the double yellow ball is the standard ball.

The ball characteristics dictate the warm-up between the players prior to a match. The warm-up shots of each player heats the ball to make it more responsive to shots made during the match.

During the course of play in the relatively close quarters of the squash court, if one of the payers is not able to reach a ball to make a shot due to the body position of the opponent, the hindered player is permitted to call "let," which, if legitimate, results in a replay of the serve.

As with other racquet sports, the fundamental tactic employed by a successful squash player is to seek control of the center of the court. In squash, given the location of the markings on the court, this desirable center position is called the "T." In this position, the player can respond more efficiently to any shot placed by the opponent.

Squash is a sport that requires continuous and effective movement. The successful squash player builds a strong aerobic base of fitness, to both support the player in a sport where the rallies are often demanding, as an aid to player recovery between serves. Squash is a sport that lends itself to a periodized approach to training, with a preseason focus upon building aerobic capacity, coupled with plyometric training to enhance explosive movement on the court, particularly in a lateral direction. The squash preseason may also include circuit training to develop overall muscular strength. The bending and turning motions associated with squash place a premium upon flexibility and optimal range of joint motion in every player. Comprehensive stretching programs are essential for this purpose in squash.

**SEE ALSO** Badminton; Handball; Racquetball; Tennis serve mechanics.

# Stationary bicycles, elliptical trainers, and other cardio training machines

Stationary bicycles are one of a group of machines commonly used for the purpose of cardiovascular exercise and training. Elliptical trainers, rowing machines, and a multitude of equipment variations that incorporate features from each type are all classed as cardio training machines. While possessing a similar fitness purpose, these total-body cardio training machines differ from the treadmills and stair climbing machines that are designed for leg exercise only.

While the various cardio training machines each permit the user a distinct physical workout due to its unique construction, all possess similar features. The intensity of the workout is both variable as well as being entirely within the control of the athlete. Most advanced models of these machines have sophisticated computer programs that assist the user in the control and direction of workout intensity level. The machines all provide the athlete with an opportunity to closely monitor and regulate performance. The assessment of various biofeedback indicators, such as heart rate, can be connected directly to the machine's built-in workout indicators, such as time, intensity level, caloric output, and others. For persons with preexisting cardiovascular problems, the cardio training machine permits them to exercise safely within their known permitted limits of exertion.

Cardio training machines generally, and the stationary bicycle and the rowing machines in particular, offer the athlete an opportunity to simulate aspects of competition. Either alone, or with the aid of computer programs that regulate the intensity associated with a race course or practice, the athlete can practice stroke or cadence in a regulated fashion.

All cardio training machines represent an excellent cross training tool that can be utilized by an athlete regardless of weather conditions. These machines are widely used as an effective rehabilitation tool, especially for those persons recovering from leg injuries who wish to gradually rebuild both strength and range of motion. The motion associated with all variations of the cardio training machines is one of low impact on the musculoskeletal system; the lower extremities, and particularly the ankle and knee joints, are exposed to less stresses than those of conventional running-oriented sports activity.

Stationary bicycles are manufactured widely throughout the world, each with its own specific features. Some models are equipped with levers that permit the athlete to exercise the biceps, triceps, and shoulder structure in a manner that does not occur with a regular bicycle. The bicycles most suited to the simulation of a road bicycle are those with a variable resistance where the rider can keep track of the rate at which the bicycle is being pedaled. A variation of the stationary bicycle that achieves the same effect is the mounting of an actual bicycle on a trainer that provides resistance to the rear wheel, simulating the effects of a ride.

An elliptical trainer positions the athlete on two parallel foot pads, usually fixed or mounted on ramps, with the leg action mimicking either a running motion or a classic cross-country skiing action, depending on the angle to the floor at which the parallel foot ramps are set. Most elliptical machines permit the athlete to vary the inclination of the ramp, and thus control the intensity level of the exercise. Some elliptical machines, like the stationary cycles, have arm levers in place of a handle bar for an additional upper body workout, as the athlete is required to pull on each lever in concert with the leg motion. The elliptical machine is not capable of providing a precise replication of the physical motion associated with the mechanics of a particular sport. The elliptical's chief training benefit is the ability of the user to reverse the motion of the machine, creating a mechanized form of retro running. This feature permits the athlete to build greater strength and to develop optimal balance between the desired strengths of the hamstring and quadriceps muscles, an important factor in the limitation of upper leg and knee injuries. The generally accepted ratio of strength between these two muscle groups is a 3:2 proportion in favor of the quadriceps; when a specific weakness in either muscle is identified in an athlete, the reverse motion of the elliptical trainer will form a part of the training solution.

Rowing machines are used in two different formats. The first are simple rowers with a fixed seat,

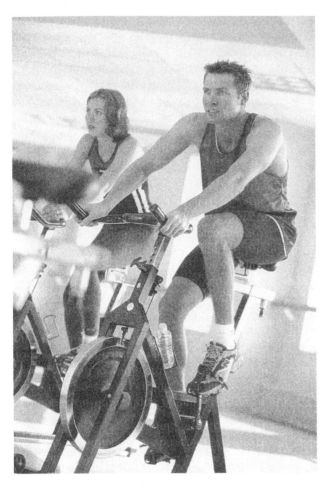

Stationary bikes are used for cardiovascular exercise and can be adjusted to meet the training needs of the individual athlete.
© JIM CUMMINS/CORBIS

usually built into a stationary weight training machine. The simple rowers are limited in their benefit as, absent the seat sliding action, they do not replicate a true rowing motion. The second and far more useful sport training device is the ergometric rower. This machine takes its name from the ergometer, a device that measures the amount of work done by a group of muscles. It is equipped with a sliding seat and a motion that is very similar to that experienced by a sculler (two-oar rower). These rowing machines are also designed with variable intensity, allowing a very accurate simulation of the rowing motion. Rowing machines are also an excellent cross trainer; over 50% of the power in a properly executed stroke will be derived from the rower's legs.

**SEE ALSO** Cross training; Jump rope training; Treadmills.

# Stimulants

Stimulants is a generic term used to describe various substances that are ingested by athletes into the human body for the purpose of increasing alertness or general physical performance. Common stimulants that have been typically utilized by athletes in various disciplines are caffeine, amphetamines (including benzedrine, ephedrine and methamphetamine), and cocaine in its various forms.

Stimulants may be legally prescribed by a physician to counter medical conditions such as narcolepsy, a disorder where the subject sleeps uncontrollably, as well as certain brain dysfunctions occurring in children.

Caffeine is a mild stimulant that occurs naturally in numerous types of plants, the most common of which is coffee. Caffeine has been scientifically determined as effective in reducing fatigue in athletes, as well as having a role in the slowing the rate of glycogen depletion in the body in the course of endurance events such as the marathon, thus potentially increasing the efficiency of the athlete. Caffeine is also a powerful diuretic, reducing the body's ability to retain fluid during performance.

Amphetamines increase the heart and respiration rates, increase blood pressure, dilate the pupils of the eyes, and decrease appetite. These substances will tend to reduce fatigue over a short term period, as well as tending to increase the self confidence of an athlete during competition.

Cocaine is a powerful central nervous stimulator, manufactured through extraction from the naturally occurring coca plant. Although more commonly used as a recreational drug, it has been used by athletes seeking additional mental sharpness and concentration. A notable example of cocaine use in elite competition is that of Cuban high jumper Javier Sotomayor, the world champion who was stripped of a Pan American Games championship in 1999 after testing positive for cocaine.

All stimulants tend to be psychologically addictive, which will cause pronounced "down" periods when the athlete ceases taking the stimulant. Other side effects, which vary from person to person, include anxiety, blurred vision, sleeplessness, and dizziness. Abuse of amphetamines can cause irregular heartbeat and even physical collapse; a number of deaths in long distance cycling have been attributed to the abuse of stimulants.

All amphetamines and cocaine are banned substances in any amount if detected in the blood of an athlete at virtually any type of international competition. Caffeine is prohibited in amounts greater than 12 mcg/ml in athlete urine samples at Olympic competition, an amount approximately equal to the ingestion of eight cups of coffee in a two hour period.

**SEE ALSO** Caffeine; Doping tests; Ephedra.

## Stitch SEE Runner's stitch

## Strains SEE Sprains and strains

## Strength, muscle SEE Muscle mass and strength

## Strength training

The development and maintenance of musculoskeletal strength are essential to athletic performance and the overall fitness of any individual. In general terms, fitness is achieved through the combination of strength, speed and lateral quickness, power, endurance (both cardiovascular and muscular), and flexibility, represented by the optimal range of motion in the joints. Different sports may demand greater or lesser proportions of each of these fitness components.

The fundamental principles of strength training are tied to both the role that strength plays in the overall fitness and performance capabilities of an athlete, as well as the connection to the biology regarding muscle growth. Muscle fibers contract in response to a nerve impulse directed to a muscle through the network of the central and peripheral nervous systems. Each muscle fiber contraction is the means by which the muscle produces movement; the rate of contraction is dependent on the muscle type and the activity to which the muscle energy is being directed.

Strength training is intended to develop three separate but interrelated types of muscle strength: maximum muscle strength, which represents the greatest amount of force that a person is capable of generating in a single muscle contraction; elastic strength, which is the ability in the muscle to contract quickly in response to a event; and strength endurance, which is the ability to repeat an action

or to sustain a force through a greater number of repetitions.

The development of each of these three types of muscle strength is achieved through the principle of overload training. Overload is the taking of a muscle past its present capacity without damage to the structure. In overload training, the muscle fibers will sustain minor injury, which the body naturally repairs by directing the formation of myoblast cells, which thicken and strengthen the damaged fiber when the body is at rest. The repeated breaking down and building up of muscle fiber will lead to larger and more powerful muscle fibers over time.

Overload training can be achieved in several ways. The first method is the increase in the number of repetitions of any strength exercise. The second aspect of overload training is the increase in the amount of weight lifted or resistance otherwise applied to the muscles. The third overload tool is the increase in the intensity of the work being done by the targeted muscles, through a reduction in the recovery interval between the repetitions.

Strength training that employs the overload principle will tend to achieve a number of musculoskeletal and neuromuscular results. The first are those known as myogenic changes; these are structural changes to the dimension and composition of the overloaded muscle. These changes induce a state of hypertrophy, meaning the muscle becomes larger and denser. The second results are neurogenic changes, when the rate of response by the nervous system is increased due to repetition of each muscular effort. Overload training will also create capillarisation in the vicinity of the muscle, where the increased workload imposed upon the muscle forces the body to increase blood flow to the region through the formation of new capillaries, which results in a greater ability in the muscle to store both adenosine triphosphate (ATP), the energy fuel in each cell, and glycogen, the cellular storage form of glucose.

There are a number of training methods that will develop each of the three different types of muscular strength. Weight training, using both resistance machines and free weights, is the type of strength training that has the broadest application, as it will aid in the development of maximum strength, elastic strength, and muscle endurance. Elastic strength is also enhanced through a combination of plyometrics, Swiss ball routines that stress core body strength, and flexibility exercises. Muscle endurance can also be achieved through circuit training, where the athlete does series of exercises that stress different muscle groups in sequence, as well as running that emphasizes resistance, such as hill workouts or running with a harness or parachute.

Strength training must also be tailored to the sport for which it is intended to be applied. All sports require a measure of strength, to put the body into balance; the strength requirements and resultant strength training for an American football lineman, who is responsible for the generation of explosive forces to be directed against opposing players, will be entirely different than the strength training of a marathon runner or a tennis player. Sports where maximum muscle strength is of primary importance include American football, rugby, wrestling, and ice hockey. Elastic strength is essential in baseball, volleyball, and cricket. Sports in which all three of the strength aspects will be relied on are those that require the athlete to master a number of differing techniques, such as the triathlon and cross-country skiing, when the entire body is engaged in the propulsion of the athlete.

**SEE ALSO** Dietary supplements; Muscle mass and strength; Resistance exercise training; Strength training for children and young athletes; Strength training: Nutrition.

# Strength training for children and young athletes

The involvement of young athletes in strength training programs has attracted a significant degree of commentary in the world of sports science in recent years. With young athletes seemingly more physically able to perform at a higher athletic level at ever younger ages, there is often an assumption that strength training will make the talented young athlete even more effective. There are significant physiological and emotional factors that affect youth strength training that are not present in similar adult programs. Strength training for young people must be approached with caution.

Defining who is a young athlete is a variable proposition. The age of puberty, the phase in physical development when a person grows to physical and sexual maturity, has been determined to have fallen significantly over the past 100 years, particularly among females in North America. A modern female can begin to exhibit the physical changes associated with puberty as ages as young as eight years old, or as old as 13. The modern age for the onset of male puberty ranges from 10 years of age to 14 years.

The determination of puberty is fundamentally important to the consideration of what, if any, weight training a young athlete may safely undertake. Puberty is a genetically determined process for every individual; it is the period when the body grows faster than at any other time in a person's life, other than during infancy. Puberty may last between 18 months and four years or more. During puberty, as the bones grow, the stresses on both the bone structure and the connective tissue in the related joints can become significant. The long bones of the body, particularly the tibia and fibula (lower leg), femur (thigh), and the humerus (upper arm), have growth plates located at the epiphysis, a segment located near the end of each of these bones. The growth plate is fundamental to the healthy and orderly growth of the bone to maturity. Until adulthood, the growth plate remains softer than the other regions of the bone, and it is far more vulnerable to physical damage from a direct trauma, as well as that caused by repetitive stress or the application of excessive forces that may occur through weight training, excessive training mileage, or other forms of resistance.

During puberty, there are also significant imbalances in the body between bone and connective tissues growth rates in specific places. The well-known adolescent knee ailment, Osgood Schlatter disease (OSD), occurs when the growth of the tibia is at a different rate than that of the patella (kneecap) tendon to which the tibia is connected. OSD causes swelling and pain in the area below the patella because the repetitive extension of the tendon through running takes place with an imbalance between the tendon and the tibia, causing strain on the tendon. OSD will often make running or weight-bearing exercise difficult until the relative growth of the two structures is equal.

Strength training in adults is usually intended to develop the three separate but related aspects of strength: maximum strength, the greatest amount of force that can be produced in a single muscular contraction; elastic strength, which is the ability of the muscles to respond and contract quickly; and strength endurance, the ability to sustain a level of force through a number of repetitions. Overload training is the most common form of strength training in adults, where muscles are built up and sustained through a repeated cycle of overload and recovery.

For children who have not yet reached puberty, any form of weight training is dangerous to the child's long-term musculoskeletal health. There is little benefit to be derived from such programs until puberty has determined more definitively the adult shape and characteristics of the person. Focused stretching and flexibility exercises will benefit all active persons of any age; the introduction of resistance and weight training is of little benefit to a child.

Training to develop maximum strength is a dangerous process for a pubescent athlete. Overload resistance training, plyometrics jump programs, intense resistance running, or any repetitive weight-bearing training activity carries with it significant structural risks. Sports science research confirms that any strength training done by persons whose bodies have not reached maturity should be confined to the exercises that focus on endurance and elastic strength; strength training should not be maximal weight training for these persons. The components of a healthy and useful strength training program for a young athlete will include a number of components, all of which emphasize athlete safety and long-term physical development.

Any youth training program must entail active supervision; young people will test themselves when permitted, and risk injury by lifting an excessive amount of weight or otherwise attempting a resistance movement that is dangerous to them. There must be a focus on instruction and the development of technique; the young athlete must have detailed instruction regarding any weight-bearing motion, with the emphasis at all times on smooth movements that take the weight or object through a full range of motion in the applicable joints. The companion to smoothness of motion is control of motion, to permit the young athlete to proceed with safety and confidence. To best enhance the range of motion desired in these programs, stretching and flexibility exercises should be incorporated with the strength training.

SEE ALSO Growth plate injuries; Musculoskeletal injuries; Strength training; Youth sports performance; Youth sports training.

# Strength training: Nutrition

Strength training is a component of every athlete's training regimen. Strength training also places additional nutritional demands on the body; the extent of those demands will depend on the intensity and the volume of the strength training program.

Strength training has three essential aspects: the development of maximum strength, the ability to generate the greatest possible force in a single repetition; the building of elastic strength, the ability to direct the muscles to respond quickly and dynamically; and endurance strength, which will involve the promotion of both cardiovascular and muscular endurance.

Proper nutrition, the nourishment of the body through foods and dietary supplements, is essential to general health and well-being. Athletes must pay particular attention to nutrition, given that the body requires a steady, properly proportioned supply of macronutrients, including carbohydrates, proteins, and fats, as well as numerous micronutrients, substances essential to the function of many human systems, including all vitamins and most of the minerals absorbed into the body. The maintenance of proper fluid levels, dependent on the mineral electrolyte sodium, and the absorption of sufficient calcium and vitamin D for bone maintenance are two examples of areas where a nutritional deficit will have a negative impact on strength training.

Strength training imposes stresses and impacts on the body that must be addressed through careful attention to nutrition. The most fundamental of these impacts is the need for additional energy to participate in the training itself. Whether strength training is the only form of athletic activity undertaken by a person, or when it is supplemental to other sports training, strength training carries with it the need to ensure that the body has sufficient energy to train and to properly recover. Most persons will obtain sufficient energy from a diet that is proportioned as 60–65% carbohydrates, 12–15% proteins, and less than 30% fats.

Protein consumption is another aspect of nutrition that is of particular interest in strength training, as dietary proteins, and their constituent amino acids, are the building blocks of muscle. There are 20 different amino acids, 10 of which are produced within the body, 10 of which must be obtained through diet. These dietary amino acids are also known as the essential amino acids. Unlike carbohydrates, stored as glycogen, and fats, stored as triglycerides, amino acids cannot be stored within the body and must be replenished on a daily basis. Myoblasts, the muscle cells that repair the cellular damage caused by training, are created from amino acids. Conventional sports science wisdom once held that extra protein consumption would speed muscle development; modern science supports the view that while there may be circumstances in the case of an individual athlete to support short-term increases in protein consumption, these are exceptional circumstances; the typical strength training athlete requires only fractionally more than the protein requirements of a healthy non-athlete.

All protein sources do not provide an equal protein value when ingested into the body. The amino acid pattern in an egg is the standard for the measurement of protein quality in all foods. Plant proteins are generally inferior in amino acid quality to dairy, soya, and meat products.

The healthiest and the surest way to ensure that the optimal amount of micronutrients are absorbed into the body is through diet; dietary supplements are a second choice, to be utilized when a dietary source is not available. The exceptions to this rule are with regard to the consumption of sport drinks and creatine supplementation.

Sport drinks are useful to assist a strength training athlete to maintain carbohydrate, sodium, and potassium levels, especially as a recovery tool after a hard workout. Creatine is a supplement that attracted wide ranging attention in the 1990s when notable professional athletes, including baseball homerun hitter Mark McGuire and English sprinter Linford Christie, were adding the substance into their training diets. Creatine is a naturally occurring chemical, found in every cell in the body as creatine phosphate, or phosphocreatine. Creatine is essential to the production of energy through an electrochemical reaction involving the creation and reduction of adenosine triphosphate (ATP).

Creatine supplementation, when conducted according to manufacturer specification, has been proven to assist athletes in the maintenance of the short-term energy stores essential for the explosive movements in strength training. Excess amounts of creatine are not known to produce any toxic effect on the body, as creatine is processed and excreted through the urine by way of the kidneys. Creatine does not contribute to the building of muscle, as might an anabolic steroid or human growth hormone; creatine supplementation is directed to the production and storage of the fuel the body needs for anaerobic activity such as strength training.

SEE ALSO Diet; Dietary supplements; Free weights; Nutrition; Resistance exercise training; Strength training.

## Stress SEE Mental stress

## Stress fracture of the foot

A stress fracture is a localized area of bone damage where the cells that comprise the bone have become damaged due to repeated forces. The forces effect is cumulative, creating a circumstance where the speed with which the body produces bone-building cells, osteoblasts, is less than the bone-reducing, or osteoclastic, activity. Next to stress fractures of the lower tibia (shin bone), the stress fracture of the foot is the second most common location for this type of injury, accounting for approximately 25% of all such fractures.

The most common location among the 26 bones of the foot and ankle for a stress fracture are the five metatarsal bones, the structures that are the skeletal connection between the tarsal bone (ankle) and the toes on each foot. The second and third metatarsals are the most common bones of the foot to sustain a stress fracture; the fifth metatarsal (the bone connecting the ankle to the little toe) is the least common location for a stress facture of the foot.

There are number of factors that inevitably lead to the creation of a stress fracture of the foot in an athlete. Stress fractures of the foot occur slightly more often in female athletes than in males, a fact that is attributable to the difference in the shapes of male versus female athletes. The proportionately wider pelvis and shorter femur and tibia in a female athlete lead to a proportionately different distribution of forces throughout the female musculoskeletal structure. For both men and women, there is often more than one risk factor operating to produce the fracture, many of which are tied to the concepts of either overuse or repetitive motion.

Sports that involve repetitive motions such as running (particularly on hard surfaces) and jumping, or training on angled surfaces, where the force of each foot strike is distributed unevenly, are a leading contributing factor in the cause of stress fractures in the foot. Similarly, when the athlete has suddenly increased either training intensity or training volume, or when the athlete embarks on a running or training program that is too vigorous for the current level of fitness, the foot is the recipient of forces to which it is unsuited.

Physiological and nutritional factors also play a role in the formation of these fractures. When the athlete has a previously undetermined dietary mineral deficiency (calcium, vitamin D, or phosphorus) that has created a corresponding bone density deficit, the bone becomes more vulnerable to injury. Structural imbalances such as unequal leg length will result in forces being generated when the athlete's foot strikes the ground. Footwear that is inappropriate to the foot strike motion of the athlete will accentuate all structural deficiencies present in the lower

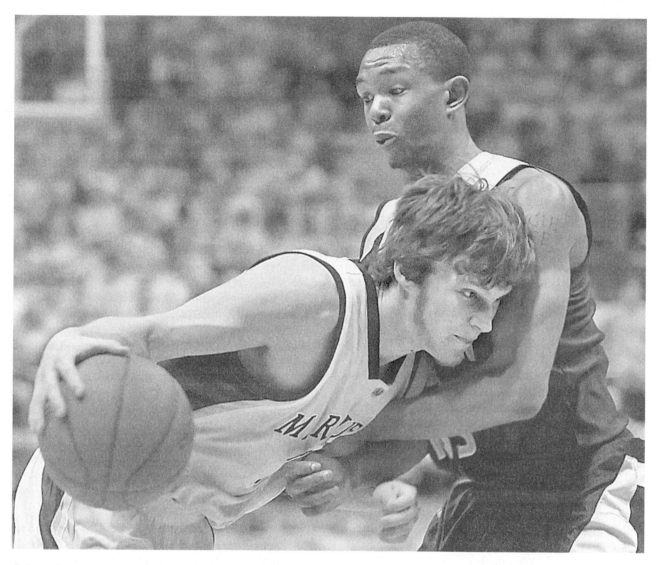

College players during basketball game; defense play resulted in broken foot of one of the players. AP PHOTO/MORRY GASH

limbs of the athlete. An example is the wearing of a running shoe that is suited to a runner whose foot pronates (the ankle rolls inward) on impact, when the foot of the runner in fact supinates (rolls outward) on impact. This footwear will improperly absorb the forces and may permit the force of impact to be excessively directed into the foot.

Athletes with poor flexibility tend to be more susceptible to stress fractures of the foot because their bodies do not move as fluidly or as responsively as those athletes who possess a greater range of motion in the joints.

From a psychological perspective, athletes with a strong desire to reach or exceed their training objectives, the so-called type A personality, often fall victim to stress fractures. These athletes are the most

likely individuals to return to training too quickly after an injury, or to excessive training intensity. These circumstances often do not permit a previously injured metatarsal bone to heal properly, resulting in a recurrent stress fracture of the foot.

Stress fractures of the foot are first noticeable through the development of a sharp, almost debilitating pain at the location of the fracture. A stress fracture will often not reveal itself while the person is at rest, but only in the course of the sports activity that caused the fracture. A regular x ray will often not reveal the location of the injury; a nuclear bone scan will almost always reveal the location of the fracture. Magnetic resonance imaging (MRI) is another technology that will usually reveal the location of the fracture.

The treatment of a stress fracture of the foot is similar to that sustained at any other bone: rest and a complete cessation of the sport for a period of at least six to eight weeks. The RICE (rest/ice/compression/elevation) treatment is also often recommended, as are the use of nonsteroidal anti-inflammatory drugs (NSAIDs) to reduce inflammation. In more extreme cases, the foot may be placed in a cast for approximately six weeks.

The preventative measures to reduce the risk of recurrence of this injury to the foot are primarily a very gradual return to training, with careful attention paid to the elimination of the stress fracture risk factors noted. High level young athletes, who move from sport to sport throughout the year, are especially vulnerable to stress fracture, because the young athlete is not provided with a period of rest and general down time from high level training.

SEE ALSO Bone, ligaments, tendons; Lower leg injuries; Musculoskeletal injuries; Recurrent stress fractures.

## Stress fractures SEE Recurrent stress fractures

## Stretching and flexibility

Stretching and flexibility are a cornerstone to building and maintaining athletic success. Without a properly stretched musculoskeletal structure, sports performance will be hampered and the risk of injury to muscles and connective tissues of the athlete is greatly increased.

While the concepts are used interchangeably, stretching and flexibility are the beginning of a sport continuum; a strong and focused stretching program that emphasizes the principle of balance between the various parts of the body will create greater flexibility in the body of the athlete. Flexibility itself over time produces a greater range of motion in the joints of the athlete; these structures permit the body to move and react, while under control, with increased dynamism and explosiveness, all with a reduced risk of injury as the flexible joint is better equipped to bear and distribute the stress of athletic movement than is a more rigid, poorly, or infrequently stretched joint.

There are numerous examples of the relationship between poorly stretched regions of the body and performance. In most sports, the athlete must adopt a version of the "athletic crouch," a position where the athlete's legs are slightly bent to permit the athlete to move quickly in any direction. The body's center of gravity is also lower and positioned above the feet, which are approximately shoulder width apart, to provide greater balance in movement. The head of the athlete is level and the arms are slightly extended for balance and participation in movement. The basketball dribbler and defender, the American football and rugby tackler, batsmen in both cricket and baseball, and all runners and skiers perform the movements necessary to their respective sports in a variation of this fundamental athletic position.

In moving from the fundamental athletic stance, an athlete with poor flexibility and correspondingly limited range of joint motion will experience limitations on performance. The first such limitation is a reduced ability to jump; if the lower leg muscles and joints are not properly stretched, the muscle power created in the calf muscles will not be completely converted to the jumping action. The second restriction on athletic movement will be observed in the stride length of the athlete; runners with inflexibility in their hips and lower back tend to have a shorter, less economical stride than do more flexible athletes. The third impact of reduced range of motion is noticed in the reduced ability of the athlete to move laterally, a fundamental aspect of all ball sports. Lateral movement becomes limited through the lack of flexibility in the groin, upper leg, and the abdominal muscles and tissues.

Impaired or ineffective throwing motions are also a common result of poor flexibility and resulting range of motion. Any limitation or impingement on the range of motion in the shoulder, elbow, or wrist joints will result in a reduced ability to throw an object.

The companion benefit to a stretching program is the reduction of the risk of injury due to muscle and structural imbalance. All joints in the body are powered by pairs of muscle groups, one of which is responsible for the extension of the joint, the opposing pair being responsible for the flexion, or bending, of the joint. The most prominent example of such muscle group pairs is the knee joint, where the quadriceps is the extender and the hamstring is the flexor. Inflexibility between muscle pairs will often create a circumstance where one muscle will overpower the actions of the other, creating an imbalance and injury. Imbalances due to inflexibility can also occur in a structure such as the lower leg; if the calf muscles and the Achilles tendon are not in balance, an overextension injury to one or the other is likely.

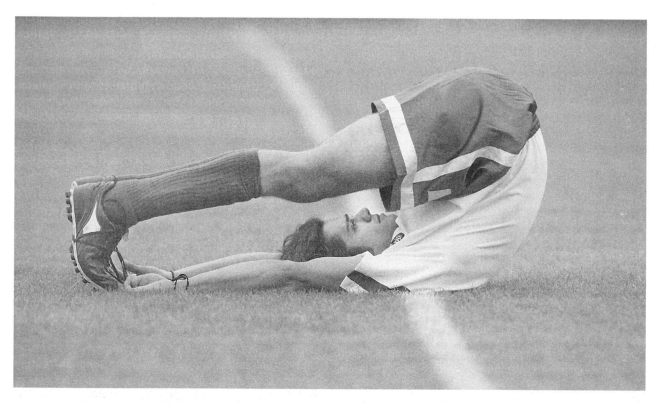

Without proper stretching prior to activity, athletes run a higher risk of injury. © DAVID MADISON/CORBIS

Similar harmony between the muscle groups of the lower back, groin, and abdominal muscles is necessary to prevent strains and tears in these tissues.

To be effective, stretching must form a part of the daily athletic routine. A series of stretches aimed at loosening the entire body is an essential part of every athletic warm up. In sports that emphasize the effectiveness of the leg function, such as distance running, the athlete will often run very easily for a short period, to generate increased heart rate and blood volume into the muscles before beginning the serious stretches. Hard, vigorous stretches should not be attempted at the beginning of the warm up; as with all athletic preparation, the body must move progressively from passive stretching, where the athlete stretches using the effect of his or her own body weight and gravity, to active stretches where the body is manipulated to achieve a particular desired result, the most demanding aspects of any routine.

Stretching is equally important as a cool down mechanism in both the completion of a training session as well as a competition. To return to a normal and rested state, the body requires a bridge from the higher intensity levels created by the demands of the sport. Stretches that stimulate all muscle groups will have such an effect; to stop the sport activity "cold" will promote muscle and joint stiffness.

Stretching and resulting flexibility are inherent in all calisthenics programs, yoga, and pilates. Each of these disciplines is both a self-contained exercise program, as well as a complement to the development of increased flexibility in any other sport.

**SEE ALSO** Calisthenics; Fitness; Hamstring injuries; Hip and groin injuries; Lower leg injuries; Quadriceps pulls and tears; Range of motion; Swiss ball training techniques; Yoga and Pilates.

# Stroke, heat SEE Heat stroke

# Substance, classification

The term restricted substances is one that is widely employed throughout the sports world; there are a number of meanings given this expression, depending on the sport and the substances referred to. The use of the expression is more common in everyday speech than it is in the formal regulations passed by national and international sports governing bodies. Restricted substances may also be variously described in the media as banned substances, prohibited substances, or controlled substances.

Each of the terms used for restricted substances has a distinct meaning, including:

- Restricted substance: A drug, chemical, or other performance-enhancing compound that is not generally permitted for use by athletes, but which may be used if advance permission is obtained from the appropriate sport governing body by the athlete. The World Anti-Doping Agency (WADA) has a protocol for the obtaining of such permission, known as the Therapeutic Use Exemption. A positive doping test for a restricted substance that is used by an athlete without the requisite permission is treated for sanction purposes as a positive test for a prohibited substance.

- Prohibited substance: Such substances are illegal in every respect, with no allowance available in any circumstances for their use by an athlete. Anabolic steroids are the most well-known prohibited substance pursuant to the WADA Prohibited List, published on an annual basis. Prohibited substances may also relate to a prohibited procedure such as blood doping, which is a process that includes the ingestion of the hormone erythropoietin (EPO), itself a prohibited substance.

- Banned substance: This expression has the same meaning in the context of performance-enhancing substances as prohibited substance. The National Football League drug policy refers to "banned substances"; Major League Baseball references "prohibited substances," both to the same effect.

- Controlled substance: These are generally pharmaceutical products whose availability is subject to government regulation, as opposed to the rules of a sports governing body. Most countries have a statutory framework governing the distribution of such drugs similar to that of the United States' Controlled Substances Act, which defines, by way of schedules, the manner in which various substances are to be legally possessed and consumed. The schedules move progressively from the most controlled and ostensibly the most dangerous of substances, such as heroin (which has a medicinal use as a painkiller), to the least controlled substances, prescription medications such as hydrozodone, an active ingredient in the nonsteroidal anti-

inflammatory drugs (NSAIDs) that include Cox-2 inhibitors in their formulation. Restricted substances in sport are similar as a concept to the government controlled substance legislation.

WADA is now the dominant regulatory agency in the battle against performance-enhancing substances as directed by all international sports bodies. The WADA Prohibited List, which is adopted as the law by all national Olympic organizations and virtually all international sports bodies, is comprehensive in its scope. An athlete must submit the Therapeutic Use Exemption to obtain permission to use an otherwise prohibited drug. A prominent example occurred prior to the 2006 Winter Olympics when a dispute arose regarding American skeleton racer Zach Lund, who used a hair restorative product that contained the prohibited substance finasteride, a prohibited steroid-masking agent.

Although the WADA rules make no specific mention of the term restricted substance, proof of the universal understanding of this shade of meaning is found in a number of national governing body interpretations of the WADA rules. The U.S. Track and Field Association (USTAF) guidelines refer to the WADA Therapeutic Exemption as "required for athletes who use Restricted Substances."

One of the most common restricted drugs approved for athletic use in international competition are the asthma medications, including beta-2 agonist, medications that assist in opening the airways to permit ease of breathing for the athlete. Glucocorticoids, a powerful class of painkilling medications that have other therapeutic uses, impact many of the human systems; these drugs are frequently the subject of exemption.

**SEE ALSO** Anabolic steroids; Diuretics; Doping tests; Ephedra; Glucocorticoids; Stimulants.

## Substances, restricted SEE
Restricted substances

## Sumo

Sumo is an ancient form of Japanese wrestling that traces its history over many centuries. It is the national sport of Japan, a contest originally intended as an earthly entertainment to appease the gods of the Shinto religion. Sumo today continues many of the traditions that are rooted in religious observance,

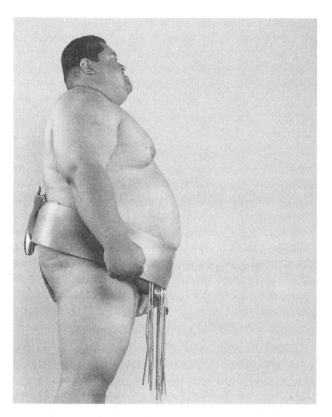

Sumo wrestler. © PATRIK GIARDINO/CORBIS

such as, for purity, the tossing of salt onto the ring surface by the competitors before the match begins.

Unlike the familiar forms of Olympic wrestling, each with rules that govern how the competitors may physically engage one another, sumo is a very simple sport. The two wrestlers face one another in the designated ring, the *dohyo*. The ring is approximately 15 ft (5 m) in diameter. Each competitor wears only a loincloth, and the hair pulled back into a ceremonial top knot. At the start of the match, the first wrestler who touches the floor of the ring with any part of his body other than the soles of his feet or the first wrestler who leaves the ring by any means is disqualified. The most common means of winning a match is to execute a hold using the opponent's loincloth to propel the opponent from the ring. The wrestlers are not permitted to punch, choke, or kick one another. Sumo has only one category for competition, with no distinct weight divisions.

A sumo champion holds an exalted status in Japanese society. Sumo wrestlers are ranked in a strict hierarchy, the *banzuke*; the grand champion of sumo is a *yokozuna*, a title that is retained by the champion at the conclusion of the wrestler's professional career. The sumo wrestler training and life-

style is of legendary strictness, where the young trainees or less accomplished sumo wrestlers are expected to be subservient to the more experienced wrestlers within their training group until they have achieved a measure of success in competition.

At first appearance, the typical sumo wrestler is the antithesis to a fit, accomplished athlete. Most champion sumo wrestlers weight over 350 lb (155 kg), with large and pronounced stomachs and heavy thighs the physical norm. Success in sumo is an application of the basic laws of physics: the lower the center of gravity of the wrestler and the more powerful the initial drive into the opponent, the more likely the opponent will be knocked out of the ring. Most sumo matches are concluded within 30 seconds. Sumo training is directed to the strengthening of the low back to support the very large body mass of the athlete and to facilitate the short two- to three-step explosive burst made by the wrestler at the start of the match to engage the opponent.

**SEE ALSO** Judo; Karate; Taekwondo; Wrestling.

# Supplement contamination

A supplement is any product that is added to an existing formulation to address a deficiency. In sports science, the expressions dietary supplements, nutritional supplements, sports supplements, and similar terms are often used interchangeably. Whatever expression may be used, supplements are consumed for one of two reasons: nutritional benefit or to enhance performance.

Nutritional supplements are sometimes added to a diet to ensure that the athlete is consuming the proper quantities of all of the dietary macronutrients (carbohydrates, proteins, and fats) and micronutrients (chiefly vitamins, minerals, and phytochemicals) essential to both general health and optimal physical performance. An athlete may also consume supplements to obtain a training or performance advantage.

The commercial market for sport-related dietary supplements is immense. It is expected that the global revenues from the sale of such products will reach in excess of $4.5 billion by 2007. The extent of this market, coupled with uneven regulation of manufacturers and distributors of supplements directed at the athletic market, is a significant contributing factor to the problems associated with supplement contamination.

Contamination of a supplement can occur in one of two general ways. Some manufacturers adulterate their product with what they know to be illegal performance-enhancing substances to create a seemingly greater beneficial impact of the supplement on the user. A common example of supplement adulteration has been the addition of unlisted or hidden stimulants such as caffeine or ephedrine to various herbal tonics to enhance supplement effect. In other cases, protein supplements, intended for purchase by athletes seeking to build muscle or to gain weight, have been contaminated by steroids.

The second type of contamination is through the carelessness of the manufacturer. Many supplement producers do not make any of the constituent ingredients of the supplement, but instead they purchase these substances in bulk and mix them into a desired formulation, with little or no testing beforehand as to the exact chemical composition of the mixture.

A number of international studies have confirmed the likely extent of supplement contamination and the consequent risks to athletes, both in terms of their health as well as the legal consequences of an inadvertent positive doping test. An International Olympic Committee-approved laboratory at the University of Cologne, Germany, determined in a 2004 study that between 14% and 25% of the supplements that were tested were contaminated with either steroids or other illegal performance-enhancing substances.

There is no question as to the efficacy of sports drinks that are directed to rehydration, mineral and electrolyte replacement, or carbohydrate source. Similarly, a number of supplements, such as those that contain creatine, vitamin and mineral complexes, or other well-defined nutritional compounds have been proven as either beneficial to general health or mildly helpful to athletic performance. Beyond these types of supplements, there is considerable difficulty in ever being certain as to the composition of the supplement formulation, due to an absence of strict labeling guidelines throughout the world. An example is the United States Dietary Supplement Health Education Act, 1994, which does not impose specific legal obligations on the manufacturers of supplements aimed at the sports market so long as no claims are made concerning the impact on athletic performance.

A lack of knowledge as to the presence of substances such as ephedrine or steroids poses a significant health risk to the consumer. Each of these substances has a significant effect on the function of the body. Stimulants such as ephedrine are intended to increase heart rate and blood volume; for such events to occur without the athlete intending them is a dangerous circumstance. If an athlete is not aware of an anabolic agent such as steroid being consumed, the athlete would be unprepared for the many side effects of those substances, including mood swings, weight gain, and decreased sexual function.

There are also significant competitive risks posed by contaminated supplements. The World Anti-Doping Agency (WADA) has identified supplement contamination as a serious concern in sport. WADA officially consider that athletes who counter a positive doping test with the defense that they were unaware of the precise contents of the supplement due to improper labeling or contamination are guilty. In the resolution of any dispute as to whether the athlete ought to have known the composition of the supplement, WADA will seek adherence to the legal principle of strict liability as the correct standard, entirely shifting to the athlete the responsibility for what he or she ingests.

SEE ALSO Creatine supplementation; Dietary supplements; Ephedra-free supplements; Glutamine supplementation; Protein supplements.

## Surfing

Surfing is a sport whose origins may be traced to the ancient Polynesian cultures of the Pacific Ocean. In 1788, Captain James Cook, the English explorer, observed the indigenous people of both Tahiti and the Hawaiian Islands using long wooden boards to move through the waves near shore. American author Mark Twain described his own adventures with Hawaiian surfing in his book *Roughing It* published in 1871. California, the place most often associated with surfing, first became a hotbed of the sport in the 1920s and 1930s. The California surfing community helped propel the sport into the cultural mainstream in the late 1950s; surfer expressions such as "stoked," "hot dogging," and "wipeout" became a part of modern speech.

Surfing has attained a worldwide appeal due in large part to its utter simplicity. A surfer paddles out into the ocean on a surfboard, and awaits a suitable sized breaking wave on which to ride back to the shore using the wave's energy for propulsion. The more ambitious and talented the surfer, the larger the wave or the greater number of tricks the surfer can execute as the wave travels towards the shore.

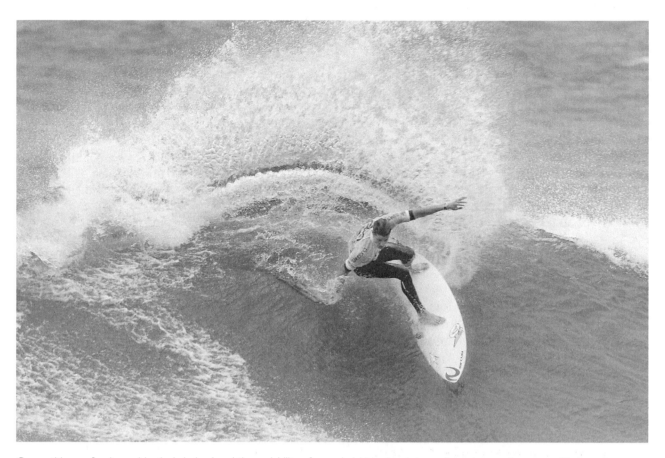

Competitive surfing is a subjectively judged and the variability of wave height and speed may impact upon the competitive result.
**PHOTO BY PIERRE TOSTEE/ASP VIA GETTY IMAGES.**

Although surfing pre-dates the popularity of extreme sports, surfing's inherent physical dangers and its potential for high levels of personal satisfaction, as opposed to achieving a competitive result, warrant its inclusion in the extreme sports category.

The modern surfboard has undergone many changes since the days of the Polynesians. Early surfboards were often as long as 16 ft (5 m), weighing over 100 lb (45 kg), and each was built to support the surfer. Modern surfboards are constructed from synthetic materials such as epoxy, fiberglass, and carbon fiber composites and the boards are usually a shorter length, designed to suit the style of the surfer but also intended to be highly maneuverable in the water. An inexperienced surfer is often directed to a wider and longer board, as the greater the surface area in contact with the water, the greater the stability of the board.

In colder weather or water temperatures below 68°F (20°C), surfers will often wear a wetsuit to protect themselves from the combined effects of cold water and cold air.

Surfing is unique among sports in that the ride on a surfboard is powered by water and the resultant force of gravity alone. The physical object of surfing is to slide down the surface of the wave at the same speed at which the water is moving upwards. If the surfer moves took quickly along the wave surface, the surfer proceed to the bottom of the wave and end the ride as the surfer will no longer be affected by the wave motion. If the surfer moves slower than the wave, the wave will out run the surfer, creating a wipeout. It is for this reason that a surfer can maintain a stable position while riding below the crest of a mammoth ocean wave.

The surfer and the surfboard are balanced on the water surface when the force of gravity acting downwards upon the surfer is precisely equal to the hydrostatic effect, or buoyancy, directed upwards. The center of mass of the board is its balance point; when the surfer moves towards the front or the rear of the board, the board will become oriented accordingly, with the nose or back moved upwards or down to reflect to shift in position by the surfer. A surfer executes a turn on the board by shifting body position to the rear of the board, a movement that creates torque (twisting effect in the motion of the board). The forces of gravity and buoyancy are now directly under the surfer, permitting the turn to be executed. When the surfer pushes downwards on the board, the force of the push is greater than the force of gravity, causing the turn to occur more quickly.

As the surfer moves through the water on the board, the surfer maintains a low, bent leg position, to maximize balance on the board and to respond to any forces directed against the board with subtle changes of position.

A shorter surfboard provides the surfer with greater maneuverability, as the shorter the board, the shorter the axis upon which the surfer is required to turn. A longer surf board possesses an inherently greater moment of inertia, the time period within which an object resists the forces directing it to turn. Conversely, a longer surfboard will tend to travel faster across the surface of the water, due to the relationship between drag and the volume of water displaced by the board. The fins attached to the rear of the surfboard, known as the "skeg" act in a similar fashion to that of a keel on a sail boat, as the fins extending downwards into the water aid in preventing the surfboard from being pushed too far sideways by the force of the moving water.

The International Surfing Association (ISA) is the world governing body of surfing; surfing is also a member of the International Olympic Committee, although surfing is not an Olympic sport. There are also various professional surfing events held in various parts of the world on an annual basis sanctioned by the ISA. Competitive surfing is a subjectively judged and the variability of wave height and speed may impact upon the competitive result.

SEE ALSO Sailing; Sailing physics; Windsurfing.

## Sweat secretion SEE Eccrine sweat secretion

## Swimming

Swimming is one of the world's oldest forms of competitive sport. Swimming ability was valued in a number of ancient cultures, including Greece and Japan.

As swimming became established as a sporting activity in the early 1800s in Europe, the most com-

mon type of swim stroke employed was a variation of the breaststroke, where the swimmer used both arms below the water and the head positioned above water. In 1844 at a competition held in London, a number of Native American entrants from the United States used a stroke that was similar in style to the modern front crawl, where the swimmer's head was submerged from time to time and the arms directed in a windmill motion. Although superior to the breast stroke, the Europeans saw the innovation as undignified and did not adopt it at that time. The first successful attempt to swim the English Channel, a distance of 21 mi (32 km) occurred in 1875.

Swimming pools were built in London, and in other European cities, prior to 1900 and the first European swimming championships were held in Vienna in 1889. Swimming was included as a sport in the first modern Olympic Games in 1896 as a men's sport; the first women's Olympic swimming was contested in 1912. The most famous of swimming strokes was developed in the early years of the twentieth century by Australian Frederick Cavill (1839–1927), who adapted the Native American overhand swim stroke and added a flutter kick (a repetitive kicking motion). This stroke was known as the Australian crawl; it is now designated in international swim rules as the crawl, the stroke used in freestyle swimming events.

Swimming has produced some athletes who became the subject of international recognition. American Johnny Weissmuller (1904-1984) won a total of five Olympic medals in the 1924 and 1928 Summer Games. Weissmuller parlayed his swim fame into a Hollywood movie career as "Tarzan." American Mark Spitz won seven gold medals in the 1972 Olympics. Australian Ian Thorpe, the 6 ft 7 in (1.98 m) "Thorpedo," won a total of nine medals in the 2000 and 2004 Olympics, the most ever by an Australian athlete. Yona Klochvova of the Ukraine won successive gold medals in the 2000 and 2004 Olympics, in addition to being named the world's top 400-m medley swimmer for seven successive years.

The Federation Internationale de Natation de Amateur (FINA), was founded in 1908. FINA is one of the widest ranging of the international governing bodies in sport, as it is the authority in the distinct disciplines of swimming (races up to 10,000 m staged in swimming pools), water polo, open water swimming, diving, and synchronized swimming. The global popularity of swimming is illustrated by the fact that over 200 national swimming associations comprise the FINA membership. Swimming is the most popular of the sports directed by FINA; there are state, regional, intercollegiate, national, and international swimming competitions, in a number of different formats and age groups, available in every region of the world in a given calendar year.

Swimming competitions are held in one of two settings sanctioned by FINA. A short course is a swimming pool 25 m in length; a long course is a 50-m pool. The 50-m facility is the standard distance for international and Olympic competition. The pool is divided into lanes, typically eight in total, with each lane divided by floating markers extending the length of the pool; to assist the swimmers in maintaining their orientation and to permit them to swim in as straight a line as is possible, the center line beneath each lane is marked along the bottom of the pool. In North America and Europe, most competitive swimming competitions are held in indoor facilities; in countries such as Australia, a world power in the sport, the climate permits the extensive use of outdoor swimming pools.

Swimming races range in length from the 50-m sprint (one length of the pool in Olympic competition) to 10,000-m events. The physiological demands of swimming are similar to those of running, in the sense that a 50-m sprint specialist will not likely succeed in a long distance race, and the various distances and specialized strokes demand specialized training approaches. There are four general types of swimming races, each defined by the stroke that the swimmer is required to employ–, freestyle (where all swimmers use the crawl), the breaststroke, the backstroke, and the butterfly. One event, the individual medley, requires the swimmer to use each of the four stroke types for a designated portion of the course. There are also relay races at various distances, including the medley relay where the four team members use a different stroke in their successive relay legs.

All types of swim strokes have five general components: the arm stroke, the kick, the timing and coordination of the body movements, the body position relative to the surface of the water, and the breathing rhythm. All swim performance theory is predicated on the fact that the human body and its composition (over 90% water), is only slightly less buoyant that the substance in which the athlete is racing.

A swim race has three distinct components, the start, the swim, and the turns. Each aspect has its own distinct technique, founded upon a body of practical racing results and scientific research as to the most efficient methods to move through and over water.

Swimmers are permitted to wear a variety of different styles of swim suits during competition. For many years, the standard was a tight fitting suit that exposed most of the body to the water; the tighter the fit, the less likely air bubbles would become trapped between the skin and the suit, causing a less sleek profile in the water. Swimmers would remove all body hair, to reduce the resistance of the water upon their skin, including the wearing of a tight race cap and hydronamically contoured swim goggles. There have been several advances in swim suit technology. One notable example was the development of the Speedo "Fastskin," a material modeled to a significant degree after the skin characteristics of sharks. The swim suit material, like the shark skin, has a series of dermal denticles, which form a series of V shaped ridges across the surface. The denticles reduce the drag that otherwise occurs from the passage of any object under water, by creating a series of tiny deflection points that force the water to pass more readily over the suit surface. These suits are often worn as a full body device, with the arms and feet uncovered.

Freestyle swimming is the fastest form of competitive swimming, as the combined function of the arms moving in an over hand and a constant kick keep the body on a relatively even and efficient plane as it moves through the water. By rule, the swimmer may only remain under water for 15 m (50 ft) at the start and at each turn; otherwise the swimmer must be on top of the surface.

The breaststroke is a swimming stroke performed with the swimmer facing downward on the water. The swimmer's shoulders must remain in line with the water at all times. With their head above the surface, the swimmer extends their arms directly ahead, with the palms facing outwards, making a sweeping stroke with both arms remaining underwater at all times. On the repeat of the stroke, the arms are permitted, by FINA rule, to break the surface of the water. The swimmer performs a "frog kick," where the legs are brought towards the torso, and then extended outwards underwater. The swimmer's arms and legs must move in unison; flutter kicks, dolphin kicks, and scissor kicks are prohibited, as are flip ("tumble") turns.

The butterfly evolved as a swim form from the breaststroke, when swimmers brought their hands and arms out of the water to drive themselves forward. The butterfly, as the name suggests, is executed by a sweeping motion of the arms above the water, accompanied by a dolphin kick. The swimmer is face down on the water, coordinating breath with

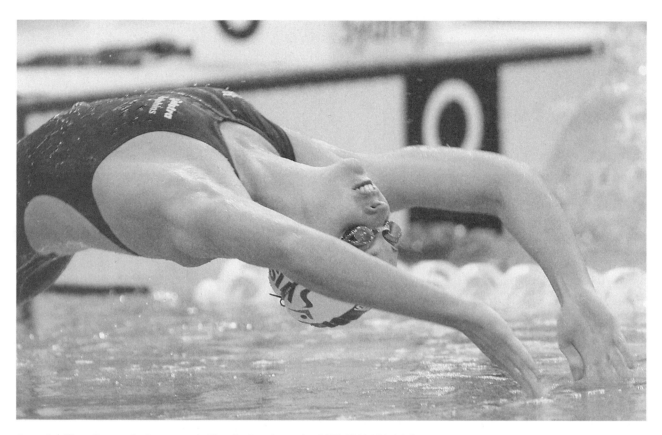

Australian Giaan Rooney in the women's 50-m backstroke at the 2005 FINA World Cup. **PHOTO BY MATT KING/GETTY IMAGES.**

the arm strokes. The butterfly is a very physically taxing event. The swimmer is permitted to be underwater for 15 m at each turn and at the start.

The backstroke is performed with the swimmer's head and stomach facing upward in the water. The stroke is an alternating windmill type motion with each arm, as the swimmer drives their body forward with a flutter kick.

Swimming is a sport that requires the athlete to develop total fitness–cardiovascular endurance, muscle strength, flexibility, and power. A schematic analysis of a typical swim race illustrates why each of these fitness elements is important. The race start requires an explosive entry into the water, employing a measure of body control and finesse to enter the water at an optimal angle for efficient movement. A powerful leg drive at the start will translate into significant benefits for the racer; if the start takes the swimmer either too deep into the water, or so shallow that additional water resistance is create by their body on entry, the benefits of a powerful start are lost.

As the swimmers move in their lanes, they seek a stable and efficient position. In shorter races (200 m and under), the demands placed upon the body's energy systems are primarily anaerobic; in the longer races, the body utilizes its aerobic systems, with anaerobic capability needed at the swimmer's drive to the finish.

On the approach to the opposite wall to make the turn, the swimmers will seek to maintain their speed by timing the execution of the turn. Each swim discipline has specific rules about the type of turn that may be employed (either open, where the swimmer changes direction at the wall, or a flip turn, where the swimmer executes a somersault and uses the wall to obtain a push in the opposite direction). Similarly, there are limits as to how long a swimmer may remain underwater after executing a flip turn; it is a general principle of swim mechanics that the body tends to move most efficiently under water as opposed to on the surface.

Swimming is a sport where the body's entire musculoskeletal system is engaged. For this reason, swim training is directed to the building and maintenance of all muscle groups. Swimming presents a lower risk of musculoskeletal injury than many sports; the chief causes of injury are related to

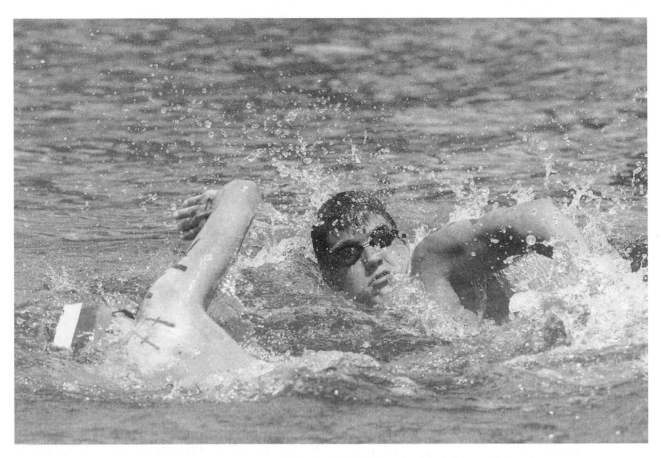

Competitors at the men's 25-m open water event at the 2005 FINA World Championships in Montreal, Canada. **PHOTO BY ALEXANDER HASSENSTEIN/BONGARTS/GETTY IMAGES.**

training, and the repetitive nature of the swim strokes which may lead to a variety of over use syndromes. Shoulder injuries, particularly those in relation to the function of the rotator cuff (the small four muscle and tendon structure positioned at the top of the shoulder, the tissues that control the amount of rotation possible in the joint), are relatively common.

The nature of swimming and the timing of the competitive swim schedule for any athlete make the development of a periodized training schedule a priority for a swimmer. As with a competitive runner, there will be readily identifiable events in the year that will be of greater importance to the athlete. It is these events that should be identified as ones for which the athlete will "peak," with training intensity adjusted accordingly. Dry land training particularly focused stretching programs to enhance optimal range of motion in the joints, weight training, and plyometric work to build explosive leg drive in both kicks and starts, will be components of this aspect of training.

The generally low incidence of injury, and the popularity of swimming generally has fostered a vibrant international master's competitive swimming community. Master's swimming is sanctioned by FINA, and master's competitive events, commencing at age 35 for both men and women, are staged throughout the world.

**SEE ALSO** Diving; Swimming strength training and exercises; Synchronized swimming; Triathlon.

## Swimming: Open water

Open water swimming is one of the five aquatic sports governed by Federation Internationale de Natation de Amateur (FINA). Swimming, water polo, synchronized swimming, and diving are the others within FINA's mandate. Open water swimming is defined by FINA as any competition that takes place in rivers, lakes, or oceans. Open water swimming is also an important part of both the Olympic triathlon (swim/cycle/run segments, with the swim 0.9 mile (1.5 km) in length) and the longer version, the Ironman, which has a 2.4 mile (4 km) open water swim.

FINA sanctions two forms of open water swimming. Long distance swimming is an open water event with a maximum distance of 10 km (6 miles); marathon swims are any races of a greater distance. The open water world championships are sanctioned for distances of 5 km, 10 km, and 25 km. The FINA rules regarding the race venue are uncomplicated, with the chief requirements being a race time water temperature of at least 16°C (60°F), and a minimum depth on the course of 1.4 m (4 ft 8 in). FINA championships may be conducted in either salt or fresh water.

Open water swimmers are prohibited from using any device which may aid in their buoyancy or propulsion, including wet suits. A wet suit, if constructed from materials such as polypropylene, will add as much as 5% to the buoyancy of a competitor. Grease or other similar products may be used in a FINA event; such materials are often employed by open water swimmers to provide an extra layer of insulation to the swimmer's body in cold water.

Aside from the competitive issues relating to open water swimming, the activity is often described as having the type of relationship to swimming in a pool that trail or cross country running has with respect to track. Open water swimming permits the swimmer to move without the boundaries imposed by a pool and the consequent interruption of the swimmer's stroke and rhythm.

Successful open water swimmers, both in those FINA styled disciplines and the triathlon swims, place significant training emphasis upon efficiency, and the corresponding ability to conserve energy and maintain an even pace. The most important variables to be considered in open water venues are the potential impacts of waves or currents.

SEE ALSO Ironman competitions; Swimming; Triathlon.

# Swimming pool chemistry

Swimming pools are used recreationally and for competitive events. Since a participant is often fully immersed in the water, the water's hygiene is important. Water that is contaminated can cause illness.

In contrast to many natural water courses, the circulation and turnover of water in swimming pools can be slow. While the water in most below-ground pools is drawn, pumped through a filter and even a heater, and circulated back to the pool at a legislated rate, the time to replace the entire volume of water can still be less than in a free-flowing stream, pond, or lake. Additionally, the number of people using the limited water volume can be much greater than in a natural setting. If steps are not taken to keep microorganisms and other contaminants under control, the water can become a dangerous medium for the growth of the microbes, and for the continued presence of noxious compounds.

One approach to maintaining swimming pool water quality involves filters, which can remove microbes and larger debris from the water. The latter are removed by a filter basket that acts as a strainer. This process is purely physical; water enters the open end of the filter, and debris that is too large to pass through the mesh basket remains trapped.

A second filter utilizes physical and chemical means to trap smaller material. The filter contains a bed of special-grade sand or diatomaceous earth. Incoming pool water enters at the top of the sand. Typically, the water is then allowed to percolate down through the sand under the influence of gravity. During the slow downward journey, microorganisms and other particles stick to the sand or earth grains. The size, surface charge, and surface chemistry of water contaminants determines how avidly they associate with the sand or earth particles.

Over time, as debris collects, the ability of the filter bed to bind particles decreases. Then, by forcing water back through the bed in the reverse direction in a process called backwashing, the collected debris can be driven out. Once the sand or earth grains have settled, the filtering action of the bed is restored.

Today, the filter bed is sometimes replaced by a synthetic filtering material packaged in a cartridge that can be inserted and removed from the water flow.

Chemicals are also added to swimming pools to aid in keeping the microorganisms at permissible levels, and to maintain a balance of inorganic parameters.

Disease-causing (pathogenic) bacteria are controlled by the use of disinfectants. The most popular swimming pool disinfectant is chlorine, which is typically introduced in the form of a solid (calcium hypochlorite) or a liquid (sodium hypochlorite). (Instead of chlorine, a chemical called bromide can be used. Since it tends to be more expensive than chlorine, bromide is not the typical disinfection method of choice.) Less routinely, chlorine gas can be added to the source water. Predetermined amounts of the materials are added, based on the volume of water in the pool, to produce a final free chlorine concentration in the water when the solid dissolves and the liquid or gas disperses. The final chlorine concentration is important. If too little chlorine is added, for example, the chemical reaction that occurs can generate various forms of a compound called chloramine. Chloramines have an objectionable smell and can irritate the skin and mucous membranes such as the eyes.

Addition of the proper amount of chlorine will produce mainly hypochlorous acid in the ensuing chemical reaction. Hypochlorous acid kills bacteria by disrupting the structure of their cell walls and destroying the activity of enzymes inside the cells that are vital for life.

Hypochlorous acid is unstable and tends to lose its potency in sunlight. Thus, many outdoor pool operators will also add cyanuric acid to the water. Cyanuric acid associates with hyochlorous acid and stabilizes its structure, while not affecting its antimicrobial potency.

Another aspect of swimming pool chemistry concerns the pH level of the water—the acidity or alkalinity of the water. The level is measured on a logarithmic scale (each division on the scale is ten times different from the preceding or subsequent value) that indicates the balance between acid and alkaline molecules in the water. The pH scale ranges from 0 (extreme acidity) to 14 (extreme alkalinity). Swimming pool water should have a pH of 7.2 to 7.8; within this range, the antimicrobial action of chlorine is most efficient and the water is most comfortable to the user. Water that is too acidic can damage metal surfaces and is too harsh to skin, whereas water that is too alkaline causes build-up of deposits on surfaces and becomes objectionably cloudy.

The pH of swimming pool water can be easily measured using a number of portable devices. If necessary, adjustments to pH can be made by the addition of sodium carbonate or sodium bicarbonate, which raises the pH, or muriatic acid, which lowers the pH.

A swimming pool is an ever-changing environment. Thus, swimming pool chemistry needs to be frequently monitored and, if necessary, altered throughout the day.

## Swimming resistance

In general terms, swim resistance is the effect of water upon the motion of a swimmer. Swim resistance is a concept closely related to drag, the hydrodynamic principle of resistance created by a fluid to forward motion. The resistance met by a swimmer in their forward progress caused by the water is passive drag; the resistance against which the swimmer is exerting a force is active drag.

There are three types of resistance that affect swimming function, namely frontal resistance, skin friction, and eddy resistance.

Frontal resistance occurs when the swimmer adopts a body position that exposes a greater than necessary body surface to the water, thus increasing the effect of the water's resistance force. To limit the effect of frontal resistance, swimmers may seek to position themselves as high on the water surface as possible, to produce an effect similar to that of a hydrofoil. This technique is sometimes useful for swimmers with a smaller body mass. Alternatively, the swimmers will roll their body from side to side as the swim strokes are executed; the turning movement keep the body higher in the water.

Swimming research has established that for a freestyle swimmer, a body position of between 30% and 40% angle in the water allows the swimmer to generate optimum speed.

Swimmers keep their head as close to the surface of the water while breathing to counter act the natural tendency of the lower part of the body to sink, producing greater swim resistance, when the swimmer raises their head to breath.

Skin friction is the type of drag created when the swimmer's body and swim suit pass through water. The most time honored technique to counter skin friction is the shaving of the swimmer's body hair on any places that have contact with the water. The shaving of body hair may have a slight impact on the hydrodynamic characteristics of the swimmer's body. A similar physical result is achieved through the design of the racing suits that mimic the characteristics of shark skin. The suit surface is constructed with a series of ridges that tend to reduce the drag created when a suit passes through water, as the ridges act to deflect water away from the surface of the suit.

The full body racing suit is also designed to preserve the symmetry and sleekness of the body as it moves through the water, by limiting the amount of movement in the swimmers muscles that is not required for propulsion. The suits maintain a constant body silhouette without affecting muscle function.

Eddy resistance is caused when a swimmer creates eddies and water turbulence through poor stroke technique. Whenever a swimmer executes a front crawl stroke, an eddy, shaped as a vortex or whirlpool, forms at the water surface. If the stroke is executed inefficiently, the vortex will remain. If the vortexes accumulate around the body of the swimmer, the water resistance is increased.

**SEE ALSO** Resistance exercise training; Swimming; Swimming strength training and exercises.

# Swimming starts and turns

The starts and the turn techniques employed in a swim race are the subject of intense practice by all competitive swimmers. Starts and turns are movements that are distinct from both the strokes used by a swimmer and from one another.

The start has three components, each of which can be broken down for discrete analysis—the starting block, the dive, and the pullout (breakout). All swim events, except the backstroke, begin on the elevated starting block situated at the edge of the pool. The backstroke commences with all swimmers in the water, facing the edge of the pool, grasping handles that permit a push off into the lane. To achieve maximum speed from the start block, the swimmers seek to keep their center of gravity as close to the edge of the block as possible. At the sound of the start, the swimmers employ a combination of explosive leg drive and a push with the toes from the surface of the block.

The dive is intended to be one that creates as little water resistance on entry as possible. The swimmer, depending upon the stroke to be employed during the race, will endeavor to take an angle of entry that balances speed through the water and an ability to seamlessly begin the stroke cadence. The transition between the dive and the stroke itself is the pullout, where the swimmer moves dynamically to the racing position in the water.

There are two general classifications of turns: the open turn and the flip turn, or tumble turn. The use of a particular type of turn, and the accompanying period of time in which the swimmer may remain underwater (in a desirable hydrodynamic position) after the completion of the turn, are specified in the rules of the sport as determined by FINA.

The flip turn is an important component of freestyle swimming. The turn is intended to permit a coordinated change of direction that allows the swimmers to maintain both their speed and the cadence of their stroke. A flip turn begins with a somersault, with the swimmers bringing their arms forward to create a long, slender upper body profile. As the upper body is being extended, the swimmers use the wall of the pool to push as powerfully as possible. In this position, the swimmers will often remain under the surface, propelling themselves with an efficient dolphin kick (legs together, moving in the manner of a dolphin). The distance in which the swimmers are permitted to remain underwater after a flip turn is also regulated in each swimming discipline.

The open turn is also used to preserve speed and form. In an open turn, the swimmers seek to coordinate their approach to the wall and the stroke rhythm; the swimmers use one hand to effect a push off from the wall, while bringing their feet and legs into a tuck position. The swimmers push off from the wall, with the entire body under the surface, extending from the tuck into a streamlined body position, from which they resume their stroke.

**SEE ALSO** Motor Control; Plyometrics; Swimming; Swimming timing.

# Swimming strength training and exercises

Effective strength training for the competitive swimmer requires an approach that may be summarized by the expression, "the three Cs"—careful, considered, and comprehensive.

Swim strength training must be carefully planned. The regular training required of a swimmer is demanding on its own, with many hours per week spent in the pool in a variety of endurance and sprint drills. The physical requirements of swimming are such that strength training is essential to both the improvement and the maintenance of strong swimming form. The balance between regular swim training and additional strength training can only be achieved through attention to the swimmers competitive schedule and intervals of scheduled "down time."

The swimming strength program must take into consideration the precise nature of the event to be supported and enhanced. All swimming involves the use of every part of the musculoskeletal structure, from the start of a race until the finish. Swimmers must place particular emphasis upon their shoulders, core strength (abdominal, gluteal, groin, and lower back muscles), and legs. As an example, for a free-style swimmer, the strength exercises to advance the full range of shoulder motion necessary to perform the stroke may include the pull down motions of a cable machine or an overhand medicine ball throw. Core strength muscles can be isolated using a Swiss ball or similar device to create resistance during push ups or other stretching motions that require the movement of the entire body, as does the swim motion.

The leg power utilized by a swimmer from the starting block is developed by various forms of plyometric training, techniques which aid in the development of the fast twitch muscle fibers in the legs, with a goal of more explosive movement.

Comprehensive strength exercise programs include not only specific strength exercises, but also stretching exercises that permit the swimmer to both utilize all available muscle strength developed in the gym. Stretching exercises are essential to the maintenance of the athlete's range of motion in all joints. If the athlete is hindered in the ability to take a particular structure through its natural range of motion, it is doubtful that the athlete can achieve the best athletic success. Swimming, as a sport of significant repetition of movement, requires the combined excellent joint strength and range of motion to prevent injury.

**SEE ALSO** Resistance exercise training; Swimming; Strength training; Triathlon: Exercises for triathlon.

# Swimming timing

The precise recording of swimmer's times in competition was a difficult task in the pre-electronic era. As swimmers raced to the finish in an event where there might be four or five competitors within inches (centimeters) of one another, the splash created by each racer as they drove for the end of the pool made the visual determination of whose hand touched first to be a very difficult and occasionally inaccurate exercise.

In 1967, the Omega company of Switzerland developed the first electronic timing system for swimming that attempted to coordinate the physical position of the individual swimmers in the pool with the recorded time. This new system placed contact pads (known as touch pads) in each lane of the pool, calibrated in such a fashion that the incidental water movement of the competitors or wave action did not trigger the pad sensors; the pad was only activated by the touch of the swimmer at the end of the race.

The touch pad technology was refined after 1967. The pads themselves are now constructed from a series of very thin vertical sheets, which extend underwater the width of a competitor's lane, so as to permit a recorded touch no matter where in the lane the swimmer may finish the race.

The starting block is also integrated into the overall timing system. The starting block is equipped with a speaker system to permit the starters horn to be directly communicated to each competitor as they await the start. When the swimmer leaves the starting block, the motion of the athlete signals the individual start by its registration on a sensor device in the block. The timer and the judge of the race can instantly determine, through the coordination of the starter's signal and the athlete movements as recorded on the block, whether there was a false start, and in which lane.

In the same fashion, the timing system is coordinated with the video recording of each race, to permit judges by replay to determine the order of result in the event of any dispute.

Swimming results in international competition are now resolved to an accuracy of one thousandth of a second. In the 1988 summer Olympics at Seoul, six competitors in the men's 100-m breaststroke finished within 0.5 seconds of one another. Since 2000, the results of most major international swim meets have been available in real time by the Internet.

**SEE ALSO** International federations; Sport performance; Swimming.

# Swiss ball training techniques

The Swiss ball, also known as an exercise ball or a gym ball, is a training aid aimed primarily at the stretching and strengthening of the abdominal, groin, lumbar (lower) back, and upper leg muscles of the body. The development of these structures is often referred to as the building and maintaining of core strength, an important stabilizing feature in any sport.

Swiss balls are inflatable, and they are typically filled approximately 80-90%. The ball is constructed from a thick rubberized compound, available in differing sizes. For optimum effect, a Swiss ball should stand approximately 2 in (5 cm) above the user's knee from the surface.

The Swiss ball permits a range of exercises that are based on the ability of the user to move with the motion of the ball while performing the exercise, using the ball to both support the body during the movement as well as to provide a measure of resistance to the muscles employed in the movement. The classic Swiss ball exercises involve the abdominal muscles, with corresponding responses from the groin and the stabilizers of the lower back, the oblique muscles that run parallel to the spine above the pelvis. The athlete, positioned on top of the Swiss ball, can take the abdominals through a complete range of motion through the performance of crunches (a motion that brings of the upper thighs and the sternum [breastbone] toward one another, to strengthen the abdominals); twisting crunches, where the upper body twists in opposite directions during the crunch to extend the muscular effect across the abdomen; and the flexion of the thoracic spine, the vertebrae of the mid-back to improve overall flexibility.

Swiss ball movements require a greater degree of coordination by the user than do conventional floor stretches. The Swiss ball also permits the execution of both static stretches (where the target body part is fully extended), as well as more demanding dynamic stretches, where the user directs force into or through the extended joint.

While a Swiss ball routine may have both aerobic and anaerobic benefits, depending on the intensity, duration, and the frequency with which the exercises are performed, Swiss ball training is not a substitute for either type of exercise. The Swiss ball is an ideal supplement to an existing training program, such as yoga or Pilates, which promote greater strength and flexibility in a safe and controlled physical setting.

SEE ALSO Calisthenics; Stretching and flexibility; Yoga and Pilates.

# Synchronized swimming

Synchronized swimming is a water sport that combines elements of swimming, ballet, and gymnastics that are performed by individual athletes as well as by teams of athletes that perform as a coordinated unit. The swimmers complete a program of movements choreographed to music that are executed both on the surface and underwater. Like sports such as figure skating and rhythmic gymnastics, the aesthetics and the grace of synchronized swimming disguises the significant physical demands of competition.

Synchronized swimming was publicly demonstrated for the first time in 1907; the first organized synchronized swimming competition took place in Montreal in 1923. A series of Hollywood films produced in the late 1930s and early 1940s that featured former United States Olympic swimmer Ester Williams in a variety of choreographed swimming displays publicized the sport in North America. After a protracted campaign to secure Olympic status for the sport, women's synchronized swimming became a part of Olympic competition at the 1984 Summer Games. Men's synchronized swimming is a regional competition only.

Synchronized swimming is one of the five aquatics disciplines governed on a world basis by Federation Internationale de Natation de Amateur (FINA). FINA convenes annual world synchronized swimming championships, and it sanctions a variety of events on a regional basis. Synchronized swimming is organized on a club basis in most countries, as opposed to organization in school or university programs. Competitions are staged in Olympic standard swimming pools, with underwater cameras to permit viewing of the movements of the swimmers from all angles.

The competitive categories of synchronized swimming are solo, duet, team, and free combination. Synchronized swimming requires the athletes to complete a series of routines, some of which are predetermined, and others of which are performed in the manner determined by the athlete or the team. A typical competition will include a series of performance segments that represent a progression from "figures"—a series of "required elements," concluding with a free routine, where the routines contain FINA approved figures choreographed to music as selected by the team or the athlete. The team competitions (with up to 10 swimmers permitted on the team) may commence with the first portion of the routine on the pool deck, with a progression of movements to take the team into the water for the next segments of the team's presentation.

The judging of synchronized swimming is subjective. Judges are provided with various guidelines established by FINA as to the respective difficulty of certain figures and required elements. Judges use two general categories within which performances are assessed—technical merit (including degree of difficulty, degree of synchronicity, and execution of the movements) and artistic expression (choreography and manner of interpretation by the athletes).

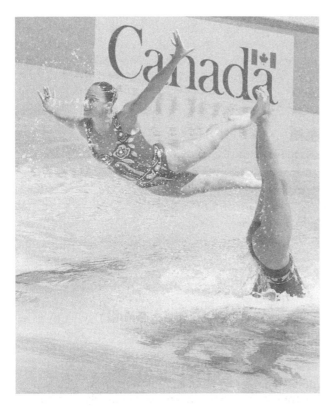

Team synchronized swimming was first added to the Olympic Games in 1996. AP PHOTO/GERRY BROOME

Technical marks represent 60% of the score awarded, with artistic marks accounting for the remaining 40%.

Competitive synchronized swimming routines vary in length. The shortest routines, the figures portion of the competition, are 2 minutes long; the team free routine may be as long as 5 minutes. It is the nature of the sport that the swimmers may be underwater performing various choreographed movements for as long as 1 minute at a time, with some routines creating a cumulative underwater period of up to 3.5 minutes for each athlete. The sport imposes significant demands upon the athlete's cardiovascular and energy systems, both aerobic and anaerobic. In addition to the often attention attracting swim suits worn by the competitors, the most important item of equipment worn by the synchronized swimmers are their nose plugs, to prevent water from entering their nose and lungs as they spin underwater.

Balance and motor control skills are of prime importance to the synchronized swimmer. The swimmers are constantly changing their body posi-

tions in time with the music and the movements of their teammates. The athletes swim with their eyes open to both assist in maintaining their balance, and to maintain their orientation to both the walls of the pool and to their teammates. Muscle memory, also known as proprioception, is a physical skill developed by the synchronized swimmer through repetition of each element to a routine. When a particular routine has been practices hundreds of times, the athlete acquires an internal sense of where all parts of the body should be in relation to one another without significant conscious thought about each movement.

The demands associated with the execution of gymnastics movements in a water environment poses unique training challenges for the synchronized swimmer. To build for a competitive season, the athletes must develop a broad range of cardiovascular and musculoskeletal strength. Running, cycling, and free swimming are the aerobic sports that satisfy this aspect of the training demands of synchronized swimming. Many athletes engage in Pilates or Swiss ball training that focuses upon the development of the strength and the flexibility of the core area of the body, as the abdominal, lumbar (low back), groin, and gluteal muscles are subject to constant stresses in a synchronized swimming routine. The ability of the athlete to maintain perfect balance and physical symmetry while executing underwater somersaults and flips requires significant core strength.

Off season weight training, using free weights, machine circuit training, and plyometric routines to enhance leg strength prepare the athlete to move decisively and explosively in the water. Many synchronized swim routines require dynamic movement, where the athletes must power themselves from a significant distance below the water surface to perform a movement at the surface, and descend as quickly to the next element. Stretching and flexibility training is a year round essential to all synchronized swimming training programs; the sport demands optimal range of motion in the body's joints, as every musculoskeletal structure will be utilized in a synchronized swimming routine.

SEE ALSO Balance training and proprioception; Stretching and Flexibility; Swimming; Swimming strength training and exercises.

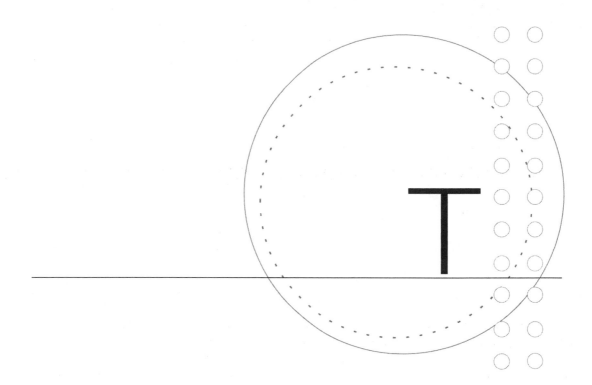

# Table tennis

Table tennis, sometimes known as "ping pong" is a miniaturized version of outdoor or lawn tennis. A dynamic indoor racquets sport played world wide, table tennis had an inauspicious beginning; the sport had its origins in England in the late 1800s as a parlor game known as "Whiff Waff," an activity played on dining room tables for recreation. The first table tennis balls were fashioned from champagne corks. In the late 1920s, the popularity of table tennis led to the formation of the International Table Tennis Federation (ITTF). Various national associations were also founded, such as the United States Table Tennis Association (now USA Table Tennis), established in 1933.

Table tennis is played today in virtually every country of the world, with sanctioned competitions in age group categories ranging from under 10 years of age to 80 yeas and over. Table tennis is an official Paralympics wheelchair sport. As with tennis, there are men', women', doubles, and mixed doubles categories of play.

The rules of table tennis have been standardized for many years. The playing surface is a 9 ft by 5 ft rectangular table (2.7 m by 1.5 m), usually dark blue or green in color. The surface of the table is positioned 30 in (76 cm) above the floor; the playing surface is divided by a 6 in (15 cm) high net. Each half of the court is marked with a white line to create the two equal surfaces used in doubles play. The table must be constructed of a material that pos-sesses a high coefficient of restitution, to ensure that the ball is sufficiently lively when it is struck off the table surface.

The ball used in table tennis is very light weight and hollow, manufactured from celluloid material. The ball measures 1.6 in (4 cm) in diameter, with an approximate weight of 0.1 oz (2.7 g). The table tennis racquet is most commonly called a paddle. The paddle is oval shaped, covered on both sides by a thin layer of rubber, sponge, or other similar synthetic material. There are no restrictions placed upon the size or weight of the paddle by the ITTF; the type of paddle surface will dictate the nature of the spin that can be generated by the player on the ball.

The rules of table tennis are relatively straight-forward. Play commences with a serve—the ball must strike on the serving players side of the court first, and then make contact with the any part of the surface of the opponent's court. The serve must be made from behind the edge of the serving player's side of the table. The ball must be fully exposed to the sight of the opponent during the serve, with a toss that travels a minimum of 6 in (15 cm) in the air. The server is not permitted to impart any spin on the ball as it is tossed into the air to commence service. The opposing player must return the ball using the paddle only, where the ball makes contact with any portion of the opponent' side of the playing surface, including the corners and sides of the table. A point is scored if the serve fails, or where one player fails to return the ball onto the opponent's court, or if the ball is struck into the net.

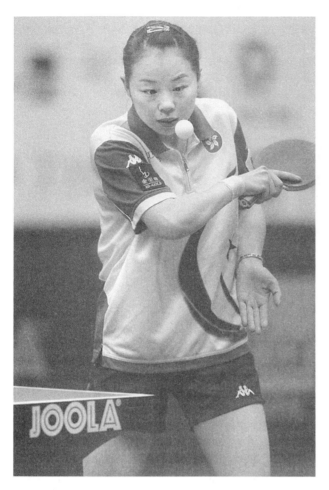

Tie Yana of Hong Kong competes against Fukuhara Ai of Japan, during the women's the 2005 Women's Table Tennis World Cup. PHOTO BY CHINA PHOTOS/GETTY IMAGES

Table tennis games are scored to 11 points, with the players alternating serves every two points scored. A typical table tennis match will be either a best of five games or a best of seven games series.

The athleticism of the modern elite table tennis player is light years removed from the old English parlor game. Players routinely deliver the ball at speeds approaching 100 mph (160 km/h), often with significant spin. The shape of the paddle permits a great deal of player creativity with respect to both imparting spin as well as the placement of the ball. The players will at times be in very close quarters, separated only by the 9 ft (3 m) length of table; in other circumstances, such as responding to a lob shot or a smash delivered at high speeds, the players might be 20 ft (6m) or more behind the table surface. Rallies in table tennis for this reason are often very high paced and dynamic segments of the game. Attacking shots are generally struck with a top spin

motion to produce speed, and defensive shots carry backspin to counter the offensive shot.

Table tennis is a sport that does not require significant athletic size or strength; many world champion caliber players achieve success through the development of their quickness, hand eye coordination, balance, and a sophisticated tactical appreciation of the game. The physical training needed to support a competitive table tennis player will include significant focus on footwork, especially through workouts that have elements of lateral movement and plyometric training. A degree of strength training, to create over all body balance, is also helpful in table tennis training. The athlete must build their aerobic fitness levels to enable the athlete to shorten recovery times in a long match or series of matches. Table tennis players also must devote significant time to stretching and flexibility exercises, both to achieve the ability to move and react explosively, as well as to prevent injury; table tennis players spend a great deal of time running and moving on les absorbent hard surfaces that place greater stress on the player's lower legs, ankles and feet. Table tennis players are vulnerable to over use injuries to these structures, such as plantar fasciitis and muscle strains.

SEE ALSO Motor control; Racquetball; Squash; Tennis.

# Tackling, soccer SEE Soccer tackling mechanics

# Taekwondo

Taekwondo is a form of empty hand martial arts combat that requires the athlete to use all parts of the body in competition. Taekwondo is a self defense discipline; the name is derived from the Korean words "tae", meaning kick, "kwon", a punch or other blow with the hand or fist, and "do", which is a way or method of operation. Among the general public, taekwondo is distinguished from other martial arts by its high speed, sweeping kicks and emphatic punches. As with judo, taekwondo was developed as a sport that is also representative of a moral code, where principles of loyalty, faithfulness, respect and the preservation of an indomitable spirit form a significant part of taekwondo training.

Taekwondo is a sport that originated from the ancient Korean forms of martial arts. It was significantly influenced in its development by elements of the Japanese martial art of karate, which were

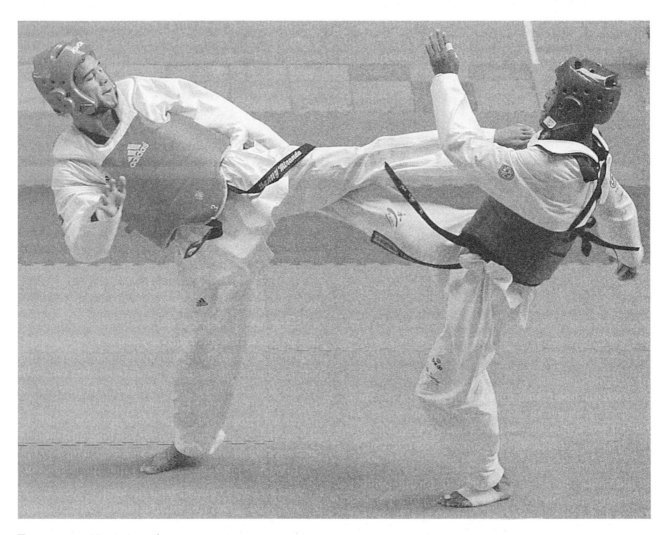

Two men practicing taekwondo. LUIS ACOSTA/AFP/GETTY IMAGES

reflected in taekwondo after the occupation of Korea by Japan in 1910. The sport was exported to the United States after the Second World War through its exposure to American military personnel who had observed taekwondo in Korea. Taekwondo became popular as a global sport. The World Taekwondo Federation, the sports international governing body, has a membership of over 150 national bodies. There are an estimated 35 million taekwondo participants world wide. Taekwondo was made an official Olympic sport in 2000, with four weight class categories of both men and women. World championship taekwondo competitions have eight separate weight categories.

Taekwondo proficiency is recognized through the award of different classifications of belt, with each belt color signifying a level of taekwondo ability. As with the sports of judo and karate, the black belt classifications are the highest levels that may be

attained in taekwondo. There are four aspects to competitive taekwondo—sparring, style, self defense, and a break test, where objects are shattered through a blow delivered with the hand or foot.

The basic competitive uniform worn in taekwondo is the *dobok*, a loose fitting white colored jacket and trousers. Athletes wear protectors to shield the torso, groin, shins, forearms, as well as a helmet for head protection. Footwear is not permitted in taekwondo.

A taekwondo match (or bout) commences with two competitors facing one another across the mat surface. The match is scored by officials, who assess points for both particular types of blows delivered as well as the style of execution by a competitor. Points are awarded for kicks delivered to the front or side of the head, and for punches to the head or the body of the opponent. Throwing or attempting to hold an opponent will attract the imposition of a penalty, as will any attack with the open hands to the head of the opponent.

Each bout in taekwondo is three rounds in length (three minutes each for men, two minutes in length for women); a winner is determined through either the accumulation of points or by scoring a knockout (defined by the inability of the athlete to resume their fighting stance within 8 seconds of being knocked down).

The dynamic punches and kicks delivered in taekwondo represent the application of different physical principles, the most important of which is the generation of force, which is a product of the mass of the object used to deliver the blow, and the acceleration of the object towards the target. Punches delivered both at a human opponent as well as in the breaking of a board must be precisely executed; the arm and hand will produce maximum effect if the hand is still accelerating at the time of the impact.

The successful breaking of a board or a brick in taekwondo is directly correlated to the speed and the precision of the strike. Depending upon the size of the hand of the taekwondo practitioner and the material being struck, the hand must strike the object at a speed of approximately 20 ft per second (6 m per second) to produce the force necessary to shatter a 1 in (2.5 cm) board. Experts who are able to break five boards simultaneously strike the targets with hand speeds of over 40 ft per second (12 m per second).

Unlike boxing, where the fighter endeavors to punch through the target to cause maximum damage to an opponent, the taekwondo expert seeks to deliver a blow with maximum speed and no appreciable follow through. This technique means that the force of the strike to the object is directed without interference to the surface. Studies conducted with respect to why a taekwondo expert is able to readily break one or more boards or bricks have centered on the concept of oscillation —if the blow is delivered as if the hand is directed through the board, like a boxer, to a point on the opposite side of the board, the target material will oscillate, which tends to negate the impact of the force intended to break the target. With a precise taekwondo strike, the hand or foot does not follow through, eliminating oscillation in the target and permitting the force of the strike to pass unimpeded through the target, creating the fractured target.

SEE ALSO Boxing; Judo; Karate; Sumo.

# Taping techniques SEE Wrapping and taping techniques

# Anatoly Tarasov
12/10/1918–6/23/1995
RUSSIAN
ICE HOCKEY COACH

Anatoly Tarasov is widely regarded as the father of modern Russian ice hockey (Russian ice hockey also describes the sport as played in the Soviet Union, or USSR, until 1989). Tarasov began coaching in the Russian club leagues in the late 1940s, at the conclusion of his successful playing career. As a young man Tarasov had also been a well regarded soccer player as well as a proficient bandy player, a game with some similarities to field hockey. Tarasov first attracted the attention of the leadership of the national Soviet ice hockey program through his success as the coach of the Moscow club team CSKA in the early 1950s. Tarasov became the national team coach in 1958, a position he held until 1972; he continued to coach CSKA until his retirement in 1974.

In the early 1950s, Canada was recognized as the dominant world ice hockey power. Canadian teams comprised of second- and third-tier ice hockey talent had regularly won both world championships and Olympic gold medals both before and after the Second World War (1938–1945). During this period, the team sent to represent Canada at a world championship was the men's senior amateur championship team from the previous season. National Hockey League professionals were prohibited from participating in these events due to the strict rules in that era concerning the division between amateur and professional international sports.

The first inkling that USSR teams had moved to a position where Canadian hockey dominance could be successfully challenged was at the World Championships in 1954, when the Soviet national team won a decisive victory over the Canadian representatives. By the time Tarasov assumed control of national team in 1958, the foundation had been established for a powerful international Soviet hockey presence. The political leadership of the Soviet Union had determined that ice hockey success would be a primary objective of the national sport program.

Tarasov was one of the first hockey coaches to appreciate the importance of the comprehensive physical condition of his players to achieve team success. In the 1950s, the standard fitness program for North American ice hockey players was to "skate their way into shape" at a preseason training camp in September, in advance of the October start to the professional season; little or no attention was paid by athletes or coaches to the concept of year-round fitness. Tarasov believed that dry-land training, the general expression for all physical training conducted away from the playing surface, was the most important part of his program. Tarasov incorporated various forms of aerobic and anaerobic exercises into the team practices through out the entire year. The players were provided specialized weight training programs, customized for the individual, and there was formal practice time devoted to sports such as soccer and handball, because Tarasov believed that the cross-training benefits of these sports were ideally suited to the development of hockey excellence.

Tarasov also furthered the interest of his own club, CSKA, throughout this period. CSKA had strong ties to the Soviet Red Army. Through Tarasov's active recruitment of hockey players who would first be drafted into the army, high-quality hockey talent was directed by the Red Army to the CSKA. Tarasov won a further 16 national championships with CSKA during his coaching career.

Between 1958 and 1972, the methods of Tarasov paid remarkable dividends to Soviet hockey. The national team won Olympic ice hockey gold medals in 1964 and 1968, in addition to the nine world championships captured during that period; Tarasov was deposed as national team coach when the Soviets failed to win gold at the 1972 Olympics. The hallmark of Tarasov-coached teams were the speed and the skating ability of the players, combined with a precision passing style that valued the creation of quality scoring opportunities, as opposed to simply taking as many shots as possible at the opposing goal. Tarasov's methods are proof that the sincerest form of flattery is by imitation; his revolutionary approaches to hockey training in the 1950s are now standard procedure today throughout the entire ice hockey world.

The coaching influence of Tarasov became evident in a different direction when his coaching career ended in 1974. His daughter, Tatiana Tarasova, is regarded as one of the most successful Russian figure skating coaches in the history of that sport. Tarasova has coached skaters who have won a total of eight Olympic gold medals in various figure skating disciplines.

Trasov's coaching brilliance has been recognized throughout the world of ice hockey. He was inducted into both the International Ice Hockey Hall of Fame

(1977) and the Canadian Hockey Hall of Fame (1974). Tarasov was also named a Master of Sport, the Soviet Union's highest athletic honor.

**SEE ALSO** Cross training; Ice Hockey; Ice hockey strength and training exercises.

# Target heart rate SEE Heart rate: Target heart rate

# Charles H. Taylor

6/24/1901–6/23/1969
AMERICAN
BASKETBALL PLAYER

Chuck Taylor became one of the most famous names in the history of basketball, not through his play, but through his contributions to the development of the Converse All Star basketball shoes for over 40 years.

Chuck Taylor achieved fame as the name associated with Converse basketball shoes without ever playing college basketball. Taylor had been a capable high school player in Indiana, and foregoing university, Taylor embarked upon an undistinguished professional playing career with a succession of teams in the Midwestern United States in 1919 that ended in 1930.

In 1917, Marquis Converse, a shoe manufacturer located in Chicago, Illinois, developed the first in a line of rubber-soled basketball shoes. Prior to the entry of Converse into this market, there were few shoes specifically available for any particular sport. The shoes worn for indoor or gymnasium pursuits tended to be constructed from lightweight products that did not stand up to excessive strain, such as thin leather. The Converse shoes were unusual for the time in that they had a relatively thick sole. In 1921, Taylor attended at the Converse offices to discuss their basketball shoe; Taylor had worn the shoes in his games and he had suggestions as to how the product might be improved.

As a result of this meeting, Converse hired Taylor to run a series of basketball clinics to promote the shoe; ironically, Taylor playing for a team called the Akron Firestone Non-Skids at the time he was hired by Converse. The first of the Taylor clinics on behalf of Converse was held at North Carolina State University in 1922; Taylor would subsequently organize Converse clinics for over 30 years. Unlike notable sports products spokesmen of the modern age, such as basketball legend Michael Jordan, Taylor was at best a journeyman-level player in his time.

Basketball grew significantly in popularity throughout the United States into the 1930s. The demand for basketball shoes increased dramatically during this period. In 1932, Converse added the signature of Chuck Taylor to its existing Converse All Star five-star logo. The precise reason for adding the name of Chuck Taylor to the Converse label is now unclear, given his lack of acclaim as a player. For the next 40 years, 'Chucks.' as the shoes were known, were the best selling basketball shoe in the world. In 1936, Converse All Stars became the official basketball shoes for the Olympic Games, a distinction Converse would hold until 1968.

Taylor became involved in all promotional aspects of the Converse operation. He spearheaded the Converse All Star yearbook, an annual publication highlighting the year in basketball in the United States. Taylor edited the Converse yearbook from 1932 until 1968. Beginning in 1932, Taylor was a selector of the annual collegiate All-American teams. On the first team that he selected, Taylor chose John Wooden, the UCLA coaching legend and member of the Basketball Hall of Fame. Taylor was himself enshrined in the Hall of Fame as a contributor to the development of basketball in 1969.

The style and the construction of Converse All Stars were not significantly varied until after 1970. By modern standards, the shoe is a decidedly low technology product; during the time of its greatest popularity, Converse All Stars were considered well suited to the game of basketball. The original versions were available in one of two styles, high top or low top, and in one of two colours, black or white. Players would note the distinctive rubber smell that attached to the Converse All Stars long after they had been purchased and significantly used.

The most significant feature of the shoe was its double reinforced rubber sole that was designed to provide traction in the various kinds of quick multi-directional movement required in basketball. Converse All Stars were shoes with a deserved reputation for having the uppers wearing out before the soles. The high top models were especially valued for providing ankle support without restricting the movement of the joint. The canvas uppers were relatively light weight.

Taylor was the face of all Converse basketball shoe marketing until the time of his death in 1969. Converse built upon the success fostered by Taylor's clinics and promotional work to introduce other sport specific shoes, in the sports of football, track, and wrestling.

Converse All Stars were supplanted as the best selling basketball shoe by the combined effects of improved basketball shoe technology and the growth of Nike, and the influence of its advertising campaign built around Michael Jordan. Today marketed as a retro-styled shoe, the Chuck Taylor Converse All Stars are sold worldwide, bearing the signature of Chuck Taylor.

SEE ALSO Basketball; Basketball shoes; Running shoes.

# Temperature regulation SEE Thermoregulatory system

# Tendinitis and ruptured tendons

Tendinitis (also spelled tendonitis) is one of the most common and debilitating of musculoskeletal injuries, in both the athletic world and among the general population. Given the structure of the human body—where tendons are engaged in the execution of virtually every type of muscular action—tendons are subjected to ongoing physical stress rendering them vulnerable to injury.

Tendons are the strong, fibrous, connective tissues that are the linkage between skeletal muscle and the bones that are powered by muscular contraction. Tendons are primarily constructed with collagen, which comprise 85% of the mass of the tendon. Collagen is a form of protein that provides the tendon with its elasticity in movement. Most tendons are constructed so that the structure glides over the adjacent bone, synchronized with the extensions and contractions of the powering muscle.

Tendinitis is an inflammation of the fibers that form the tendon, resulting in pain in varying degrees, and often some restriction of movement, usually most noticeable during and immediately after the activity. Tendinitis is a condition that may be caused through a number of mechanisms, including overuse of the of the tendon, commonly the result of a repetitive motion; an absence of "glide" between the tendon and the bone; and inflexibility in either the tendon or the connected muscle. In older athletes, collagen tends to lose some of its elasticity, causing the tendon to be more vulnerable to injury.

A ruptured tendon is a more serious and debilitating event than a strain. In a rupture, the tendon fibers will be either partially torn or completely severed, creating the rupture. The injury will be immediately apparent to the athlete as the rupture, either partial or full, will produce sharp and significant pain in the region of the injury, as well as immediate swelling. This injury will either significantly reduce or eliminate the function of the tendon. A ruptured tendon most commonly occurs through an explosive movement by an athlete, such as a jump, or a very sudden pivoting or accelerating movement.

The common musculoskeletal regions for tendon injuries are vulnerable to both the onset of tendonitis as well as ruptured tendon. The wrist is one such area, at the point where the tendons that connect the forearm muscles meet the bones of the wrist. These tendons that assist in the rotation, flexion, and extension movements of the wrist are particularly vulnerable to tendinitis, especially in sports that require the throwing of an object, or repetitive grappling and grasping movements.

The elbow is susceptible to tendon injury at both the medial (inside) and the lateral (outside) epicondilytis, the tissues that surround the elbow joint, providing a connection between the humerus (upper arm) and the radial and ulnar bones (forearm). In sports that involve considerable repetitive motion, such as tennis, golf, and baseball pitching, these structures are exposed to overuse and resulting tendinitis.

The rotator cuff is an assembly of four muscles connected by tendons to the bones of the shoulder joint, the humerus, and the scapula (shoulder blade). The rotator cuff tendon is vulnerable to both tendinitis through repetitive strain, as well as a rupture in a single act of excessive force. The rotator cuff, positioned at the top of the shoulder mechanism, is also particularly susceptible to damage due to imbalances between the muscles surrounding the shoulder, particularly the biceps and the muscles that power the movement of the scapula.

The patellar tendon and the quadriceps (thigh muscles) tendon are tissues that connect the patella (kneecap) above and below the knee. Repetitive jumping, as in basketball, volleyball, or the high jump, can result in a tendinitis known as jumper's knee. In more rare occasions, often when the tendon has been already weakened through tendinitis, either of these tendons may rupture in the course of a single movement.

Achilles tendon injury is of particular athletic concern. The longest and the strongest tendon in the body is the connection between the gastrocnemius and soleus muscles (calf muscles) of the lower leg, and the calcaneus (heel bone). The Achilles tendon is particularly vulnerable to injury because this structure is exposed to stresses with every upright movement of the body. All sports where the athlete walks, runs, or jumps can create circumstances where tendinitis may arise. The Achilles tendon is the most vulnerable tendon in the body for tearing or rupture, given its length and the frequency of movement. With the Achilles tendon, complete recovery from a rupture, in the sense of healing in the tendon fibers, will often result in a degree of permanent loss of some flexibility in the tissue.

A tendon rupture will usually involve surgical repair, and the requirement of a cast on the damaged area for a number of weeks following. Tendinitis is treated in a variety of ways, subject to the severity of the condition. All types of tendinitis benefit from the RICE (rest/ice/compression/elevation) treatment, which serves to reduce the swelling and the inflammation of the injury. In some circumstances, lightweight and inflatable air casts have been used to assist with protection and the rehabilitation of the injury. The return to activities must be gradual, with stretching and a focused effort to ensure balance between the adjacent musculoskeletal groups essential. The use of nonsteroidal anti-inflammatory drugs (NSAIDs) such as ibuprofen will often assist in managing pain. For a jumper's knee condition, an infra-patellar strap, an orthotic that is a flexible band-shaped device wrapped securely around the patellar tendon to support the jumping movement, is also used.

There are a number of preventative measures to be taken by athletes regarding the onset of tendinitis. Shoe selection is important. A proper fit, suited to the characteristics of the athlete, will reduce the structural problems that may lead to the development of Achilles tendinitis. For runners, scouting out the training surfaces is important. Running intervals on hard, angled, or hilly routes without proper buildup or stretching may magnify the risk of Achilles tendon injury.

**SEE ALSO** Achilles tendon rupture; Achilles tendonitis; Elbow injuries; Hamstring pull, tear, or strain; Lower leg injuries; Musculoskeletal injuries; RICE (rest/ice/compression/elevation) treatment for injuries.

## Tendonitis SEE Achilles tendonitis

## Tendons SEE Achilles tendon rupture; Bones, ligaments, tendons

# Tennis

Tennis is a sport played within a defined rectangular zone called the court. The court is divided into two equal portions by a net that runs across the width of the court. Tennis is played between two players (singles) or between two teams each consisting of two players (doubles). The object of the game is to hit the ball over the net into the opposition zone such that the ball is not successfully returned. The player or team that has hit the un-returnable shot scores a point. A game is decided by a set number of points, with a determined number of games constituting a set, and a defined number of winning sets determining the overall winner of the match.

In its present form, tennis originated in France in the sixteenth century. A precursor to the modern game, which used a racquet that was more similar to a squash racquet, was played even earlier. Records date back to the twelfth century.

Once a game restricted to the wealthy and privileged, the appeal of tennis grew in the twenty-first century. Now, municipally operated and maintained tennis courts are a recreational mainstay of most communities. Tennis is a medal sport of the Summer Olympics and the various professional tours are a popular spectator pastime. As with the sport of golf, professional tennis has four tournaments that are considered to be paramount in prestige to the others. Winning one of these tournaments is a career accomplishment. Winning all four of the tournaments in the same competitive season—a feat called the "Grand Slam"—has been accomplished by only a handful of players.

The tennis court can be made of different surfaces, including concrete or wood ("hard court"), grass, or pressed clay. The surface affects the way the game is played. The tennis ball will rebound with greater energy off a hard court, since less energy is absorbed on impact. Conversely, a ball that is hit so that it spins through the air after it leaves the racquet face will tend to move more following impact with clay or grass, whose increased friction grabs the ball more than a hard court. As well, the surface character of concrete will be much more uniform than either grass

or clay, whose surfaces can be marred during play. The changing character of the latter surfaces can add to the appeal and challenge of the tennis match.

The set-up of a player for a shot will be different on concrete, where he or she cannot slide into the shot, versus grass or clay, where sliding to meet the ball is the desirable way to achieve the best shot. Players who are successful on the various surfaces must have an ability to alter their style of play to match the conditions.

Of the four Grand Slam tournaments, the United States Open and Australian Open are hard court competitions, the French Open utilizes a clay court, and Wimbleton (an English tournament) is a grass court event.

Whatever the composition of the playing surface, the dimensions of a tennis court are standard. In a singles match, the rectangular surface is 78 ft (almost 24 m) long and 27 ft (slightly over 8 m) wide. For a doubles match, the length of the court is the same, but the width increases to 36 ft (almost 11 m). The different widths are denoted by an outer set of lines running the length of the court and two other lines parallel to these that define the width of the singles area.

Another line runs parallel to the length of the court. This line begins at the center of the court and extends 21 ft (6.4 m) to either side of the net. This line helps create the zones where the first shot of each point (the service) must land.

Horizontal lines are also present. A central line divides the court in half. A mesh-like net with a reinforced top is placed over this line. A rope strung through the top of the net connects the net with support posts at either side of the court. A properly positioned net should be 3 ft 6 in (slightly over 1 m) off the ground at each post and 3 ft (slightly less than 1 m) high at center court. Two other horizontal lines positioned 21 ft (6.4 m) on either side of the net join the central line to complete the service zones (which, if viewed from overhead, look like four smaller rectangles positioned within the main rectangle of the court). Finally, two other horizontal lines (the baselines) define either end of the court.

In singles play, one competitor is on either side of the net. In doubles play, the two teammates are on the same side of the net. Typically, one of the doubles teammates will be closer to the baseline, with the other teammate positioned closer to the net. Play begins in the same way in singles or doubles competition, with the server, who is positioned behind the baseline, hitting the ball to the receiver. Recreational

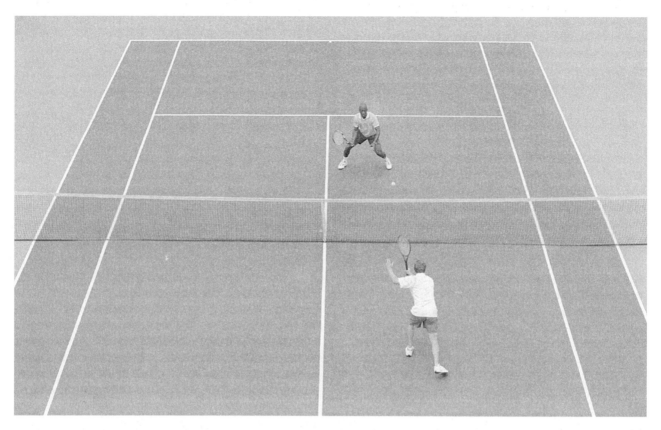

Tennis has broad appeal as a recreational and competitive sport. © JOE MCBRIDE/CORBIS

level players may elect to hit the ball with an underhand motion or after tossing the ball slightly up into the air to improve their changes of making contact with the ball. Elite players will toss the ball about 10 ft (3 m) above them, giving time to position their body to make an aggressive movement toward the descending ball in such a way that a great deal of energy from the body movement and swinging of the racquet is transferred to the ball. If properly done, the ball can rocket off the racquet face at over 100 mph (160 kmp).

If the ball does not land in the same rectangular service area on the other side of the net, or does not make it to the net, or hits the net on its way to the other side of the court, the server must hit another shot. If the second shot is unsuccessful, the competitor is awarded the point for that part of the game.

The receivers' task is to make contact with the ball and send it back over the net before or after it has bounced. Only one bounce is allowed. If the ball bounces twice or more before being returned, the server is awarded the point for the play. Sometimes the ball moves so fast that contact is not made. This is called an "ace" and is worth a point to the server. Sometimes the receiver is successful in sending the

ball back to the server's side of the court. Play then continues, with the ball being hit back and forth across the net (a rally) until one player is unable to return the ball. Then, the other person or team is awarded the point for that portion of the game.

A complete tennis game is called a match. The match is divided into sets, and each set consists of games. Finally, each game is decided by the number of points accumulated. Each player begin each game with zero points (also called "love"). As serves are won, a player or team accumulates points in the order 15, 30, 40, 41, 42 (game point). One player or team serves for an entire game. The next game, the service shifts to the other player or team.

As one or the other competitor wins games, a point is reached where one player or team has won the predefined number of games necessary to win the set. A new set then begins, with the tally of games won shifting back to zero. A complete match is won when a player or team wins a defined number of sets.

Depending on the experience and athleticism of the competitors, a match can be relatively sedate and relaxing, or a fast-paced and serious contest. Recreational contests typically involve just the players, who govern play and interpret results by themselves. More competitive contests may involve an umpire (who is the ultimate authority should disputes arise and who sits in an elevated seat, permitting a view of the entire court), other umpires who determine if serves and other shots land in bounds or out of bounds, and helpers who retrieve the balls and keep play moving at a brisk pace.

Tennis is played using a specially designed racquet and a ball constructed of rubber that is hollow and is covered by a felt layer. The felt imparts some resistance to the ball, allowing it to be hit so as to give it spin, and so it will not bounce wildly high or wide on impact. Elite players can hit the ball such that it rotates clockwise or counterclockwise while moving through the air, or has a vertically oriented, downward spin (topspin). The different spins will cause the ball to move differently on contact with the court.

In top-flight tennis, the felt is worn out quickly, and a new ball will be put into play after a designated number of games (typically nine) or when both players or teams agree that the ball in play is worn out.

In singles tennis, each player must roam over the entire half of the court to try to return shots that have landed close to the net, far back on the court, or near each sideline. In doubles competition, the teammates will coordinate their movements so that they most efficiently cover the territory of the court. This is important since, in doubles, the play can be very fast, with the ball often cannoning back and forth over the net without touching the ground.

A tennis ball can be hit with a forehand or a backhand motion, and can be returned very close to the net at higher speeds or high up in the air at a slower speed (a lob). The choice of shot depends on the player's ability and the position of the competitor. For example, if a competitor is very close to the net, a prudent shot can be to hit a lob that lands far back in the court, since it may be difficult for the competitor to reach the shot and return it.

Part of the appeal of tennis is that it can be played for a lifetime and by people of all physical abilities. Millions of people around the world are active participants and millions more enjoy the thrill of watching the game.

SEE ALSO Badminton; Racquetball; Squash; Tennis racquet construction.

# Tennis racquet construction

The sport of tennis has been played for centuries. Over hundreds of years, the technology of the game has changed dramatically. In the fourteenth century, a tennis racquet was more like a present-day squash racquet, having a long handle and small hitting surface shaped like a teardrop. Furthermore, with strings made of animal gut, the racquets' construction was quite different from their modern-day counterparts.

By the end of the nineteenth century, the shape of the tennis racquet head was more similar to the present-day design, although the head was flatter at the top rather than being rounded. Also, the size of the head was smaller than the present-day racquet head.

This design did not change appreciably until almost a century later, during the 1960s. Structural innovations that were introduced prior to the 1960s included laminated construction (where thin layers of wood are glued together, instead a using a single piece of wood to form the racquet) and the use of fabric strings instead of sections of gut.

A metal racquet existed prior to the twentieth century, but it was considered a novelty and was not well-received. In 1967, the Wilson sporting goods company introduced a steel racquet that proved to be popular. The racquet was lighter and less cumbersome than the existing wood racquets. Use of the racquet by Jimmy Connors—then a top-flight professional—brought the metal tennis racquet into the mainstream.

In 1976, Howard Head designed a racquet whose hitting surface was over 50% larger than the existing racquets. The use of aluminum as the frame material allowed the increased hitting surface to be incorporated into a racquet that was as light as the existing versions. The Prince Classic and Prince Pro racquets immediately became popular among recreational players, who found the greater hitting surface made it easier to make contact with the ball.

However, elite players found that the larger surface area could make the ball more difficult to control, as the racquet head would pivot slightly during the hitting stroke and at the point of impact. In contrast to strings, which rebound to their original configuration very quickly after contact with the tennis ball, the aluminum racquets required several milliseconds to resume their original shape. This reduced the energy that is transferred to the ball, and affected the accuracy of the shot.

To remedy this, a racquet material that was light but more resistant to torque, and was more efficient as energy transfer was needed. The answer proved to be a combination of carbon fibers and plastic resin that was dubbed graphite. One of the well-known tennis players who helped popularize the composite racquet was the late Arthur Ashe.

Tennis racquets are now constructed either of graphite or aluminum. Wooden racquets are a rarity.

Beginning in the 1980s, racquets with thicker frames were marketed. Designed to lessen the vibration felt when hitting a tennis ball, "wide-body" racquets did not achieve great popularity as they felt very stiff. However, some present-day players still prefer the increased power that these racquets produce.

During the 1990s, a tennis racquet was introduced that, at 28 in (71 cm) in length, was 1 in (2.5 cm) longer than the conventional racquet. The extra length enabled a shorter player to stretch slightly higher at the moment of impact with the tennis ball during the serve, producing a harder shot. Now-retired tennis professional Michael Chang used the longer racquet with great success.

Another aspect of tennis racquet construction that has changed over time is the grip—the portion of the racquet that a person holds to make a shot. The grip was originally made of wound leather. However, this material would become slippery when covered with sweat and would become brittle with age. Modern-day grips are synthetic, which provide moisture absorption and cushioning.

Strings have also evolved. Modern-day strings are also synthetic. Nylon is a popular material. Some strings are made of synthetic threads of material that are spun together to produce a string that is very strong yet flexible. These strings are very elastic; they deform when contacting a ball but quickly resume their normal length. This transfers a great deal of energy to the tennis ball very quickly, causing the ball to rocket off the racquet face. The tendency of the strings to deform is beneficial to the recreational player, since even an off-center shot will still tend to rebound back in the intended direction. Elite players will stretch the strings tauter and under greater pressure, to produce a harder return. This reduces the deformation of the strings, increasing the need for a player to precisely and accurately strike the ball.

Some strings are not of uniform diameter along their length. Instead, strings that run parallel to the racquet handle can increase in diameter from the bottom of the racquet to the racquet central region and then taper in diameter towards the top (or toe) of the racquet face. This acts to direct the most efficient hitting zone (the "sweet spot") more to the toe, which is the region where most recreational players tend to make contact with the tennis ball. By altering the string design, tennis racquet manufacturers can produce a racquet that is easier and more pleasurable for a recreational player to use.

SEE ALSO Badminton; Golf: Why graphite-shafted clubs produce longer drives; Racquetball; Tennis serve mechanics.

# Tennis serve mechanics

The tennis serve is the most important single shot in the game of tennis. The serve permits the player to assert control over how the game unfolds, as the serve dictates how a particular return shot must be made. The successful service of the tennis ball is the product of a kinetic linkage that begins with the player's feet, extending through the legs, hips, shoulders, and wrist to the racquet on impact with the ball.

The first step in the proper mechanics of a tennis serve is the establishment of proper footwork. The player must begin the serve sequence from a stable position, where at the conclusion of the serve the player will be in a stance that permits an effective response to the next shot from the opponent. For a right handed player, the left foot will be placed immediately behind the boundary line, and the right foot behind. The player will ideally assume a balanced stance with the knees bent as the player prepares to execute the serve.

The most effective serve is one where the ball is struck by the player with elbow slightly bent, but the arm otherwise fully extended, making contact with the ball directly above the server's body. As the ball is tossed in the air to begin the serve sequence, the body is positioned to uncoil itself, with the full extension of this imaginary coil being achieved at contact with the ball. To achieve maximum power through this uncoiling mechanism, the twist of the player's torso, the swing of the racquet, and the drive upwards of the legs towards the ball all combine to generate greater speed in the racquet. As a general proposition of physics, the faster the racquet is moving upon impact with the ball, the faster the tennis ball will travel, as the greater racquet velocity translates into greater force directed into the ball and consequent velocity achieved by the ball on impact.

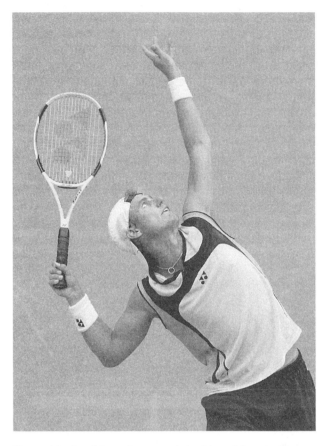

Lleyton Hewitt of Australia serves during his match against Jurgen Melzer of Austria. PHOTO BY CAMERON SPENCER/GETTY IMAGES.

The racquet must be held securely but not tightly in the wrist and hand of the player. If the player grips the racquet too tightly, seeking to apply significant muscle power from the arm to the serve, the effective flow of energy generated by the movements of the rest of the body to the racquet will be defeated.

The precise point at which the ball is struck is also an important aspect of the mechanics of a tennis serve. If the ball is tossed too low, the player will not be able to fully extend the arm at impact. An incomplete extension of the arm and racquet decreases the amount of force directed into the ball on impact. A further consideration of a low service toss is that the lower the point of contact between ball and racquet, the greater chance that the ball will be delivered into the net. If the ball is tossed too high, studies have shown that the player will also hit the ball at a lower than optimal point; in visually tracking the ball thrown to a point above them, players tend to allow the ball to fall too far before striking it with the racquet. To preserve serve mechanics, the ball should be tossed to the desired height and struck on its

ascent, at the moment the ball has reached the peak of its flight.

The concluding position of the player is also an important mechanical issue. As the player strikes the ball, the right foot of a right handed player will power through the stance, taking the player inside the court surface. The player must complete the serve in a bent knee (crouched) stance, in order to best react to the next shot of the opponent.

SEE ALSO Stretching and flexibility; Tennis; Tennis strength and training exercises.

# Tennis strength and training exercises

Tennis strength and training exercises are directed to a number of distinct but interrelated physical aspects of the sport. Tennis is primarily a game of short, dynamic bursts of running action and lateral movement, separated by brief recovery intervals. These anaerobic features of the sport are coupled with game and practice situations where the player might be active for two to three hours at a time, a circumstance that requires the promotion of cardiovascular endurance.

The mechanics of the tennis serve and the various types of volleys executed by a player place an emphasis upon the development of balance and coordinated movement, to both move laterally and to deliver effective shots from a variety of positions. Tennis does not require overwhelming upper body strength, but the ability to combine shoulder and arm strength with an effective core muscle structure (abdominal, gluteal, groin, and lumbar muscles) is required to strike the ball with power.

As with any sport, a proper tennis exercise program will be periodized; the competitive, pre season and off season periods should be identified with training organized accordingly. As tennis is a sport that is played year round by many athletes (the tennis year is often divided between the outdoor and the indoor seasons), elite players will identify those competitions or those periods of the year in which they will seek to achieve their competitive peak, with other periods designated as the off season, or periods of recovery and rebuilding.

It is in the preseason that a tennis player can pay most particular attention to cardiovascular training, to develop endurance. Exercises such as running, cycling, indoor cardiovascular machines, and swimming all achieve the necessary goal for the tennis player. A failure to develop a reasonable level of endurance will limit the ability of the player to recover between rallies and between the sets of a match. Where the cardiovascular training takes the form of running, the athlete can also achieve a degree of acclimatization to the heat of outdoor competitive tennis. Tennis not only taxes the body's ability to maintain a healthy fluid level through the exertions of competition, the outdoor surfaces typically radiate additional heat into the player's environment, a circumstance which accelerates the dehydration of the athlete. Acclimatization to warm weather tennis can occur within approximately 10 to 14 days of the commencement of warm weather training.

Pre season anaerobic fitness can be developed in a variety of methods for tennis. Footwork exercises that replicate the length and the intensity of court movements are ideal. The shuttle drill is one such device, where the player moves in distances that replicate the distance from baseline to net and back in a number of sequences; the drill can also be executed moving laterally, sideline to sideline, or backwards. Tennis training is also ideally suited to ladder drills, which are similar to hopscotch, the children's schoolyard game. Ladder drills require the player to move explosively from square to square, all while maintaining balance and focus upon the next part of the drill. Given that tennis court surfaces are often constructed from hard and unyielding material, continuous play presents a greater risk of stress injuries to the feet or lower legs of the athlete. Hard running drills of this nature can be performed on any softer surface.

Core strength exercises will contribute to the effective delivery of a serve and the making of a return. Exercises that include the simplicity of sit ups and abdominal crunches, to more involved Swiss ball routines, where the body's own mass is the resistance provided to the muscles, are all effective.

In tennis the body is subjected to a significant range of movement. In a single sequence of shots, a player may be required to run in every direction, lunge from side to side, and to reach up or jump to play overhand shots. Stretching and the development of maximal joint flexibility is essential to tennis success. Of particular importance is the preservation of the range of motion in the shoulder, elbow, and wrist of the player's dominant hand, as these joints in particular are subjected to the repetitive stresses in every swing of the racquet.

Increased muscle mass is not usually a desired goal in a tennis player, as increased mass may hinder the important qualities of quickness, balance, and lateral movement. Tennis players will use strength training to maximize shoulder strength and to ensure that they have a reasonable balance between all muscle groups. Circuit training, with the emphasis upon high repetition, low weight routines, is commonly employed to achieve this result.

SEE ALSO Stretching and Flexibility; Tennis; Tennis serve mechanics.

# Terrorism SEE Sports security and terrorism

# Testosterone

Testosterone is the male sex hormone. Testosterone is a steroid hormone, with a chemical structure closely resembling that of the anabolic steroids used to produce increases of mass and strength among athletes. Testosterone is chemically classified as an androgen, one of the group of hormones that promote the growth and development of the male body characteristics, including greater muscle mass. The contrasting female growth hormones are estrogens, chemically similar to the male hormone. Because testosterone promotes the growth of male characteristics, it has been long desired as a muscle and strength building agent. While testosterone is essential in the creation of the physical distinctions between the male and female structures, the female endocrine system also produces testosterone, though in much lesser quantities than males.

Like all steroids, testosterone is constructed from four carbon rings; it is the location of various oxygen and hydrogen molecules within the ring structure that distinguishes testosterone from other well-known steroids used by athletes, including stanozolol, dianabol, and nandrolone.

Testosterone formation begins within the body as a process-utilizing cholesterol, itself a byproduct of the fats ingested through diet and absorbed for storage within the body as triglycerides. Within the body, cholesterol is used to form testosterone and numerous other hormones. As a hormone, testosterone is a product of the body's endocrine system, a sophisticated series of glands that are subordinate to the functions of the thyroid gland, which is itself directed in its actions by the region of the brain known as the hypothalamus. The hypothalamus/pituitary gland/testes glandular relationship is referred to as the gonadal axis. The testes produce between 4 mg and 7 mg of testosterone each day in a healthy male.

Hormones function as chemical signals directed by the brain to compel bodily organs or systems to function in a particular way. The release of adrenaline when a threat to the body is perceived and the production of the growth hormone during the period of adolescence are two common examples of hormone secretion and function. With testosterone, any disruption of the signals delivered along the gonadal axis will interfere with testosterone production.

Within the endocrine system, the primary source of testosterone production is the testes, the pair of male glands located inside the scrotum. The adrenal glands, positioned above each kidney, are a secondary source of this hormone. Testosterone is of fundamental importance to human function in a number of areas. Testosterone influences the development of all primary and secondary sexual characteristics in males, including their sexual function, and appearance attributes such as voice characteristics and the growth of body hair. The general speed and quality of male tissue growth is influenced by testosterone, as is the overall development and maintenance of muscle mass and strength. Adequate levels of testosterone production are necessary for the formation and preservation of bone structure and bone density. Testosterone contributes to effective brain activity, including learning and memory skills. Finally, testosterone contributes to the maintenance of the body's general energy levels necessary for effective function in all physical activities.

For males over 50 years of age, there is a natural decline in the amount of testosterone produced by the testes. This decline can present a significant difficulty for older male athletes, as reduced testosterone production will contribute to muscle weakness, a potential decrease in sexual function, as well as the decreased bone density that typically contributes to osteoporosis, the bone-thinning disease. The most widely used treatments for testosterone deficiency involve a hormone replacement therapy, which provides replacement testosterone to the body either through a transdermal (skin-applied) patch, or intramuscular injection.

In international athletic competition governed by the World Anti-Doping Agency (WADA), testosterone is specified as a banned substance on the Prohibited List of all illegal performance-enhancing substances. Testosterone is classed as an anabolic androgenic steroid, an illegal steroid that is intended to produce or facilitate male growth and physical characteristics in an athlete. Prior to the ascendancy of WADA in the late 1990s as the foremost drug regulatory agency in athletics, a number of notable world-class athletes had been the subject of positive testosterone tests, among them American sprinter Dennis Mitchell, American middle distance runner Mary Decker Slaney, and Dutch shot putter Erik de Bruin. Unlike other chemically produced performance-enhancing substances, testosterone is present in the body of all athletes in varying degrees. Testosterone testing is based on whether the hormone appears to be present in an unnatural amount, beyond the range that would typically be expected in that person. The WADA standard for the testosterone range is generally where the amount of testosterone present through testing is greater than 4:1 ratio to the expected levels; at those levels, a positive drug test is deemed to have resulted.

WADA have developed similar testing standards for all potentially endogenous substances (like testosterone, those capable of originating within the body), as opposed to the stricter limits defined for exogenous substances (those that can only originate outside of the body, such as most anabolic steroids and stimulants).

**SEE ALSO** Anabolic steroids; HGH; Hormones; Nandrolone.

# Therapeutic Use Exemption

The Therapeutic Use Exemption (TUE) is a part of the comprehensive anti-doping strategy developed and promoted by the World Anti-Doping Agency (WADA) for implementation in all Olympic sports, Paralympics and international athletic competition.

Upon the founding of WADA in 1999, a series of protocols were developed by WADA to assist in the world wide combat of doping in sport. A cornerstone of the anti-doping campaign has been the creation and the maintenance of the *WADA Prohibited List*, which sets out in a definitive fashion every substance that is prohibited for use by athletes in WADA compliant events. The Prohibited List is published annually, after consultation with sports scientists, sport administrators, and national anti-doping agencies. Many of the substances included on the Prohibited List have legitimate medical and therapeutic uses, often available as prescription medication.

WADA established the TUE to allow athletes to participate in competition who were required to take an otherwise prohibited substance for a legitimate medical purpose. A successful TUE application has three aspects: one, that the athlete would experience significant health problems if the subject medication were not taken; two, the athlete would obtain no significant performance benefit from the prohibited substance; three, there is no reasonable therapeutic alternative to the prohibited substance. The athlete's national anti-doping agency is responsible for the determination to grant or refuse the TUE application, with WADA reserving its right to either review the grant of the exemption, or to consider an appeal from an athlete who was refused a TUE. The Court of Arbitration for Sport is usually the final venue of appeals made in relation to TUE applications.

TUE applications are commonly advanced by athletes who use substances such as beta-2 agonists, the active ingredients in the bronchodilator medications used to treat conditions such as upper respiratory tract infections and asthma.

In the lead up to the 2006 Winter Olympics, two prohibited substance cases received prominence in the international media. Jose Theodore, a Canadian ice hockey goaltender, and American skeleton racer Zach Lund each tested positive for the use of a banned substance, finasteride, which each had ingested through their use of a hair restoration product, Propecia. Both Theodore and Lund had used the restorative for a number of years; had these athletes availed themselves of the TUE process, the likelihood of an exemption being granted was high, given that finasteride is only a prohibited substance through its other uses as a diuretic, the substances frequently associated with the masking of steroid use. As neither had applied for a TUE, each was subject to sanction as the WADA philosophy is that athletes must know what they are placing in their bodies, and a failure to take all reasonable steps to confirm the nature of all substances consumed in any fashion, or alternatively, a failure to us the TUE process, will not constitute a defense to a doping allegation.

SEE ALSO Athlete Location Form; Out-of-competition testing; World Anti-Doping Agency (WADA).

# Thermoregulation, exercise, and thirst

Thermoregulation is the manner in which the body is able to maintain a consistent internal temperature, notwithstanding significant fluctuations in external temperatures caused by the environment. Thermoregulation is a primarily involuntary function,

with the controls centered in the hypothalamus, the region of the brain that controls many other important systems, including the production of hormones, the chemical signals generated throughout the body in the endocrine system, as well as the function of the heart. Humans have evolved to function best at an internal temperature that can be maintained at approximately 98.6°F (37°C).

Exercise may be broadly defined as any exertion of the musculoskeletal system that goes beyond the involuntary functions of basic human metabolism, such as eating, breathing, or sleeping; exercise levels will naturally place a correspondingly greater impact on the body's ability to regulate temperature. The impact of exercise on the thermoregulatory system will also vary subject to the presence or absence of environmental conditions such as heat or humidity.

Thirst is a universal human experience. All humans, when their fluid levels are low, will crave water or other fluids. The thirst mechanism is also progressive in its signal from the involuntary system to the human senses, a sensation that cannot be shut out or deactivated through any means. It is the timing of the activation of the thirst mechanism that is of interest. Unlike other mammals, the human thirst mechanism does not activate until the body supply of water is depleted by approximately 15 oz (500 ml). Although a person cannot survive for more than three or four days without water, it is ironic that a person may survive as long as 30 days without food, even though the hunger craving is a more powerful one than that of thirst.

There is a crucial component of the osmoregulation of the body, the control of the body's levels of water and mineral salts, particularly those of sodium and potassium. Osmoregulation, thermoregulation, and the maintenance of the body's blood glucose levels, are the three main aspects of homeostasis, or the balance achieved by the body in its involuntary operating functions.

The thirst mechanism must also be considered in contrast to the daily fluid requirements of the body. Of the water consumed daily in various forms, a sedentary person will eliminate 45 oz (1,500 ml) as urine, 15 oz (500 ml) through evaporation and perspiration, 10 oz (300 ml) through the lungs, and 6 oz (200 ml) through the digestive and other gastrointestinal processes. An athlete engaged in a demanding workout or who is active in a warm weather environment may lose between 1 qt (1 l) and 4 qt (4 l) of fluid through perspiration in less than 90 minutes of activity. The fluid losses in such circumstances outpace the thirst mechanism, putting athletic performance and athlete health in jeopardy. It is entirely possible for an athlete to begin to sustain the adverse effects of dehydration, which include impaired cardiovascular function, impaired muscle function, and loss of coordination and motor control, before the thirst mechanism has been signaled.

The gap between the triggering of the thirst mechanism and fluid levels is also a factor at the beginning of the activity. If an athlete relies on the thirst sensation to determine hydration, the athlete will often begin the activity in a mildly dehydrated state.

The warm weather activation of the anti-diuretic hormone (ADH) is also an important factor when assessing the function of the thirst mechanism. ADH is released when the body senses, through the hypothalamus, that it is becoming dehydrated and that the blood volume has been reduced through additional perspiration. ADH is the signal conveyed to the kidneys to produce less urine, and to direct greater amounts of water into the blood. This process also may be triggered in advance of any thirst experienced by the athlete.

Because the thirst mechanism is an unreliable indicator of the body's true thermoregulatory and osmoregulatory condition during exercise, an athlete must develop a fluid replacement/hydration strategy that permits optimal function irrespective of the thirst sensation. The consumption of water in the period prior to, during, and subsequent to performance is essential. When the athlete will be involved in significant exercise for periods greater than one hour, the consumption of sport drinks that will assist in maintaining the sodium level, a key component in how the body maintains fluid levels, is important. In warm weather circumstances, the consumption of water to address dehydration, absent proper sodium levels, can lead to a state where the water will not be absorbed into the body as the involuntary systems strive to maintain a desired sodium balance with the sodium remaining. This condition is hyponatremia, a state of water intoxication.

Urine color is a useful general indicator of hydration. When urine is a light yellow color, it signals a proper fluid level; when urine is dark yellow, it is evidence of dehydration, as the urine is too concentrated, a result of the body is secreting greater amounts of ADH to limit fluid outflow.

**SEE ALSO** Cold-related illnesses and emergencies; Heat stroke; Hydration.

# Thermoregulatory system

Thermoregulation, and the bodily system that performs this function, is the maintenance of a consistent internal body temperature, even when there are significant fluctuations in the external environmental temperature. The thermoregulatory system operates within two general boundaries: hypothermia, the condition where the body becomes so cold that its systems will not properly function, and hyperthermia, the corresponding opposite physical state where the body is overheated.

The thermoregulatory system performs one of the three major homeostatic, or overall balancing functions within the body, all of which are interrelated. Osmoregulation is the internal mechanism that controls the level of water and mineral salts, chiefly sodium and potassium, within the body. The third of the key homeostatic functions is that performed by the liver, through the operation of the cardiovascular system in the maintenance of glucose (blood sugar) levels.

Thermoregulation is primarily achieved through physiological processes, as a function of the autonomic nervous system. The processes of the body are controlled involuntarily through various stimuli transmitted through the body that originate at the hypothalamus, the region of the brain that regulates much of the body's functions, such as heart rate and hormone production in the endocrine system. The brain processes the multitude of external signals that it receives through the sensory organs to direct the bodily systems in appropriate ways to control temperature.

Body temperature is automatically regulated in one of four ways: conduction, convection, evaporation, and radiation. Conduction is the process whereby a warm surface transfers heat to an adjacent cooler surface. If a warm body dives into a colder lake while swimming, there will be a conduction of some of the heat on the surface of the person's body to the surrounding water. Convection is created when a passing air current removes heat from the surface of the skin as it passes over it.

Evaporation occurs with respect to the perspiration produced through the actions of the capillaries, the small vessels of the cardiovascular system located near the surface of the skin. As the body releases the perspiration, a byproduct of the body's increased internal temperature raised by the energy created to produce movement, the conversion of the fluid perspiration from liquid into a gas as it evaporates on the surface of the skin tends to produce a cooling effect on the body. The extent of the cooling effect achieved through perspiration is subject to both the temperature and the level of the humidity in the surrounding air.

Radiation is the effect on body temperature as a result of heat received from external sources, primarily solar radiation. Heat may also radiate from the body to a limited extent.

Thermoregulation can also be achieved through the voluntary regulation of human behaviors; the seeking of shade on a warm day or shelter on a cold one are examples.

The mechanism of thermoregulation is centered on the fact that the ideal temperature for the healthy function of the internal organs of the body is approximately 98.6°F (37°C); the body will not tolerate significant variation from this standard, as hypothermia begins at approximately 95°F (35.5°C) or below; hyperthermia will begin at 103°F (40°C) and above. Both conditions can cause irreparable damage to the internal organs if not remedied quickly, as the body's involuntary response in each situation is to shut down organ function.

The involuntary mechanisms triggered when either hypothermic of hyperthermic conditions are sensed by the hypothalamus begin at the surface of the skin. When the body seeks to maintain body heat, the small hairs at the skin surface will be pushed into an upright position to better retain heat; if the body temperature is too high, the hairs will lie flat on the skin surface as a heat-release mechanism.

The subcutaneous glands (sweat glands) are located in the dermis, the second of the layers of the skin, a part of the endocrine system responsible for the release of perspiration. The sweat glands will be activated when the body seeks to cool itself.

The blood vessels located next to the surface of the skin are also activated whether the body seeks to cool or to warm itself. When the body is overheated, the cardiovascular system automatically directs the flow of additional blood into these vessels to permit the blood warmed by the body activity to be cooled. The vessels expand to accommodate the additional blood flow, a process known as vasodilation. In circumstances where the body senses an unhealthy low temperature, blood flow closest to the surface is restricted to permit all available blood to be directed to the internal organs and the brain, which is the contrasting process of vasoconstriction.

It is the action of vasoconstriction that renders the warming of the extremities for a person who has sustained hypothermia. When a person has suffered this cold weather illness, there is the temptation on the part of the helpers to quickly warm the feet and hands of the victim. This action upsets the body's thermoregulatory efforts and results in a potential wave of cold blood from those extremities flooding into the heart and internal organs. This cold blood can cause a shock to the heart function and trigger a heart attack. The thermoregulatory function is a powerful one and, in such circumstances, the entire body must be warmed slowly.

SEE ALSO Acclimatization; Cold weather exercise; Hydration; Thermoregulation, exercise, and thirst.

# Thermotolerance SEE Exercise and thermotolerance

# THG

THG is the acronym for tetrahydrogestinone, an anabolic steroid first developed in the early 1990s. THG came to prominence as a so-called "designer" steroid, a steroid formulation that was alleged to have been specifically created to defeat the then-current testing processes available in international sport.

The existence of THG was first confirmed in 2003, when an individual anonymously provided the United States Anti-Doping Agency (USADA) with a used syringe containing traces of a product that was ultimately linked to San Francisco-based BALCO (Bay Area Laboratory Cooperative). BALCO was operated by Victor Conte, a sports entrepreneur who sold athletic supplements and training aids to a number of prominent professional athletes, including American shot putter C.J. Hunter, sprinters Marion Jones and Tim Montgomery, and baseball slugger Barry Bonds. There was evidence gathered in the subsequent investigations into the legitimacy of THG which suggested that THG was being represented and marketed as a legitimate supplement.

One such claimant was European sprint champion Dwaine Chambers of Great Britain. He received a two-year suspension from international competition as a result of a positive doping test that revealed the presence of THG in his system. Chambers stated that Conte and BALCO had expressly represented to him that the purported nutritional supplement was compliant with all international standards regarding its formulation. World Anti-Doping Agency (WADA) has long taken the position that positive drug tests invoked the legal doctrine of strict liability, where the burden of proof to establish innocence was very high and rested entirely with the athlete; innocent error as to the supplement content, in the eyes of WADA, is no defense.

In 2003 the WADA released a formal statement indicating that THG was not a supplement, but a banned anabolic steroid. It has the same four-ring carbon structure of all steroids, and THG bears a close chemical similarity to nandrolone (a WADA-prohibited substance). THG and variants of the substance are expressly listed on the WADA Prohibited List. Professional sports leagues, including the National Football League (NFL) and Major League Baseball (MLB), also moved to ban THG in 2003.

The revelations concerning BALCO and THG usage raise the issue of retrospective drug testing in sport. When an athlete has provided a blood or urine sample that has been preserved by the testing authority, and a performance-enhancing substance that the athlete may have consumed at the time prior to the testing is subsequently determined to be illegal, the question is whether the athlete should be punished retrospectively. In 2003 and 2004, international rugby, track and field, and swimming bodies all determined that retrospective testing was appropriate, even if the substance was not determined to be illegal at that time of testing.

SEE ALSO Anabolic steroids; Nandrolone; Testosterone; World Anti-Doping Agency (WADA).

# Thigh and upper leg injuries

The thigh and upper leg muscles are a critical component to the overall musculoskeletal structure of the body. The upper leg is composed of the femur (thigh bone), the longest and the heaviest bone in the skeleton, which forms a part of the hip joint at one end, and the knee joint at the opposing end. The femur supports the quadriceps (thigh muscles), a group of four powerful muscles positioned on the front of the thigh that are primarily responsible for the extension motion of the knee. The quadriceps is attached at the knee joint to the tibia (shin bone) by way of the quadriceps tendon.

The muscle and tendon that are responsible for the knee's opposing flexion (bending action) are the hamstrings. The hamstring tendon is also connected to the tibia, immediately below the rear of the knee joint. In most sports, the ideal ratio in the relative strength of the quadriceps to the hamstring is 3:2.

Significant imbalances in this strength ratio can lead to significant injury in one or both of the muscle groups.

The upper thigh muscles are connected to the abductors (located at the upper and inner aspect of the thigh) and the groin muscles of the lower abdomen, which assist in both the stabilization of the body and the movement of the upper legs; the strength in these muscles forms a significant part of the core strength of any individual. At the rear of the upper thigh, the femur and connective tissues are supported by the gluteal muscles (buttocks). From the illiol bone of the hip to the tibia of the lower leg, the iliotibial (IT) band extends, constructed of a fibrous and thickened soft tissue material, called fascia, that provides stability to the entire upper leg.

One of the most common upper leg and thigh injury is a muscle or tendon strain, which can occur in any of the large muscle structures between the knee and the hip. A strain is an overextension of the muscle fibers that comprise the muscle organism, caused by either a repetitive movement or an imbalance in the relative strengths of the hamstring and the quadriceps. A strained tendon, often referred to as a "pull," frequently occurs in the hamstring, especially when the athlete moves explosively to accelerate. In some cases, certain of the long, cylindrical muscle fibers, which may number in the thousands, may be microscopically torn, without a rupture or other more serious damage to the muscle. Muscle strains are categorized according to their severity. A grade 1 strain produces a cramping or tightening sensation in the affected muscle. An athlete can often continue in a competition if the injury is immediately treated, provided that the athlete understands that the strain may become aggravated with continued stress directed into the tissues.

A grade 2 muscle strain will produce an immediate and pronounced pain in the region of the injury, and the athlete will usually not be able to continue in competition after the injury is sustained. A grade 3 strain is characterized by an immediate and direct stabbing sensation in the injured muscle. This injury will incapacitate the athlete until the damage to the tissue is healed.

Another common injury to the quadriceps is caused by a direct blow to the muscle. As a large prominent structure, the thigh is exposed to a considerable variety of traumas, most of which result in a contusion, creating swelling, bruising, and a limitation of movement and flexibility. Athletes in sports that involve the blocking or tackling of an opponent, and those sports that create incidental contact between opponents, such as soccer and basketball, frequently sustain these injuries.

All soft tissue injuries in the thigh or upper leg can be effectively treated in their initial stages with the RICE (rest/ice/compression/elevation) treatment method. Given the size of the quadriceps and hamstrings, the compression element to the RICE progression must be especially thorough. It is estimated that over 90% of these injuries can be resolved conclusively through RICE, or using the treatment in conjunction with the administration of a nonsteroidal anti-inflammatory drug (NSAID) to relieve pain and inflammation.

The most serious injury to the thigh or upper leg is a facture of the femur. In an adolescent person, this injury can be particularly worrisome if it affects the growth plate, the soft area of bone located at the epiphysis near the head of the femur, as the fracture may interrupt the proper growth of the bone. In an adult, a fracture is a debilitating injury that will often require surgery to insert one or more pins into the bone to provide it with support. Both injuries are caused by significant force being directed into the bone, such as may occur in a high speed collision.

Sports science research regarding the incidence of thigh and upper leg injuries has repeatedly identified a lack of stretching and flexibility in the athlete as a significant contributing factor to their causation. Stretches that promote harmony between the quadriceps, hamstrings, IT band, gluteal muscles, and groin will provide both greater inherent stability in movement and reduced risk of musculoskeletal injury in the structures.

**SEE ALSO** Groin pulls and strains; Hamstring injuries; Iliotibial (IT) band friction; Musculoskeletal injuries; Quadriceps pulls and tears; Tendinitis and ruptured tendons.

# Thirst SEE Thermoregulation, exercise, and thirst

# Frank Edward Thomas

5/27/1968–
AMERICAN
PROFESSIONAL BASEBALL PLAYER

Frank Thomas is one of the most effective and most feared baseball hitters in the history of the sport. His nickname, "The Big Hurt" is an accurate description of the damage that he has directed against opposing pitchers throughout his major league career.

At 6 ft 5 in tall (1.95 m) and a weight of approximately 265 lb (120 kg), Thomas was a much sought after American football player at the conclusion of his high school career. He accepted a football scholarship to Auburn University in Alabama; after playing both varsity football as a tight end and baseball in his freshman year, Thomas devoted his athletic attentions to baseball for the balance of his university career. Over 50 major league baseball players at one time played for Auburn; the university has a reputation as a collegiate baseball powerhouse.

While at Auburn, Thomas was named the South East Conference baseball player of the year among other athletic distinctions in 1989. After being selected the seventh player overall in the 1989 baseball amateur draft by the Chicago White Sox of the American League, Thomas opted to sign with the White Sox and end his college playing career.

Most major league baseball players serve an apprenticeship in the American minor leagues, no matter how talented they may be. Thomas minor league career was short and emphatic, as he impressed the Chicago White Soc management with his power hitting abilities. Thomas was called up to the major league team in 1990, where he made an immediate impact against major league pitching. By 1992, Thomas was established as one of the most potent all round hitting threats in all of baseball. Thomas played first base when in the field, but his defensive play was never more than average. Later in his career he would seldom be called upon in a defensive role, as he was usually listed in the lineup as a designated hitter, the player who may be entered in place of any other player as a hitter, with no obligations in the field.

Thomas was the rare slugger who could consistently get on base through the drawing of a walk from the opposing pitcher. A number of baseball experts, including those known as sabermetricians, regard the performance of Thomas throughout the 1990s as one of the finest periods of sustained offensive play in the history of baseball. Sabermetrics is the analysis of baseball performance through statistical means; the term was coined using the acronym for the Society for American Baseball Research, SABR, an organization made famous through its promotion of a better understanding of baseball performance through statistics. The SABR was founded by baseball writer and statistician Bill James in 1977.

Thomas's level of play, as supported by his statistics through the 1990s was remarkable. Using the sabermetrics statistical device known as Runs Created, Thomas was the most dominant hitter of this decade. Runs created is a statistical measure of baseball performance, expressed by the equation (Total Hits + Total walks [Base on balls]) × (Total bases) ÷ (Total number of at bats + Total walks). Sabermetricians believe that the runs created calculation is the most accurate assessment of a player's true offensive value to a team, as the more runs a player creates (as opposed to scores), the greater the player's contribution to the overall offensive success of the team.

Using the more conventional baseball standards of batting average, runs scored, walks, and home runs, Thomas established a major league record in the 1990s, with seven straight seasons where he exceeded .300 in batting average, drew more than 100 walks, scored over 100 runs, and hit more than 20 home runs. Thomas broke the record of five consecutive seasons at this level of excellence, established by the legendary Ted Williams in the 1940s.

In the 1993 and 1994 seasons, Thomas became only the second first baseman in the history of the game to win successive Most Valuable Player awards. The 1994 season remains one of the great speculative questions about precisely how much Thomas might have been to achieve had the season not been shortened by almost 50 games in mid-August of that year by a player strike. At age 25, Thomas was entering his physical prime and through 113 games (of a 162 game regular season), Thomas had posted a .353 batting average and amassed 38 home runs. He also had 101 RBIs, leading the league with runs scored (106), walks (109), slugging percentage (.729), and on-base percentage (.487). *Sports Illustrated* was one of a number of sports publications that concluded, barring the strike, Thomas may have broken Babe Ruth's long standing records for runs, walks, and extra-base-hits in a single season.

Given his demonstrated skills as a hitter, it is not surprising that Thomas was a hero to the Chicago White Sox faithful through out the early and mid-1990s. Off the field, Thomas made contributions to charity, particularly those directed to his own foundation established in honor of his younger sister, who had died of leukemia at an early age. Thomas was periodically bedeviled by weight problems, as he weighed close to 300 lb (136 kg) on occasion. He was injured in April of the 2001 season and did not play for the remainder of the year, after which the White Soc exercised a clause in his contract where by he could be released as a free agent if certain performance standards were not attained by Thomas.

After Thomas re-signed with the White Sox in 2002, he was frequently injured, missing most of both the 2004 and 2005 seasons. The most serious of his injuries was sustained to his left foot, which was fractured. In 2005, the Chicago White Sox won the major league World Series for the first time since 1917; the greatest irony of the White Sox triumph was that Thomas, the White Sox best offensive player in the club's over 100-year history, was on the disabled list and did not play any of the championship games.

**SEE ALSO** Baseball; Baseball Bat Speed; Baseball Bats: Sweet spots and tampering; Baseball Injuries.

# Tinea pedis SEE Athlete's foot (tinea pedis)

# Title IX and United States female sports participation

Title IX is the most influential legislation ever passed in the United States with respect to female sport. Title IX is a freestanding section of the United States Civil Rights Act, passed by the United States Senate in 1975, with a built-in implementation date of 1978. Title IX has been the subject of considerable litigation, all of which has turned on the interpretation of the following fundamental statement of Title IX principles: "No person in the United States shall, on the basis of sex, be excluded from participation in, to be denied benefits of, or be subjected to discrimination under any educational program or activity receiving Federal Assistance."

By definition, American professional sports leagues were exempt from Title IX. From the outset of the passage of the legislation, the notion of athletic equality between the sexes contemplated by Title IX was most prominently debated in the context of inter collegiate athletics, the largest part of which is governed by the National Collegiate Athletic Association (NCAA), which has over 1,000 institutions competing at three different competitive levels; a smaller number of schools are members of the National Association of Intercollegiate Athletics (NAIA). The issues concerning the usefulness and impact of Title IX remain most keenly felt at the NCAA level. It is to be noted that the NCAA, in its corporate capacity, is not liable for the actions of its member institutions concerning Title IX compliance; the United States Supreme Court ruled in 1999, in the case of *National Collegiate Athletic Association v. Smith*, as the NCAA only receives dues from some members that are recipients of federal funds and therefore these institutions would attract responsibility, the NCAA cannot be sued for any purported Title IX breach.

"Equal" in the context of the legal relationship between an academic institution and its male versus female athletic programs pursuant to Title IX has been determined to possess three distinct aspects in its meaning. The first meaning is equal in the number of athletic scholarships granted to women as opposed to men, proportionate to enrollment. The second branch of intercollegiate athletic program equality is equal participation in the sports offered at individual institutions, in both the total numbers of participants, as well as the number of opportunities, specialized athletic programs, and experiences available to female athletes. The third equality marker is that regarding the treatment and benefits available to female athletes at a given institution.

Further policy directives from the federal government in the period following the enactment of Title IX clarified the government position as to what precise measures would be expected of an educational institution to achieve compliance with Title IX; these directives have often included a number of specific examples. The key features of the federal government position regarding the specific components of Title IX compliance have both subjective and objective components. The first specific requirement is that an institution must have sports programs that accommodate both sexes. As an example, where a school prior to 1978 had a 90-member football team, a 15-member men's basketball team, a 20-member men's baseball team, and a 15-member men's volleyball team, the institution would be required to offer either the same sports to female athletes, or more commonly, offer female sports that permitted female participation proportionate to the total enrollment of women in the institution. A parallel expectation is the provision of the same quality of equipment and supplies to both male and female sports participants.

It is also expected that institutions will ensure that both men's and women's teams have similar competitive scheduling, as far as could be accommodated, both in terms of games scheduled and quality of competition. Further, female teams should have the same quality of travel arrangements as the men's teams, with similar arrangements for the per diem expenses for all athletes.

There exists an expectation of administrative equality as well. Both the athletic coaching as well as any related academic tutoring provided to scholarship athletes would be of an equal quality for both male and female athletes. The policies regarding the hiring, selection, or assignment of coaches to work with female teams would be equitable. The locker room facilities, practice fields or gymnasiums, and competitive facilities used by female athletes would be of the same quality as those used by male athletes. It was stressed by the federal government that Title IX assures that female athletes would have the same access to medical, rehabilitative, and training services as the male athletes at the institution. Equality of the quality of student athlete housing and dining facilities for female athletes to those of the male athletes was stressed. Lastly, when the institution publicized its athletic programs, the publicity generated would equally reflect the male and the female sports programs at the institution.

Raw participation data regarding female sports participation in the United States since the passage of Title IX confirms that there are far greater numbers of women active in sport that were participating prior to its enactment. A 2005 study confirmed that since 1975, there had been an 875% increase in sports participation levels in American female high school athletics, and a 435% increase in corresponding college athletics. ("College" is the American term used to describe all four-year, post-high school, degree-granting institutions, including those designated as colleges and universities. An American junior college is a two-year program institution).

The quality of play in women's sports has increased dramatically through the period in which Title IX has been in force. Female teams have full-time coaching staffs in many sports, with a corresponding attention to year-round training and fitness.

The same study revealed additional data that tends to suggest that Title IX's implicit purpose has not yet been achieved. While female athletes constitute over 45% of all student athletes (210,000 male athletes to 150,000 female athletes), only 37% of athletic scholarship monies and 33% of institutional expenses devoted to recruitment of prospective student athletes are directed towards female athletes. These figures become more starkly outlined when other demographic information is considered. As of 2006, female students represented approximately 55% of the general college student population in America. In addition, female student athletes had on average higher Scholastic Aptitude Test (SAT) scores (the SAT is prerequisite to college admission in the United

States), as well as higher grade point averages upon graduation from high school than did male student athletes.

Some of the disparity between the expenses associated with each gender can be explained through the nature of the sports typically played by male and female NCAA athletes. In team sports, women compete in the greatest numbers in volleyball, basketball and soccer. Each of these sports is far less expensive a proposition than a sport such as football, where the cost to equip a single player may exceed $2,000; a typical NCAA Division I football team may have as many as 80 players.

The commercial issues surrounding Title IX are more difficult to incorporate into an analysis of whether Title IX has achieved its equality goals. NCAA-organized men's sports championships such as those in football and basketball are remarkably profitable events for both the NCAA and its member institutions. Each of these sports enjoys massive media coverage, supported by multi-billion dollar revenues generated by television. Female sports do not receive any comparable coverage, nor do they generate any significant commercial benefits for either the NCAA or the participating institutions. No matter what Title IX may dictate to any entities in receipt of federal monies, the marketplace, as reflected by consumer demands, has plainly stated that male sports are a far more profitable venture than those involving female athletes at the college level.

Critics of Title IX have repeatedly argued that the legislation is simply an effort to alter basic human nature. The impact of Title IX has also been felt in an ironic fashion: some traditional and non-revenue-producing male sports have been eliminated at a number of American colleges, to reduce the number of male teams or athletes, to create a more desirable ratio of male to female athletes without adding more female programs. Male sports such as wrestling, tennis, and gymnastics have been casualties of this approach to Title IX compliance since the 1980s.

An equal irony flowing from the substantial increase in the total number of female college athletes since the passage of Title IX is the well-documented upwards spiral in obesity rates among young people, accompanied by parallel increases in serious eating-related diseases such as diabetes. While greater- than-ever numbers of female athletes compete at an elite college level, there is no conclusive evidence that the overall health of American society has benefited.

One significant area of litigation has been with respect to equality of facilities available to female athletes in public high schools. A notable example was the action initiated by Alabama high school teacher and girls' basketball coach Roderick Jackson, who sued his school for wrongful dismissal in 2001, when he complained that the high school provided significantly inferior equipment and practice resources to his female team than those enjoyed by the boys' program. The Supreme Court of the United States ruled that Jackson was entitled to continue with his action, citing the need to protect those like Jackson, who was a whistleblower on a Title IX discrimination issue. There have been a number of successful Title IX actions initiated against local town and municipal governments over the quality of girls' municipal softball diamonds versus comparable boys' baseball facilities. Another common issue at the municipal sports level has been equality of access by girl's team and boy's teams to publicly owned facilities during the most desirable practice and games times. American courts have generally been sympathetic to Title IX claims advanced on these issues.

**SEE ALSO** Female exercise and cardiovascular health; Women and sports: Exercise data, goals, and guidelines.

# Topical corticosteroids

Corticosteroids are a commonly prescribed class of medications used to treat a wide variety of inflammations occurring within the body. The most prescribed corticosteroids are those used to treat asthma, the inflammation of the airways and lungs. In a topical formulation, corticosteroids are used to treat and to resolve inflammations and related skin conditions.

Corticosteroid substances include both natural and synthetically produced hormones, the chemicals employed within the body through production in the glands that form the endocrine system. Hormones are primarily messengers, whose glandular secretion and directions throughout the body are controlled in the hypothalamus, a region of the brain responsible for many of the body's involuntary regulatory actions. Natural corticosteroids are an end product of a system described as the hypothalamus/anterior pituitary/andrenocortical axis (the HPA axis); these hormones are manufactured within the adrenal glands, each located above a kidney. Corticosteroids in general have a similar chemical composition to that of the male sex hormone, testosterone.

Corticosteroids are also known as glucocorticoids, as they impact the utilization and metabolism of the fats ingested into the body through diet. Cortisol, the natural hormone that gives it name to the group, is referred to as the stress hormone. When the synthetic form of the hormone, cortisone, is injected into the body, it is converted into cortisol for effective anti-inflammatory use.

Steroids are naturally occurring, fat-soluble substances, chemically defined by the 17 carbon atoms that form four carbon rings in the structure. The word steroid was invented in the 1920s to better describe the sterol group of proteins, of which cholesterol is the most prominent. In contrast to muscle-building anabolic steroids, whose notoriety through their performance-enhancing use by athletes has skewed much of the popular perception as to how a steroid functions, the steroids' designation is a part of a very broad classification, including substances as diverse in their function as vitamin D, testosterone, and the phytosteroids, the steroids present in plants and consumed in food products.

The skin is the body's largest and most exposed organ, comprising approximately 15% of body weight. The skin functions as a component of immune system, the frontline defense against the entry of a multitude of pathogens into the body. The skin is composed of two distinct parts: the epidermis, which is the thin, flexible outer layer, and the dermis, the thicker second layer, where the subcutaneous (below skin surface) glands, such as the sweat glands and sebaceous (oil) glands, and hair follicles are located. The epidermis does not have any direct supply of nutrients by way of the capillary network of the cardiovascular system; the epidermis receives its necessary nutrition through the diffusion of these substances from the dermis.

Inflammatory skin conditions tend to affect the epidermis only. The conditions commonly treated by way of a topical corticosteroid include eczema, a non-contagious skin disease that may persist for an indefinite period, which presents as an uncomfortable itching, a red rash, and, in some instances, lesions on the epidermal surface. Psoriasis is a similar skin condition in its effect on the skin to that of eczema. The precise cause of psoriasis is undetermined; psoriasis is evidenced by a red-colored inflammation with a rough, uneven surface, which in some cases starts with the appearance of silver-colored scales formed on the skin surface. Various forms of psoriasis affect the elbows, knees, groin, and the fingernail structure.

In addition to the discomfort caused to the skin through the presence of the infection, the rubbing and chafing of sports equipment, coupled with the effect of perspiration and drying of the skin make sports participation an often uncomfortable proposition for the athlete. As many inflammatory skin conditions are unsightly, a long-term visible infection can also present psychological problems.

Topical steroids are manufactured in a variety of formulations, including ointments, creams, gels, and lotions. The type of topical application will be determined by the nature of the skin where the inflammatory condition is present. The anti-inflammatory properties of the topical corticosteroids are not universal in strength; the potency of these medications is rated in seven separate categories, from those with ultra-high potency to the lowest potency. An example of a low potency topical corticosteroid is hydrocortisone, used to treat the sensitive skin of young children or the facial or groin areas of adults. The ultra-high potency formulation is often prescribed to counter inflammations such as chronic eczema lesions on the thicker skin of the elbow or palms of the hand.

Topical corticosteroids have a number of well-known side effects, each of which must be considered at the time of the prescription. It is for this reason that topical corticosteroids are not available as over-the-counter (OTC) medications, but by prescription only. These effects include two types of temporary skin damage, reversible skin atrophy (a loss of health in the epidermis), and striae, the formation or lines or marks on the surface of the skin. These medications may also cause a distension of the capillaries in the area of the application of the corticosteroid, the appearance of bruising, and temporary acne. In a naturally dark skinned person, the corticosteroid may cause hypopigmentation, a temporary lightening of the natural color of the skin.

**SEE ALSO** Abrasions, cuts, lacerations; Anabolic steroids; Glucocorticoids; Nonsteroidal anti-inflammatory drugs (NSAIDs); Prescription medications and athletic performance.

# Total daily energy expenditure

The total daily energy expenditure (TEE) is an important calculation in the determination of the overall dietary and exercise practices of any person. The amount of energy needed by anyone to meet the daily physical demands will have two components: the amount of energy needed to maintain the body's needs at rest, the basal energy expenditure, expressed as the base metabolic rate (BMR), and the needs generated by the daily activity levels, which include employment, sport, and any other activities.

In general terms, the body will function at a reasonably efficient level where the amount of energy-producing foods consumed is equal to the amount of energy expended. The macronutrients consumed in all diets are the carbohydrates, proteins, and fats present in varying amounts in all foods. As a rule of thumb, a healthy diet will be approximately 60–65% carbohydrates, 12–15% proteins, and less than 30% fats; this standard is subject to deviation to suit individual dietary requirements necessitated by the particular demands of a sport or an existing physiological condition, such as diabetes.

In calculating the total energy expenditure for a given person or the impact of a particular dietary practice on the energy value of the foods consumed, different types of foods have differing values. One gram of a carbohydrate will produce four calories of energy. One gram of a protein will also produce four calories of energy. One gram of fat produces nine calories of energy.

The BMR represents the total daily energy requirements to permit the function of all of the essential body systems, including heart rate, brain function, cardiovascular function, and the work of the thermoregulatory system. The BMR is the energy used by the body at rest. A component of the BMR is the thermic effect, the energy consumed through the ingestion and digestion of food.

Five critical factors will most significantly influence the BMR value for any individual. The first such factor is the body type and body composition of the individual. Heredity plays a role in the determination of the metabolic rate of every person. The second BMR factor is the presence of lean muscle within the body. The body's lean muscle mass has an inherently greater level of metabolic activity than does corresponding body fat tissue. Age is the third factor; the BMR slows by a rate of approximately 2% per decade after age 30. Gender is the fourth factor; females, primarily due to the fact of their typically greater percentage of body fat than males, tend to have a BMR approximately 10% lower than males of similar age and level of fitness. The final BMR factor is a reduction in the body's caloric consumption. When the body is forced to operate on a reduced calorie diet, the body becomes more efficient in the use of the energy sources available to it.

There are a number of methods to determine how many calories of food energy a person requires to simply maintain their BMR. One method, the Harris-Bennet calculation, provides an equation that factors height, weight, and age into a fixed formula, with certain constants provided, calculated in metric measure. This calculation is premised on the fact that a larger person will tend to consume a greater number of calories at rest than would a smaller person. For example, using the Harris-Bennet calculation, a 47-year-old male who is 6 ft 4 in (1.93 m) tall and weighs 190 lb (86 kg) could estimate his BMR as: $66 + (13.7 \times 86) + (5 \times 193) - (6.87 \times 47) \cong 2,660$ calories per day.

While the BMR will vary from person to person, the daily physical activities of an individual are the greatest single factor in energy expenditure. It is an indisputable factor of human function that the more active the individual, the more energy will be expended and the more calories burned from the body's dietary stores. There is significant evidence that the BMR, which is elevated by exercise, will remain elevated from a period of time after the exercise has ceased, causing the body to use more energy than it would otherwise require at rest.

The amount of energy expended during an athletic activity will be determined by the size of the person, the duration, and the intensity of the activity. The total daily energy expenditure will be significantly influenced by these factors. When a person seeks to maintain a particular weight, the total daily energy expenditure can be variable, so long as the caloric consumption remains no greater than the BMR and the TEE combined. One pound of stored body fat (0.5 kg) represents 3,500 calories of potential energy, thus any increase in the TEE or decrease in the daily physical activities that represents a net difference of 500 calories will result in a 1 lb weight loss per week (500 calories per day over seven days).

**SEE ALSO** Carbohydrates; Diet; Fat utilization; Low-carbohydrate diets and athletic performance; Nutrition; Weight gain; Weight loss.

# Tour de France SEE Cycling: Tour de France

# Track and field

The various disciplines that come under the umbrella of the sport of track and field are among the oldest of the world's athletic contests. Track and field is a North American term; these sports are better known in most of the world as athletics; the original athletes were those who competed in the events governed by the motto of the ancient Olympics, "higher, faster, stronger." The events staged in the venues of the equally historic Scottish Highland Games were conducted with the same simple goals and passions.

The Olympics Games have retained the most prominent connection with track and field competition of any sports event. When Baron Pierre de Coubertin (1863–1937) revived the modern Olympic Games in 1896, the track and field events were the most prominent of the competitions. To be crowned an Olympic champion in any athletics discipline remains the most prestigious prize that a track and field athlete can capture. The gold medalist in the 100-m sprint or the decathlon at the Olympics is inevitably dubbed the World's Fastest Human, or the World's Greatest Athlete, respectively, each with considerable justification.

Track and field also enjoys international prominence by virtue of the biennial World Track and Field championships, as governed by the International Amateur Athletics Federation (IAAF). The IAAF also sponsor an annual world championship that is based on the participation of athletes in a Grand Prix competition circuit, with event venues primarily centered in Europe, where track and field competitions enjoy a considerably greater public following than is the norm in North America. Track and field on an international level has two seasons, the outdoor summer season where competition takes place in large outdoor stadiums, and the winter season, where the events are modified to accommodate the smaller confines of the indoor arenas.

National track and field championships are held in virtually every country of the world on an annual basis. The National Collegiate Athletic Association (NCAA), the governing body for most college and university sports in the United States, sanctions an extensive series of yearly competitions, in both indoor and outdoor formats. With necessary modifications given the nature of athletes who compete in spite of physical or mental disabilities, track and field forms a very important part of both the Summer Paralympic Games, as well as the quadrennial Special Olympics competitions.

Track and field includes all of the events that are designed to take place either on the standard 400-m outdoor track, or on the track infield. The distances that define the Olympic and international track and field events have been calculated exclusively in met-

ric measure since 1976, with the exception of the one-mile race. The disciplines that comprise track and field may be broadly grouped into the running, throwing, and jumping events.

The running events span a significant range of distances, ideal body types, and requisite training approaches. The sprints include the 100 m, 200 m, and 400 m races, as well as 110 m, 200 m, and 400 m hurdles. The sprint relays include the 4 × 100 m, and the 4 × 400 m races, where each runner of the team passes a baton to the next runner within a prescribed passing area on the track. Sprint racing is a combination of tremendous power, an ability to accelerate explosively, coupled with a smooth and efficient stride.

The middle distance events in track and field span the 800 m, the 1,500 m (often referred to as the metric mile), and the 5,000 m events. In these races, speed, especially as it is generated by the runner to deliver a closing "kick" over the final 200 m to 300 m of these races, is of significance. However, pure running speed is one of a combination of talents required of the middle distance runner. The nature of the distances to be run requires that the successful runner combine muscular strength and optimal weight, a proposition known as the strength to weight ratio. For this reason, middle distance runners are generally lighter with a more slender build than that of the powerful sprinters.

The only track and field race that is categorized as a long distance event is the 10,000 m competition. Marathon running is sometimes classed as a track event, as the marathon competition usually begins and ends at the 400-m track in an Olympic competition, with the balance of the race contested over the roads of the host city. The event that is a running event and yet an exception to the other track disciplines is the steeplechase, a 3,000-m race where the athletes are required to negotiate both hurdles and a water jump over the 7.5 lap course.

The various running disciplines of track and field are the subject of continuous changes in the training techniques used by the athletes. The constant refinements in technique lead to incremental improvements in performance. Some of the most notable scientific advances in sport have arisen in the context of track and field competition. As an example, in 1964, at the Tokyo Olympics, electronic timing was first used in track racing at the finish line, replacing the less reliable hand-held stop watch.

The most profound technical developments in track and field centered on the nature of the running

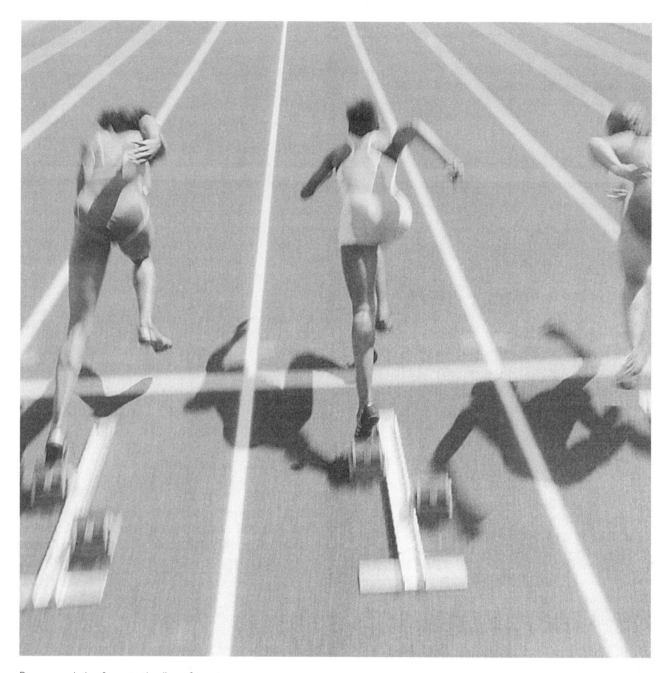

Runners sprinting from starting line of event. © MICHAEL WONG/CORBIS

surface of the track itself. Until the 1960s, most running surfaces used in track and field were composed of cinder, a coal residue, or clay materials. In wet weather, these surfaces were very difficult to maintain. Plastic and rubberized surfaces began to be developed in the 1960s, and the modern tracks used for most national and international competitions are built from a combination of plastic rubber, principally styrene and polyurethane. These composite tracks are resistant to ultraviolet light radiation damage and maintain both their qualities of traction and compression in poor weather. Most importantly to the runner, the plastic composite surface provides a much better return of the runner's energy that is delivered with each stride into the track surface. This rebound effect tends to produce greater running efficiency and faster times.

The throwing competitions in track and field share a number of similarities in both training approaches and the physical type in their respective successful athletes. The discus, the javelin, the shotput, and the hammer throw each place a significant premium on muscular strength and power. Each sport has relatively simple mechanics within which to deliver the requisite object; it is the honing of those mechanical features that ultimately determines competitive success in each of these sports. In simple terms, many athletes can become incredibly strong through weight training, but success in the throwing events comes with a combination of strength and a mastery of the footwork, weight shifts, and release points unique to each discipline.

The jumping events in track and field competition, the high jump, the long jump, the triple jump, and the pole vault, are the most dissimilar among the track and field groupings. While each of the sports requires jumping ability, the body types best suited to each sport and the training required to achieve success in each sport are quite distinct. The high jump, a test of vertical leaping ability and technique, and the long jump, a measure of the furthest horizontal leap, are as simple to perform as any sports that have ever existed. The triple jump, while similar to the long jump in its execution, requires greater attention to the mechanics of the "hop, skip, and jump" routine that is at the heart of a successful jump. The pole vault is the only track and field event where the athletes use an object to assist themselves in self-propulsion.

The pole manufactured for use in the pole vault is another example of sports science development. The first poles used in the Olympics by vaulters were made from bamboo or steel. The modern pole, manufactured from fiberglass and other composite plastics, permits the vaulter to transfer the energy in the speed of the run-up into the lift toward the bar when the pole is planted.

There are two track and field events that encompass the entire range of running, jumping, and throwing. The men's decathlon is a two-day, 10-event competition, including the 100 m, 400 m, 110-m hurdles, and the 1,500 m as its running events. The high jump, long jump, and the pole vault are the jumping events. The shotput, the javelin, and the discus are the decathlon field events. The seven-event women's heptathlon is also contested over two days, with the 100-m hurdles, the high jump, the shotput, and the 200-m race the events of day one; the long jump, the javelin, and the 80-m race are contested on the second day. Each of these competitions demands all-round athletic technical brilliance with strength, speed, and endurance.

Track and field at the highest level is the pursuit of excellence, usually measured by razor-thin margins of distance or time. It was the pursuit of those tiny advantages that led to the widespread use of anabolic steroids and other performance-enhancing substances by a wide range of track and field athletes. The publicity that surrounded the positive steroid test of Canadian sprinter Ben Johnson in the 1988 Olympics served to make the steroid issue a far more important matter to both government and national sports governing bodies than had previously been the case. A large measure of the efforts of the World Anti-Doping Agency (WADA) and its national representative agencies continues to be directed to track and field athletes.

**SEE ALSO** Decathlon; High jump; Pole vaulting; Shotput.

# Trampoline

The trampoline is a gymnastics device, constructed from a very strong, tightly stretched material, attached with springs to a frame. The trampoline was invented by American George Nissen in the period after 1930, when as a 16-year-old he observed circus performers rebounding from their nets after performing an acrobatic stunt. Prior to any athletic applications, trampolines were used by World War II pilots, and later astronauts, to simulate the movement of their bodies in a weightless environment. In recent years, trampolines built for recreational and home use have increased in popularity, both as a recreational device and for fitness training.

Trampoline became a popular part of gymnastics training, and later established itself as a distinct competitive sport. The first world championship in Trampoline was held in 1964. Trampoline competition made its debut as an Olympic sport in the 2004 Summer Games; the sport is governed under the international umbrella of FIG, the Federation Internationale de Gymnastiques, where trampoline is a separate division of the gymnastics competition, along with artistic and rhythmic gymnastics.

Trampoline is organized as an individual competition. The trampolinists are required to execute a number of pre-determined movements in each routine, with no set time limit prescribed within which to perform. Competitors generate sufficient height from the surface of the trampoline within which they perform somersaults, flips, and other movements where they are subjectively judged on their technical execution of each movement and their presentation.

Trampoline has acquired a reputation as one of the more dangerous sports available, especially among young people. Most trampoline accidents arise where there is either a lack of supervision over young people using the device, or where a trampolinist lands on the supporting framework to the trampoline and not the landing area within the trampoline. The trampoline poses special risks of young persons under the age of 15, given the stresses of landing on a musculoskeletal structure that is not fully mature.

In addition to the aesthetic qualities of Olympic styled trampoline competition, the trampoline has a number of positive physical training benefits. The actions associated with bounding from the trampoline surface are a form of resistance exercise, meaning that the musculoskeletal structures associated with the bounding motion are subjected to weight bearing stress that tends to strengthen the human frame. Various studies have determined that a persons exercising upon a trampoline uses approximately 15% more energy per minute than does a runner.

The trampoline and its associated exercises are also useful tools to develop better balance and proprioception (muscle memory). As the athlete is both rising and falling in a bounding movement, they are weightless. In this state the athlete can practice different body positions and thus condition the body to move instinctively through the course of a rehearsed routine. Athletes who participate in gymnastics vaulting, aerial skiing, ski jumping, and snow boarding all use the trampoline as a part of their training programs for this reason.

**SEE ALSO** Balance training and proprioception; Gymnastics; Gymnastics landing forces.

# Treadmills

A treadmill is a stationary exercise machine designed to promote cardiovascular fitness and leg strength. Treadmills are commercially available in a number of different designs, all of which accommodate both walking and running at a variety of speeds. The stair climbing machines, often referred to by the Stairmaster trade name, are similar in their training purpose to the treadmill, as each provides for continuous forward motion.

Treadmills were first developed in the 1800s as a means of producing power; animals were employed on treadmills to power grain threshing machines and other agricultural equipment. The first treadmill designed for an athletic purpose was built in the early 1950s in the United States, so that medical doctors could perform accurate heart monitoring on patients with known cardiovascular problems. Modern treadmills and stationary exercise bicycles are the most common method for performing electrocardiogram (ECG) and blood-pressure testing on persons at risk for heart disease.

A treadmill is typically constructed with a set of rollers or other repetitive motion devices overlaid with a rubber compound running surface. The modern treadmill is equipped with a computerized digital screen and various monitors that display the controls that govern the speed and the incline or decline of the running surface. Most treadmill control mechanisms are compatible with various brands of heart monitors and biofeedback devices, which permit the treadmill users to obtain a comprehensive reading as to their workout quality. It is for this reason that the highly controlled exercise obtainable through a treadmill is very useful for persons with a predetermined cardiovascular condition, where the user can operate the device at a rate consistent with a known safe limit.

The treadmill is not a low impact exerciser in the fashion of an elliptical machine or a stationary bicycle, in that the running motion performed on a treadmill is identical to that of an athlete running anywhere. The surface of the treadmill, as a rubber construction, is often more forgiving than that of the roads used by distance runners, but there will be significant forces directed into the lower legs and feet in a treadmill running session.

More sophisticated treadmill models will permit both the significant adjustment of the ramp elevation on which the user runs, as well as a reverse motion, which permits forms of running training. Reverse action on any stationary machine is most effective in maintaining the proper distribution of muscle power between the quadriceps and the hamstrings of the upper leg; an imbalance in their typical optimal ratio of quadriceps to hamstring, 3:2, is a primary factor in the cause of muscle pulls and strains in these structures.

Stair climbing machines are often used by persons seeking general cardiovascular fitness benefits as well as a more specific cross training effect. Stair climbers are built with similar computerized control equipment to those provided on treadmill machines, permitting the user to vary the speed and the intensity of each workout. Stair climbers also have a reverse motion available in their operation, for the same benefits as created by the treadmill reverse feature. Other than the day-to-day act of climbing a

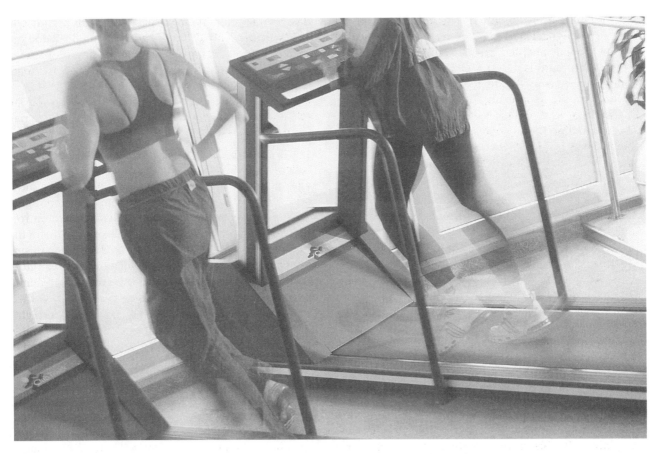

Exercising on a treadmill can be good cardiovascular exercise and is an alternative to running outdoors. © PETER BARRETT/CORBIS

set of stairs, the stair climbing machine does not replicate the movements of any particular sport.

The chief distinction between the treadmill and the stair climber is the true low impact nature of the stair climber exercises. On a stair climber, the contact between the user's foot and the machine is constant, limiting the impact directed into the foot and leg to those of the force generated in the climbing motion. On all such devices, hand rails are constructed along the area where the user is positioned to perform the exercises. The most demanding workouts on both a treadmill and a stair climber are those where the user does not hold the handrail during exercise. The less external balance provided to the user by the rigid machine, the more reliance that the user must place upon the abdominal, lumbar (low back), and groin muscles to maintain balance. The development of these muscle and tissue structures is the building of the core strength of the athlete. Both stair climbers and treadmills provide a beneficial resistance training effect for the musculoskeletal structure of the legs, hips, and pelvis.

There are differences in the fitness benefits obtained between running outdoors and a treadmill workout. All other factors being equal, a runner exercising outdoors will expend a greater amount of energy than a similarly situated athlete on an indoor treadmill. The treadmill, in a controlled, indoor environment, eliminates external factors such as cold air and wind resistance. For an outdoor runner, wind resistance may account for up to 5% of the energy expended by the runner. The treadmill runner derives a benefit from the manner in which the machine operates, as the rotating motion of the treadmill will pull the runner's feet slightly backwards with every stride, reducing the energy the runner requires to push off the running surface with each step. At greater running speeds, the outdoor runner will expend as much as 9% more energy than the treadmill runner.

For runners who desire a controlled environment, either for health reasons or to avoid adverse environmental conditions, the treadmill and the stair climber are excellent cardiovascular options.

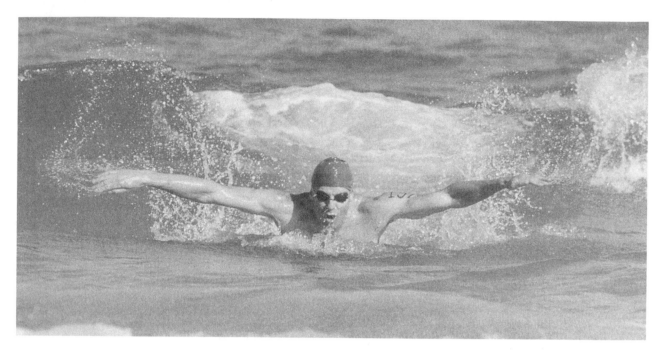

Tri-athlete in the waves. © RICK GOMEZ/CORBIS

**SEE ALSO** Cross training; Fitness; Health; Stationary bicycles, elliptical trainers, and other cardio training machines.

# Triathlon

While three sport athletic competitions had been held prior to the 1970s, the first triathlon that included a sequence of swim, bicycle, and run events over set distances took place in Mission Bay, California, in 1974. With its easy access to the Pacific Ocean and excellent bicycling opportunities, the Mission Bay event had grown as a natural extension from the local athletic training scene. The triathlon became a fast-growing international sport, especially after the longest of the triathlon-styled events, the Hawaii Ironman, achieved international prominence in the early 1980s.

The ever-expanding number of races spurred the growth of a corresponding triathlon bureaucracy. The sport's governing body in the United States, USA Triathlon, was founded in 1982, with the corresponding international federation, the International Triathlon Union (ITU), formed in 1989. The world wide popularity of the triathlon was confirmed when the sport was made an Olympic event for both men and women in 2000. The ITU has over 150 nations as members, and hundreds of participatory as well as elite-level triathlon competitions are held annually throughout the world.

The basic swim/bike/run pattern is essential to the triathlon; there are five recognized distance formats used in official triathlon competitions. The swim portion is contested over an open body of water, and the cycling and running sections utilize open roads or, less frequently in the run stage, cross-country courses. The first type of triathlon is more informal, an introductory level race where each of the three segments are short, so as to encourage participation in the sport. Introductory level triathlon events are sometimes held in conjunction with a longer-sanctioned triathlon competition. A typical entry level triathlon will consist of race segments comprised of a 250-yd swim (250 m), a 5-mi (8 km) bicycle segment, and a 2-mi (3 km) run.

The remaining four triathlon distances are sanctioned by the ITU and each is subject to the ITU rules regarding the nature of the race course in each segment and other similar regulations. The sprint triathlon is a 0.5-mi swim (800 m), a 13-mi cycle (21 km), and a 3.2-mi run (5 km). Sprint triathlons are attractive to athletes both as a progression from an introductory triathlon, as well as a training mechanism for more advanced competitors in which to work on their speed in each segment. The Olympic triathlon is the most popular international format, representing the standards used at the Olympic

Games; it is a 0.9 mi swim (1.5 km), 24.8 mi cycle (40 km), and a 6.2 mi run (10 km).

The longest of the triathlon competitions are the Ironman events, which take their name from the original Hawaii Ironman competition. The full Ironman competition is a grueling 2.4 mile (4 km) swim, 112 mile (180 km) cycle, and a marathon run of 26.2 miles (42.2 km). Where the Ironman originated, on the big island of Hawaii, the heat and prevailing winds are as demanding an environmental factor as a triathlete would ever likely face. The half Ironman event is precisely 50% the length of the Ironman: 1.2 mile (2 km) swim, 56 mile (90 km) bike, and 13.1 mile (21 km) run.

Triathlon training is limited by fitness level, not age or gender. While an elite triathlete is usually very strong in one of the disciplines (most commonly, swimming, the most technically demanding of the three sports, where 70% of all ITU champions had their competitive sports background), successful triathlon participation will be built primarily on an understanding of the principles of cross training. Triathlon training will combine the development of muscle balance, as all musculoskeletal groups within the body must function optimally.

Implicit in effective triathlon cross training will be the enhancement of the flexibility of the joints and muscles through a focused and consistent stretching program. The majority of injuries sustained in triathlon are overuse or repetitive strain injuries, particularly in the legs and shoulders, given the nature of the triathlon's three components. Effective and consistent stretching, and a corresponding greater range of motion, serve to protect from overuse conditions to a degree; strains and other minor muscle or tendon ailments are a natural risk of the sport.

With the rise in the international popularity of the triathlon, there have been a number of sport-specific technological developments designed to increase athletic performance. In 1984, the Timex Ironman, a relatively inexpensive and durable timepiece, was created to assist the triathlete in the digital management of the split times in all three segments of the race, coupled with elapsed time capability. Hydrodynamic neoprene wetsuits were also developed to provide both additional buoyancy to the athlete (within permitted ITU regulation), as well as reducing the effect of drag created by the water on the swimmer. These suits are also built with closures to permit the swimmers to make a speedy exit from the suit as they prepared to proceed to the cycling portion in the transition area.

The triathlon also sparked changes in the design of bicycles built for triathlon racing. The high mounted seat and lowered handlebars of the "tri bikes," with the addition of aerodynamic extensions from the bars, permit the cyclist to take an extremely low and aerodynamic position on the road. With gear shifts mounted at the end of the extension, the rider is not required to change body position as often during the course of the race. The rider gains the additional advantage of being able to rest the upper body against the longer handle bars, a significant benefit to the athlete after the conclusion of the swim portion and the resulting demands on the upper body.

**SEE ALSO** Cross training; Cycling; Environmental conditions and training; Ironman competitions.

# Triathlon: Exercises for triathlon

Like the decathlon and the heptathlon, the triathlon represents an ultimate cross training, multidisciplinary challenge for the athlete. The individual triathlon segments of swimming, cycling, and running each present distinct training issues: swimming requires strength, endurance, and an adherence to proper, efficient technique; cycling also demands efficient form and stamina; and running training will be directed to optimal stride, running form, and cardiovascular fitness. Integrated with these macro-training features will be triathlon-specific race training, such as interval training in each discipline, and hill workouts necessary for cycling and running success.

It is the nature of the sport that every part of the musculoskeletal system must be trained if the athlete is to be a successful triathlete. In the Olympic distance, the most popular of triathlon competitions, the 1.5-km (1 mile) swim, 40-km (24 mile) cycle, and the 10-km (6.2 mile) run are relatively equal in their relative importance to overall race success. The training time devoted to each event at a base level should also be equal, subject to the preexistence of a greater level of ability or training in one or more of the events.

The demands of the three triathlon events creates the ultimate training requirement to develop each of the foundation parts of total fitness: speed, power, endurance, flexibility, and strength. Exercises that integrate more than one of these components will be an asset to the triathlete.

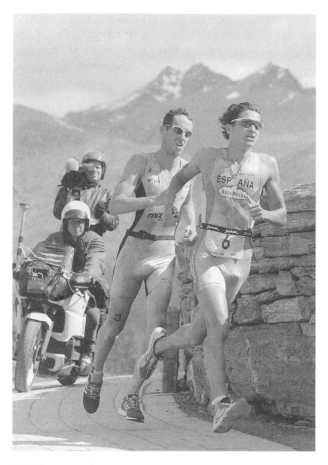

Triathlon competitors. PHOTO BY BARRY HARCOURT/GETTY IMAGES.

Much of triathlon training will be directed to the three principle activities. The training exercises must support the athlete with respect to the development of the basic parts within each event, but in the advancement of the athlete's overall abilities. A fundamental aspect of the training in each event segment is that of overload, the universal sports training theory that an athlete must do more training than he or she may expect to face in competition. The cycling training is an example of how overload principles apply to the triathlon. Triathletes will not train to finish 40-km on the cycle portion; they will train to finish the 40-km course in a physical condition that they may easily move to the next segment, without undue fatigue. The overload can be accomplished in two ways: the triathlete will organize a training program where distances in excess of 40-km are easily covered in single training sessions, coupled with weekly or monthly mileage totals that build significantly greater endurance over time.

The second of the fundamental approaches to triathlon exercises will be the development of max-imum flexibility and corresponding range of motion in each joint. The triathlete can utilize specific exercises drawn from basic calisthenics stretches to ensure the proper extension of the working tissues, coupled with flexibility-enhancing stretch routines common to yoga and gymnastics. The shoulder is an example of the importance to enhanced joint flexibility in triathlon. In the swim, the triathlete will be using the shoulder in a rotational motion to power through the water. During the cycling portion, the shoulder will assume a relatively rigid position, absorbing the forces of the road through the handlebars and upper body. In the 10-km run, the shoulders are part of the balancing mechanism needed to offset the power of the legs driving forward. Exercises that put the shoulder through the full range of those anticipated motions will assist in triathlon performance.

The third fundamental is the development of training intensity. Intensity will be a factor in both the event training as well as general strength, training, and flexibility sessions. Interval training, which can occur in swimming, cycling and running training, is an excellent intensity developer. It is impossible for an athlete in any sport, particularly one as demanding as the triathlon, to continually train at a lesser intensity level and compete at a higher intensity level. The enhancement of physiological qualities such as oxygen uptake, the ability of the body to process oxygen efficiently (expressed as $VO_2max$), require periods of maximum training intensity.

Much of the event training in the triathlon is geared to the overall development of the triathlete's aerobic fitness. However, there are a number of instances in a triathlon where anaerobic fitness, in support of the ability to surge or sprint, is of critical importance. The start of the swim, often in a mass start, with hundreds of swimmers attempting to get away quickly, is an example of where sprinting speed is important. To be able to sprint up hills on the bicycle or to finish the run section with a kick are also examples of anaerobic fitness requirements. Hill-training on both foot and bicycle and the swimming of 100 m to 200 m repeats both develop this capability in each of the three competition segments.

Weight training or other resistance training is an essential component to a well-rounded triathlon program. While the swim portion requires a measure of upper body strength, it is the maintenance of an optimal strength to weight ratio that will best assist the athlete, the balancing of the desired amount of mass versus the requisite power and necessary energy to move the body efficiently. In both cycling and running, the development of the athlete's core strength, the capacity of the interconnected muscles of the gluteal (buttocks), abdomen, groin, and upper legs will assist in the provision of both balance and stability in movement. Circuit weight training—emphasizing sets comprising a high number of repetitions using lighter weights—tends to achieve the desired balance, as does vigorous Swiss ball workouts, which combine the resistance of the ball and stretches of these muscle groups through exercises such as abdominal crunches and extensions.

A training exercise unique to triathlon competitions is that of transition, where the triathlete practices the steps necessary to transform from swimmer to cyclist, and from cyclist to runner. Each of these transitions requires the triathlete to change or remove clothing and footwear in a designated area known as the transition area. The competitor's time to complete a triathlon begins when the swim race portion commences, and ends when the triathlete crosses the run course finish line; all time in transition is counted, and the faster the competitor can move through the transition stages, the more efficient the athlete shall be. Triathletes will specifically rehearse how they will move from one event to another, with all requisite equipment carefully organized at the transition station for ease of access. Modern triathlon clothing such as wetsuits and cycling clothing has been designed to be removed with greater ease for this reason.

SEE ALSO Cross training; Cycling strength training and exercises; Ironman competitions; Running strength training and exercises; Swimming.

# Tribulus

The puncture vine is the green climbing plant known as tribulus, the abbreviated form of its botanical name, *Tribulus terrestris*, a leafy green climbing plant that grows in various parts of the United States, as well as in warm weather climates such as those of India and Sri Lanka. The tribulus is regarded as a noxious weed for agricultural purposes in most U.S. states.

Tribulus, or its regional variations, has been held in high regard in the ancient medical practices of India (where the herb is known as Gokshura in the Ayurveda holistic medical teachings) and the traditional Chinese medicines for many centuries. In both cultures, tribulus leaves were valued for their use in herbal formulations and tonics for the purpose of elevating mood, as well as to ease the discomfort caused to the digestive and urinary tracts by conditions such as colic. Tribulus was also believed to act as a remedy for male impotence in both cultures, as well working as an agent to alleviate the symptoms of menopause in women.

It is the connection believed to exist between the ingestion of tribulus and the increase in male sexual potency that has fueled a more recent interest in tribulus as a weight training supplement. The active chemical ingredient contained in the leaf of the tribulus plant is steroidal saponins, also known as furostanol. There has been a significant analysis of this chemical with respect to its impact, if any, on increased levels of testosterone within the body. Testosterone, the male sex hormone, is a key regulator of many important functions within the body, including the formation, development, and maintenance of muscle mass. Taken as a freestanding supplement to build greater strength, testosterone is a banned performance-enhancing substance in almost all international athletic competitions. Testosterone, when ingested as a training supplement, is classed as an illegal anabolic steroid by the World Anti-Doping Agency (WADA), given its muscle-building properties.

Tribulus and its active ingredient furostanol are not anabolic substances, as tribulus itself does not directly affect the growth of human muscle. The tribulus research has been focused on the relationship between tribulus ingestion and its impact on the chemical that occurs naturally in the human body, the luteinizing hormone (LH). LH plays an important role in the regulation and maintenance of testosterone levels in the body, which provided the theoretical basis for the proposition that a positive impact by tribulus on LH might itself increase levels of testosterone production. There has not been any conclusive scientific research to support the proposition that tribulus consumption will definitively increase testosterone production within the body. The chief difficulty with any determination that tribulus consumption raises testosterone levels is connected to the fact that all exercise will temporarily increase the production of testosterone. It is therefore difficult to scientifically differentiate between the purported effect of tribulus and the known effect of the exercise.

Tribulus adherents believe that the herb functions within the body in a similar fashion to that of creatine, in the sense that each substance acts as an agent that works to stimulate or precipitate a positive physiological effect in training, without acting directly on the targeted body system. No side effects have been identified in research with respect to tribulus usage. Many bodybuilders and strength athletes consume tribulus in a formulation known as a "stack," where it is believed that a number of supplements, taken together, will produce a beneficial effect where the sum is greater than its constituent parts. A well-regarded stack in the strength training community consisted of tribulus, DHEA (dehydroepiandosterone, a hormone-building raw material within the body), and androstenedione (or andro, a substance known as a prohormone, and one which will be converted into testosterone within the body, a muscle-building supplement). Andro was proven to cause significant side effects among its users, including cardiovascular problems, and it has somewhat fallen from favor in the strength training and fitness community.

Persons engaged in strength training who use tribulus are now more likely to stack tribulus with a mineral supplement known by the acronym ZMA, a compound that is commercially available in several formulations. The most popular ZMA mixture is generally constituted with zinc, magnesium, and vitamin B-6; zinc is a component of over 3,000 different proteins within the body, and magnesium is essential to both nervous system function and bone formation. The popularity of this tribulus stack is rooted in word-of-mouth endorsements from users than it is supported by hard science. There are few side effects that have been identified from the use of the combination of tribulus and ZMA.

**SEE ALSO** Dietary supplements; Ephedra; Herbs; Muscle mass and strength; Strength training.

# Triple jump

The triple jump is one of the most exacting and physically demanding of the field events in modern track and field competition. The triple jump has been a part of the modern Olympics since its inception in 1896, and it has also been a part of the competitions sanctioned by organizations such as the International Amateur Athletics Federation (IAAF) and the National Collegiate Athletic Association (NCAA) of the United States. As with many sports that form the broader world of athletics, the triple jump does not enjoy a significant public appeal except at a world championship or at the Olympic Games.

The triple jump is also known by the simple expression that defines the mechanics of the sport,

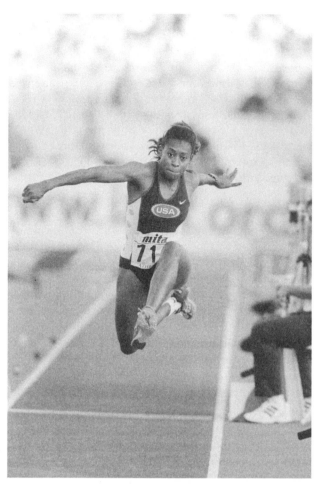

The triple jump is also known by the simple expression, the "hop, step, and jump." © JEAN-YVES RUSZNIEWSKI; TEMPSPORT/ CORBIS

the "hop, step, and jump." The object of the sport is to travel the furthest along a straight line that begins at a defined takeoff board, culminating with a landing in a jumping pit, using the hop, step, and jump footwork pattern of the sport. The successful triple jumper must seamlessly mesh the distinct physical attributes of running speed, strength, and explosive jumping capability, and a well-developed sense of balance and coordination. For this reason, triple jump training exercises are employed to develop a wide range of athletic skills.

The triple jump is divided into four distinct phases for training and coaching purposes; these phases are the approach, the hop, the step, and the jump. In the approach, the athlete seeks to develop as much speed as possible, much as a long jumper will sprint with maximum power to spring from the jump. As with the long jump, the athlete must make the initial movement from behind a predetermined mark, typically a takeoff board.

The second phase begins with the athlete making a hop as a takeoff. The jumper will maximize lift in the hop through the full extension of the takeoff leg, followed by a powerful drive through the air with the second leg. Much of the focus in triple jump coaching and training is the precise coordination of this movement; the more supple and smooth the takeoff, the greater the amount of approach energy directed into the hop. The athlete will also seek to be as streamlined in the air as is possible, with the legs positioned as nearly one behind the other in flight as is possible to emphasize maximum forward movement and to reduce drag.

The landing of the hop phase is the essential linkage to the step phase. The athlete will seek to drive the landing leg on the hop downward with force, to create a steady landing and to ensure the maximum return of energy to the landing foot from the ground that will power the step phase. As the athlete enters the step, there is again a powerful drive forward with the planted leg and a corresponding stride in the air with the second leg. The second leg will be the landing leg to provide a takeoff for the jump phase. To create an effective jumping lever, the athlete will extend this lead foot as far forward as is possible.

The jump phase commences with the takeoff leg being extended by the athlete as forcefully as possible, accompanied by a drive with the second leg forward to the waist height of the jumper. This movement is designed to ensure a maximum forward thrust of the body as the jump continues into the landing area. In a coordinated motion, the jumper will seek to drive the arms forward and upward, with the legs positioned in a seeming kneeling position in the air. As the athlete prepares to complete the jump, the arm and the legs simultaneously drive forward, with the hips elevated as far as possible.

Triple jumping is a sport where there is an increased importance in the core strength, the body's ability to balance the action of the muscles of the abdomen, gluteal (buttock), lumbar region (low back), groin, and upper legs. The weight training typically used to develop the core strength of a triple jumper includes shoulder presses, abdominal crunches, and squats. Plyometrics and bounding drills are essential to develop leg strength as well as the explosiveness required in the approaches and takeoffs between each triple jump phase. It is not uncommon for a male triple jumper to possess a vertical jump exceeding 30 in (0.7 m).

Effective triple jump drills will also emphasize the rhythm necessary to coordinate the four phases of the sport. Exercises that incorporate continuous hops or bounding in various sequences achieve this end.

SEE ALSO Cross training; Muscle fibers: Fast and slow twitch; Plyometrics; Stretching and flexibility.

# Two-a-day practice sessions

The two-a-day practice session is a part of both the folklore and the reality of American football training camps. It is a regimen and a rite of passage imposed on players competing at the high school level through to the professionals of the National Football League. At every competitive level, the American football season begins in September. Given the intensely physical nature of the sport and the technical demands of integrating distinct positions into a team concept, it is common for the preseason practices to provide both training volume and training intensity, all of which tends to occur in the warm weather months of July and August. Two-a-day practice sessions are designed to achieve those sometimes disparate training objectives.

The purpose of the two-a-day practice must first be considered with respect to the larger concept of season planning, known as the periodization of training. All competitive teams and individual athletes cannot train at a constant maximum level for an entire calendar year; the athlete and the team perform best when they are trained to peak for certain periods during the year, with an appropriate build-up to the peak performance, and a recovery and rebuilding phase to follow.

To properly account for the physical demands of American football, a properly periodized training schedule for a football team will consist of three general subdivisions: the preseason, the competitive season, and the off-season. Each of these segments will be further subdivided to address specific training or competitive issues that are anticipated to arise within each individual training period. As an example, an American college football team will commence its competitive season on approximately September 1 of a given year; the team may have aspirations of playing in a season-ending championship game in late December or early January, a competitive period of approximately four months. Once the season is completed, the players will be encouraged to reduce the level of their physical activities for four to six weeks to permit physical recovery. The players will then be expected to begin ever-increasing weight training and running workouts in preparation for spring practice in May. The players would return to individual weight and running workouts in the summer, to commence the preseason two-a-days in early August, with a new season beginning in September. The lead-up to the beginning of the two-a-day workouts would include a period of acclimatization to any expected warm weather conditions at the practices.

Heat acclimatization is usually achieved for an individual player within 10 to 14 days of commencement of the player's exposure to unaccustomed warm weather conditions. If plotted on a graph, the training periods would reflect both the amount of time and the intensity to be devoted to each workout segment.

With proper periodization of training, one of the key dangers of two-a-day football practices is reduced: the dramatically increased risk of injury due to improper conditioning leading up to the commencement of such practices. The second danger, a failure on the part of both athletes and coaching staff to ensure the proper hydration of the athletes during practices, is also one that may be minimized, if not prevented, through adherence to basic hydration principles. It is essential that the athletes engaged in such vigorous exercise be encouraged to consume water or appropriate sport drinks before, during, and after practice. The body's thermoregulation system is constructed in such a fashion that the thirst mechanism, located in the hypothalamus region of the brain, is activated after the body has become dehydrated. Encouraging athletes to consume fluids even where they are not thirsty combats this mechanism. The death of Minnesota Vikings football lineman Kory Stringer in 2003 at a two-a-day practice session as a result of heat stroke served as a warning to all teams conducting any type of warm weather training.

As a general rule, water, water with sodium or other electrolytes added, or sports drinks with a maximum of 6% to 8% carbohydrate are the most effective fluid replacement products in two-a-day practice environments. Sport drinks with greater than 8% carbohydrate tend to be absorbed more slowly in the body through the small intestine. The consumption of caffeine or alcohol during or after the practice period will contribute to dehydration as each of these substances acts as a diuretic, creating additional urine production and fluid loss. Urine color is a useful indicator as to whether the body is properly hydrated; light yellow urine is an indicator of proper fluid levels, and dark-colored urine is a symptom of dehydration, as the urine is overly concentrated.

The total amount of fluid to be consumed as a part of a sound hydration strategy at a two-a-day practice schedule will vary from person to person. As a general rule of thumb, most players should consume between 28 oz (800 ml) and 40 oz (1.3 l) of fluids for every hour they are involved in a practice or a game in the course of such workouts. Two-a-day workout effects are also reduced if the players have access to a cool area between practices, where they can reduce their body temperatures.

Two-a-day practices are not unique to American football; many endurance athletes, such as marathoners and triathletes, will train twice a day. Sports that are popular in warm weather countries, such as soccer, cricket, and rugby, will engage similar training issues. The football two-a-day in American football is of particular interest, given the inherent combination of intense physical contact, overall exertion on the part of the athletes, and warm weather environments.

**SEE ALSO** Acclimatization; Heat exhaustion; Hydration; Warm weather exercise.

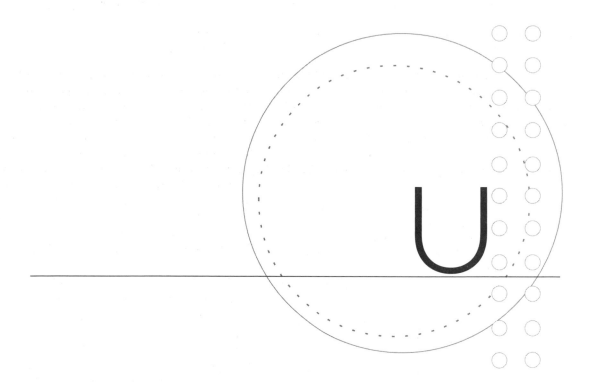

# U.S. Anti-Doping Agency (USADA)

The U.S Anti-Doping Agency (USADA) was formed in October 2000, as a part of a concerted worldwide effort to combat drug cheating, popularly known in sport as "doping." The founding of the USADA was of acute importance to the credibility of drug testing and enforcement mechanisms in the United States, as the international sport community had been vocal concerning the perceived lack of interest in American sport to police the use of steroids and similar performance-enhancing products.

The USADA is legally associated to the World Anti-Doping Agency (WADA), through the WADA Anti-Doping Code, to which the United States Olympic Committee (USOC) is a signatory. Through this relationship, it is the stated mission of the USADA to preserve the well-being of Olympic sport. The USADA seeks to advance this mission on four separate bases: research, education, the conduct of doping tests (both in-competition and out-of-competition), and the provision of an adjudication system, where disputes as to the outcome of a particular test may be arbitrated on the model provided by the Court of Arbitration for Sport (CAS). From October 2000, the USADA has possessed the full authority to regulate all aspects of the United States Anti-Doping programs.

In its most visible function, the conduct of doping tests, the USADA conducted 8,175 tests in 2005, of which almost 5,000 were a part of the USADA's comprehensive out-of-competition testing program. Most out-of-competition tests were conducted at either the home or the training facility of the athlete. All such tests were conducted in accordance with the protocols developed by WADA. Approximately 25% of the out-of-competition testing was performed as a lead-up to the 2006 Winter Olympics in Turin. Most of the testing conducted was with respect to American athletes; the USADA also conducted tests at the request of other national anti-doping agencies or WADA. Of the tests conducted, 22 produced a positive result—either directly determined through scientific analysis or through the refusal of the athlete to provide a sample—resulting in a deemed positive result.

The second most prominent aspect of the work of the USADA is the research that it funds into new or improved methods of performance-enhancing substance detection. Two recent projects have included the refinement of a steroid-detecting technology, a gas chromatography/combustion/isotope ratio mass spectrometry, and the development of a marker for the enhanced detection of the presence of a synthetic human growth hormone (hGH) in bodily fluid test samples.

The USADA mandate extends to United States Olympic team athletes, athletes who are seeking a place on the Olympic team, athletes participating in the Pan American Games, and athletes who are a part of the quadrennial Paralympics teams. The other prominent aspects of the American sports landscape, such as the National Football League (NFL), the

National Basketball Association (NBA), Major League Baseball (MLB), or the National Collegiate Athletic Association (NCAA), each provide for their own anti-doping procedures, to which the USADA is not necessarily a party.

The most high profile illegal substance case in which the USADA has been involved did not involve any tests conducted by the organization. In 2003, an anonymous party forwarded a used syringe to the USADA that was subsequently determined to contain the so-called designer steroid nandrolone, a steroid formulation that had been distributed by the San Francisco-based athletic supplement company, the Bay Area Laboratory Cooperative (BALCO). The investigation conducted by the USADA linked a number of prominent American athletes to the illegal use of this anabolic steroid.

As an agency with a direct relationship to WADA, the USADA has endorsed the principle that the defense of "mistake," as it may be advanced by an athlete in a positive doping test scenario, will be difficult to maintain. The "I didn't know" has been routinely dismissed by WADA as a legitimate answer to a positive test since the late 1990s. The 2006 case of American skeleton racer Zach Lund tested this issue. Lund tested positive for the presence of a drug known as finasteride, a substance contained in a hair restoration formulation used by Lund for a number of years. In 2005, finasteride was added to the WADA Prohibited List, rendering it a banned substance; finasteride is often employed as a steroid-masking agent. After Lund was initially suspended by the FIBT, the international federation that governs bobsled and skeleton racing, he appealed to the USADA to permit his reinstatement to the American Winter Olympics team for 2006. The USADA took the unusual step of warning Lund, as opposed to imposing a suspension from international competition. WADA appealed the USADA decision to the CAS, which handed Lund a one-year suspension, while criticizing WADA for the manner in which finasteride appeared on the Prohibited List.

**SEE ALSO** Doping tests; International Olympic Committee (IOC); Prohibited substances (competition bans); World Anti-Doping Agency (WADA).

# United States Olympic Committee (USOC)

Baron Pierre de Coubertin of France announced his plans to revive the Olympic Games in 1892, with a projected date for the staging of the first modern Games in the summer of 1896. The International Olympic Committee (IOC) was created in 1894 to lead the organization of the Games. As countries around the world came to embrace the notion of an international sports festival, national organizations within the participating Olympic nations were created to advance the Olympic dream in their respective countries. The American Olympic Committee (later known as the United States Olympic Committee, or USOC) was founded in 1894. The future USOC was the American product of this initial revivalist effort, and the USOC has remained the official voice of the Olympic movement in the United States since that time.

The IOC is the ultimate authority in all matters pertaining to the conduct of both the Summer and Winter Olympic Games. Although the IOC is the ultimate authority in all aspects of the governance of the Olympic Games, the structure of Olympic administration is best understood as a series of concentric rings of authority emanating outward from the IOC, with each successive outward circle representing the national Olympic committees, the Olympic Games organizing committees, and the international federations responsible for every individual Olympic sport. National committees such as the USOC have a measure of influence in the overall conduct of the affairs of the IOC.

In its role as the official representative of the Olympic movement in the United States, the USOC seeks to provide leadership and guidance to athletes, sports organizations, and the public at large regarding Olympic competition. The USOC is bound by the principles enunciated in the Olympic Charter, which stress the role of sport in the advancement of a peaceful world, emphasizing friendship, solidarity, and fair play in international sport. The USOC operates a number of training centers throughout the United States, chiefly those located at Colorado Springs, Colorado, Lake Placid, New York, and Chula Vista, California.

The most notable member of the USOC to occupy a position of influence in the IOC was Avery Brundage (1887–1975), elected to the IOC in 1936, and assuming its presidency from 1952 to 1972. Brundage is the only American ever to preside over the IOC. Brundage was famed for his many pronouncements regarding the role of professional athletes within the Olympic movement. He was a lifelong opponent of any form of Olympic professionalism. It was Brundage who determined that the 1972 Summer Games competitions in Munich would continue notwithstanding the terrorist capture in the Olympic Village and the subsequent murder of 11 Israeli athletes, a decision that remains controversial today.

An example of the nature of the leadership lent to American sport in general by the USOC is the 2005 publication of its comprehensive *Coaching Code of Ethics*. This document emphasizes the overarching coaching principles of competence, integrity, and professional responsibility. The Code develops the notion of "responsible coaching" in the context of respect for all participants, the elimination of harassment in all of its forms, and an understanding of the potential negative influence that poor coaching may have on impressionable athletes.

The USOC *Coaching Code of Ethics* makes particular reference to the obligation of coaches to seek drug-free sport. It is this issue that caused the USOC particular difficulty in terms of the international reputation of American sports in the late 1980s and early 1990s. In the period between scandals created at the 1988 Summer Olympics when Canadian sprinter Ben Johnson tested positive for the steroid stanozolol and the creation of the World Anti-Doping Agency (WADA) in the late 1990s, the USOC administered the Olympic drug-detection program. The USOC was widely criticized for its maintenance of an ineffective anti-doping program. Dr. Wade Exum of the USOC, who was responsible for the direction of the program, was terminated from his position in 2001. Exum revealed at that time that the USOC had recorded 18 positive drug tests among its tested athletes between 1984 and 2000, but it had not published the names of these athletes nor had the USOC imposed any sanctions regarding the participation of the offending athletes in international competition. The positive tests ranged from the presence of stimulants such as ephedrine, as well as banned steroids. These athletes were permitted by the USOC to participate in the Olympics; Carl Lewis, gold medalist in the 1988 Olympics 100 m, was among those that tested positive.

Since 2000, with the creation of the international anti-doping strategy that is headed by WADA, the national anti-doping agencies work with their respective Olympic committees to advance the goal of drug-free sport. The United States Anti-Doping Agency (USADA) performs that function in the United States, providing information to the USOC of relevance to selection of athletes.

SEE ALSO International federations; International Olympic Committee (IOC); Prohibited substances (competition bans); U.S. Anti-Doping Agency (USADA).

# Upper respiratory tract infection

Upper respiratory tract infections (URTIs) are defined as non-specific infections of the breathing mechanism of the body. The upper respiratory tract includes the nose, mouth, sinus, throat, and the upper portion of the bronchial passages that lead to the lungs.

The respiratory tract is a common location for the entry of pathogens by way of airborne microorganisms. It is estimated that as many as 10,000 such foreign bodies enter the body in this fashion each day. Most of these organisms are trapped by the immune system's first line of defense, the layer of sticky mucus that lines the interior of the nasal and throat passages. Most of the particles are stuck to the mucus layer, and ultimately swallowed and destroyed in the stomach.

The second line of defense in the immune system located in the upper respiratory system are the adenoids and the tonsils. Positioned at the back of the throat between the nasal passages and the larynx, these small organs are a part of the lymphatic system, designed to protect the body from harmful organisms by trapping any such bodies that pass over them. URTIs generally occur when either bacteria are able to bypass the immune system defenses, or by airborne virus.

The most frequent of URTIs is the common cold, which is transmitted by way of viruses that are spread from person to person, with a greater frequency in the winter months. The typical adult person in North America will develop between two and four colds in the course of a year. The most severe form of these viruses is influenza, which can cause significant communitywide health problems. Nasal congestion, sneezing, a sore throat, and a generalized feeling of weakness are the most frequent symptoms of the common cold. Although a cold by itself is rarely a completely debilitating event, the negative effect of a cold on athletic performance can be dramatic.

The mouth may be the means by which a cold virus enters the body. The URTIs that affect the mouth specifically are trench mouth (a very painful and progressive infection of the lining of the mouth and throat) and herpes simplex type 1 (an infection that causes lesions and sores inside the mouth). This condition is unrelated to herpes simplex type 2, a sexually transmitted disease.

Pharyngitis is the term that includes a broad range of infections of the throat. The sore throat is a condition linked to the presence of a common cold. Because the condition is viral in nature, the sore throat cannot be eradicated in the body through antibiotics, which are only effective against bacteria-based conditions. The bacterial agent that does cause a serious throat infection is the streptococcal organism, the precipitator of strep throat. Strep throat is a progressive condition usually accompanied by fever and significant headaches.

Infections can also attack other specific locations with in the upper respiratory tract. The most common of these are sinusitis, laryngitis, and tonsillitis. Sinusitis is an infection that presents itself with symptoms of facial pain in the area of the sinus passages, toothache as a result of excess pressure from the infected passage upon the upper teeth, and large amounts of discolored mucus from the nose. Laryngitis is an infection of the larynx, commonly referred to as the voice box, which impairs the person's ability to speak clearly.

Tonsillitis is a condition affecting the tonsils, whose function as a part of the lymphatic system is to filter bacteria out of the body; tonsillitis occurs when the tonsils become overwhelmed by the bacteria. When the condition is caused by bacteria, such as streptococcal, antibiotics are prescribed and the typical course of healing is between 10 to 14 days. In severe cases, the tonsils are surgically removed.

The tracheobrochial area, located between the trachea (throat) and the bronchial tubes leading to the lungs, is another common site for URTIs. Tracheobronchitis is an infection that causes a significant cough and wheezing sensation in the person; this condition can persist for one to three weeks.

The mechanism by which bacterial agents are able to establish themselves within the upper respiratory tract is complex. The nasal passages have a natural complement of bacteria, which compete with any bacterial invaders for space within the passages. Without such space, the foreign bacteria cannot multiply sufficiently to pose any threat to the healthy function of the respiratory system. To infect the upper respiratory system, the invading bacteria must be both airborne and alive at the time that it enters the body. The bacteria must then be deposited in a susceptible host tissue, and once established in the respiratory tract, the variant illness will be developed within anywhere from 12 to 36 hours, depending on the speed with which the condition spreads.

**SEE ALSO** Asthma, exercise induced; Cardiorespiratory function; Immune system.

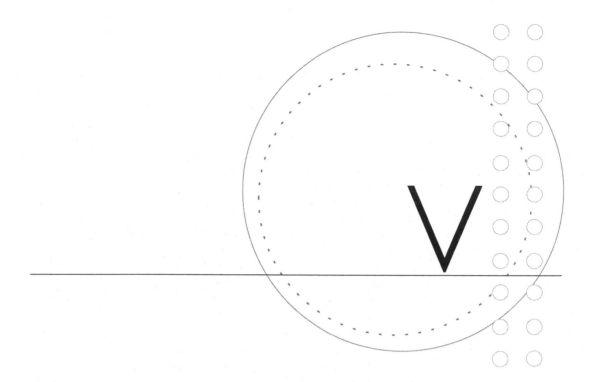

# Variable resistance exercise

Muscular strength is defined as the maximum force that can be developed by a muscle or muscle group against resistance. Resistance can take one of two forms in athletic training: constant resistance or variable resistance.

Constant resistance is a form of training where the resistance directed against the target muscle or muscle group does not vary through the range of athletic movement. The lifting of free weights is an example of constant resistance. In an exercise involving constant resistance, the muscular power generated and the effect of the resistance on the muscle are not constant. An example of the effect of constant resistance is found in the simple curl of a free weight using a conventional dumbbell. At the start of the exercise, the muscles of the arm, primarily the bicep, pull the weight upward. There is a point, as the dumbbell is lifted, where the resistance on the muscle is greatest; at the movement before and after that maximal point, the resistance force is much less. At the conclusion of the exercise, there is little or no resistance being applied to the bicep.

Variable resistance requires differing degrees of force to be applied to the target muscle to create constant resistance, compelling the muscle to work harder to meet the demands of the exercise. In a variable resistance arm curl, the forces applied to the bicep are variable at each stage of the curl in order to maintain the same resistance throughout the trajectory of movement.

Variable resistance exercise is designed to achieve maximum muscular involvement. Inherent in the effectiveness of variable resistance exercise is the relationship between the intensity required of the athlete and the volume of resistance work involved. Resistance exercises are typically carried out through the use of specialized machines that are designed to permit control of the entire force-generating movement.

The machines may be designed for the training of any muscle group in the body. Machines that isolate the pectoral muscles through a seated bench press, deltoid machines, and shoulder extension machines are three of a multitude of models commercially available. The common features of variable resistance training machines are the presence of cables, pulleys, or other devices to create variability, coupled with the placement of the user in a fixed position to ensure that the user cannot recruit other muscle groups to assist in the completion of the prescribed movements.

Variable resistance training also endeavors to capitalize on the fact that the force that is inherent in the development of greater strength has itself two aspects: the internal forces that are generated within the joint to produce strength and the external force produced by the resistance.

Variable resistance training success is predicated on the principle of regulating the amount of work per unit of training time. The variable resistance training is intended to harness the strength of the user in a coordinated movement. Repetition of those coordinated movements is a means of refining the relationship between the brain and the muscles it directs in the exercise. The repetitions also serve to help exclude the interference by external stimuli in the performance of the movement. This progression through the exercise that subjects the body to variable forces ultimately enhances athletic skill.

One of the world's best known variable exercise machines is the Universal line, developed in the early 1970s by Dr. Gideon Ariel, a specialist in biomechanics. The Universal machines are constructed on the basis of two principles that guide their application in muscle development. The first principle is that resistance exercise is most effective when a multiple number of joints are required to complete the exercise. The second principle is the notion of explosive repetitions—to achieve the maximum level of mental concentration and to obtain the maximum firing levels of muscle fiber for optimal performance.

The engagement of a multiple number of joints in resistance training requires the body develop the strength to counteract the forces applied by the machine throughout the entire range of motion in each repetition. When those repetitions must be performed as rapidly as possible, without sacrificing adherence to proper form or otherwise compromising the desired range of motion, the athlete will be compelled to react with greater speed. The faster that the athlete must react to the resistance directed into the target muscle, the faster the individual muscles will fire. This approach mirrors the other training methods that are used by athletes to develop the capabilities the fast-twitch fibers present in each muscle.

SEE ALSO Exercise, high intensity; Muscle mass and strength; Preseason strength training; Range of motion; Resistance exercise training.

## Vaulting SEE Gymnastics vaulting

## Vertical jump

The vertical jump is one of the most explosive physical movements executed in sport. In a number of sports, the higher the athlete is able to jump, the greater the prospects of success in that discipline. Basketball and volleyball are the two most prominent examples of sports where that correlation is plain. The jumping ability of an athlete is also an indicator of overall athletic ability, as there is a clear relation-

ship between the ability to jump and the running speed that the athlete will develop over short distances. The National Football League, where prospective players are subjected to various physical tests, requires every player to be tested for both vertical leaps and 40-yd (37 m) sprints, irrespective of the position played.

The vertical jump is defined as the highest point that the athlete can touch from a standing jump, less the height that the athlete can touch from a standing position. The measurement of the jump is flawed if the athlete is permitted to take one or more steps before jumping, as the athlete will convert some of the energy developed in the step taken into the force of propulsion that generates upward lift. Basketball has numerous legends and other urban myths concerning the seemingly superhuman leaping ability attributed to certain players; one such player, former University of Louisville star Darrell "Dr. Dunkenstein" Griffith, was reputed to possess a 42 in (1 m) vertical leap. It is likely that the average National Basketball Association player 6 ft 6 in (1.97 m) or shorter has a vertical leap of between 25 and 30 in (0.63 and 0.75 m); taller and heavier players will usually not be able to jump as high.

Because jumping ability is a combination of leg strength and explosive power, jumping can be developed in the same fashion as any other muscular activity. The ultimate limit to how high any athlete can jump will be determined to a significant degree by the distribution of fast-twitch versus slow-twitch fibers present in the muscles of the legs. This distribution is a genetic determination. Fast-twitch fibers are those whose governing neurons, the component of the nervous system that receives the impulses generated by the brain to direct muscular movement, fires more rapidly, which in turn creates the more rapid muscle contractions required for speed. As a general proposition, an athlete with a greater distribution of fast-twitch fibers will be able jump higher than one with a preponderance of slow-twitch fibers.

Plyometrics is the best known of the jumping development exercise programs. Plyometrics training emphasizes speed and explosive movement, and a plyometrics program will typically consist of a series of bounding, hopping, and jumping drills. The object of a plyometrics program is to perform the exercises at maximum intensity. For this reason, plyometrics training must be approached with caution, and the athlete must progress slowly from one level to the next to reduce the risk of injury. Proper rest intervals must also be incorporated in to plyometrics training, as the exercises are intended to place significant stress on the target muscle groups.

A common, low-tech plyometrics method is performing box jumps, where the athlete jumps repeatedly from the floor to the top of the box and back again. By concentrating on the mechanics of the jump, directing propulsion from the balls of the feet and thrusting with an explosive extension of the legs, the ability of the athlete to land lightly and immediately return to the floor enhances motor control over the movement.

To build strength in the legs that will be compatible with the speed developed through successful plyometrics drills, squat and lunge exercises are important components. Squats are performed with free weights, where the athlete uses a weighted bar to carry out the exercise. The additional weight will be supported by the body through the abdominal, lumbar (low back), and gluteal muscles, in addition to the legs. This form of exercise permits the strengthening of the legs in conjunction with enhancing the core strength of the body, essential to the balance necessary to have the several muscle groups involved in leaping work in harmony.

Lunges, also performed with the athlete lifting free weights in each hand that are within the athlete's capabilities, will significantly strengthen the legs, without the risk of injury that may exist in the squat or plyometrics movements.

Muscular strength and explosiveness must be developed in conjunction with flexibility if the athlete is to maximize the jumping ability and reduce the risk of injury to structures such as the Achilles tendon and knee ligaments. Flexibility, when achieved through focused stretching programs, will serve to increase the range of motion in the joints essential to jumping: the ankles, knees, and hips. A common muscular deficiency that plagues athletes who require well-developed leaping ability is a lack of flexibility and resultant strength imbalance between the quadriceps (thigh) muscles and the hamstrings, the pair of muscles responsible for the flexion and the extension of the knee. Proper stretching will assist the athlete in the maintenance of an approximate 3:2 ratio in the relative strength of the quadriceps to the hamstring. When there is a significant deviation from that proportion, the knee and the muscles themselves are at greater risk of injury.

When the athlete proceeds with caution, with emphasis on the form of the training exercise, it is not uncommon to gain between 4 in and 9 in (0.1 and 0.2 m) in vertical jumps in periods as short as three months.

SEE ALSO Basketball: Strength and training exercises; Lower leg anatomy; Muscle fibers: Fast and slow twitch; Plyometrics.

# Lasse Viren

7/22/1949–
FINNISH
RUNNER, POLICE OFFICER, POLITICIAN

Lasse Viren was a middle distance runner from Finland who won gold medals in the 5,000 m and 10,000 m races at both the 1972 Olympics in Munich, Germany, and the 1976 Olympics in Montreal, Canada.

Viren epitomized the concept of training with a specific goal and a specific competition in mind. In sport jargon, this is known as "peaking," and means that an athlete trains with the intent of reaching maximum fitness at the time of a certain competition.

In Viren's case, the competitions were the Olympics. In the years preceding the 1972 and 1976 Olympics, his running accomplishments were relatively minor. Instead, he dedicated himself to training, seldom participating in non-Olympic competitions.

Viren began to run as a hobby in his youth. His training continued after he became a police officer in Helsinki. By 1971, his running had progressed to the point where he was of international caliber.

Prior to the 1972 Munich games, Viren was a talented runner but seemingly not world-class. For example, in the 1971 European Championships, he placed seventh in the 5,000-m final and seventeenth in the 10,000-m final. However, reflecting his training philosophy, just a month prior to the start of the Olympics he established a new world record for two miles in a time of 8 minutes, 14 seconds (an average of 4 minutes, 7 seconds per mile).

His performance inspired the then 23-year-old to compete in both the 5,000-m and 10,000-m events at the 1972 games. Originally, he had intended to enter only the shorter distance.

In the 10,000 m final at the 1972 games, Viren became entangled with another competitor and fell down. Even with this mishap, he managed to win the race, finishing 6 m ahead of the next competitor. In the process, he set a new world record of 27 minutes 38.4 seconds. In the 5,000-m final, held one week later, Viren outsprinted the other runners, including the late American runner Steve Prefontaine.

Fours days later, Viren set a new world record for the 5,000 m in a time of 13 minutes 16.4 seconds.

Then, true to form, he relaxed his training regimen. At his next competition, held later that year, Viren finished nearly 20 seconds behind the winner.

By 1974, with the next Olympics only two years away, Viren's times had improved, as he began to ratchet up his training schedule.

Viren's training regimen was done alone and consisted of thousands of kilometers of runs through the woods around Helsinki. He maintained that running through the undergrowth of the forest floor sharpened his mental focus and created opportunities to alter the pace of his run.

A factor in Viren's training was his continuing obligation as a fulltime police officer. In contrast to the situation for elite athletes in 2006, athletes received little if any compensation for training and no prize money. In the spirit of the times, Olympic competition was reserved for amateur athletes; rules then in place by the International Olympic Committee (IOC) discouraged participation by those who benefited financially from their sport. Viren experienced the IOC's wrath when, after his 10,000 m victory in the 1976 games, he removed his shoes and carried them during a post-race lap of the track. IOC members felt that this action was done to display the shoes' logo. According to Viren, he had removed his shoes to relieve the pain of a blister.

In the 1976 Montreal games, Viren easily won the 10,000-m competition, finishing almost 30 m in front of the field. The 5,000 m was a sterner test, with the top six runners separated by only a few meters heading into the final stretch. Viren prevailed only by outsprinting a trio of runners that included New Zealanders Dick Quax and Rod Dixon.

Viren attempted to win the marathon after having secured gold in the 5,000 m and 10,000 m events, a feat not done since Emil Zátopek's triple gold medal performance at the 1952 games held in Helsinki. He was not successful, but finished the race in a very respectable fifth place.

Viren competed at the 1980 Olympics held in Moscow (an event that was boycotted by 65 nations, including the United States, in protest of the Soviet Union's 1979 invasion of Afghanistan). There he placed fifth in the 10,000 m and did not complete the marathon.

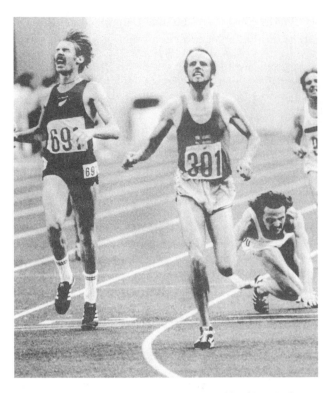

Lasse Viren wins the 5,000-m run during the 1976 Olympic Games held in Montreal, Canada.

He retired from competition following the 1980 Olympics. After his athletic career, Viren continued to work as a police officer in Helsinki. His running became confined to sporadic recreational outings. In 1999, his political interests culminated in his election as a member of Parliament in Finland's Conservative Party.

## Visualization in sport

Visualization in sport is a training technique that forms a part of the larger science of sports psychology. Visualization is also known as mental imagery and rehearsal. Visualization is used primarily as a training tool, one that improves the quality of athletic movement, increases the power of concentration, and serves to reduce the pressures of competition on the athlete while building athletic confidence.

Visualization occurs when athletes are able to create an image or a series of images relevant to their sport, without any external prompts or stimulation; the images are mentally generated by the athlete alone. Visual images are usually the most important to athletic training and may be employed as the sole mental training method. Athletes may also depend on auditory images (sounds), kinesthetic images (movements), tactile sensations (touch), and purely emotional stimulation, in combination with visualization or as freestanding training aids, as may be appropriate to the effort to elevate the performance of the athlete.

There is a powerful relationship between mental and physical performance in sport. The development of a wide range of mental powers, such as focus and concentration, elevates athletic performance; over-analyzing detracts from the athlete's ability to react instinctively, an attribute that is usually a more desirable quality than the ability to reason through every sporting circumstance.

Visualization is intended to take the athlete to an image that conveys what perfection represents in the particular aspect of the sport. During visualization, the brain is directing the target muscles to work in a desired way. This direction creates a neural pattern in the brain, a pattern identical to the network created by the actual physical performance of the movements. A neural pattern is similar to diagramming the specific wiring and circuits necessary to transmit an electrical current. Alexander Bain (1818–1903) of Great Britain was the first scientist to develop a theory as to how the brain built such patterns to direct and control repeated physical movement. Numerous researchers since that time have expanded on the concept. Visualization alone will not develop the most effective mechanisms in the brain to later perform the desired action, but physical training coupled with visualization will create better recognition of the required nervous system response than physical training alone.

During organized athletic training, sports psychologists will commonly direct the visualization techniques employed by an athlete to be utilized in a quiet, secluded area, so as to eliminate distractions. It is common for athletes who are employing visualization training to participate in three such sessions per week.

The first application of visualization tools is the mental rehearsal or practice of the specific techniques required in a sport. Every sport has such training opportunities; the mental rehearsal of the precise footwork that a high jumper will take in an approach to the bar prior to takeoff, or the steps and delivery of a soccer player attempting a corner kick can be replayed by the athlete indefinitely.

The mental replay of the image of a successfully executed maneuver is a tool used by athletes to reinforce athletic confidence. When this type of visualization is used in conjunction with other sports psychology tools, such as positive self-talk, the self-encouragement that athletes direct inward for motivation, they can connect to an actual past success as a means of enhancing their future prospects.

Visualization is also a useful tool to contemplate the appropriate tactics the athlete might employ in a given competitive situation. A middle distance runner can visualize where in a particular 1,500-m race the closing kick ought to be employed; for an ice hockey player or a lacrosse defenseman, game situations such as defending a two-on-one break by opposing forwards can be analyzed. In a similar fashion, the athlete can reenact circumstances where an error was made or a breakdown occurred, making the image an educational tool.

Visualization is also useful while the athlete is recovering or rehabilitating from an injury. Positive images of either competition or healthy athletic movement can be employed, particularly while the athlete is using a stationary trainer or otherwise exercising, to mentally remove the athlete from the mundane training room or gym to the exciting athletic life.

The beauty of visualization as a training tool is its portability; this form of mental training can be used during the athlete's off hours, during training, rehabilitation, or in the course of actual competition, particularly in those sports where there are intervals between event segments. The delivery of a tennis serve and the throwing of a javelin are acts that permit athletes to engage their powers of visualization and, when coupled with a positive mental outlook, assist in achieving their best form.

**SEE ALSO** Motor control; Sport performance; Sport psychology; Sports coaching.

# Vitamin C

Vitamin C, also known as ascorbic acid, is one of the many micronutrients consumed through diet that is essential to life. Vitamin C is an organic (carbon-based) compound, with a chemical structure expressed as $C_6H_8O_6$.

Vitamin C is a water-soluble compound, which permits it to be absorbed into the body directly through the small intestine. Unlike the fat-soluble vitamins A, D, E, and K, vitamin C is not stored for indefinite periods in the body's tissues. Vitamin C is stored for temporary periods within the liver, and any excess amounts are excreted as urine through the renal system.

Vitamin C performs two critical functions within the body, both of which are of the utmost importance to athletic performance. First, it is a facilitator in the absorption of iron by the body, the mineral necessary to the transport of oxygen within the bloodstream. Second, vitamin C is an important component in the ability of the body to manufacture collagen, the protein with elastic properties that is employed in the formation and maintenance of all bones, teeth, and connective tissues. Vitamin C also assists in the maintenance of the capillaries, the smallest vessels of the cardio-vascular system.

Vitamin C is present in large quantities in many varieties of citrus fruits, green vegetables, and pota-toes. Many of these foods are excellent sources of the vitamin, a standard often defined as one serving of the food has at least 10% of the recommended daily allowance (RDA) of the vitamin. The generally accepted international minimum standard for vitamin C intake is 90 mg per day for an adult male and 75 mg per day for an adult female, with nursing mothers requiring between 100 mg and 120 mg per day. A good dietary source for vitamin C or any other micro-nutrient is also one where the caloric content is appropriate; the benefits of excellent vitamin C content in a particular food must be weighed against the number of calories otherwise contained in it.

Vitamin C is often described as an antioxidant, as it inhibits the actions of oxygen on cells. Contact with oxygen, called oxidation, degrades human cells and tissues, much in the same fashion that bare metal will rust if exposed to the air and elements. The oxidation process creates a multitude of compounds known as free radicals, electrically charged and unstable compounds, which are possessed of one or more electrons that are not paired within the mole-cule. These compounds are so named because they will seek out otherwise chemically stable molecules from which to remove electrons necessary to bring their own structure into balance. The removal of an electron from a previously stable nearby molecule creates a chain reaction that causes cellular damage, whereby that previously stable compound will itself seek to obtain a replacement. Vitamin C acts as an antioxidant through the provision of one of its own available charged particles, giving up an electron to stop cycle of cell damage. Vitamin C also protects the fat-soluble vitamins A and E, and accompanying fatty acids, from oxidation as they are transported throughout the body.

A diet lacking vitamin C may cause various nega-tive effects including oxidative stress (exposure of the cells to the adverse effects of oxidation). Those whose bodies are subjected to greater than normal oxidative stress for various reasons, including stren-uous exercise, tobacco and alcohol consumption, dialysis, viral illness and fever, or other stressful conditions, require correspondingly greater quantities of vitamin C. Severe vitamin C deficiency may lead to scurvy, a debilitating condition, characterized by a lack of energy, tooth decay, gum inflammation, and bleeding problems, that has been generally eradi-cated in modern western society other than in alco-holics, some elderly people, or those whose diets do not contain fresh fruits and vegetables.

Care must be taken in food preparation to pre-serve the amount of vitamin C present in a particular food. Vitamin C is water soluble, so actions such as cooking a vitamin C source in water or otherwise soaking the product in water will reduce its vitamin C content. Whole food sources, such as a potato with its skin intact, will preserve greater quantities of vitamin C than processed foods.

Due to its water solubility, vitamin C is not known to create any adverse effects if consumed in larger than recommended quantities, although vita-min C dosages in excess of 2,000 mg per day are not recommended. Linus Pauling (1901–1994), Nobel prize winner in chemistry, was at the forefront of the movement advocating massive daily supplements of vitamin C (amounts in excess of 5,000 mg), as both a potential cold preventative and as an anticancer agent. It was the view of Pauling and others that, because the body does not have the ability to synthe-size its own stores of vitamin C (unlike other mam-mals), large doses would in essence fill a genetic gap. While modern research has confirmed that vitamin C's antioxidant properties will prevent and possibly counteract cell damage, evidence of any greater capa-bilities is inconclusive.

**SEE ALSO** Bone, ligaments, tendons; Diet; Liver function; Nutrition.

## Vitamin E

Vitamin E is the name given to a group of eight chemicals with similar properties that are essential to health. Vitamin E was first isolated as a distinct substance in various green leafy vegetables in 1922. Vitamin E is classed as a micronutrient, a substance that is not required in large quantities through diet but which is otherwise essential to the maintenance of good health. In all of its forms, vitamin E is an organic (carbon-based) compound, of which alpha tocopherol is the most prolific. Vitamin E is often referred to as nature's antioxidant, a testament to the important function of these chemicals within the body.

Vitamin E, as with all micronutrients, is required in trace amounts for bodily function. The recommended daily requirement for adults of this substance is 15 mg per day. The consumption of dietary supplements to ensure the ingestion of the required quantities of vitamin E is unnecessary if the person is consuming a well-balanced diet, as the best sources of the chemical are commonly available food products, such as wheat and its large number of byproducts, many green leafy vegetables, and most nuts, seeds, and their oils. Vitamin E is the least toxic of all fat-soluble vitamins; the recommended upper daily limit of vitamin E consumption is 1,000 mg.

Vitamin E is a fat-soluble compound. It is processed for entry into the body at the small intestine, where the vitamin is parceled into chemical packages made from both high density lipoproteins (IIDLs) and low density lipoproteins (LDLs) to facilitate the absorption of vitamin E into both the lymphatic system and the liver. From these locations, vitamin E then is released directly into the bloodstream.

With either its HDL or LDL transportation in the bloodstream, vitamin E is carried to various cells within the body. As a fat-soluble vitamin, vitamin E can be stored within the cell mitochondria (often described as the cellular powerhouse) of the adipose tissue, the cells designed for the storage of triglycerides (fats), for an indefinite period. Once utilized as an antioxidant, the spent vitamin E is disposed of by the body through the stomach bile; it is ultimately excreted from the body as feces.

Oxidation is a biological concept that is readily understood with reference to many daily life examples. Rusted metal, food that turns rancid, and the various aging processes observable within the body are examples of oxidation, which is the decay or the degradation of a cell due to the effect of oxygen. An antioxidant, such as vitamin E, is any substance that by its presence or its operation, serves to specifically delay, prevent, or reverse the rate of deterioration caused in the cells by oxygen. Antioxidants are classed as one of two types: metal sequestrants, which prevent metals from reacting with oxygen, and free radical scavengers, which operate to interrupt the destructive chain reactions that occur within the body that are precipitated by the compounds known as free radicals. Vitamin E and, in certain circumstances, vitamin C, are free radical scavengers within the body.

Free radicals are the most common cause of oxidation within the body. Occurring throughout the body, these chemical compounds are inherently unstable, as their electron structure is unbalanced due to one or more electrons within the structure not being paired, which creates either a positive or negative electric charge within the free radical. The free radical therefore seeks to obtain the necessary electrons to create electrical balance from nearby stable compounds. This "theft" of electrons by the free radicals renders the previously stable compound unstable and reactive. This use precipitates a chain reaction of electron use that is the essence of the oxidation that causes cell damage.

As an antioxidant, vitamin E traps the free radicals that it encounters, through its donation of a hydrogen atom to the free radical molecule, rendering it chemically neutral. Vitamin E ranges throughout the tissues of the body, and it provides its antioxidant benefits to all aspects of the cardiovascular and musculoskeletal systems. Vitamin E does not differentiate between the types of free radicals it may encounter, nor does vitamin E restrict its actions based on the place of origin of the target free radical.

There is no question from a scientific perspective that vitamin E is a very important compound within the body, as it protects the tissues from decay and degradation. The companion issue of whether megadoses of vitamin E, by daily supplement or otherwise, will provide enhanced health protection has not been conclusively determined. The actions of vitamin E must also be considered separately from the healing and repair of tissue that occurs within the body. Antioxidant function is separate from the cell repair that occurs within the body at all cell production points—bone, connective tissue, muscles, and blood cells may be degraded by the actions of free radicals. Vitamin E does not play a role in cell production.

**SEE ALSO** Diet; Free fatty acids in the blood; Nutrition; Oxygen.

# Volleyball

Invented in 1895, volleyball has grown from its roots as a non-contact recreational exercise to its current status as one of the world's most popular sports. It is a remarkable irony of sports history that volleyball's inventor, a Massachusetts Young Men's Christian Association (YMCA) instructor, William G. Morgan (1870–1942), developed this sport in same American town where James Naismith had created basketball four years earlier.

Originally known as "mintonette," Marshall intended his game to be played by an older age group, persons who sought the benefits of an exercise that did not present significant physical risks. Marshall envisioned the new game to be one that would strictly avoid any potential for body contact between opponents and thus be less demanding than the recently developed, but locally popular, basketball. The popularity of the newly named volleyball spread throughout the United States and overseas in the early 1900s due to the worldwide influence of the YMCA, which introduced the sport at its local gyms. In 1916, the style of the sport changed forever when the offensive tactic of the set and spike was first developed in the Philippines, where it was known by the colorful description, *la bomba*.

Other than subsequent technical refinements to the manner of play, the rules of volleyball have been unchanged since their codification in 1920. The United States Volley Ball Association (later known as USA Volleyball) was formed in 1928, the world's first national governing body in the sport. The first variant of volleyball, beach volleyball, was first played and developed in California after 1930. The international growth of volleyball was impeded only by World War II, and in 1946 the international federation governing the sport, Federation Internationale de Volley-Ball (FIVB), was chartered. FIVB sanctioned the inaugural world volleyball championships in 1949, and the sport was included for the first time as both a men's and women's sport in the 1964 Olympics.

The first professional volleyball league was formed in 1983, and other professional leagues were established in a number of other nations in the succeeding years. Beach volleyball developed its own following, which resulted in both a first FIVB world beach championship in 1987, followed by the inclusion of beach volleyball as an Olympic sport in 1996. Volleyball in both forms is played in every country of the world.

The rules of volleyball are relatively simple; it is the precision with which a team can execute within this uncomplicated rules framework that defines success in the sport. The object of both indoor volleyball and outdoor volleyball is to direct the ball over the net without the ball being safely returned by the opposing team. A team is permitted a maximum of three contacts with the ball after receiving the ball from the opposing team, in addition to any contact with the ball at the net if one of the team attempted to block the ball. Outdoor volleyball is played with two players per side, the indoor game with six per side. If the team can combine to deliver the ball over the net so as to prevent its return by the opposing teams, either by directing into the floor within the playing surface, or when the opponent cannot return the ball after three contacts, a point is scored. Games are scored by the first team to reach 25 points, and a match usually will consist of a best-of-five-games format. When a fifth game is necessary to decide the match that game will be played to 15 points.

Height is an important, but not determinative, physical attribute in volleyball. While tall players typically will dominate in the play at the net, smaller and more agile players are essential in covering open areas of the court, to both keep the ball in play after an opponent's attack, and to coordinate the offensive attack by putting the ball into play as a part of a set offensive sequence. The setter is such a player, the team member responsible for putting the ball into a position where it can be delivered with an authoritative spike into the opponent's court. In elite international volleyball, it is not uncommon to have male players at 6 ft 9 in (2.06 m) or taller playing in the frontcourt, and on women's teams, 6 ft 2 in or taller (1.87 m). However, unlike basketball, where the game has evolved so as to require a significant degree of muscular strength at the forward positions, volleyball players are often very lean of build, with tremendous leaping ability.

The net is positioned midway on a court that is 59.6 ft long, and 29.6 ft wide (18 m by 9 m). The net is 7.95 ft high for men's play, and 7.4 ft high for women (2.43 m and 2.24 m, respectively). The ball used for all players is constructed from synthetic materials, with a circumference of between 25.5 in and 27 in (65 and 67 cm), and a weight of between 9 oz and 10 oz (260 g and 280 g).

The court is marked by lines to define the side defended by each team. As a general rule, the ball may be hit by a player from anywhere on the team's side of the net, including what would otherwise be an out-of-bounds position. Each court has an attack line placed 9.9 ft (3 m) behind the net; this is the boundary that determines the frontcourt from the backcourt. Players in the backcourt are not permitted to attack, or spike, the ball unless they are positioned behind that line. The attack line also assists in

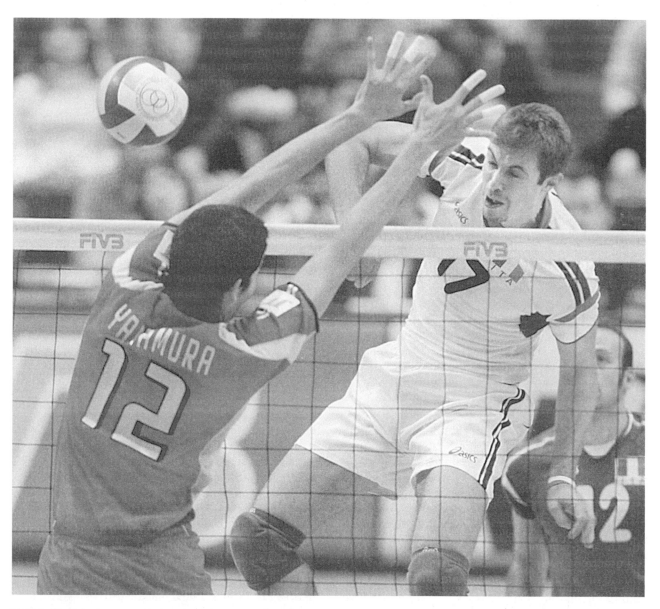

Volleyball is played at many levels worldwide. TORU YAMANAKA/AFP/GETTY IMAGES

defining the role of a specialist known as the "libero." The libero is a player who can be substituted for any player in a team's backcourt. The libero is not permitted to serve the ball nor may the libero spike the ball or rotate into the frontcourt. The libero was a position invented in the mid 1990s to create an additional role for the shorter volleyball player.

A volleyball game commences with a serve of the ball, a shot delivered from behind the end line of the court. A serve may be made with any arm action, provided that the fundamental rule of ball contact and handling is observed—a volleyball may not be thrown, lifted (typically with a cupped hand), or struck twice in one motion (double hit). A hard serve

will often be delivered as a jump serve, where the power of the jump is converted into arm speed and consequently a greater force is imparted to the ball. The manner in which the player's hand is applied to the serve will determine how the ball will travel through the air. Like a soccer ball or a baseball, the spin imparted to a volleyball creates the Magnus effect, where the ball moves in the direction of the lower air pressure created by the spin. A hard-spinning serve is a difficult ball to handle for an opposing team. A float serve is designed to achieve the opposite effect from a spike serve. The float serve is delivered with little or no spin, making its path through the air unpredictable.

There are many specific methods for handling the ball once it has been served. The basic movements are the bump, set, and spike. The bump is usually performed with both arms held together and the hands as fists held together, and the ball then directed upward; the bump is usually made to keep the ball live and to establish an offensive maneuver. The set is a pass directed by a player with the intention that it will be delivered for a score by a teammate. The setter is the person who is designated to perform the bulk of the setting duties for a team. The spike is the ultimate effort by a team to score a point, representing an attack on the ball above the height of the net. A successful spike will result in a "kill," a point for the team where the ball could not be returned. As a general rule, no player is permitted to touch the net while the ball is in play.

The rules regarding the manner in which the ball may be handled are essentially the same for the outdoor beach volleyball game. The presence of two players versus six makes the tactics of beach volleyball relatively simple; the sand playing surface makes jumping much more difficult. The outdoor court is slightly smaller than that used indoors: 52.5 ft by 26.2 ft (16 m by 8 m). In a curious way, the most significant difference between the indoor and outdoor games is the flash and the glamour that quickly became associated with the beach version. The sunny venues and the form-fitting uniforms worn by players gave the newcomer sport tremendous international television appeal at every Olympics since its introduction in 1996.

Volleyball training must be oriented to the objects of the game. It is a game that is primarily anaerobic in the manner in which athletic movement is required and energy produced in support. On any given point contested during a game, the athletic movement demanded of a player may be of between five seconds and 30 seconds duration. The typical rest interval between each point is approximately 10–20 seconds. Exercises that assist in the development of explosive leaping ability, quick lateral movement, and hand-eye coordination are of primary importance to the volleyball player.

Aerobic training is also important to overall volleyball performance. Aerobic strength will permit the players to sustain their energy levels through games that may last as long as two hours, as well as to facilitate physical recovery. Physical strength in the sense of developing maximum muscular power is not as important as the achievement of balance and flexibility. Volleyball success requires that the player possess an optimum range of motion, to permit the greatest degree of lift in the leaping required, as well as to enhance the cushioning of the forces repeatedly directed into the body through jumps and landing.

One appeal of volleyball, beyond the nature of the game itself, is that it is a sport that can be played by any body type at any age. It can also be played safely and without significant rule changes by men and women, mixed, or co-ed settings.

**SEE ALSO** Plyometrics; Stretching and flexibility; Volleyball strength training and exercises; Volleyball: Set and spike mechanisms.

# Volleyball: Set and spike mechanisms

Volleyball is a sport with a simple object: the ability to deliver a ball over a net against the efforts of an opposing team. The manner in which this object is achieved is defined by rather rigorous rules as to how the ball may be struck and handled by a player. A premium is placed on the offensive team's ball-handling efficiency by the limitations on touching the ball, particularly the maximum of three hits (including unintentional contacts) for returning the ball over the net.

The set and spike mechanism is the most effective offensive series that can be executed in volleyball. The set and spike are a progression from the simple return of that ball safely to the opposing side of the net. The set and spike are designed as an aggressive sequence of maneuvers, with the goal of striking the ball with sufficient force into the opposing court that it cannot be returned.

An understanding of the proper execution of the set and spike mechanism begins with how the volleyball is directed into a position where the mechanism may be initiated. Although there are many variations as to how the ball may be received when hit into the defensive team's court, in most cases the ball will be bumped by a defensive player. The bump is the first of the three permitted touches by a team upon receiving the ball from an opponent. In the rules of volleyball there is no prohibition against the first touch of the ball being a return over the net, but the accepted tactic to ensure the most effective attack is to ensure that the ball is handled so as to permit an optimal and powerful delivery with the spike.

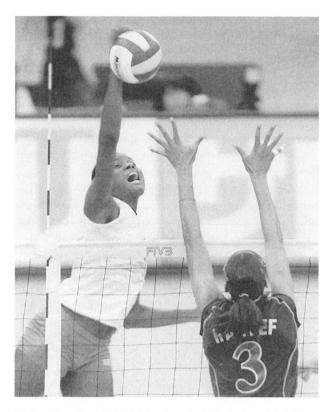

Fabiana Claudino of Brazil (L) spikes the ball. TOSHIFUMI KITAMURA/AFP/GETTY IMAGES

The bump is usually employed as a pass to the setter, the player with the primary responsibility for setting the ball up in such a fashion that the third contact with the ball will be the spike. The player who delivers the spike will usually be a hitter, predetermined in the team's offensive strategy.

The set is usually executed in one of two ways, depending on the height and the position of the ball relative to the floor. The setter must possess well-defined agility and lateral quickness to obtain the proper body position relative to the ball in order to set it. The bump set is employed when the ball is delivered to the setter at a height where the player is not able to use the fingertips to handle the ball as is permitted by the rules; the setter places both arms together to direct the ball upward for the intended spike. An attempt to place the palms of the hands under the ball in such a position will almost inevitably result in a lift violation being called by the umpire.

The second type of set performed is the overhand set. In this maneuver, the setter uses a hand to better control the direction and the spin of the ball during the set, to permit maximum control over the ball by the hitter on the spike. When possible, the setter endeavors to have the body "square to the ball" when the ball is set, moving from a crouched position to perform the set, and then maintaining a low position to anticipate a return from the opponent.

The spike culminates the offensive set piece that is the pass, set, and spike. The player designated as the hitter will start the spike mechanics before the ball has been set. The hitter will first get positioned behind the place where the ball will be set. As the ball is set and begins to move upward, the hitter begins a short run up approach and launches the body into the air, driving both arms upward to create as much lift as possible. An ideal set and spike will result in the ball being struck at the peak of the parabolic path taken by the ball. The hitter transfers the kinetic energy created by the approach to the ball with a powerful arm swing. The greater the height at which the ball is struck on a spike, the more acute the angle at which the ball will travel toward the opponent, making the ball more difficult to handle.

The spike combines the force of the leap into the spike with the more delicate hand-eye coordination demanded to place the ball where required in the opposing court. To maintain balance in the air prior to contact with the ball, the hitter's body remains relatively perpendicular to the floor throughout the jump, with the hitting hand positioned between the ear and the shoulder of the hitter. The ball is then struck with the heel of the palm at the center of the ball, with the wrist extended so as to ensure that the player follows through on the spike motion to maximize hitting power.

The Magnus effect is a physical phenomenon that occurs when a spinning object moves through a fluid (liquid or gas like air), where the spin creates areas of lower air pressure to which the ball will turn, causing a deviation in its path. The volleyball serve is subject to this principle, and, though the spike generally travels a shorter distance, the Magnus effect still occurs, but is less pronounced.

SEE ALSO Range of motion; Stretching and flexibility; Volleyball; Volleyball strength training and exercises.

# Volleyball strength training and exercises

Volleyball is a sport that involves a number of distinct strength training and conditioning considerations. As with sports such as cricket, running, and slow pitch softball, any healthy person can participate in a game of volleyball. It is generally safe, being a sport played in a regimented fashion with a limited number of contacts permitted with the ball when delivered across the net, with no physical contact permitted between the participants. It is not necessarily physically demanding in terms of exertion, as there are significant rest intervals between each point scored in a game.

Volleyball shares similarities with softball and cricket on another level. To succeed as a volleyball player in elite competition, the athlete must develop a wide range of physical skills. The ideal volleyball player is often tall and very physically limber. All players, irrespective of their height, will be agile, possessed of explosive leaping ability, a superior vertical jump, and balance. Volleyball players invariably possess outstanding reaction time and hand-eye coordination.

The techniques involved in successful volleyball play are built on repetitive drills and the simulation of various game situations to hone a combination of physical and mental skills. The distinct skills of bumping, blocking, setting, spiking, digging, and receiving the ball are those practiced at every volleyball training session.

Effective volleyball strength training is premised on building the best musculoskeletal structure possible to perfect these game skills. Volleyball training, as with any sport, will be designed through the application of the periodization of training principle. This principle is founded on the broader concept that no athlete can train at the same high level for indefinite periods, as the body requires both physical and mental down time (rest) to recover from periods of intense exertion or competition.

The training year for the volleyball player will be divided into three general segments, with further subdivisions within each segment to accommodate a particular training or competitive objective. Typical periodization would include a preseason, a competitive season, and an off-season. The physical training performed by the player will be tailored to the respective seasons.

For adolescent athletes, periodization and the specific exercises performed must also be modified to properly account for the differences in the adolescent musculoskeletal structure. When a young athlete has not yet reached physical maturity, excessive repetitions of particular exercises or excessive resistance training may cause significant damage to the epiphysis regions of the long bones of the body, which contain the growth plates. Such training may also place unhealthy stress on the growing connective tissues.

The training program, once properly segmented into training periods, will focus on four general types of physical development essential to the successful execution of the various volleyball techniques: increased jumping ability through plyometrics exercises; the core strength of the player; stretching and flexibility training; and general aerobic fitness.

Leaping ability and volleyball are inextricably linked. The ability of a player to rise above the floor, either to deliver a spike or to block an opponent's attack, is an essential of the game. At an elite level, much of the game is played well above the net, which is approximately 8 ft (2.4 m) high. Plyometrics is a collection of leaping and bounding exercises designed to stimulate the fast-twitch muscle fibers of the legs to produce a correspondingly greater and more dynamic vertical jump. The stresses placed on the leg structure through plyometrics training are significant, especially when regular volleyball training involves a significant number of jumps by a player in any given training session. Plyometrics is a common feature of both off-season and preseason training for this reason, with less focus on plyometrics drills in the competitive season.

Core strength is the generic term used to describe the functions of the abdominal, gluteal, lumbar (lower back), and groin muscles. Well-developed core strength will provide any athlete with greater balance in movement, especially in actions requiring the athlete to move quickly from a crouched position, a common feature in volleyball. Volleyball players will train aggressively in the development of core strength during both off-season and preseason training periods, with reduced intensity in the competitive period for the purpose of strength maintenance. Focused weight training, such as squats and lunges (both of which develop the upper thighs and hamstrings), and various types of abdominal crunches, including forms of Swiss ball training, are effective in the enhancement of core strength.

Stretching and flexibility exercises, both through traditional calisthenics and using devices such as a Swiss ball, are essential to performance and to the reduction of the risk of injury. Stretching is an integral part of the entire volleyball training regimen, in all three general training periods. It provides protection to the musculoskeletal structure against imbalances that often lead to muscle strains and pulls, as well as maximizing the range of motion in all joints, encouraging greater flexibility and correspondingly more effective movement. A stiff player will not be responsive on the volleyball court. Exercises that assist the player with recovery from the potential repetitive strains on the shoulder from the practice of serves and spikes are emphasized.

Aerobic fitness is a less emphasized but important aspect of volleyball training. Endurance acts as a platform on which the more spectacular leaping and athletic movements in the sport may occur. A five-game volleyball match, played in a warm gymnasium, may take two hours to complete. In the same fashion that running provides a boxer with the stamina to recover from the exertions of each round with an opponent, aerobic fitness permits the volleyball player a speedy recovery after a particularly intense series of points.

**SEE ALSO** Plyometrics; Stretching and flexibility; Volleyball; Volleyball: Set and spike mechanisms.

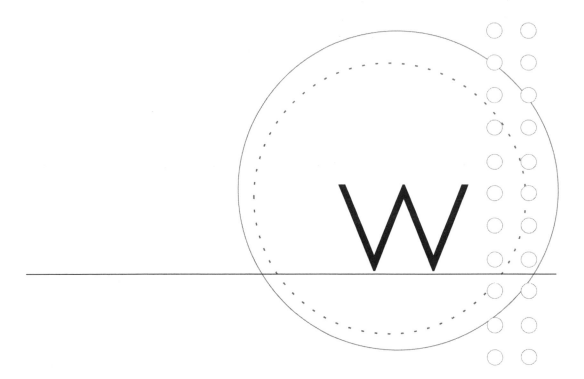

## WADA SEE World Anti-Doping Agency (WADA)

# Grete Waitz

10/1/1953–
NORWEGIAN
RUNNER

Grete Waitz is a former world-class track and distance runner. Among her accomplishments, she may be best known for her success in the marathon. Her victories included nine of the New York City Marathon.

Waitz is a pioneer in women's track events. She was one of the first women to compete at 3,000 m. Her world records attained at that distance reinforced the idea that women could successfully compete in track at a high level internationally.

Waitz was born in Oslo in 1953. Despite displaying a childhood aptitude for athletics, she was discouraged from training by her parents. At that time, athletics in general, and track in particular, were not considered a proper pursuit for a woman.

As a result, Waitz's early training was self-financed. Even when she competed at the 1972 Summer Olympics held in Munich, the first time women were allowed to compete in the 1,500-m, Waitz supported herself by studying at a teachers college in Norway. By then, she had gained her parents' acceptance for the serious development of her obvious running talent. Nonetheless, her teachers' training represented her safeguard occupation.

While at college, Waitz began to train twice a day and increased her training mileage to an average of 75 mi (121 km) per week. Her dedication and diligence paid off. Her running career blossomed and by the end of the 1970s, with the acceptance of women's running, running had become a lucrative fulltime pursuit.

In 1975, she twice set new world record times for the women's 3,000-m. Despite her success on the track, the high weekly training mileage had convinced Waitz that her calling lay in longer distances. She focused on the marathon, a 26.2-mi (42 km) event.

During the 1970s and 1980s, she enjoyed great success in the marathon. Beginning in 1978, Waitz won the New York Marathon nine times, an accomplishment that has not been matched by any other woman, or man. As well, she was victorious in the 1983 and 1986 London Marathon, and at the 1983 World Championships.

Prior to her first marathon victory, Waitz had never run more than 13 mi (21 km) in training or competition. She not only won the race, but set a women's world record in the process.

Her best showing in the Olympic women's marathon was in the 1984 Olympics held in Los Angeles, the sole time she competed, where she placed second behind American Joan Benoit Samuelson. She was denied a chance to compete in the 1980 Olympics, as Norway was one of the 65 countries that boycotted the Moscow Olympics in protest of the Soviet Union's 1979 invasion of Afghanistan.

In addition to her marathon successes, Waitz won the World Cross-Country Championships four years in a row beginning in 1978 and followed by another victory, this time in 1983.

Among the tributes accorded Waitz are "Grete's Great Gallop" (a race held in her honor each year by The New York Road Runner's Club), a statue outside Oslo's famed Bislett Stadium, and a set of stamps issued in her honor by the Norwegian government.

Although she is no longer a competitive runner, Waitz continues to contribute to the sport by participating and organizing corporate running events. Her focus now is to inspire others to adopt a more healthy lifestyle and to raise funds for charities that include CARE International and the International Special Olympics.

Her emphasis on health has become especially poignant since she began therapy for cancer in mid-2005 at the age of 51. As of 2006, her therapy continues.

# Wakeboarding

Wakeboarding is one of a number of sports that have attained world wide popularity in recent years through their association with the class of activities generally described as extreme sports.

Wakeboarding is performed using a specially designed item of equipment built to support a rider that is towed behind a relatively powerful motorboat, called a wakeboard. The equipment and the techniques employed to ride the wakeboard are a hybrid created from a number of sports, notably water skiing, surfing, and snowboarding. When wakeboarding was first developed as a water sport in the early 1980s, the signature equipment at that time was a "skurfer," built as a cross between a surfboard and a water ski.

Unlike water skiing, where the skier uses stationary ramps constructed on a water ski course to execute jumps, wakeboarding requires the tow boat to generate a large wake that the boarder uses to ride across and generate lift from the action of the wake. Similar to the construction of a snowboard, the rider's feet are attached to the wakeboard by way of non-release bindings.

The physics of riding a wakeboard are similar to both snowboarding and surfing. The rider seeks to maintain a low body position over the board, to permit both greater stability and to facilitate quick weight shifts to change the direction of the wakeboard. The wakeboard has sharp edges along its entire perimeter, permitting the rider to carve turns in the manner of a slalom skier on snow. Once airborne, as the boarder is attached to both the wakeboard and the two rope, the rider can execute any number of aerial tricks, including flips, rolls, and other sequential moves.

Wakeboarding has been a featured sport throughout the history of the X Games, the annual extreme sports festival. The World Wakeboard Association is the international body that sponsors competitions, where the athletes are subjectively judges on the quality and creativity of the tricks performed.

Although wakeboarding is itself a recently developed sport, it has given rise to another distinct sporting activity, wakeskating. Wakeskating is a form of wakeboarding that has been significantly influenced by skateboarding. The rider's feet are not attached to the board, one that is typically shorter than a conventional wakeboard. The surface of the wakeskating board is coated with a gripping material, and the rider seeks to operate the board using similar techniques to those employed by skateboarders on the ground.

Kneeboarding is another wakeboard variant, where the rider kneels on the board as it is pulled.

**SEE ALSO** Extreme sports; Snowboarding; Water skiing.

# Wall climbing SEE Rock climbing and wall climbing

# William Ernest Walsh

11/30/1931–
AMERICAN
PROFESSIONAL FOOTBALL COACH

Bill Walsh was the coaching genius behind the successes of the San Francisco 49ers football team during the 1980s. Walsh combined technological advances such as computer assisted play development to script an entire game, with his deep understanding of how to maximize effectiveness of the most important offensive player, the quarterback. These innovations were a part of the style of play pioneered by Walsh later known as the West Coast offence.

Like many successful coaches in any sport, Bill Walsh was a good but not outstanding athlete in his own competitive athletic career. As a high school and as a college quarterback, he was never regarded as a professional football prospect, and Walsh, a realist, secured his university degree in physical education.

Bill Walsh was one of the many successful NFL head coaches who served a lengthy and somewhat tortured apprenticeship before landing his desired place. Walsh began his coaching career at Monterey Peninsula College in 1959, an otherwise undistinguished California junior college program. He served in a succession of NFL assistant coaching positions before being named head coach at prestigious Stanford University.

Walsh had been pegged as a specialist assistant coach as a result of his work with various NFL quarterbacks, particularly as a result of his coaching with the Cincinnati Bengals staff. In Cincinnati, Walsh had the opportunity to serve under one of the greatest minds to ever coach in football at any level, Paul Brown. Walsh stayed in Cincinnati hoping to be appointed head coach there when Brown retired in 1975; he was passed over and Walsh was bitterly disappointed with the NFL, prompting his search for a suitable college head coach position.

Walsh's acceptance of the head coaching position at Stanford was an important bridge in his ultimate NFL success. Stanford was a major college program in the Pacific Athletic Conference that had fallen on difficult times in its football program. Walsh served for two successful years at Stanford, commencing in 1977. Walsh guided a previously lackluster Stanford team to a 9-3 season in 1977 and an 8-4 season in 1978. He also won the 1977 Sun Bowl and the 1978 Bluebonnet Bowl, further endearing him to the Stanford administration. Walsh was in a position to remain for an extended tenure at Stanford.

Walsh moved into the NFL with San Francisco in 1979, in the dual capacity of coach and general manager. Walsh's reputation in NFL circles as developed from his various assistant coaching stints around the league was that Walsh possessed a highly developed intelligence for football, that he was a thinker and a teacher, qualities that were not always held in high regard in the fast paced, results driven world of NFL football. Walsh had one advantage inherent in this new coaching position—the 49ers had been so bad for so long that very little was expected of Walsh.

The installation of Walsh as the head coach coincided with the most fortuitous player event in the history of the 49er organization, the arrival of future

Hall of Fame quarterback Joe Montana. Walsh began to assemble players who complimented Montana's controlled but aggressive quarterbacking style, and by 1981, Walsh had built the first of his three Super Bowl champions. His 49ers were a threat to win every year, and the subsequent Super Bowl victories in 1985 and 1989 cemented Walsh's reputation as one of the NFL's greatest coaches.

The West Coast offence implemented by Walsh at San Francisco has been imitated by many coaches and teams in subsequent years, at both the NFL and collegiate levels. Walsh, using first Montana and later Steve Young at quarterback, endeavored to control the ball with a short, precision passing game where the quarterback was given specific options once the ball was in play; both Montana and Young, Hall of Fame performers, were brilliant in this role. Walsh employed computer technology to assist in the breakdown of an opponent's defensive tendencies. Once the tendencies were determined Walsh endeavored to ensure that his quarterback had defined options available on every play. With pre-determined options, Walsh could limit the risks of the quarterback being sacked or otherwise forced into a decision that was not supported by the game plan.

Walsh purported to retire from football in 1989, the highest paid coach in the history of the NFL. He returned to the head coach position at Stanford in 1992 for two seasons. Walsh rejoined the 49ers as the club's General Manager from 1999 to 2001, without achieving the same level of success as he did as a coach.

Walsh was inducted into the Pro Football Hall of Fame in 1993.

SEE ALSO Football (American); National Football League (NFL); Sports Coaching.

# Warm-up/Cool-down

Proper and comprehensive athletic warm-up and cool-down protocols are essential to short-term exercise performance, as well as long-term injury prevention and general physical health. The warm-up/cool-down sequences are as important to athletic performance as the athlete's abilities in the sport itself. While each is a part of the exercise and training continuum, different principles are at play in these training phases.

A warm-up is intended to ready the athlete for either a training session or a competition. While a

WORLD of SPORTS SCIENCE                                                                                         767 warm-up routine may take many forms, subject to the sport or the training goals of the athlete, the warm-up will both physically and mentally prepare the athlete for the intended task. From a physiological perspective, the first objective of the warm-up is the increased flow of blood through the cardiovascular system, preparatory to the heart being engaged in more vigorous and demanding effort. The increase in blood flow serves to make the skeletal muscles supple and more prepared to stretch. Increased blood supplied to the muscles correspondingly increases the amount of oxygen and other nutrients available to the muscles during exercise.

The start of a warm-up is a signal to the body that exercise is about to commence, a form of mental preparation. The warm-up also is a trigger to the neuromuscular system that the linkages between the nervous system and various muscle groups will be utilized shortly. While a lack of available training time and a desire to begin the substantive parts of the training or activity are the most common reasons as to why some warm-ups are not thorough, numerous sports science studies have confirmed that a thorough warm-up will reduce the rate of injury while increasing overall athletic performance.

While the intensity and the duration of a warm-up will vary due to individual circumstances, evidence that the desired increase in cardiovascular activity and an increase in internal body temperature consistent with muscle warmth is the generation of a light-to-moderate degree of perspiration. A minimal warm-up, where the athlete is not engaging in a specific or targeted activity, will generally last from eight to 10 minutes. This warm-up might include very easy jogging or vigorous walking, with a pronounced arm swing to increase the heart rate. When the warm-up is conducted in cold weather, the body may require a longer period of time to produce the desired cardiovascular and thermoregulatory effects. The athlete may conduct some sport-specific warm-up movements to provide benefits.

Once the body has been activated through a basic warm-up, the athlete may engage in a stretching program. All skeletal muscle groups are more vulnerable to strain and tearing if the muscles are aggressively stretched without a warm-up. The most effective method of stretching, the static stretch, requires the athlete to maintain the muscle structure in the extended position for between 20 and 30 seconds. It is particularly important to conduct the static stretches for the muscles that will be primarily engaged in the activity ahead.

The primary goal of the cool-down phase is to gradually reduce the level of activity achieved by the body during either training or competition. An effective cool-down program will gradually reduce the person's heart rate to its normal level, and it will assist in the efficient removal of metabolic wastes, such as lactic acid produced by the cardiovascular system. Just as importantly, a proper cool-down will ready the muscles for the next training session or activity. There is no conclusive scientific proof that cooling down necessarily reduces a condition known as delayed onset muscle soreness. This condition frequently occurs to athletes whose muscles have been subjected to a strenuous workout, with the onset of muscle discomfort not present for between 24 to 48 hours after the event. However, overall muscle health is promoted through the cool-down process whether or not the muscle subsequently becomes sore.

A simple and effective means of cooling down is to continue to exercise at a low intensity level for approximately 10 minutes for every hour of vigorous exercise, immediately at the conclusion of the primary exercise. A gap between the higher intensity levels is counterproductive to the goals of a gradual return to resting levels. A stretching routine of the same extent and intensity level to that employed in the warm-up is also useful, as the muscles are properly warm from the activity.

SEE ALSO Calisthenics; Exercise recovery; Fitness; Musculoskeletal injuries; Stretching and flexibility.

# Warm weather exercise

Warm weather is a term familiar to most people as a phenomenon that can be defined in subjective terms—individuals have differing perceptions as to what will constitute warm versus cold weather conditions. The establishment of warm weather conditions suitable for exercise is not simply a function of temperature; it is a combination of the air temperature, humidity, wind, air pollution, and other environmental factors. The physical conditions affecting warm weather exercise are diverse. For example, the surface on which a sport is played may change with varying conditions; sports such as marathon running, in which the race is run over heat-radiating pavement, have additional warm weather factors that would otherwise be reduced or absent.

Warm weather is a training and competitive issue that must be overcome by most athletes at some stage in their careers, from those at the recreational level to elite competitors. While increased physical fitness will usually better equip an athlete to combat the effects of warm weather, the principles of warm weather exercise are applicable to all fitness levels.

The consideration of the impacts and consequences of warm weather exercise are of vital importance to sport performance and athlete safety. In the course of the long-term planning for an athlete's competitive and training season, referred to as the periodization of training, the season will be divided into the preseason, the competitive season, and the off-season. When known climatic conditions will be a factor at various points of the season, the athlete can plan the training accordingly. In the same fashion, when the athlete is aware of particular competitions in warm weather climates, specific steps can be taken in advance to best prepare for the event.

A failure to anticipate warm weather factors in training can lead to competitive disaster. When an athlete, particularly in a sport with a significant aerobic component, is unaccustomed to the impacts of warm weather and the collateral impacts of insufficient hydration and fluid replacement, it is highly unlikely that the athlete can compete effectively at the accustomed cool weather training levels.

Once the appropriate training periods are determined through preseason analysis, the athlete can progressively build warm weather exercise components into training sessions. The first step is the incorporation of acclimatization training into regular workouts. Acclimatization is the process through which the body adapts itself to the stresses of warm weather. As a general rule, when the body is exposed to warm weather conditions (often accompanied by humidity), there will be a pronounced and cumulative effect of the local environment on three interrelated bodily processes: the cardiovascular system, particularly through decreased blood volume; the thermoregulatory system, which will strive to maintain a constant internal temperature of approximately 98 °F (37 °C); and the osmoregulatory system, which preserves fluid levels in relation to the presence of sodium and other minerals.

Although individual athletes will respond in different ways to the effects of warm weather, as a general rule, an athlete'sbody will be over 90% acclimatized to the presence of heat within 10 to 14 days of first exposure to the new conditions. Acclimatization is best achieved at the location where warm weather is anticipated during competition. Warm weather can also be simulated; indoor workouts in increased temperatures are an example.

The second step to be taken by an athlete to develop warm weather exercise ability is the implementation of a hydration strategy. Hydration is the process by which an athlete seeks to maintain a relative constant fluid level within the body throughout exercise. As a general rule, hydration requires the athlete to consume fluids before, during, and after the exercise activity, sufficient to replace all fluids lost through perspiration and other bodily functions (primarily breath and urine production). It is a well-accepted sports science proposition that when an athlete loses between 1% to 2% of body weight through fluid loss (an amount that is classed as a slight degree of dehydration), athletic performance may decrease by up to 10%. As slight levels of dehydration may not necessarily trigger the body's thirst mechanism, regular fluid consumption is crucial to proper hydration.

A failure to observe proper and timely hydration will often trigger a progressive series of increasingly dangerous heat-related illnesses, including muscle cramps, heat exhaustion, and heat stroke.

There are a variety of fluids available to the athlete to achieve hydration. Water is the most common fluid used, although a significant science has developed with respect to the formulation of various sports drinks, each designed for specific sports and usages. Most sports drinks contain amounts of sodium and potassium to aid in the body's ability to maintain proper osmoregulation. For hydration, as opposed to the replenishment of carbohydrate stores, sports drinks do not generally contain more than 6% to 8% carbohydrate, to ensure ease of absorption of the fluid into the body by way of the small intestine.

During the acclimatization phase, the athlete and coaches must carefully monitor the twin performance keys of intensity and duration. Failure to observe the appropriate balance between these factors can create significant physical consequences for the athlete. It is imperative that all warm weather exercise be conducted with ready access to appropriate first aid equipment.

**SEE ALSO** Acclimatization; Heat exhaustion; Hydration; Thermoregulation, exercise, and thirst; Two-a-day practice sessions.

# Water

Water, along with air and food, is one of the three cornerstones of the physical element to human existence. In its pure state, water is transparent, tasteless, and colorless. The water molecule is comprised of two hydrogen atoms and one oxygen atom, as described by the chemical equation $H_2O$. Water is the most prominent substance found within the body, and its importance to human structure and function is borne out by the relationship of water relative to the size and the composition of the body as a whole. Water constitutes approximately 92% of the volume of blood plasma, the fluid component of blood, as well as forming 60% of the mass of the erythrocytes (red blood cells) present in the bloodstream. A further 80% of the mass of skeletal muscle tissue is water, and the water molecule constitutes over 95% of the total molecules within the body.

Water is also classified by commercial purposes as "hard" and "soft." Hard water is a fluid substance that naturally contains significant quantities of the minerals, calcium and magnesium; these minerals are absent in soft water. Depending on the geological characteristics of the location where the water originates, water may contain other minerals such as sodium and potassium, as well as compounds such as chlorides and sulphides. Many of these mineral-laden waters are reputed to possess health-giving qualities.

From an athletic perspective, water has been described as "nature's original sports drink." All persons, both sedentary and athletic, must consume water on a daily basis, preferably at regular intervals throughout the day, for the body to function properly. Water is lost from the body through the processes of perspiration, through the discharge of breath from the lungs (the breath when exhaled includes water vapor present in the lungs), and through the elimination of the waste products urine and feces. The recommended daily amount of water to be consumed will be subject to the significant variables of age, body size, level of fitness, environmental conditions, type of exercise, the duration and the level of intensity required in exercise, and other related physiological factors. For persons whose physical exercise in any given day is at a moderate level, defined as running 3 mi (4.8 km) or working out 30 minutes on a cardio machine, they will generally be required to consume approximately 3–5 qt (approximately 4 l) of water daily to maintain efficient overall bodily function.

In sports science, the terms water and fluid are often used interchangeably when issues regarding the proper approach to the hydration of athletes is considered. Fluids are those substances that are primarily water, with other substances added to create an effect on the body that is designed to assist with respect to a particular physiological or chemical function in the body. Water with minerals or other additives, milk, sport drinks, and energy drinks are all examples of fluids commonly used by athletes to maintain fluid levels. The hydration strategy referred to as fluid replacement may include consideration of the relative merits of both pure water as well as any other fluid.

The essential role of water in the function of the body is best illustrated in three systems that are central to athletic performance: the cardiovascular system, the osmoregulatory system, and the thermoregulatory system. It is a commonly stated sports science proposition that, if the body loses as little as 1% to 2% of its fluids through dehydration, athletic performance may decline by as much as 10%.

The all-pervasive power of cardiovascular function within the body is felt in every aspect of physical performance. The bloodstream, through the movement of its erythrocytes, carries oxygen and nutrients to working cells to facilitate the further production of energy. As a general proposition, when the body becomes dehydrated, the blood volumes within the system are reduced, which slows the efficiency of both the transport of oxygen and nutrients, as well as a delay in the corresponding removal of metabolic wastes through the blood. The cardiovascular system cannot function effectively if the system is dehydrated, no matter what other steps may be taken by the athlete to assist in performance in any other respect.

Osmoregulation is the built-in mechanism that seeks to ensure the levels of bodily fluids and the electrolytes throughout the body. When the ratio between water and electrolytes fluctuates too far from optimal levels, the body's ability to maintain overall fluid levels and to transmit nerve impulses into muscular action is affected. The proportion of sodium to water is the most important of the ratios sought to be maintained through osmoregulation. The sodium level directly impacts the organ functions that relate to hydration, such as blood pressure and the production of urine by the kidneys. The kidneys excrete urine in accordance with the hormonal signals triggered by fluctuations in sodium levels; when the sodium level is too low, the kidneys will tend to produce more urine to decrease the proportion of water to sodium in the body, with the converse action of limiting urine production when the sodium level is too high.

Thermoregulation is the body's control of its internal temperature in response to all external environmental forces. The most effective regulator of internal temperature is the cooling of the body through the production and release of perspiration. In warm weather exercise, an athlete may lose up to 32 oz (1 l) of fluid per hour; perspiration is not pure water, as it includes both water and minerals, primarily sodium. The body's thirst mechanism, triggered in the hypothalamus region of the brain, is not activated until the body has lost approximately 1 to 2 qt (1 to 2 l) of fluid. It is for this reason that athletes must hydrate on a regular basis during both training and competition, whether or not they have experienced thirst.

With the importance of fluid replacement paramount for every athlete, the quality and the precise formulation of the replacement fluid is a critical issue. The overall goal of fluid replacement is to replace the amount of fluid lost to perspiration and other bodily functions during athletic activity. While pure water will often provide a solution for dehydration, the consumption of large quantities of water for this purpose creates risks for the athlete. Water consumed alone may dramatically affect the desired proportion of sodium to water within the body, signaling the body to prevent the absorption of further water into the bloodstream, directing the excess instead to the tissues of the body. This condition, hyponatremia, is potentially fatal, as the person will become further dehydrated.

For longer periods of exercise, there is considerable scientific support for the proposition that a sports drink, primarily water, with no more than 8% carbohydrate, that also provides sodium and potassium in the mixture, will adequately address the hydration needs of an athlete. The carbohydrate will provide an athlete with another fuel source during exercise; carbohydrate in excess of 8% is more difficult to absorb into the body and may cause cramping.

Energy drinks are a poor hydration choice. Although most of these beverages are over 90% water, all contain stimulants that are also powerful diuretics, primarily caffeine. Recent studies have illustrated that many energy drinks contain over 120 mg of caffeine per 16 oz (500 ml) serving; the U.S. Food and Drug Administration has limited soda to 65 mg of caffeine per 12 oz (350 ml) serving. If the body has begun to sustain the effects of dehydration, the consumption of energy drinks will likely accelerate the process.

**SEE ALSO** Blood volume; Cardiovascular system; Hydration; Renal function; Sodium and sodium deficits; Thermoregulation, exercise, and thirst; Water (oxygen enhancement).

# Water (oxygen enhancement)

In recent years, water that has been treated with additional oxygen has been marketed as both a sports drink and as a general nutritional supplement. These oxygen-enhanced water products are popularly known as oxygenated water or oxygenized water, depending on the particular manufacturer. The substances are marketed commercially under a variety of trade names.

Oxygenated water is a product whose appeal can be traced to the rise of the marathon and the triathlon as mass participation sports in the late 1970s and early 1980s, developments that sparked the formation of the international sports drink industry. By the late 1990s, sports drinks had established a significant niche in the health and nutrition marketplace as a whole, with advertising campaigns that took clear aim at both athletic and non-athletic consumer targets. Sports drinks have been subsequently marketed not simply as a rehydration tool for the active athlete, but also for the inherently healthy formulations that is claimed by their producers.

In a similar fashion, oxygenated water, like mineral water, is claimed to promote better general health among its users. Its proponents also advocate oxygenated water as a supplement that will significantly enhance athletic performance, particularly in endurance sports.

Water, both in its pure laboratory form and in its natural state, is a fluid, a molecule created through the binding of two hydrogen atoms and a single oxygen atom. The chemistry of water is expressed as the formula $H_2O$. Oxygen in its elemental state is a constituent of water, but that oxygen is tightly bound to the hydrogen atoms within the water molecule; this oxygen is not capable of any release from the chemical structure in a sports drink in a fashion that the body can use in the production of energy, in the manner that oxygen inhaled through the lungs is subsequently transported by the erythrocytes (red blood cells) in the bloodstream. The oxygen added to an oxygenated sport drink is injected into the fluid under pressure and bottled.

The theory in support of oxygenated water as a training aid is the more oxygen that a person can consume, through any means, the more oxygen will be directed into the cells of the body. Once it enters the stomach, oxygenated water will be ingested through the small intestine. The cardiovascular system will transport the additional oxygen to the cells that need it, as with any other nutrient. As a result, the oxygenated water will enhance athletic performance, stamina, and overall energy levels, because the cells have more oxygen available to them to metabolize its energy stores.

A number of scientific studies conducted since the late 1990s concerning the benefits of oxygenated water have reached conclusions that counter the claims of the water manufacturers. All of these studies confirm the physiological proposition that oxygen carried into the stomach through the water consumed will not enter the bloodstream, as this oxygen will never pass beyond the membranes of the intestine. None of the studies conducted found any observable difference in the heart rate or overall cardiovascular function in persons using oxygenated water.

The American Council in Exercise was one research group to conclude that the only method by which oxygen could reach an energy-producing cell would be by way of the hemoglobin present in each erythrocyte, or by way of the tiny amounts that might be dissolved in blood plasma. Hemoglobin is the oxygen carrier present in every red blood cell. As the hemoglobin is at all times saturated with oxygen (as much 95% capacity) through the normal oxygen transport processes centered in the exchange mechanism situated in the alveoli, the tiny air sacs within the lungs, the oxygenated water has no delivery mechanism available to it.

Confirmation of the research critical of the oxygenated water industry claims is also supported, in a more oblique way, through the controversies regarding the illegal use of the hormone erythropoietin (EPO) by endurance athletes. EPO is the natural hormone that spurs the production of greater numbers of red blood cells to increase the body's oxygen-carrying capacity. The considerable body of science concerning EPO confirms that the only method by which oxygen capacity can be increased in an athlete is through increasing the number of erythrocytes available in the bloodstream.

While the athletic performance-enhancing claims made with respect to oxygenated water may be of questionable scientific validity, there is also the placebo effect of such products to be considered. Unlike many other sports supplements, pure water is not inherently harmful, and the consumption of oxygenated water is safe. The cost of these products aside, oxygenated water is a proper method with which to obtain the daily recommended water consumption levels. If the athlete believes that he or she is obtaining a physical advantage through the consumption of oxygenated water, the athlete may have created a personal psychological edge.

SEE ALSO Cardiovascular system; Hydration; Oxygen; Water.

# Water polo

Water polo has a reputation as one of the toughest, most physically demanding team sports in the world. It is a game that combines the tactical elements and the physicality of such diverse sports as swimming, soccer, basketball, ice hockey, and rugby. The object of water polo is to throw a ball into a net defended by a goal keeper and six teammates who use physical means to hinder the offensive team's attack. The ball is advanced using passing plays and other offensive tactics. All of this takes place in water that is 6 ft (1.8 m) deep. Players move in the water at all times and are without swimming aids.

Water polo was born as an aquatic version of rugby in England in the 1870s. The early versions of the game were brutal contests that permitted almost any tactic in the stopping of an opponent, including blows, kicks, and grappling maneuvers. Eventually, water polo evolved to a greater emphasis being placed on the swimming abilities of the players; speed and passing ability gained a corresponding importance in the game. Water polo has the distinction of being the first team sport included in the Olympic Games, played for the first time in 1900 as a men's sport; women's water polo was added to the Olympics in 2000.

The Federation Internationale de Natation Amateur (FINA) is the international body responsible for the governance of water polo and sponsors a popular World Water Polo League, where national water polo teams compete for an annual championship. In the United States, the National Collegiate Athletic Association (NCAA) has sanctioned a water polo championship since 1969, an event historically dominated by Californian universities.

Water polo is played in an pool that is generally between 66 ft and 100 ft (20–30 m) long, and 33 ft to 66 ft (10 m to 20 m) wide. In international play, the pool must be at least 6 ft (1.8 m) deep. There are six players per side plus a goalkeeper, who defends a net that is 10 ft (3 m) wide and 3 ft (90 cm) high.

The water polo ball has the approximate dimensions of a soccer ball; it may only be carried in, or thrown with, one hand by the players. Within the 5 m line (16 ft) of the goal, the goalkeeper may play the ball with two hands. The goalkeeper may also use a fist to strike the ball. The other players may move

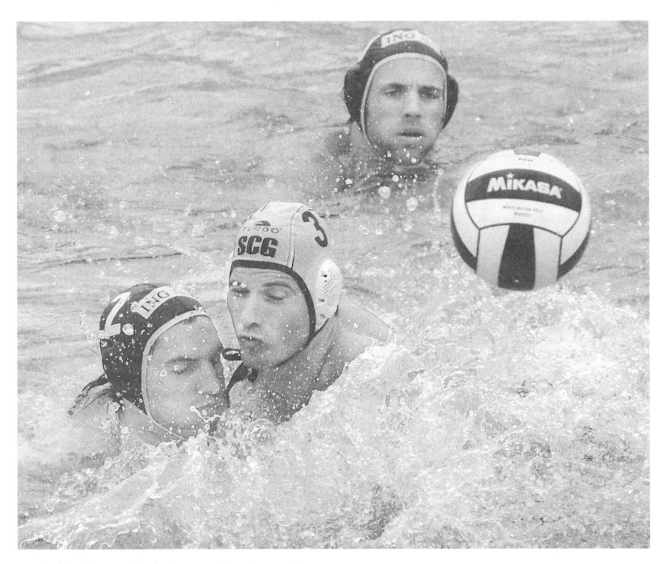

Gold match at the 2005 Men's World Water Polo Championships. STAN HONDA/AFP/GETTY IMAGES

with the ball pushing ahead of them in the water, an action described as "dribbling" the ball. The ball may be passed between the players using one hand on the throw and the catch.

To succeed in water polo, the player must have a number of physical skills, the most important of which is strong swimming ability. The player must be able to tread water using their legs only, to maintain a consistent body position above the water, for minutes at a time. The player must also have extremely well developed hand eye coordination, in order to both follow and handle the ball from a variety of angles and positions.

The offensive tactics employed in water polo require precise perimeter passing and accurate shooting. The "point" is the player with the most offensive responsibility, this player functions much like a point guard directing a basketball offence. The point distributes the ball to teammates, seeking to create advantageous angles in which a shot may be delivered. Shots in water polo may be a power shot, where the player delivers the ball with maximum velocity towards the goal, or as a skip shot, where the ball is fired to create a deflection off the water near the goal, making the ball difficult to handle for the goalkeeper.

The defensive tactics used in water polo are at the heart of its deserved reputation as a rugged, physical sport. There is virtually continuous body contact as the ball is played, much of it occurring below the surface of the water. A minor foul will result in possession of the ball to the opposing team. A major foul, such as holding or "sinking" an opponent, will result in a 20-second penalty, where the player must leave the play and remain at the side of the pool, in a fashion similar to an ice hockey infraction. If a penalty is committed against an offensive player within the 5 m area of the goal, the offensive player will be awarded a penalty shot.

The nature of water polo requires a comprehensive off season physical training regime. In an Olympic level game, composed of four 8 minute quarters, a water polo player will swim as far as 3 mi (4 km to 5 km). Elite players will usually divide their fitness programs between aerobic training, anaerobic training, and weight workouts, with stretching and flexibility training incorporated into each division. A useful training technique designed to build the player's ability to tread water for extended periods is to hold a weight over the players head while they tread water for minutes at a time.

SEE ALSO Endurance; Ice hockey; Soccer; Swimming.

# Water skiing

Water skiing is a sport that combines the grace and power of alpine skiing with the acrobatic flair of gymnastics and aerial skiing. Water skiing, the action of pulling a skier across a body of water by a motor boat, was invented by American Ralph Samuelson (1903–1977) in Minnesota in 1922. In its early period, the sport of water skiing was limited to the simple demonstration of balance by the athlete as they were transported across the water. With the development of increasingly powerful motorboats, water skiers could be pulled at significantly greater higher speeds. As skier speeds increased, water skiing expanded to include three distinct components—slalom skiing, where the skier navigates through a series of buoys set at irregular intervals on the water, creating obstacles similar to the gates used in Alpine slalom skiing; trick skiing, including the use of a single ski, barefoot skiing, and different types of acrobatic tricks; ski jumping, where the skier is pulled by a tow boat towards a ramp that is approximately 21 ft (6.5 m) long and 6 ft high (1.8 m); the ramp is anchored in a fixed position in the water. The winning jump in competition is determined by the distance achieved by the skiers, as there are no marks awarded for style or form. Elite water ski jumpers can attain distances of over 150 ft (45 m) in the air.

From its creation in the United States, water skiing was introduced to parts of Europe; it gained a particular popularity in areas such as the French Riviera. The International Water Ski Federation (IWSF) was founded in 1949. Today, water skiing is popular in all countries that possess access to any significant bodies of water. The IWSF sponsors a World Cup water ski tour that attracts professional competitors. The IWSF is a member of the Olympic movement; water skiing is not an Olympic sport.

The IWSF is also the governing body for the related sports of wakeboarding and kneeboarding. A wakeboard is a device with a construction similar to that of a snowboard, and the sport incorporates elements of surfing, snowboarding, ice skating, and waterskiing. As the name suggests, the wakeboarder rides in the wake generated by the towing motorboat; a knee boarder is positioned on their knees. Each discipline is particularly suited to the performance of tricks, including high speed turns, and a variety of somersaults and flip movements.

In water skiing, the prospective skier is generally introduced to the sport through the use of two skis. Once the skier establishes the desired degree of balance and proficiency, the skier will often develop further skills using a single ski, particularly in the execution of more demanding turns and slalom techniques.

The basic principle of physics that explain how the water skier is kept afloat while being towed is the same principle involved in the motion of the boat itself across the water. Planing is the application of the physical law that provides that all action will produce an equal and opposite reaction. With the water ski, designed with the ski tip tilted slightly upwards from the surface of the water, the water strikes the ski as the skier moves forward, creating a rebound downward from the ski. The rebound creates an upward force on the ski and the skier. So long as the upward water force is equal to the downward force of gravity (the weight of the skier), the skier must remain afloat.

When the skier is traveling in a straight line behind the boat, the two forces acting upon the skier are the force of the tow rope, as created by the movement of the tow boat, and the force of the water upon the skis. Assuming a constant tension in the tow rope, the skier will travel at the same speed as the boat when positioned directly behind the boat. When the skier endeavors to move in a perpendicular direction from the path of the tow boat (across the wake, the wave turbulence produced on the water's surface by the boat and its engine), a centripetal force is added to those forces directed against the skier.

Centripetal force means to "seek the center." The skier who moves in a path perpendicular to the

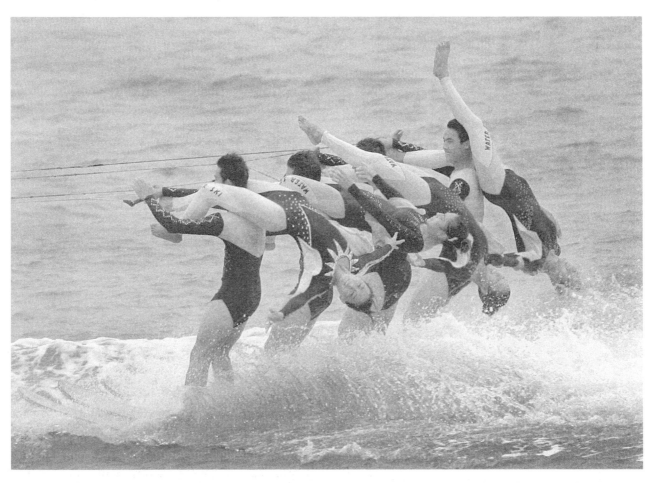

Chinese water skiing team. GOH CHAI HIN/AFP/GETTY IMAGES

direction of boat travel will be subjected to a force that produces acceleration upon the body of the skier toward to the center of the circular path, which is the boat. It is for this reason that the skier can move faster than the tow boat when all three forces acting upon the skier are combined.

Water skiers often travel at speeds in excess of 50 mph (80 km/h) if the tow boat is sufficiently powerful. If the skier falls at such speeds, the force of the impact into the water can cause significant injury.

The equipment used by water skiers in competition is regulated by the IWSF. The skis may be manufactured from wood, metal, or composite material products. Skis may not exceed 39.3 in (1 m) in length, with a maximum width of 9.75 in (25 cm). In cooler temperatures, most water skiers wear a full body wetsuit, which provides insulation to the skier as well as a degree of cushioning in a fall. A sleek, form-fitting life jacket is also mandatory.

The most common water ski injury are those sustained to the lower legs, including the knee joint. Research has established that 35% of water ski injuries occur in the lower extremities, with one half of those injuries sustained to the knee. The execution of high speed jumps and twisting movements directs significant and often irregular forces into the knee, as do the high speed falls that create awkward angles of collision between the water skier's body and the water surface.

Strength and conditioning exercises for water skiing are directed to both physical performance and the reduction of injuries. Skier leg strength is developed through exercises such as lunges or squats that assist in maintaining an appropriate strength ratio between the two sets of muscles that govern knee flexion and extension, the hamstrings and the quadriceps. A 3:2 ratio in the relative strength of the quadriceps to the hamstrings is generally accepted as one that will ensure balance in knee movement. Exercises such as calf raises develop the gastrocnemius and soleus muscles (the calf muscles) of the lower leg, which are important to maintain the skier's balance on the water.

As with many sports where the athlete operates in the air, as with a water ski trick or jump, the development of the skier's balance and perception skills is vital to competitive success. A Swiss ball is an effective tool for these purposes, as the skier can replicate many water ski movements and sensations through balance exercises with the Swiss ball; in essence, these exercises permit the skier to practice at being stable in a variety of positions.

Large muscle mass is not an essential aspect of water skiing. High repetition/low resistance weight exercises, designed to promote a well balanced physique, are an important part of the comprehensive dry land training of the water skier.

**SEE ALSO** Balance training and proprioception; Skiing, Alpine; Surfing; Windsurfing.

# Weight categories

Weight categories have been employed for centuries as a method of equalizing competition in a number of different sports. In sports where the physical strength of the combatants was understood to be crucial to their ultimate success, weight categories recognized the fundamental principle that, all things being equal, in strength sports the larger athlete was likely to be the stronger athlete. Stated in the alternative, where two athletes possess equal technical skill in a strength-oriented sport, the larger athlete is more likely to overpower the smaller athlete.

Weight categories are fundamental to the organization of competition in the individual sports of boxing, wrestling, and weightlifting. Each of these sports requires the athlete to build a dynamic, powerful body that possesses explosive power capabilities, all of which are integrated into a physical structure with a strong aerobic foundation. The only prominent team sport where weight divisions are employed is in rowing, which is divided into lightweight and heavyweight competitions.

Boxing is perhaps the best known of the sports in which weight divisions define the extent of the competition. The definition of each weight class varies slightly between those used at the Olympic Games and the common professional weight designations and some amateur competitions. The same weight categories are used with different weight limits for women's boxing. Boxers compete in divisions that range from the straw weight division for men up to 105 lb (46 kg), through the heavyweight division for men over 200 lb (91 kg). Throughout the history of professional boxing, certain weight divisions have garnered greater degrees of public attention and acclaim, particularly the heavyweight and the welterweight divisions (140–147 lb, or 66.6 kg limit).

In all sports where there are weight categories, the limits provided are not merely guidelines; they are inflexible limits. An inability on the part of the athlete to "make the weight" will disqualify the athlete from competition. Strategies have often been devised by athletes to assist in meeting a particular weight category standard, many of which compromise both the ability of the athlete to compete at the optimal level, in addition to placing significant adverse stresses on the function of many bodily systems.

There are two general approaches with respect to how an athlete should achieve and maintain a competitive weight standard. The first is the development of a training program in which the athlete seeks to develop maximum strength and fitness while at all times maintaining the target weight for competition. The second strategy is to develop maximum strength and fitness without a primary concern for the weight limit, with a concerted weight loss effort immediately prior to competition to come under the standard. The second strategy is premised on the theory that the athlete can bring a level of strength to competition that would otherwise only be attainable at a higher weight.

The number of times during a competition that an athlete will be tested for compliance with the weight category limits varies from sport to sport. In amateur boxing and wrestling, in which the competitions may span a number of bouts over a period of several days, the athlete will be weighed at the beginning of the competition and then prior to each succeeding match. Once the athlete has achieved a desired weight, it must be maintained throughout the competition.

All weight category sports place significant demands on the body during both competition and in training with respect to sufficient caloric intake, proper nutrition, and hydration. Whatever strategy is employed concerning the achievement of the requisite weight standard, sports scientists and nutritionists generally recommend that the athlete maintain a year-round weight that never exceeds the competitive weight limit by more than 10%. The management of weight targets is another

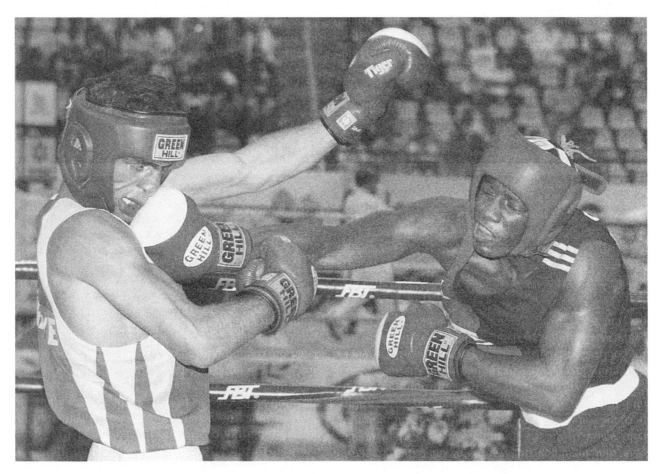

Weight categories have been established in boxing and other sports to equalize competition. SAEED KHAN/AFP/GETTY IMAGES

aspect of how the athlete will plan the training for a competitive season, a process known as the periodization of training. In these sports, weight management is as important to athletic success as the development of sport-specific technique, for without making the proper weight, there is no competition.

There are no additional risks to an athlete who maintains competitive weight year-round. Athletes who must dramatically cut weight before competition create potential physical and psychological risks that must be carefully considered. Weight cutting strategies should first be implemented in the dietary choices made in training, where nutrition-rich, and relatively low-calorie, low-fat foods will reduce the accumulation of excess weight. The body's ability to repair itself during the rest intervals between workouts is founded on its nutritional intake; when athletes are monitoring their weight, they must seek maximum nutritional return for reduced caloric value.

When the athlete seeks to lose weight through a "crash" diet in the period leading up to competition,

nutrients that are not stored in the body, including the water-soluble vitamin B complex and vitamin C, may not be present in sufficient quantities to perform their respective maintenance and repair functions. Vitamin C, as an example, is essential to the production of collagen, a building block of bone, ligaments, and tendons.

When the athlete must lose 5 lb (2.2 kg) or more on the eve of competition, it is common to dehydrate to make the desired weight. The sudden loss of fluids, which must be maintained through the entire competition, will likely impair the performance of the athlete. The loss of significant quantities of body fluid will directly impact blood volume, which limits the ability of the cardiovascular system to function at peak efficiency. When the athlete competes in successive bouts at reduced fluid levels, the risk of a heat-related illness triggered by dehydration is significant, as the body's thermoregulatory system will not be able to cool itself as efficiently through perspiration.

Peak athletic performance will require a complete commitment to the employment of competitive strategies and the execution of demanding physical maneuvers. The additional stress imposed on the competitor to make weight or be disqualified may serve as a significant distraction to the efforts of the athlete to maintain competitive focus prior to the event.

The most common dehydration techniques used in weight category sport are the use of "sweat boxes," or similar artificial heating of the athlete to induce perspiration, and taking diuretics. The use of diuretics is a time-honored practice in sports such as boxing; these are substances that stimulate the increased production of urine by the kidneys. Many diuretics are prohibited in international competitions that are regulated by the World Anti-Doping Agency (WADA), although this ban is aimed more at the use of diuretics as a steroid-masking agent than for their use by athletes to achieve a weight. Diuretic use for any purpose will lead to disqualification.

In some youth sports, weight categories are a means of ensuring safety for all participants; American football for players below high school age is an example.

SEE ALSO Boxing; Rowing; Weight gain; Weight loss; Wrestling.

# Weight control SEE Body composition and weight control

# Weight gain

Humans have had a fascination with their weight throughout the course of history. The perfect weights, ideal weights, and optimal weights of the human body have been the subject of both social and scientific study for centuries.

For non-athletic people, weight is not determined with reference to science or physiology, but by the appearance of the individual. "If you look good, you feel good" is a rule of life for many throughout the world, and these people view ideal weight as one at which they can function as they wish, in terms of the clothing that they may comfortably wear and the daily activities in which they may participate. Ideal weight from a social or personal perspective is unrelated to science.

Sports science approaches weight considerations from a far more rigorous perspective. Ideal weights are not determined with any reference to appearance, but are tied to the analyses of human performance and capabilities achievable at a particular weight to achieve a desired result. The scientifically sanctioned ideal weight for an individual may engage a multitude of physiological, nutritional, training, and competitive considerations, a product of analysis as opposed to personal preference.

Weight gain is a physical process that is diametrically opposed to that of weight loss. These two familiar concepts are positioned on either side of a flexible standard that represents the ideal body weight of an individual. A weight gain strategy is not effective if it later results in the implementation of a corrective weight loss strategy. Western society in general, and North American culture in particular, has been swamped with weight loss strategies in seemingly ever-increasing numbers, with a paradoxical rise in levels of obesity and the numbers of overweight persons; weight gain is a less common concern for the general population.

Weight gain among athletes will be observed in one of three general scenarios: an intentional weight gain, as a part of a structured training and dietary program to achieve a defined athletic goal; a careless or negligent weight gain, when the athlete fails to pay proper attention to diet and nutrition relative to the body's physical demands; and unavoidable or involuntary weight gain, such as those triggered by prescription medication or pregnancy. It is the intentional and the carelessly triggered weight gains that are of prime concern in sports science.

From a scientific perspective, weight gain and weight loss are straightforward scientific propositions. When the attainment of a particular body mass, without reference to physical performance or athletic capability, is the goal of any individual, weight gain or weight loss is readily achievable. One pound of excess body fat represents the storage of 3,500 calories of unused and convertible energy in the body. If a person increases the amount of calories consumed over the amount of energy expended by an amount of 500 calories per day, whether through increased food consumption, decreased physical activity, or a combination of these actions, the individual will gain one pound of body mass per week (7 days × 500 calories), where all other physiological factors remain constant. The same proposition, calculated in reverse, applies to weight loss.

For an athlete, the stark mathematical calculation in support of weight gain is not so straightforward.

WEIGHT GAIN

Ideal weight in any athlete must first be broadly considered with reference to the physical attributes of the athlete with reference to the broader demands of the sport. To reference an extreme example, an 18-year-old female athlete stands 5 ft 6 in tall (1.67 m), and is a strong and fit 135 lb (61 kg). This athlete enjoys throwing the shotput, and wishes to pursue this sport in university competition. An understanding of both the physics of the shotput, and the type of physique needed to compete at a higher level would suggest that the 40–50 lb (20–23 kg) weight gain this athlete would have to achieve to continue with her competitive objectives is likely a physical impossibility. If the athlete wished to be a shot putter for her pleasure, she could do so at her present healthy weight. The ideal weight for this athlete relative to the desired activity is unlikely to be achieved through healthy means.

Once the ideal weight for the specific athlete to compete in the sport has been broadly determined, a number of factors are engaged. The first is the physical composition of the athlete. It is common for persons in the general population and athletes alike to possess a body weight that falls within the apparent ideal range for their participation in a sport. The amount of that ideal weight that is useful lean body mass versus body fat is an important consideration.

The lean body mass is the weight of the musculoskeletal structure; the total mass of an individual less the amount of body fat provides the total musculoskeletal weight. Body fat has been the subject of considerable scientific study. It is generally the fat, stored in the form of triglycerides, that is contained within the specialized adipose tissues of the body; excess fat is simply mass that creates an additional physical demand on the body in the course of athletic performance; leaner bodies tend to be more efficient. The best assessment as to the impact of body fat on performance is to determine the percentage of body fat.

A general tool to predict body fat percentages is the body mass index (BMI). The BMI is a formula that estimates the percentage of body fat in an individual through a consideration of the current height, weight, and age of an individual. The BMI is depicted as a chart that permits people to place themselves accordingly. The BMI is not a determinative measure of body fat.

A more accurate analysis of body fat percentage is achieved through the physical examination of the person. Measurements of the skin folds at the upper arm, abdomen, thighs, and buttocks (the most

common storage areas of fat), and submersion in a specially designed water displacement tank will provide accurate measurement of body fat.

The other physiological issues that must be considered in the development of a weight gain strategy are any pertaining to the underlying health of the person. Preexisting conditions, such as diabetes, including prior physical injuries, may influence the manner in which the weight gain program is implemented.

Weight gain will occur whenever the amount of food energy consumed through diet exceeds the amount of physical energy expended. On the simplistic level, an increase in food intake will result in a weight gain. It is the well-managed and carefully directed weight gain program for an athlete that will create a stronger, fitter, more capable athlete. It is for this reason that, once the needs and the person of the athlete has been properly assessed, the diet and the training schedule of the athlete can be coordinated.

Examples of the managed weight gain for a specific athletic purpose are common in elite sports, particularly among athletes seeking to achieve a future professional career. The style of play in the National Football League (NFL) of the United States requires very large and very strong linemen, both in the offensive and defensive formations. Modern football has spawned an evolutionary process at this position, where the offensive linemen are often tall, at heights in a range of 6 ft 4 in to 6 ft 7 in (1.82 m to 1.90 m), with an average weight of over 300 lb (135 kg). The long arms and significant weight permit the linemen to extend their arms to drive back to the somewhat smaller but faster defensive ends; conversely, the most desirable interior defensive linemen outweigh their offensive counterparts, and the defenders seek to secure the lowest possible position and leverage in line play against their opponents.

It is common in NFL football for an aspiring offensive lineman competing at the college level to be encouraged to gain as much as 30 lb (14 kg) in the six months between the end of university football and the commencement of the NFL training camps. Unlike the example of the high school female shot putter, this encouraged weight gain for an athlete 6 ft 4 in and 280 lb (127 kg) is readily achievable. With careful attention to body fat and other efficiency factors, the prospective football player will combine intense resistance training, a moderate amount of cardiovascular conditioning, and balanced diet to manage a weight gain where there is also an increase in his muscle mass.

Careless or unstructured weight gains are often problematic for an athlete. At the conclusion of a long and demanding competitive season, many athletes enjoy a period of deliberate and unfocused rest away from the demands of training. This phenomenon is of particular interest in sports where the athlete competes in a defined weight category. In these circumstances, if the athlete overindulges, consuming food in excess to the regular diet, with a lesser nutritional value, the resumption of training will be hindered by the dual presence of possible nutritional deficiencies and excess weight. Numerous sports scientists and nutritionists advocate that the weight of an athlete who competes in a defined weight class sport should not vary by more than 10% from the ideal competitive weight; these athletes include boxers, lightweight rowers, wrestlers, and many martial arts athletes.

Once an ideal weight has been attained through a healthy and focused weight gain program, it must be maintained at a consistent level. When the athlete no longer competes at either the same competitive level, or on retirement, the basis on which the weight gain was sought will no longer exist. The ideal weight for the athlete will likely be reduced, with appropriate strategy to manage the healthy reduction of body mass to the new desired level.

**SEE ALSO** Diet; Eating disorders in athletes; Fat burners; Metabolic response; Muscle mass and strength; Weight loss.

## Weight loss

Weight loss and the strategies advertised as achieving weight loss are a remarkable example of human nature at its most capricious. It seems that a large percentage of the adult population of modern Western culture is prepared to seek and pursue a weight loss solution, in the midst of societies where fast foods rich in saturated fats, sugared beverages, and generally unhealthy physical habits reign supreme.

The advertising campaigns in support of commercially advocated weight loss schemes that regularly appear in North America appeal primarily to the vanity of the individual. The scientific imperatives behind weight loss are far starker and far more compelling than if one looks attractive. Excess body weight impacts human performance in a multitude of ways, all of which are serious. There has been a flood of statistical data in recent years to support various campaigns aimed at addressing the lack of fitness people of all ages. Governmental and private organizations throughout the world have highlighted the rise in the incidence of overweight and obese children, and the predicted crippling public cost of the additional health care that will be necessitated by the consequences of obesity in adults.

Weight loss strategies are compelling in the face of this data. Aircraft, movie theater, and sports stadium seating is now too narrow to accommodate the typical modern North American adult. The incidence of diabetes, osteoarthritis, cardiovascular illnesses (including high cholesterol), coupled with the doubling of rates of adult and juvenile obesity (generally defined as when the percentage of body fat in a given individual exceeds 30%), have lead researchers to conclude that the present generation of young people (those born after 1985) may be the first generation in recorded history to experience a shorter lifespan than that of their parents.

The Office of the Surgeon General of the United States estimated in 2006 that 300,000 Americans die every year as a result of complications stemming from obesity, with childhood obesity increasing 230% since 1980. It is further estimated that 62% of all Americans are overweight.

From a physiological perspective, weight loss is a simple proposition, and the negative health consequences of excess body weight are consequently significantly reduced. The body has two basic structural components when assessing the ideal weight for any individual. Lean body mass is the weight of the body's skeleton, organs, and muscle. Body fat is the product of the food consumed through diet that is not immediately required by the body for energy. Stored as triglycerides in the specialized fat storage cells known as adipose tissue, body fat plays an important role as a reserve energy source, as well as insulation for the more vulnerable internal organs. While excess body fat is an unhealthy physical state, small percentages of body fat are desirable; healthy males, depending on their age, physical build, and the nature of sports activities, will possess a body fat percentage of between 10% and 15%, while females naturally possess greater amounts of body fat, and a healthy woman may possess between 16% and 20%.

One pound of body fat represents stored energy in the body of 3,500 calories. To lose weight at a rate of 1.5 lb per week (a figure often cited as a safe rate of weight loss), the person must either reduce food consumption or increase the level of physical activity by a total of 750 calories per day ($5,250 \div 7$).

The weight loss issues faced by athletes are not generally as dramatic as those for members of the general population. Most athletes who perceive a need to reduce their weight have a specific athletic objective that is measurable, such as being able to finish a training run, or lift a specific amount of weight. When the athlete is actively engaged in a sport, but seeks to reach a perceived ideal weight for competitive purposes, the formulation of a weight loss plan must include the following components: targeted ideal weight; current weight; and level of fitness, including body fat and lean muscle mass, physical conditioning factors (such as preexisting health concerns), and the anticipated competitive schedule.

For active athletes seeking to achieve a reduction in their current weight to a desired weight, rapid reductions in weight are usually not healthy nor do they enhance their present athletic ability. To maintain a minimum level of fitness, the athletes must continue to train at their current level, or even harder during an active period of weight loss. Training requires careful attention to the athletes' nutritional needs, and a reduction in food intake. Additionally, increased training creates a risk of nutritional deficits. Using the calculation of the energy contained in one pound of body fat, an athlete could continue with a normal diet (subject to an analysis of the nutritional issues that may have lead to the weight gain), and lose weight through increased training alone.

The multitude of commercial diets, particularly those that promote low carbohydrate intake, must be approached with considerable caution by an athlete seeking to lose weight. In a typical balanced diet, the body will receive 60–65% of its energy sources in the form of carbohydrates, 12–15% as proteins, and less than 30% as fats. Carbohydrates are the preferred energy source for many types of human functions, including those of the brain and the nervous system. Purported low-carbohydrate diets proceed on the proposition that when the body has limited carbohydrates available, it will naturally turn to its fat stores as an alternative. If the only concern were the accessing of fats, this diet might operate as intended. However, athletes and the energy pathways (anaerobic, anaerobic alactic, and aerobic) used by the body to power muscular function only operate optimally when the energy stores are compatible.

A further difficulty for the athlete on the low-carbohydrate diet is the fact that many micronutrients (including all vitamins and most minerals) and phytochemicals tend to be most prolific and readily absorbed into the body through carbohydrates such as fruits and vegetables. Weight loss without a corresponding maintenance of nutritional health is an undesirable state of any athlete.

There are a number of specific weight loss scenarios that carry significant psychological issues. Eating disorders are prevalent among young females, a demographic where concerns over body image are often a motivation to extreme diets. Among female athletes, the sports of gymnastics, diving, and figure skating emphasize physical presentation and appearance, to the extent where, in some circumstances, the athletes will convince themselves that their body is inadequate for competition. The mental illnesses of bulimia and anorexia nervosa are the best known of these disorders. Bulimia is a condition where the athlete will commonly eat and purge, apparently consuming regular quantities of food, but eliminating meals through either vomiting or the use of laxatives. Anorexia nervosa is a self-imposed starvation to achieve thinness; anorexia can be fatal.

Weight loss supplements, fat burners, and so-called diet pills are sometimes touted as fast-acting remedies to assist in the elimination of excess weight. As with many of the products sold commercially as weight loss supplements, there are nuggets of factual science-based material buried among the claims of speedy, effortless weight loss. The first of the common and truthful representations made is that the determination of the basal metabolic rate (BMR) for every individual is important in the development of a weight loss strategy. The BMR is an expression of how much energy an individual consumes in a given day. The BMR will fall within a range for all persons, generally in relation to their body type. There are three generally recognized body types: the ectomorph (thin, smaller bones build), the endomorph (the rounder, stouter build), and the mesomorph (larger, more muscular build).

Many of the fat burner supplements have thermogenic qualities, meaning that they will increase the BMR of an individual to a limited degree by increasing the energy generated by the body and stimulate the metabolism. As with any nutritional supplement, knowing exactly what is contained in the formulation will indicate whether the product will promote or assist in weight loss in a safe manner. A number of weight loss products include known stimulants such as ephedra or ma huang (containing ephedrine), caffeine (including herbs such as guarana), bitter orange, and similar substances. Stimulants tend to act as an appetite suppressant through their action

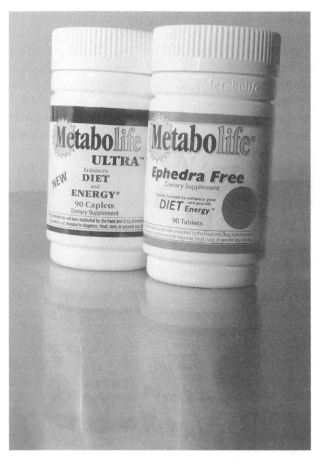

In 2003, the popular dietary supplement/weight-loss aid, Metabolife 356, was shown to cause potentially dangerous heart effects. **PHOTO BY JUSTIN SULLIVAN/GETTY IMAGES.**

# Weightlifting

The origins of weightlifting as a sport are primal, with the main goal the ability to lift more weight than an opponent. The competitive sport of weightlifting is a separate discipline from the athletic training that is defined by the umbrella term weight training. Weight training is used by athletes to build muscle mass, strength, and endurance; to improve performance in a particular sport; or to generally enhance overall fitness.

In weightlifting, as in boxing and wrestling, there is a well-defined correlation between the size of the athlete and the amount of weight that the athlete is capable of lifting. Competitive weightlifting is a sport in which the competition is organized into weight categories, with defined limits that are confirmed by a weigh-in of each athlete prior to competition.

Weightlifting competitions were known to have occurred in both the ancient Olympics as well as the traditional Scottish Highland Games. Weightlifting has been a part of the modern Olympic Games since 1896. Women's weightlifting, using similar principles in the determination of weight categories, became an Olympic sport in 2000. The eight categories used in Olympic men's weightlifting begin at 123 lb (56 kg), continuing to the heaviest category for competitors weighing more than 231 lb (105 kg). The women's categories range from 105 lb (48 kg) to those competitors heavier than 165 lb (75 kg).

Olympic weightlifting includes two different forms of competition at each of the weight categories, the snatch and the clean and jerk. All Olympic weightlifting is conducted using a bar that is loaded with the requisite weight to be attempted in the lift. Each event has a prescribed technique that the athlete must apply; each technique serves as proof that weightlifting is far more than an exercise in simple brute strength.

Successful lifters in the snatch event will endeavor to generate maximum muscle power with their hands grasping the bar, the back held erect, and legs bent in a low, crouched position in front of the bar. With a movement that coordinates the entire musculoskeletal structure, athletes first generate maximum possible force with pushing their feet and calf muscles into the floor to act as a counterbalance to the lift of the bar upward. Lifters then bring the bar approximately level to the thighs, at which point they lift the weight with a powerful coordinated thrust to move the bar above the head. At this position, the bar is thrown slightly upward, to permit the lifters to place their body directly under the bar; when the bar is judged to have been held in a steady position, the lift is deemed legal.

on the central nervous system, with a corresponding elevation of blood pressure and heart rate. An athlete engaged in physical activity must be cautious regarding the consumption of such products, given the stress produced by training alone on various bodily systems. Ephedrine has been the subject of worldwide controversy in all manner of herbal formulations, as there is considerable evidence that ephedrine played a role in a significant number of cases involving heart attacks, increased high blood pressure, and strokes. It is clear that ephedrine and caffeine consumed together heighten user risk.

There is little question from a scientific standpoint that the best weight loss programs are those that simply combine exercise and a reduction of calories in diet, without compromising nutrition.

**SEE ALSO** Diet; Eating disorders in athletes; Fat burners; Metabolic response; Muscle mass and strength; Obesity; Weight gain.

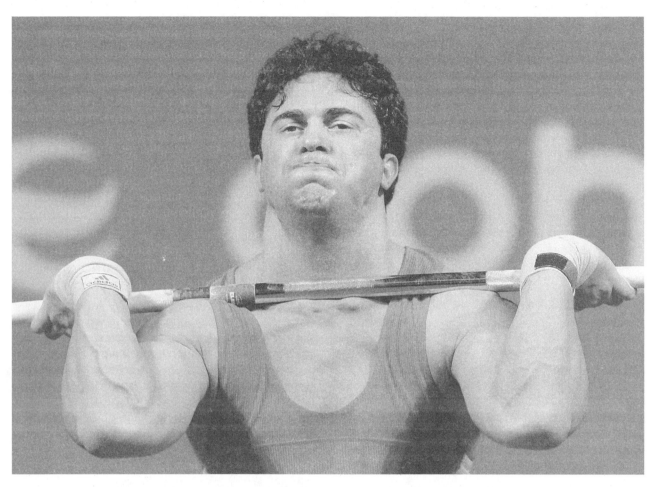

Iranian Ibrahim Asghar competes in the 94-kg weightlifting category at the 2005 West Asian Games. KARIM JAAFAR/AFP/GETTY IMAGES

The clean and jerk is a two-step maneuver. The clean portion of the lift refers to the lifting of the bar from the ground. The bar is lifted into a position where the athlete may then crouch with the bar approximately across the chest in a pronounced squat position, with the weight of the bar directly above the lifter's hips. The jerk sequence requires the lifter to forcefully drive the legs and hips upward, and with a coordinated exertion of the arms, the bar is lifted above the head. The closer to a perpendicular body position the lifter can maintain, the more efficient the action of the muscles employed on the bar.

A form of competitive weightlifting outside the Olympic format is power lifting. Power lifting is comprised of the individual disciplines of the bench press (the traditional technique of lifting a weighted bar while lying on a training bench), the squat (a maneuver similar to the first part of the clean and jerk event), and the dead lift, the lifting of a weighted bar off the floor.

As with many strength disciplines, such as the shot put or the hammer throw, the successful weightlifter is the athlete who can harness great muscular strength with efficient technique. As weightlifting requires all muscle groups to work in a coordinated effort, the weight training required to support competitive weightlifting must develop all muscle groups. No sport places greater importance on the development of core strength, the ability of the abdominal, lumbar (lower back), and groin tissues to stabilize the body during a lift, particularly as the weights are moved forcefully upward in both the snatch and the clean and jerk. Significant portions of weightlifting training are devoted to the stretching, flexibility, and development of these core strength structures.

As weightlifting requires explosive movement in the execution of all lifts, especially in the legs and hips, plyometrics training is also an important tool. Unlike the plyometrics that would be employed by a basketball player or a long jumper, the weightlifter seeks to develop the fast-twitch muscles fibers to move the bar upward once positioned.

In the 1970s and 1980s, weightlifting was perceived by many observers as a sport much corrupted by anabolic steroid use. As a strength sport, there is no question that anabolic steroids could create a significant competitive advantage for a user. Weightlifters are now subjected to the same types of performance-enhancing substance testing as all other athletes. As a sport where adherence to weight categories is required, weightlifters must also comply with the prohibitions concerning the diuretics that are listed on the World Anti-Doping Agency (WADA) Prohibited List; diuretics mask anabolic steroid use, and they are an illegal method by which to lose weight in advance of competition to meet a required weight limit. Whether the sport has been entirely made clean of the use of anabolic agents is unclear. At the 2006 Commonwealth Games, the world's second largest sports festival after the Olympics, a large cache of doping paraphernalia was found; its use was attributed to the members of the Australian weightlifting team.

**SEE ALSO** Anabolic steroids; Free weights; Muscle mass and strength; Muscle protein synthesis; Protein supplements; Resistance exercise training; Weight categories.

# Weights, free SEE Free weights

# Wetsuits

The wetsuit is a protective garment worn by athletes who participate in any water sports where either warmth or greater buoyancy are desired. Wetsuits are constructed in a variety of styles, with neoprene rubber the common construction material used. A wet suit provides insulation to the wearer in two separate ways. Neoprene is a compound that contains tiny air bubbles in its structure, a characteristic that insulates the wearer against the effect of cold water or air. As its name suggests, the wetsuit permits water to enter between the wetsuit material and the skin of the user. The thin layer of water created is warmed by body heat, forming a second insulating layer between the skin and the neoprene. In contrast, a *drysuit* is constructed with rubber seals at the neck, wrists, and legs of the suit, to prevent water from contact with the skin.

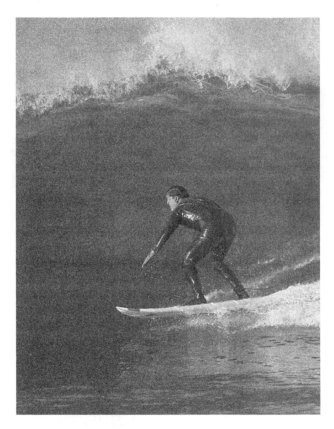

A surfer in a wetsuit rides a wave. **PHOTO BY ROY TOFT/ NATIONAL GEOGRAPHIC/GETTY IMAGES.**

The originator of the wetsuit cannot be determined with absolute precision. The weight of historical evidence suggests that Hugh Bradner, a physicist employed at the University of California Berkley developed the first wetsuit for use by United States Navy "frogmen" in 1952. Bradner hoped to make these divers more efficient in their underwater movements through his one piece wetsuit. After manufacturing a few prototypes, the project was abandoned and Bradner never patented his creation, which employed neoprene its design.

Wetsuits are worn by participants in virtually every outdoor water sport; the protective properties of the wetsuit are of particular importance to surfers, water skiers, kayakers, and other athletes who are exposed to the effects of cold water and air for a considerable period. In the triathlon and Iron man competitions, the wetsuit affords both protection to the athlete in cold water, as well as providing an extra degree of buoyancy in swim segments that may be as long as 2.4 mi (4 km). In internationally sanctioned competition, a triathlon wetsuit may not exceed 5 mm in thickness to prevent an athlete from gaining an undue buoyancy advantage with the suit.

Swimmers who compete in the traditional Olympic races held in a 25-m or a 50-m pool may also utilize wetsuits of a highly specialized nature. These suits are designed not for protection or buoyancy, but to provide the swimmer with a more hydrodynamic profile in the water. Designed to mimic the effect of a shark's skin in water, these swim wetsuits are manufactured with tiny v-shaped ridges that create differing regions of water pressure across the suit surface, reducing the effect of drag on the swimmer as they move through the water.

Wetsuits are now manufactured in specific styles for particular sports; the triathlon wetsuit, as an example, has a number of carefully positioned zippers and releases to permit the athlete to remove the suit very quickly as they make a transition to the bicycle segment of the events. Wetsuits are generally available in three distinct styles—a full coverage suit that exposes the head, hands, and feet; the "Farmer John", where the shoulders and arms are also exposed for greater freedom of movement; the "shortie", styled to expose the legs as well as the arms.

SEE ALSO Ironman competitions; Swimming; Triathlon; Water skiing.

# Wheelchair sports

The first organized sports competition for persons competing in wheelchairs was a part of the Stoke-Mandeville Games, the forerunner to the modern Paralympics movement, held in England in 1948 for persons with physical disabilities. The wheelchair technology then available to the competing athletes was crude; the wheelchairs were not modified from their intended purpose of basic hospital transport for persons who lacked motor control of their legs.

Modern wheelchair design and the ever-increasing range of sports available to disabled persons create a symbiotic relationship. As sports in which a wheelchair can be adapted for athletic use have been proposed and developed, technology and design have kept abreast of athletic interests.

The modern international Paralympics movement, supported by the efforts of over 150 national Paralympics organizations, has created a structured wheelchair sports environment that continues to grow with every Paralympic Games. The Summer Paralympic Games provide for wheelchair sports across a range of disciplines, the best known of which are within those sports that comprise track and field. Wheelchair athletes compete in a variety of races, ranging from the 100 m track event to the marathon (26.2 mi, or 42.2 km).

The wheelchairs currently used by disabled athletes are remarkable feats of engineering. The sleek frames are composed of a combination of lightweight titanium and composite carbon fiber materials. The two larger rear wheels and the smaller lead wheels are configured for both aerodynamic effect as well as the propulsion efficiency of the athlete. The athlete is usually tightly strapped into the wheelchair, to eliminate any bounce on the part of the body that would detract from the efficient forward motion of the wheelchair. The combination of wheelchair technology and the muscular power developed by the racer has resulted in the elite wheelchair-powered racers being faster than able-bodied runners at all distances greater than 800 m.

The wheelchair team sports of the Summer Paralympics represent both modified traditional Olympic summer sports and adaptive events. The best known of the wheelchair team sports is basketball, which has been played in various parts of the world since the late 1940s. Wheelchair technology has greatly improved the range of techniques available to the wheelchair basketball player; a three or four wheel, lightweight chair is now used, with two built-in anti-tipping devices used to stabilize the chair on contact with another competitor. The wheelchairs used by forwards are constructed with an elevated seat; those used by the guards are lower seated, permitting the player to move and react more quickly to the play.

The other summer Paralympics team sports employ wheelchairs specifically modified for each event. Dance sport, fencing, rugby (an indoor variant of the outdoor game), and tennis could not be performed without the technological benefits in modern wheelchair construction. As an example, the lightweight tennis wheelchair employs a pivoting front wheel to permit the player to move quickly in any direction to make a return to an opponent.

The Winter Paralympics do not provide as many competitive opportunities for the wheelchair athlete, given the presence of snow and the nature of the Alpine terrain. Curling was introduced as a winter wheelchair sport at the 2006 Winter Paralympics, with specialized chairs adapted to permit both the throw of the curling stones as well as to facilitate the sweeping of the ice to control the speed and the direction of the stones.

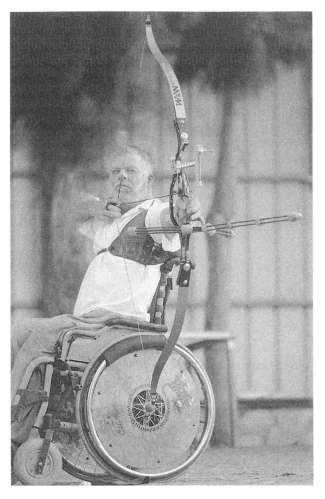

Israeli archer Amit Dror, 50, practices from his wheelchair.
PHOTO BY URIEL SINAI/GETTY IMAGES.

Wheelchair racing has continued to enjoy popularity beyond the scope of the Paralympics. Many international marathon races have provided for a wheelchair division for many years. These specialty machines are built with larger than typical wheels for propulsion, and a small lead wheel built on an elongated structure extending from the wheelchair. The athlete is seated as low to the ground as is possible, while still permitting the athlete to direct maximum muscular power to the wheels. The large wheels are very thin, to create a more aerodynamic profile. Many competitors also race with the wheels of the chair aligned in a negative camber, where the top of the wheel is angled toward the chair. This alignment permits the racers to corner more aggressively at high speeds, a significant benefit on marathon road courses with a number of turns, as well as permitting the athlete to direct maximum muscular power from the arms positioned as closely as possible to the wheel.

In recent years, there have been incursions into the realm of extreme sports by wheelchair athletes. Examples of these activities include hang gliding and use of a wheelchair that approximates the all-terrain experience of mountain biking, using a very durable, well-cushioned frame equipped with a braking system.

**SEE ALSO** Endurance exercise; Exercise, high intensity; Hydration strategy in distance running; Paralympics.

# Whole-body heat cramping

Whole-body heat cramping is a progressive and debilitating physical state, one that tends to afflict athletes who are training or competing in warm weather conditions. Cramping that affects the function of muscle groups throughout the entire musculoskeletal system is a result of the same mechanisms that trigger more localized and painful muscle cramping, which is typically isolated in the calf and hamstrings.

Muscle cramps are caused by the combined operation of sodium deficit, muscle fatigue, and dehydration. The primary cause of muscle cramps is a deficit in sodium, the essential mineral and electrolyte that is obtained from a variety of dietary sources. In hot weather, sodium is lost through the increased levels of perspiration generated by exercise, as the body endeavors to maintain a healthy internal temperature through the cooling release of sweat. When the body perspires, sodium (and trace amounts of other minerals, such as calcium and magnesium) and water are passed together from the body.

Muscle cramps rarely occur in a strong and rested muscle. Cramps invariably become a factor in athletic performance after the muscle has endured significant stress.

When the factors of sodium depletion, dehydration, and muscle fatigue are combined, muscle cramping is a real risk. The cramps occur because the body requires sodium to perform two critical tasks that are especially relevant to warm weather athletic performance: the maintenance of fluid levels, particularly blood volume, throughout the body (the process of osmoregulation), and the ability of the nervous system to transmit the nerve impulses that are required to initiate the muscular contraction necessary to produce movement. The ratio between total body fluid volume and sodium is the key marker relied on by the body to determine how much fluid should be present. When the proportion of sodium to body fluid is too low, the body will resist the absorption of further water or other fluids, which can initiate a dangerous physical condition known as hyponatremia. When there is too great a level of sodium relative to fluids present in the body, the body senses that it is dehydrated, which will signal the kidneys to reduce the production of urine. The thirst mechanism is also activated at this time.

The athletes most prone to whole-body cramping are those who have a relatively low body fat percentage, with a relatively high proportion of fast-twitch muscle fibers. All athletes who become dehydrated to the relatively modest amount of 2% of their total body weight during the course of a warm weather activity are at risk of developing muscle cramps.

Muscle cramping that occurs to any extent in the body, also referred to as heat cramps, is the least serious of the well-recognized heat illnesses that may befall athletes in warm weather conditions. Heat exhaustion is the cumulative effect of heat exposure that prevents the body's thermoregulatory mechanism from effectively dispersing the internal heat generated by exercise. Heat stroke is the most serious and the potentially fatal failure of the body to prevent overheating, leading ultimately to a shutdown of organ function, and a significant risk of permanent damage to the heart or liver.

Sodium depletion that leads to whole-body cramping takes place even though most athletes consume far in excess of the required and recommended daily allowance of dietary sodium. The body does not store sodium for indefinite periods, as it does fat-soluble substances such as vitamin D. Excess sodium, while capable of unduly stressing the cardiovascular system, primarily through the high blood pressure that is a byproduct of the osmoregulatory process in sedentary persons, is excreted as urine.

The first line of defense to whole-body heat cramping is built in the period prior to the start of warm weather sports. The introduction of any athlete to an unaccustomed warm environment must be gradual, both in terms of training volume and training intensity, to permit the acclimatization of the athlete to the environment. For most athletes, the heat acclimatization process will be over 90% complete within 10 to 14 days of its commencement. The more efficient the function of the cardiovascular system in warm weather, the better the body will maintain the necessary blood volumes during exercise, subject to proper hydration practices.

The second component to the prevention of debilitating whole-body cramps is the implementation of a rigorous hydration strategy. Athletes must be directed and encouraged to consume appropriate levels of fluids prior to, during, and subsequent to all training and competitions. Fluids that contain sodium, or water consumed along with a salt tablets (regular salt is 40% sodium by weight), are a preferred rehydration choice to that of water alone during warm weather, due to the actions of the body to preserve its desired osmoregulation.

A defined hydration strategy is of supreme importance in sports that employ a two-a-day practice regime in warm weather training. American football is a prime example; football carries with it an additional cramping risk, due to the full equipment, which has a significant additional weight and covers the body from the knees to the top of the player's head, preventing heat from dissipating.

The most effective remedy for whole-body cramping is immediate rest from the activity, the placement of the athlete in a cool environment, and the consumption of appropriate replacement fluid. Playing through these often-debilitating cramps is likely impossible, and if the athlete attempts to force further strenuous movement from tissues that have sustained sodium depletion, the athlete is at risk of causing more serious muscular injury.

**SEE ALSO** Cramps; Heat cramps; Muscle cramps; Sodium and sodium deficits; Thermoregulation, exercise, and thirst.

# Wild yams

Wild yams are a trailing vine whose natural habitat includes most of the eastern and southern United States. The roots of this plant were valued by ancient cultures for their medicinal properties. Wild yams were also known as colic root and rheumatism root among the early American settlers of these regions in the 1800s. This herbal form of the wild yam has no horticultural relationship to the sweet potatoes and yams sold as vegetables in North American food stores.

The root of the wild yam is typically harvested in autumn. It is consumed either as a tea made by boiling the dried root, or from a manufactured fluid extract.

Wild yam has been reputed to possess powerful curative properties with respect to female reproductive system disorders of all kinds, including menstrual pain, the regulation of the menstrual cycle,

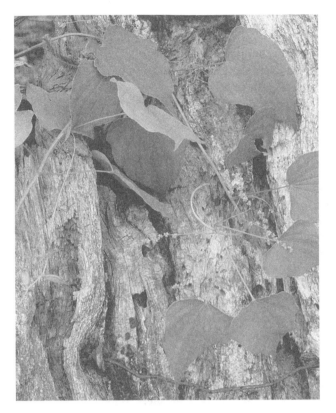

Wild yam fruit and flowers. © HAL HORWITZ/CORBIS. REPRODUCED BY PERMISSION.

and the pain caused through child birth. These particular medicinal effects are connected to the presence of chemicals in the wild yam root that possess anti-spasmodic properties. The herb is also valued as a general revitalizing agent for both men and women; it is used to treat joint inflammations, stomach cramps, and it is effective as a vasodilator (chemicals that stimulate opening of the blood vessels to promote greater blood flow, and a resultant lowering of blood pressure).

Much of the recent scientific interest in wild yams stems from the presence of a number of different steroid saponins, substances which may be converted to hormones, as well as a number of phytochemicals that assist in the promotion of good health when ingested into the body. Diosgenin is a steroid saponin that is easily converted to the female hormone progesterone; for a considerable period diosgenin was extracted from the wild yam root to manufacture progesterone and female birth control pills. There is no scientific evidence in support of the proposition advanced by some commercial promoters of wild yams as a herbal remedy that the human body will naturally convert diosgenin into progesterone.

Recent scientific study has provided some support for the proposition that wild yams may assist in the reduction of low density lipoproteins, the cholesterol that contributes to the clogging of blood vessels. Diosgenin increases the rate of stomach bile production. Stomach bile requires cholesterol, which in turn reduces the amount of cholesterol that otherwise would remain a danger to the effective function of the blood vessels.

The properties of wild yam have been shown in some settings to alleviate the symptoms of joint inflammation and menstrual difficulties. The amount of benefit to be derived from the consumption of wild yam products will vary from person to person. Unlike many herbs and dietary supplements, there are no known significant side effects or potential for harmful interaction with other substances when wild yams are consumed.

**SEE ALSO** Dietary supplements; Herbs; Phytochemicals; Tribulus.

# Wind tunnel testing SEE Cycling: Wind tunnel testing

# Windsurfing

Windsurfing (also known as boardsailing) is a sport that evolved from a desire to combine the exhilaration and the freedom of movement inherent in surfing, with the precision and the techniques of wind powered sailing. In a remarkable historical development, three groups have at one time or another laid claim to the invention of the windsurfer. Peter Chilvers of Great Britain developed a prototypical windsurfer in the late 1950s, Pennsylvania inventor Newman Darby first published his designs for a windsurfer in the early 1960s, and Californians Jim Drake and Howard Schweitzer had independently designed and patented their craft, featuring an articulated mast and featuring a u-joint attachment between mast and board in 1968.

The windsurfer became a very popular recreational device, as it was very portable and less cumbersome to transport and assemble than a conventional sail boat. Windsurfing is also not particularly restricted to any particular type of water body, as a windsurfer is nimble enough to navigate larger rivers, lakes, and oceans. With the rise in the popularity of the windsurfer rose the number of opportunities to race these craft. Racing brought significant

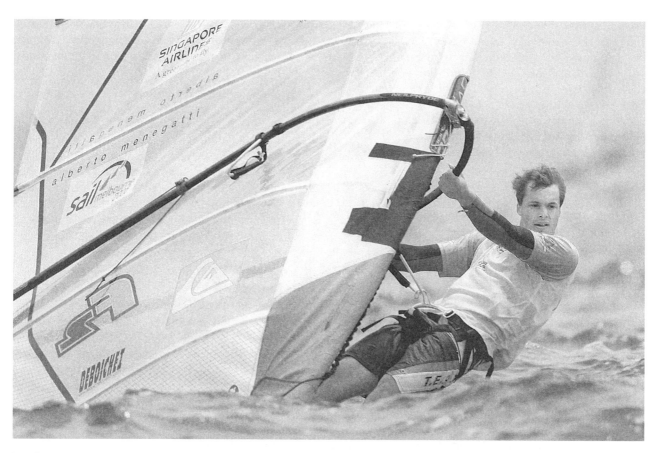

The Sail Melbourne 2005 Formula Windsurfing World Championships, Melbourne, Australia. **PHOTO BY MARK DADSWELL/ GETTY IMAGES.**

technological developments to both the boards and the sails used by elite and recreational competitors. A modern windsurfer can attain speeds of over 50 mph in the appropriate winds.

The world wide popularity of windsurfing prompted the formation of various national and international windsurfing organizations. The International Sailing Federation (ISAF), is the world body responsible for the convening of world championships in various windsurfing categories. Windsurfing has been an Olympic sport since 1984.

A windsurfer is a very simple type of boat. A standard windsurfer is constructed with a mast, a sail, and a board. The board has foot straps built into its surface to provide the surfer with a stable base upon which to maneuver the craft, and all boards are equipped with a skeg, a type of fin positioned on the rear that provides additional stability to the craft while it is being steered. Some models of windsurfers are equipped with a daggerboard that functions much as a keel operates in relation to a sailboat, as a stabilizing force to counter the force of wind, which

might otherwise send the windsurfer sideways. The upper portion of the windsurfer is the sail, mast, and boom, a wishbone shaped attachment fixed perpendicular to the mast, the primary means used by the windsurfer to control the craft.

The U-joint is the hardware component that is critical to the function and the maneuverability of the windsurfer. In many ways, the u-joint is what distinguishes the windsurfer from any other sailboat, as the surfer can manipulate the mast in any direction, permitting the windsurfer to be turned quickly in any weather.

There are two basic types of wind sailing boards. Long boards are approximately 10 ft (3 m) long, and sufficiently wide that the sailor can stand on the board when the board is at rest and remain afloat. This type of stable board is popular among persons learning how to windsurf. The predominate competition board in use today is referred to as a short board, with a length of less than 10 ft, but a significant width, featuring large fins at the rear of the board and no daggerboard.

Sailing a windsurfer requires the application of many of the principles involved in sailing a boat.

When the wind is directly behind the intended path of travel of the windsurfer, the sails of windsurfer can be positioned to perpendicular to the path of the wind, thus capturing the maximum wind effect. When the surfer intends to travel in a direction generally into the wind, the windsurfer can be tacked in the same fashion as a sailboat, where the sail, positioned at approximately 45° angle to the direction of the wind, operates as a foil, creating two different wind speeds on each side of the sail. The result is the creation of high pressure and low pressure effects on the sail, and the windsurfer is pulled in the direction of the lower pressure. Tacking will take a windsurfer along a zig zag path across the surface of the water.

A windsurfer can also jibe to steer the craft, when the wind is from the rear of the windsurfer. The boom is maneuvered from side to side to permit the maximum amount of wind to be captured the sail. The surfer changes body positions during both the tacking and jibing techniques to balance his or her body weight with the effect of the wind to keep the craft on an even plane. The windsurfer design is such that the craft will readily plane in the water in relatively light winds (some models will plane in winds of less than 12 mph (20 km/h). The board can plane is achieved when the nose and forward portion of the windsurfer rises above the water surface, reducing the friction between the bottom of the board and the water. It is for these reasons that the windsurfer is the fastest of all sailing craft.

While windsurfing is usually raced as a competitive event on marshaled courses, it has an extreme sport edge. Many windsurfers seek out the worst wind and weather they can find to challenge themselves to conquer the elements and to attain the highest speeds possible. Other windsurfers have taken on extreme endurance challenges, such as windsurfing around the British Isles, or sailing the huge waves that form off the island of Maui in the Hawaiian Islands.

**SEE ALSO** Sailing; Sailing and steering a sailboat; Surfing.

# Women and sports: Exercise data, goals, and guidelines

The history of the participation of women in sport is long, extending at least to the female competitions established in Greek mythology by Hera as an alternative to the male-only Olympics of Greek antiquity. Yet, as with many histories of activities that were regarded as secondary to the more publicized male sports events, hard data concerning female sports participation in many athletic disciplines prior to 1900 is nonexistent.

In many respects, the 1928 Summer Olympics are a point of commencement in the data and goals of women in sport. This event represented the introduction of female sports at the world's most prestigious athletic event. The competition was as global as the era could have ever permitted, and the athletes who competed in the relatively limited number of track and field events open to women at the 1928 Games set definable standards for the women who followed.

The women's sports that further entered the public consciousness in the decades that followed the 1928 Olympics were an extension of individual competitions that served as the trailblazers in 1928. Figure skaters such as Sonja Henie of Norway and tennis players like American Althea Gibson became prominent athletes, although there is no particular evidence that their successes attracted greater female athletic participation in either sport. Until the 1960s, female athletics on the prominent national stages of the United States and Europe, and that of the Olympic world, tended to be those engaged in individual sporting events only.

Significant data concerning female sports began to be accumulated in the 1960s, when women began to participate on a larger scale in team sports. Volleyball was introduced for both men and women at the 1964 Olympics; basketball was introduced as a women's sport in 1976, and field hockey, a popular women's competition in Europe and Asia, was added in 1980.

The advancement of female sports in the United States paralleled Olympic developments. In 1972, the federal government of the United States passed an amendment to its existing civil rights legislation that became universally known as Title IX. Title IX established a legislative framework that mandated that all institutions in the United States that received federal funding for sports of any type were obligated to offer equal athletic opportunities for women as were offered for men. Title IX has proven to be a significant stimulus to the expansion of female sport in America, with its influence felt at every level and sports age group. The most profound example of Title IX's effect on athletics has been in the growth of female participation at the intercollegiate level; in 2005, the National Collegiate Athletic Association published the results of its own studies that illustrated an increase in intercollegiate female sports participation of over 825% since the passage of Title IX.

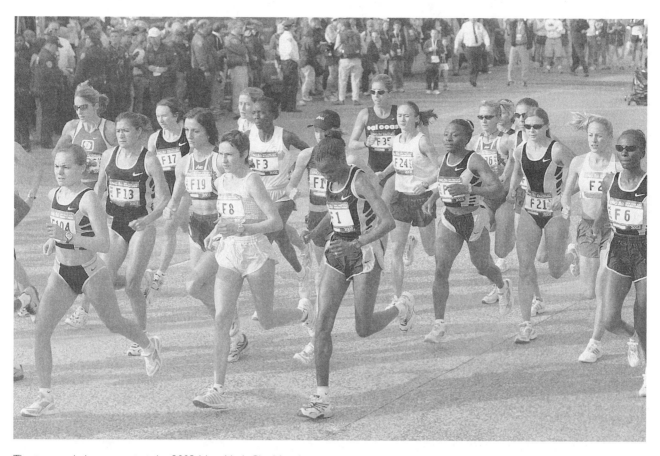

The top seeded women start the 2003 New York City Marathon. © MICHAEL KIM/CORBIS

Studies conducted in nations such as Great Britain and Australia confirm that, like the United States, there are more women participating in competitive sports than ever before. Canadian studies identified a similar trend in the numbers of competitive female athletes. Yet since 1990 there was a parallel reduction in recreational female sports participation for women over the age of 18 years, from 61% to 48%; participation was broadly defined as an exercise or sporting activity in which the person participated at least one time per week.

The running boom of the late 1970s and the early 1980s sparked a corresponding increase in female running participation on a recreational and fitness level. The United States Track and Field Association (USTAF), the sanctioning body for all marathons held in the United States, determined that in 1980, approximately 10% of all marathon participants were women; by 2005, over 40% of marathoners were female, in an environment where overall marathon participation had increased by over 300% over the 25-year period. An example of the significant growth of the marathon as a female sport of choice is the 2005 Nike Marathon for Women, held in San Francisco, where 15,000 female runners entered the race.

Of statistical interest is the median finishing time for the 1980 female marathon group versus the modern runners. In 1980, the USTAF determined that the median female time to be approximately 4 hours, 3 minutes. In 2005, the median was determined to be over 4 hours, 20 minutes. It is clear that marathon participation has been fueled by female interests other than seeking to improve performance as measured on an absolute scale.

When the examples of increased Olympic participation and increased female participation generally are considered together, there is no ready conclusion as to whether increased participation has proven to be indicative of a widespread desire to achieve better female fitness or sport competence. Australia and other nations have identified a persistent gap, often referred to as an under representation, of females in sports coaching, officiating, and administration.

Paradoxically, the increased rate of female competitive sports participation has been paralleled by the rapid global rise in chronic health problems in both genders at all ages. In the Western world especially, poor dietary habits and a lack of exercise are significant contributors to obesity, diabetes, osteoarthritis, and various cardiovascular diseases, and each are as great a health risk for women as they were traditionally for men. The impact of each of these identified conditions is significantly reduced by exercise and good nutritional practices, which suggests that while a minority of the female population participates in sport to a significant degree, increasing numbers of women may lead entirely sedentary lives.

SEE ALSO Female exercise and cardiovascular health; Genetics; International Olympic Committee (IOC); National Collegiate Athletic Association (NCAA); Sport performance.

# Women's ice hockey

Women's ice hockey is a relative latecomer among the female sports to achieve internationally sanctioned status. Played informally in Canada since the latter part of the nineteenth century, and in various other northern cold weather nations as early as 1920, women's ice hockey did not attract a significant following outside of North America until the 1980s.

The International Ice Hockey Federation (IIHF) is the governing body for ice hockey played on an international level, including the women's game. The first sanctioned women's IIHF championships were held in 1990 in Ottawa, Canada. From 1990 to 2005 the dominance of the United States and Canada was so profound that either the Canadian or American team won the gold medal, with the other taking the silver, at each championship event. During these years, no other team ever mounted a significant challenge in any single game to either program, despite the competition including the same countries that traditionally have very strong mens' international and Olympic championship entries, including Sweden, Finland, Russia, and the Czech Republic. The respective women's teams from these nations were never competitive at the world championships.

A similar competitive imbalance has been evident in the shorter history of women's Olympic ice hockey, introduced at the Nagano Games of 1998. Going into the 2006 Winter Games, Canada and the United States had only one another country as rival for the gold medal. In a 2006 semi-medal game, Sweden beat the United States in what was the greatest upset in the history of women's ice hockey.

It is difficult to determine what the future of international competition will hold in women's ice hockey. Canada has both a definitive hockey culture (where ice hockey is the national winter sport) as well as established women's elite-level leagues within which to develop a pool of national talent that is both broad and deep. The United States does not have women's leagues that rival the Canadian examples, but National Collegiate Athletic Association (NCAA) women's ice hockey continues to expand, especially as athletic scholarships are offered by many hockey–playing institutions. The Swedish upset in 2006 notwithstanding, the prospect of the competitive level of women's ice hockey rivaling that of the men's game, where at least eight nations can enter an international championship with a reasonable chance of success, is likely remote in the years to come. Other than Canada, the United States, Sweden, and Finland, no other nation has any system of organized national training camps or coaching hierarchy for the women's game.

The reasons as to why women's ice hockey has lagged in apparent popularity, even in countries with a strong hockey tradition, are difficult to ascertain. The speed of the women's game does not compare to that generated by larger and stronger male athletes, but in relative terms to virtually every other team sport, women's ice hockey is a very fast and dynamic game. Like men's ice hockey, passing, the ability to move up and down the ice in transition from offense to defense, and strong goalkeeping are essential to success. The premium on hand-eye coordination generally, and shooting and playmaking ability specifically, are also consistent in both versions of the sport.

The only significant rule difference between men's and women's ice hockey is one regarding body checking. In men's ice hockey, a body check is defined as the general physical contact permitted by a defensive player against an offensive player who has control of the puck, or who has, immediately prior to the contact, lost control of the puck. A body check may be delivered with the hip or shoulder, and it is a devastating defensive tactic. In women's ice hockey, body checking is prohibited; a defensive player is permitted to angle an offensive player off the puck through the body position and skating motion, which leads to incidental contact between the players. For this reason, the women's game does not include the physical features that often excite hockey spectators. Conversely, the deemphasizing of physical contact in the women's game would theoretically make the game open to players of more disparate sizes, provided they possessed strong skating and playmaking skills.

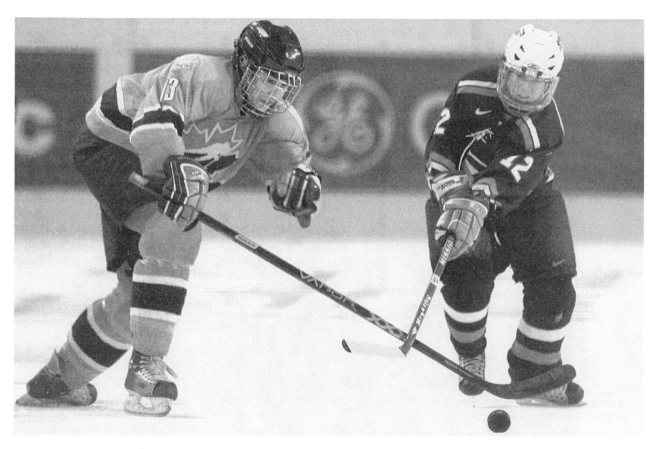

The U.S. women's ice hockey team won the silver medal (to Canada's gold) during the Torino Ice 2005 playoffs match. MONTEFORTE/ AFP/GETTY IMAGES

Two female ice hockey players made history when each secured a place on a competitive men's teams. Goaltender Manon Rheaume earned a well-publicized tryout with the National Hockey League Tampa Bay Lightening in 2001; Hayley Wickenheiser, a forward regarded as the finest female ice hockey player ever produced in Canada, played for a season in the second tier of the Finnish men's professional league in 2003. Neither player was able to sustain a career with either male team, and the criticism of both Rheaume and Wickenheiser was that their efforts to participate in men's hockey served to detract from the perceived strengths of the women's game.

SEE ALSO Female exercise and cardiovascular health; Ice hockey; Ice hockey strength and training exercises.

# Women's sport clothing and protective equipment

Specialized women's sports clothing is an indus-try that has sustained a growth paralleling the rise in the number of women engaged in both competitive sport as well as numerous other forms of exercise activities such as aerobics, yoga, and Pilates.

The growth of the women's sport fashion indus-try is also related to an increase in marketing exer-cise clothes specifically made for women, in terms of both style and the intended specialized fit for the female body. Items such as shorts and tights for exercise or training purposes are designed to take into account the wider female pelvis relative to leg length; additional clothing items, such as sports bras, take other female physical characteristics into account.

The breasts are a region of the female athlete's body frequently exposed to injury. The inadequate covering of and lack of support for the breasts are also common causes of physical interference in ath-letic performance. The human breast is composed primarily of fatty tissues, which enclose the mam-mary glands (designed for nurturing an infant), and the capillary network that supplies nutrients to the breast tissue. There are thin ligaments that inter-sperse the breast tissue and provide a limited

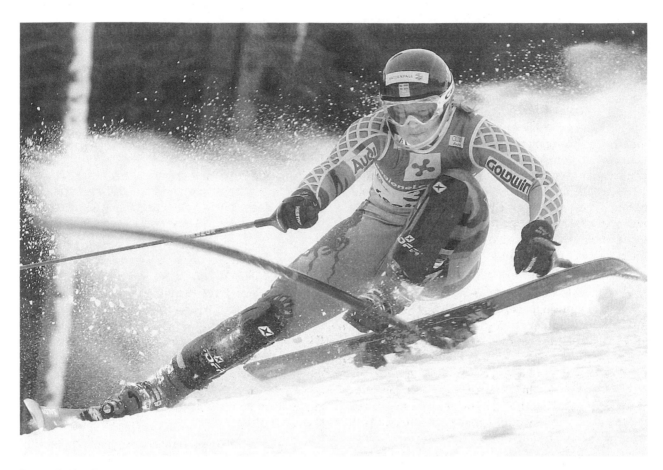

Sports clothing for women is a growing industry, paralleling the rise in the number of women engaged in both competitive sport (such as skiing) and specialized exercise (such as yoga, aerobics, and Pilates). © ANDREAS MEIER/REUTERS/CORBIS

measure of support to the breast; these ligaments are not strong enough to provide structural support to the breast during athletic movement. The muscles that underlie the breasts are not constructed to assist with the support of these tissues during movement.

As a general physical proposition, the larger the athlete's breasts, the greater the forces that will be directed into the supporting muscle structures of the shoulder, upper back, and upper chest through the undulating movements of the breasts. This repetitive movement can cause significant discomfort for the athlete if the breasts are not properly supported, as the result will be an imbalance between the breasts and the function of the upper back and shoulder muscles.

The female breasts are often a source of irritation and interference in the desired athletic function. If breasts are incorrectly supported or placed in repeated contact with material that creates irritation, the condition known as jogger's nipple (intense soreness, dryness, inflammation and/or bleeding of the

nipple) will occur. This condition may also occur in male athletes for the same reasons. Additionally, with the female athlete, the risk of a permanent stretching of the ligaments in the breast tissue is present.

For these reasons, the sports bra is the most important female sports clothing essential. The specialized bra did not exist until the 1990s; previously, female athletes typically improvised a supportive bra from commercially available products. Popularized by the successes of the 1996 U.S. women's soccer team, the sports bra is a product of both form and function. The most important aspect of the selection of a sports bra is the fit; the bra must be tight to the athlete's body, without being constricting, and sufficient to ensure that the breasts have minimal movement during exercise.

There are hundreds of different sports bra styles; for all sports where the athlete will be perspiring to any extent, sports bras are constructed of a variety of polypropylene and Lycra -based fabrics, which permit both stretching and the ability of the material to "wick" away moisture (remove perspiration from the skin surface through the material) to keep the skin relatively dry through competition.

The type of support required by the sports bra is a function of the breast size of the particular athlete. Support is provided in varying degrees in each of three general types of construction. A compression sports bra is designed to pull the breasts into the body during motion; the compression model is best suited to women with smaller breasts. An encapsulated-style sports bra fits around each breast to secure the tissue against excess movement; this model is usually recommended for women with larger breasts. Underwire sports bras are the third type; this construction is found as a distinct style or it can be used in combination with the encapsulated style.

The breasts are also vulnerable to injury in sports where a direct trauma is possible. As a sensitive glandular structure, a direct blow can cause a contusion, with resultant discomfort, swelling, and bleeding within the tissue. Some models of sports bras have additional padding that can be inserted into the bra cups for protection. In a number of sports, including martial arts, fencing, boxing, and rugby, specialized chest guards can be worn by female athletes. In both rugby and soccer, some jersey manufacturers have designed built-in chest protectors for female athletes

In sports such as ice hockey, field hockey, and lacrosse, where players, particularly the goaltenders, are exposed to an object directed at them at high speed, female athletes can wear a specialized groin protector (known as a "jill," in contrast to the well-known male equipment used to protect the genitals, the "jock" strap). This protector is fashioned consistent with the structure of the female body.

**SEE ALSO** Athletic shoes; Female exercise and cardiovascular health; Heart rate monitors; Jump rope training; Orthotics; Yoga and Pilates.

# John Robert Wooden

10/14/1910–
AMERICAN
COLLEGE BASKETBALL COACH

John Wooden is regarded as the quintessential basketball coach in the history of American college competition. Wooden's achievements at the University of California at Los Angeles (UCLA) are the standard by which all college basketball coaches are likely to be judged for many decades to come. Wooden's success stands as an example that a challenging

practice environment, rigorous attention to the execution of fundamentals, and cohesive team play will produce champions.

As a coach, John Wooden was the sainted Wizard of Westwood, a name bestowed in reference to the location of the home court of his dynastic UCLA Bruins. It is sometimes forgotten that Wooden was first an accomplished high school player in Indiana, leading his team to a coveted Indiana state championship in 1930. Wooden then proceeded to Purdue University in Indiana, where he led Purdue to a 1932 national championship, a season in which Wooden was named national player of the year.

After a brief stint in the poorly organized professional basketball leagues that endeavored to secure a foothold in the consciousness of the American sporting public in the 1930s, Wooden became a high school basketball coach. Wooden built a scholastic coaching record of 218-42 at Dayton, Kentucky, and South Bend, Indiana, before taking the head job at Indiana State University, a school later famous as the alma mater of Hall of Fame player Larry Bird. Wooden achieved a record of 47–14 over two seasons at Indiana State before moving to the head coaching position at UCLA in 1948.

One of the most remarkable features of the career of John Wooden at UCLA is that while Wooden won ten national championships, more than any other college basketball coach in history, he did not win any national championships during his first 15 seasons at UCLA. Wooden, in those first seasons at UCLA, was undeniably successful, winning the accepted benchmark success, 20 games, on six different occasions. Wooden achieved employment stability in a position that by modern standards would represent a remarkably lengthy tenure.

It was during this period that Wooden laid the groundwork for what would become the dynasty of all dynasties in American college basketball. Wooden was an advocate of lengthy practices for conditioning and endless drills to perfect fundamental skills. Wooden placed the athletic principles of conditioning, skill development, and teamwork at the core of any team's success. Wooden preached a mantra that basketball is a game of threes: forward, guard, center; shoot, drive, pass; and ball, you, man. Wooden was pleased to develop outstanding individual basketball talents, of whom Lew Alcindor (later known as Kareem Abdul-Jabbar) and Bill Walton are two of the best known. However, Wooden never permitted individual player excellence to overshadow or to skew his team-centered approach to tactics and execution at both ends of the floor.

When Wooden and his UCLA teams captured their first national championship in 1964, the UCLA roster did not have a starting player taller than 6 ft 5 in (1.95 m). UCLA compensated for its lack of frontcourt size with a stifling zone press defense; Wooden's players had the physical conditioning to execute it effectively.

The 1964 national championship title gave the Bruins a national visibility in an era that preceded all-sports cable networks, 24-hour access to game stories and the innumerable sport recruiting resources of the Internet. In 1964, scores from the West Coast seldom made the following day's morning newspapers in the East. Two seasons after repeating as champions in 1965, the Bruins corralled the most prized recruit in the United States, Alcindor, out of Power Memorial High School in New York. With Alcindor in the middle, the Bruins sported an 88-2 record from 1968 through 1970 and won three consecutive national titles. One of the losses was arguably the most publicized college basketball game to that point in the game's history. UCLA fell in a memorable 71-69 defeat to the University of Houston Cougars and its standout player, Elvin Hayes, before a record crowd of 52,693 at Houston's Astrodome. Basketball games played in domed stadiums are commonplace today, but the UCLA/Houston clash was the first such contest. UCLA avenged this defeat later that season, routing the Cougars 101-69 in the NCAA semifinals.

In the nine championship seasons that followed, Wooden's coaching genius is best illustrated by the fact Wooden and UCLA were successful playing a variety of different styles, as dictated by their available manpower. When UCLA had Alcindor, they could utilize the most dominant player in the game, a lithe and athletic 7 ft 2 in (2.15 m) presence who was virtually impossible to defend with a single opponent. In the latter period of the Wooden dynasty, UCLA had the 6 ft 11 in (2.08 m) Bill Walton, who was less of a power player than Alcindor but a formidable defender and passer. Each of these players was ultimately named to the National Basketball Association Top 50 players of all time list.

With success came an almost inevitable desire on the part of UCLA's rivals to discredit the hyper successful program. In the early 1970s, the activities of UCLA supporter, or booster, Sam Gilbert were subjected to the most significant of these attacks. Gilbert, a Los Angeles area businessman, was regarded as a father figure by many UCLA players and sat at a prominent courtside seat during the Bruins' home games at Pauley Pavilion. Rival coaches such as Jerry Tarkanian and Dale Brown called UCLA's program corrupt, citing cash and gifts from Gilbert to UCLA players, though the NCAA investigated and cleared Wooden's program and Wooden personally of any wrongdoing or impropriety.

The stark statistical summery of Wooden's career at UCLA is remarkable. Between 1948 and his retirement in 1975, Wooden directed UCLA to an overall record of 620–147, with four undefeated seasons. In the midst of that success came an 88 game undefeated streak, a record never likely to be matched in modern Division 1 college basketball, as no other team has enjoyed even a single undefeated season since the 1976 Indiana Hoosiers, let alone the equivalent of almost three straight seasons.

The UCLA run of 10 national championships between 1964 and 1975 is also unlikely to be duplicated. In part, this accomplishment is a testament to Wooden and his UCLA teams. It is also a reflection of the greater number of Division 1 programs now competing at the NCAA level (there are now over 330 Division 1 basketball programs, an increase of over 70 schools since Wooden retired). The increase in the number of talented players leaving university before the expiration of their college eligibility to seek an NBA career has also dramatically limited the ability of any team to dominate in the fashion of Wooden and UCLA for even a two- or three-year period. There are few records in sport that may be said to be unassailable; the UCLA national championship record may be the exception.

Wooden's coaching genius has been recognized both by his peers in the basketball community and the American sports media. Wooden is one of only two players to be inducted into the Basketball Hall of Fame as both a player and a coach (the other is Atlanta Hawks star and NBA coach Lenny Wilkins). Wooden was named NCAA coach of the year on six occasions. The sports television network ESPN named Wooden the Coach of the Century in 1999.

SEE ALSO Basketball; National Collegiate Athletic Association (NCAA); Sports coaching.

# Lynette Woodward

1959–
AMERICAN
BASKETBALL PLAYER

Lynette Woodward is one of the most successful female basketball players in the history of the sport. Born in 1959 in Wichita, Kansas, Woodward's first brush with fame occurred during her high school playing career, when she lead her team to a Kansas state championship. Woodward then attended the University of Kansas from 1978 to 1981, where she was one few athletes in the history of National Collegiate Athletic Association (NCAA) competition in any sport to be named an All-American for all four years of her collegiate career. In addition to graduating as the NCAA's all-time career female scoring leader, Woodward lead the nation in the key statistical categories of points scored, steals, and rebounds in at least one of those four seasons.

On graduation from the University of Kansas, Woodward was recruited to play in the Italian women's professional basketball league, where she starred. In 1984, Woodward was named captain of the United States Women's Olympic basketball team, which won a gold medal at the Los Angeles Summer Olympics. In 1985, Woodward made history as the first female player ever signed to play by the Harlem Globetrotters, the famous African-American basketball team that traveled the world playing exhibitions. Woodward was a member of the Globetrotters until 1987. The Globetrotters mixed a measure of showmanship, comedy, and basketball tricks in their games, and Woodward participated as a full member of the Globetrotters entourage.

After her tenure with the Globetrotters, Woodward returned to Italy where she played professionally for an additional two seasons and led the league in scoring. Woodward also played for one season in the Japanese women's professional league. At the age of 38, Woodward joined the newly established Women's National Basketball League (WNBA) as a member of the Cleveland Rockers. Woodward retired after completing two seasons in the WNBA in 1998.

Woodward was never the biggest or the strongest competitor. But her natural athleticism, leadership, and floor sense were the attributes that separated Woodward from her contemporaries. Woodward was inducted into the Basketball Hall of Fame in Springfield, Massachusetts, in 2004. She was also named by *Sports Illustrated* magazine as one of the greatest athletes in the history of the state of Kansas.

SEE ALSO Basketball.

# World Anti-Doping Agency (WADA)

The World Anti-Doping Agency (WADA) was founded in 1999 as a result of what had been a growing international effort to counter the effects of performance-enhancing substances in sport. Headquartered in Montreal, Canada, WADA is the supreme international authority with respect to both doping test procedures and the determination of what substances will be the subject of athletic sanction when detected.

The stated mission of WADA is the international monitoring, promotion, and coordination of the international fight against doping in sport in all of its forms.

The use of various substances by athletes to improve performance is likely as old as competitive sport itself. Competition has often spurred athletes to seek any edge—however slight, and at their own physical risk—that might separate them from their rivals. In 1928, the International Amateur Athletic Federation (IAAF) banned the use of doping, which in that era was primarily the use of stimulants such as amphetamines and strychnine (also a well-known poison).

The history of formal doping tests can be traced to the late 1960s, when the properties of certain substances, particularly anabolic steroids and stimulants, began to raise concerns among athletic governing bodies that a level competitive field be preserved. In 1968, the International Olympic Committee (IOC) formally banned a wide range of performance-enhancing substances from Olympic competition and established formal doping tests. In 1976 the IOC was able to formally ban anabolic steroids as a test had been developed to detect the presence of these compounds in the body.

As the IOC did not possess the comprehensive or foolproof detection technologies necessary to rigorously enforce the doping rules, both the Olympic movement and international sport generally remained the subject of significant public concern regarding drug use in sport in the following 20 years. Doping became a more serious problem, with the rise of professionalism in many previously amateur disciplines, such as track and field. The testing procedures employed by the IOC became more accurate and more reliable, as was evidenced by the disqualification of Canadian sprinter Ben Johnson in the 1988 Summer Olympics for a positive anabolic steroid test, after he won the 100-m sprint final. However, the competitions held in a number of international sports, most notoriously cycling, appeared to be significantly affected by doping practices. A police seizure of various doping products during the 1998 Tour de France gave further publicity to the use of both stimulants and the then-recently synthesized

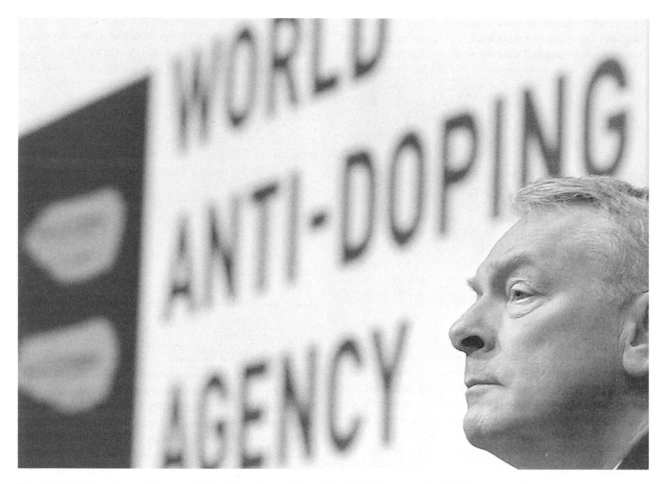

World Anti-Doping Agency Chairman Richard Pound at podium during WADA symposium, 2004. © ARC/DOMINIQUE FAVRE/ REUTERS/CORBIS

hormone, erythropoietin (EPO), which was administered to increase the ability of the body to produce a greater number of erythrocytes (red blood cells), which permitted a correspondingly increased transport of oxygen in the bloodstream during competition.

In 1999 worldwide public concerns regarding doping culminated in the creation of WADA, established with the full support of both the IOC and numerous national governmental and sport-governing bodies. Through the regulatory instrument known as the WADA Anti-Doping Code, a worldwide sport consensus was forged in the years following the founding of WADA. International sports federations, national sport-governing bodies, national Olympic committees, and independent sports leagues that agreed to be bound by the terms of the WADA Code became correspondingly obligated to enforce all of the WADA rules concerning the administration of doping tests (both in-competition and out-of-competition), to abide by the enforcement of the WADA Prohibited

List (the annual publication of all illegal performance-enhancing substances), and to participate in comprehensive doping education strategies.

The influence of WADA and the efforts of its constituency to create a drug-free sport have resulted in an international sport climate where the failure of a sport to properly administer transparent anti-doping practices will ensure that the sport will not be included in the Olympic Games. In 2006, baseball was removed from the roster of sports to be contested at the 2012 Summer Games by the IOC. The International Baseball Federation (IBF) was vigorous in both its objections to the removal of its sport from the Summer Games, as well as advancing its claim for reinstatement in advance of the 2016 Olympics, and beyond. WADA investigated the dope-testing practices of the IBF, particularly as they applied to Major League Baseball (MLB), whose professional players would be eligible for participation in an Olympics; MLB is not a signatory to the WADA Code. WADA determined that unless the IBF demonstrated compliance with WADA practices, WADA would declare the sport noncompliant, an act that would all but eliminate baseball from any Olympic reinstatement.

Over 200 countries, through their national sports-governing bodies, are signatories to the WADA Code. In addition, most of those countries have created a national anti-doping agency as the instrument to further the work by WADA on their national level; the United States Anti-Doping Agency (USADA) is an example. The chief work conducted by the national agencies is the coordination of national doping testing among all of the national sports federations in a particular country. In virtually all sporting nations, both the ability to participate in international competition as well as the receipt of government or private sponsor funding will be dependent on the athletes' compliance with all doping testing as mandated by the national anti-doping agency, consistent with overall WADA direction.

The most visible aspect of WADA is the combined effect of the annual Prohibited List and the resultant competition bans that are imposed when a positive doping test is registered. The Prohibited List is updated by WADA on an annual basis to reflect any scientific developments with respect to newly discovered substances that are deemed to represent drug cheating. The emergence of nandrolone in 2003, the so-called designer anabolic steroid, is an example of a discovery that resulted in its inclusion on the List. WADA, through various accredited laboratories, actively researches what it anticipates as the next cutting edge in the battle against doping. An effective system to determine whether an athlete has participated in gene doping, the modification of the athlete's genetic structure to develop better muscle structure, is an example. Another recent area of WADA-authorized research has assisted in the creation of a marker to be used in urine tests to prevent the switching of urine samples for the purpose of deceiving a test administrator.

The sanctions imposed by WADA are generally significant: a two-year ban from all competition for a first offense positive doping test is common. In many cases, the athlete advances a defense that centers on either his or her personal ignorance of the substance (often as a component in a dietary supplement), or that he or she was advised by a coach or trainer that the substance was legal for use. The general position of WADA is one of strict liability, an application of the legal proposition that the responsibility rests with the atheletes to ensure they know at all times that anything they ingest into their bodies is both safe and legal for use.

SEE ALSO Anabolic steroids; Doping tests; International Anti-Doping Agreement; Nandrolone; Prohibited substances (competition bans); Stimulants; U.S. Anti-Doping Agency (USADA).

# World Cup Soccer SEE FIFA: World Cup Soccer

# Wrapping and taping techniques

Wrapping and taping are terms that are often used interchangeably in the consideration of athletic training and sports injury rehabilitation, though each has a distinct meaning.

Wrapping is the procedure used both in administration of first aid to an injury, as well as ongoing treatment. Wrapping is the compression aspect of the RICE (rest/ice/compression/elevation) treatment commonly administered in the event of a soft tissue injury. RICE treatment is designed to immediately limit the consequences of injuries such as an ankle sprain, a strained hamstring, or groin pull, or a shoulder joint injury. Any strain, sprain, or suspected tear or tissue rupture should be treated with the RICE technique.

Wrapping a soft tissue injury is often done in conjunction with the application of ice. The wrap is applied to permit the ice bag or cold pack to be properly positioned on the surface of the injury, and also provide the desired compression to the surface. Compression, when properly administered, will be tight without restricting blood flow. The compression is used in combination with the application of ice to prevent the joint from swelling, a natural process that tends to lengthen recovery.

While any material could be used as a wrap in an emergency, first aid wraps are typically made of an elastic substance, to permit the wrap to be stretched over the injured joint and any ice being applied. The technique used to apply the wrap will depend on the location of the injury; the wrap must be applied in a fashion that ensures compression, but permits some degree of movement.

Taping is generally a preventative measure taken to protect an athlete from further injury to a previously damaged joint or tissue. Taping is a temporary device, where the applied material functions in the same fashion as an orthotic, providing support and a

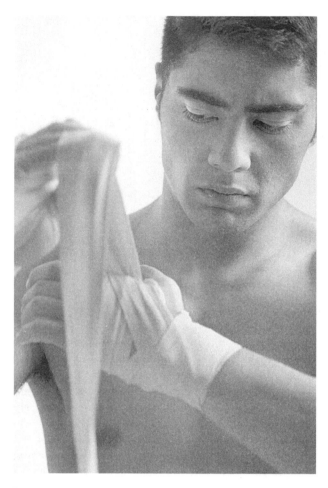

Boxer wrapping his wrist with athletic tape. © ROYALTY-FREE/ CORBIS

measure of protection to the desired area. Tape is generally applied in two stages; the first is an underlay of a thin, porous, and foam-like material, often referred to as pre-wrap. The tape, an adhesive, is then applied over the pre-wrap in thin strips. There are a multitude of taping methods, each individually designed to suit a specific athletic need. As a general proposition, the primary goal of athletic taping is to provide additional support for the specific joint, while not unduly hindering the degree of movement. Taping seeks to achieve the same physical result as a brace. Due to the combined effects of movement and perspiration, the athletic tape will not maintain its degree of rigidity for extended periods; it is not uncommon to see an athlete being re–taped at a break in play to ensure that the joint is still well supported.

SEE ALSO Ankle sprains; First aid kits for sports; Hamstring injuries; Knee injuries; Orthotics; RICE (rest/ ice/compression/elevation) treatment for injuries; Sprains and strains.

# Wrestling

Wrestling is one of the world's oldest forms of athletic competition. Many cultures had forms of wrestling as a component of their military preparation. The ancient Olympics included wrestling, with the competition first recorded as taking place in the Games of 708 BC.

The recognized sport of wrestling is an athletic event, sanctioned by the International Federation of Associated Wrestling Styles (FILA), and it is included as both an international and Olympic competition. In North America, a variant to the FILA-styled competition is popular in both high schools and at a university level. In a number of countries in the modern world, wrestling, referred to as pro wrestling, is the name given the entertainment exemplified by the shows staged by the World Wrestling Federation, but this type of wrestling is not FILA-related.

Wrestling is a sport involving two athletes engaged in a physical competition that is limited to a specified area defined on a mat. The general object of all types of wrestling is one wrestler attempts to force the shoulders of the opponent to the floor in a prescribed manner. The contest, a bout, is generally two rounds, each three minutes in duration. A wrestler wins a bout by either scoring a fall against the opponent, or by accumulating points through the successful execution of various maneuvers. In all forms of wrestling, a referee will supervise the contest, and judges positioned near the mat will score the progress of the contest. The two different types of wrestling competition are freestyle (in which men and women compete in separate divisions) and Greco-Roman.

Freestyle wrestling is the most popular form of the sport throughout the world. In freestyle, the wrestler is permitted to use his entire body in the execution of any of the permitted techniques. Holds of the opponent, including the use of the legs and the tripping of an opponent, are a part of freestyle. The Greco-Roman discipline restricts the competitors to holds applied to an opponent from the waist up, and the use of the legs to hold or throw the opponent is prohibited. North American collegiate freestyle wrestling is similar to that of FILA competition; the chief differences are variations in the rules with respect to the definition of a fall and the length of a bout.

In all forms of wrestling, there are a variety of methods in which to score against an opponent. When the wrestler places the opponent in a position in which the opponent's back is pressed to the mat, points are scored. In the course of a maneuver that

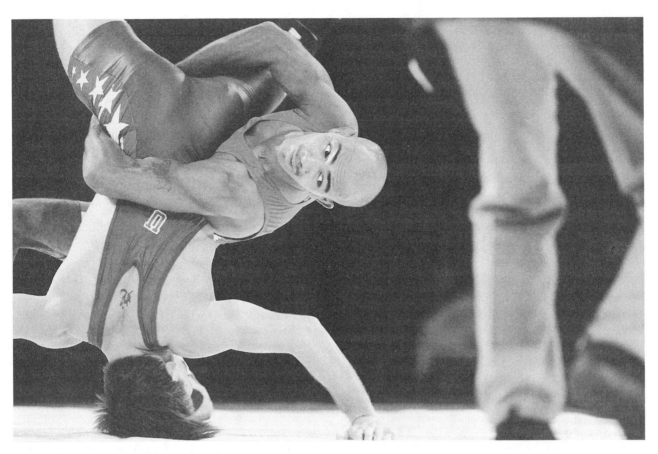

Competitors wrestling at the 2003 Titan Games. © DAVID MADISON/NEWSPORT/CORBIS

appears to have the wrestler in a position of control by the opponent, the wrestler will score if he is able to execute an escape from the disadvantageous position. A reversal is scored when a wrestler turns a scoring position for the opponent into a scoring position for himself. The best-known wrestling maneuver, a takedown, is when the wrestler takes the opponent from a standing position to the mat.

Wrestling in all of its forms is a demanding and highly athletic sport. As with many sports where physical strength and size are important competitive factors, wrestling competitions are divided into specific weight categories. Wrestling training must be comprehensive to produce a successful athlete, and all of the traditional attributes of complete physical fitness are engaged in the sport: strength, power, speed, flexibility, and endurance. The primal nature of wrestling, and the requirement that a single opponent be conquered, also demand the development of a very rigorous mental approach to training and competition.

The foundation of successful wrestling training is the development of a strong cardiovascular system. Like boxing, wrestling places demands on both the anaerobic energy system, due to the short, intense nature of the competition segments, as well as the aerobic system, necessary to facilitate recovery by the athletes. Traditional means of developing anaerobic fitness, such as interval training, are of benefit to the wrestler. Most comprehensive wrestling programs will ensure that the athlete obtains significant aerobic exercise, including running and cycling or the use of cardio machines when the athlete wishes to minimize the stress directed into legs, since they are the subject of very pronounced stresses in other aspects of training and competition.

The development of core strength is perhaps as important to a wrestler as any other physical attribute. Successful wrestling techniques each apply basic principles of physics, especially those relevant to the establishment of leverage, necessary to successfully throw an opponent, and the maintenance of a low center of gravity, to ensure stability in all movements. Successful wrestlers seek to develop their core strength to permit the maximum utility of the muscles of the abdomen, lumbar (lower back) region, groin, and gluteal area.

A characteristic of all successful wrestlers is the combined effect of flexibility and agility. Wrestling is a dynamic sport where the athlete must be able to respond to an opponent's attacks from a variety of physical positions. The rules of wrestling permit a multitude of different applications of force in which the greater the flexibility and resultant range of motion in the joints of the athlete, the more likely a positive response can be made and the less likely an injury will be sustained.

SEE ALSO Exercise, high intensity; Muscle mass and strength; Stretching and flexibility; Weight categories.

## Wrestling, Sumo SEE Sumo

## Wrist injuries

The wrist is a joint that is vulnerable to a wide variety of injuries, due to its exposure to an equally broad range of potential impacts, both with respect to trauma received from external forces, as well as the considerable extent of damage sustained through flexion, extension, and compression of the nerves radiating through the structure.

The wrist is a joint that if considered with respect to its bone alignment alone, the structure would be regarded as a rather delicate and vulnerable joint. The chief bones that create the wrist joint are the bones of the forearm (the ulnar and the radial bones), which meet the carpal bones (the assembly of eight small bones that separate the hand from the forearm at the joint). The various bones of the hand, including the metacarpals, which extend from the wrist to the fingers, are connected to the wrist through a series of ligaments at each metacarpal bone. There are also ligaments that connect the ulna and the radius to the carpal bones, and the resulting joint is capable of 360° movement. The main nerve root that passes through the bones of the wrist to coordinate the movements of the hand and the fingers is the carpal nerve, which radiates from the forearm into the palm of the hand through the tunnel created by the assembly of the bones and tendons of the wrist.

The most common athletic injury sustained to the wrist is a sprain, in which one of the ligaments of the wrist is either overextended or twisted. Sprained wrists are caused in a number of different fashions. When the ligaments of the wrist are subjected to a force applied by the hand being pushed backwards in an emphatic fashion, the ligaments may become stretched. Similarly, when the wrist is engaged in a grappling or grasping movement, such as often occurs in sports such as wrestling, American football, or rugby, and the forces directed into the wrist joint exceed the strength of the joint, the ligament will become stretched or, in a worst case scenario, the ligament will tear.

The same mechanism that produces a sprain of the wrist joint may also lead to a fracture of a number of different carpal bones. Most fractures of the wrist are caused in one of two ways: a direct blow to the joint, usually centered in the top of the wrist, or when a fall causes a force to radiate from the hand into the joint.

In sports such as lacrosse, hockey (both ice and field), or baseball, where the wrist is exposed to a forceful blow from an object such as a stick or a ball, the bones of the wrist are consequently vulnerable to fracture. There is very little covering muscle or tissue on the top of the wrist, and all significant external forces are absorbed by the underlying bone.

A common cause of wrist fracture is any circumstance in which the person falls and puts out the nearest hand to prevent the body from striking the ground. These types of falls, which often occur without warning, frequently occur in sports such as cycling, where the athlete moves instinctively to break a fall. When the hand and arm are thrust out from the athlete's body, the force sustained will radiate into one of three joints: the wrist, the elbow, or the shoulder. As the smallest of the joints of the arm, the wrist is least capable of bearing a weight that produces a force that often exceeds two times the mass of the athlete. The small bones of the wrist are most vulnerable to this injury, particularly the scaphoid bone (located directly below the thumb), also known as the navicular bone. The scaphoid bone is often extremely slow to heal, and fractures of these small components of the wrist are not always readily observed in a regular x ray. Bone necrosis (a death of the bone cells in the vicinity of an untreated fracture) is a risk more often associated with scaphoid fractures than any other type of fracture, as the injury disrupts the blood flow to the bone.

A fall can also produce a condition known as triangular fibrocartilage complex (TFCC). The small cartilage that acts as a spacing device between the ulnar bone and the carpal bones can become torn in a fall where the hand is extended, causing both pain and a lack of mobility in the joint.

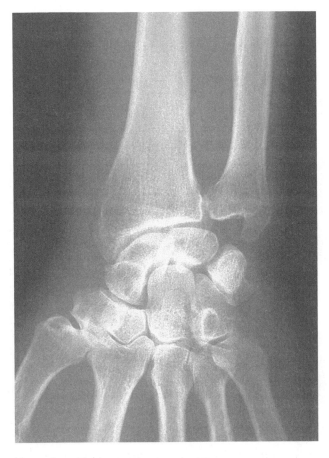

X-ray of a wrist. © ROYALTY-FREE/CORBIS

usually require any manipulation to straighten the bone; healing will occur if the joint is immobilized for a period of weeks.

The most frequent injury to the nerve roots that pass through the wrist is the condition known as carpal tunnel syndrome. The causes of this syndrome are varied, but the most prominent of these is the irritation of the nerve in the bone and tendon tunnel immediately adjacent to the palm of the hand, accompanied by significant repetitive use of the hand. Rest and immobilization of the wrist are the first line of attack to resolve this injury, coupled with the appropriate use of anti-inflammatory medications to reduce pain and swelling. In severe cases, when the wrist cannot be used for any significant period without pain and limitation of movement, surgery may be employed to create additional space between the radial nerve and the tunnel.

The tendons that assist in the operation of the muscles of the hand extend from immediately below the elbow to connect with the muscles at the wrist. Tendonitis is a common wrist injury. The mechanics of its causation may be those that would otherwise lead to a sprain of the wrist. In most cases, the tendonitis is caused through repetitive strain of the tissue that causes the fibers of the tendon to both overstretch and to become the subject of micro tears. In rare cases, the tendons may rupture; given their relatively small size and the fact that all tendons work in concert through the wrist, forces sufficient to tear the tendon are rare. Tendonitis of the wrist occurs with frequency in athletes playing sports such as tennis, baseball pitching, cricket, bowling, wrestling, and various martial arts, which require strong and constant wrist action.

As with any other soft tissue injury, wrist sprains and tendonitis are most effectively treated with the application of RICE (rest/ice/compression/elevation); a failure to quickly and aggressively address a wrist injury of any kind is an invitation to the onset of a chronic wrist condition. It is for this reason that wrist orthotics, particularly supportive sleeves and partial splint-type braces, are required.

**SEE ALSO** Bone, ligaments, tendons; Hand injuries; Musculoskeletal injuries; Sprains and strains.

Falls or other impacts in which the thumb is forcibly separated from its normal spacing on the hand will often result in a tear of the ligament connecting the thumb to the base of the wrist. Skier's thumb, so named to reflect a common cause of the injury, can also result from a ball or object being directed into the thumb. This injury may commonly require surgery.

In young athletes whose bones are not fully developed and hardened (the process known as ossification), when the athlete sustains a fall and extends an arm, the bones of the wrist are exposed to a specific type of fracture known as a buckle or greenstick fracture. In this injury, the bone does not break, due to the softness of the still-developing structure; the bone bends on impact. Such fractures do not

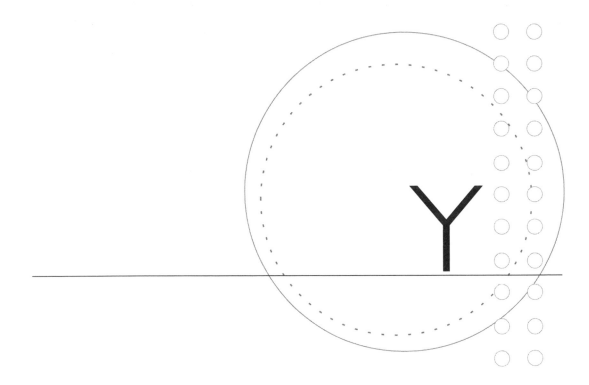

# Yams SEE Wild yams

# Yoga and Pilates

Yoga and Pilates are two separate forms of exercise that share common origins and philosophies. Both yoga, and to a lesser extent, Pilates, are popular worldwide as both freestanding health and conditioning programs and as components of comprehensive stretching, flexibility, and injury rehabilitation techniques employed by physical therapists.

The principles of yoga developed as a part of the Buddhist religion in India over 5,000 years ago. Yoga incorporated eight different philosophies, of which physical training was only one part; yoga adherents were also directed to abstain from violence, to develop an inward focus, to work in harmony with the universe as whole, and to practice meditation. The physiological aspects of yoga included the execution of the physical exercises and the development of breath control. Yoga formed a part of a number of the traditional alternative medicines of India and was believed by its adherents to assist in the progression along a pathway to better spiritual enlightenment.

The essence of yoga exercises is the emphasis on the use of the entire musculoskeletal system to perform the movements. Yoga is predicated on the body supporting its own weight in the course of all of the positions, both standing and prone, where multiple muscle groups must act in unison to successfully sustain the movement. The resistance against which the muscles must act is constant, given that the individual's body weight is the source of the resistance; the longer that the particular movement is sustained, the greater the potential muscular development and corresponding anaerobic effect. In a one-hour yoga session, the practitioner may require the expenditure of as many as 600 calories, subject to the difficulty of the movements. Yoga stresses correct posture, precise movement, and efficient breathing that assists the body in controlling both heart rate and mental control.

Because yoga places emphasis on tranquility and peacefulness in the exercises, it has a deceptively gentle appearance. Most yoga beginners find that it takes a significant measure of practice in a number of the established yoga positions before any of the more demanding yoga routines is attempted. It is common in a yoga position to stretch a muscle group in a static fashion (body weight only generating the resistance), and then to move to a dynamic stretch, where the subject is generating greater resistance through the movement.

Pilates, the exercise program named for its developer, Joseph Hubertus Pilates (1880–1967), is rooted in similar physical principles to yoga. Pilates originally named his program contrology to stress his determination to enhance mind, body, and spirit through his system. Pilates looked to the traditions of yoga, the calisthenics associated with gymnastics training, and his own research to develop a series of over 500 exercises, with progressive increases in

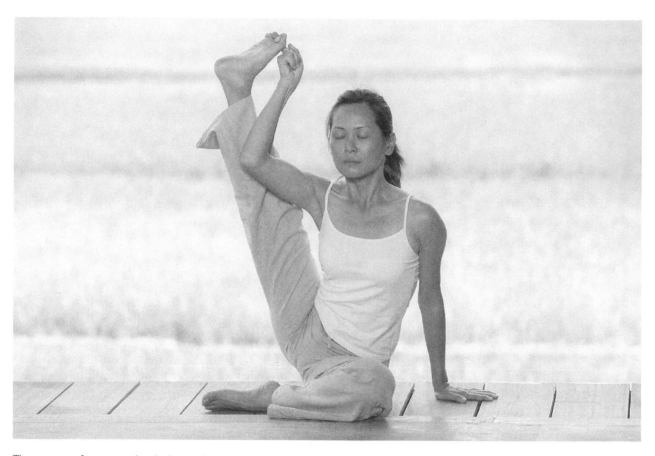

The essence of yoga exercises is the emphasis on the use of the entire musculoskeletal system to perform the movements. © SIMON TAPLIN/CORBIS

difficulty. He intended his program to function primarily as a set of therapeutic movements; Pilates's first clientele were dancers working in the New York entertainment industry in the 1950s. Pilates exercises employ either a floor mat, a simple roller/pulley machine, called a Reformer, for the extension of the arms and legs, or a Swiss ball, sometimes referred to as a fit ball.

All Pilates exercises emphasize the building of core strength, the ability of the body to maintain balance, flexibility, and control of movements through a strong abdomen, groin, and lumbar (lower back) structure. These muscle groups tend to work in a coordinated fashion in most forms of human movement, and a demonstrated imbalance in any single aspect of core strength will generally impair efficient and capable movement. Like yoga, a vigorous Pilates session carries a low risk of injury to the user, and may require the expenditure of over 600 calories per hour of training.

There are no competitive forms of either yoga or Pilates. Yoga is commonly enjoyed by people as a primary means of fitness, and Pilates is a popular feature in North American health and fitness clubs. The beauty of both yoga and Pilates is that once the user is introduced to and is comfortable with the required movements, the exercises can be performed anywhere that there is space to spread out a mat. There are numerous video presentations available for both yoga and Pilates to be used for programs in the home.

**SEE ALSO** Bone, ligaments, tendons; Calisthenics; Range of motion; Stretching and flexibility; Warm-up/cooldown.

# Yohimbine

Yohimbine is a product made from the bark of the yohimbe tree, a species native to west Africa. Yohimbine is an alkaloid, one of a group of nitrogen based compounds present in plants that acts as a base, a substance that combine with acids to form salts. Many alkaloids have a pronounced effect upon the function and performance of the human body;

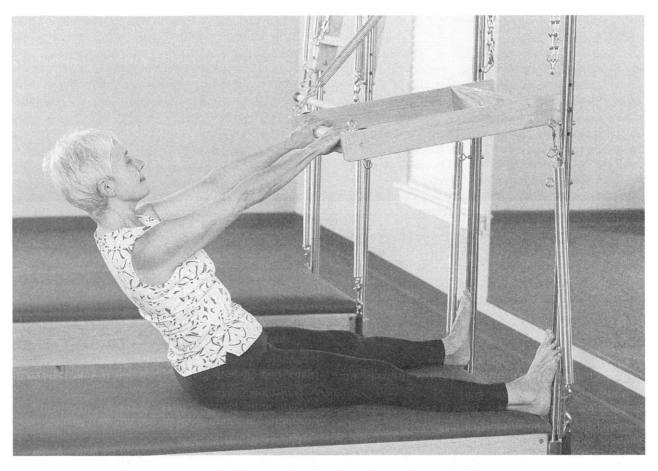

Pilates is a strenuous activity that increases flexibility, strength, and cardiovascular capacity. © ROB & SAS/CORBIS

prominent alkaloids include caffeine, cocaine, and nicotine. Yohimbine has a chemical composition that is expressed by the equation $C_{21}H_{26}N_2O_3$.

Among native African cultures, the bark of the yohimbe tree was renowned as an aphrodisiac. Modern medical science has recognized the value of Yohimbine in the treatment of erectile dysfunction.

Yohimbine is classed as one of the medications known as sympatholytics, those drugs or other pharmaceutical agents that act against the sympathetic nervous system, the portion of the autonomic nervous system that regulates the "flight or fight response", as well as the function of various glands.

Yohimbine is a vasodilator, a chemical that causes the blood vessels to expand. This action results in an increase in the amount of blood flowing to the peripheral parts of the body. In a similar fashion, yohimbine acts to trigger the release of noradrenalin from the adrenal gland, a hormone which produces an accelerated heart beat and tends to dilate the airways in the lungs, making breathing easier.

Modern scientific research has focused on the potential use of yohimbine as an anti-oxidant, the molecular scavengers that operate within the body to neutralize the effects of free radicals, those substances that are electrically unstable and consequently seek to balance themselves by preying upon otherwise stable cells within the body. Free radical activity is a contributing factor to the spread of cancers within the body. Similar research has also illustrated the potential for yohimbine as a weight loss product. When consumed, yohimbine tends to increase the conversion of stored fats to triglycerides, the fatty acids used by the body as an energy source.

Yohimbine has few side effects; given its effect upon heart rate, it is not recommended for use by persons with a prior history of heart disease or other known cardiovascular irregularities. The most common side effect attributed to yohimbine in an otherwise healthy person is dizziness.

SEE ALSO Dietary supplements; Herbs; Sexual and reproductive disorders.

# Youth sports injuries

Youth has a variety of meanings in the world of sport. As a description of the relative physical maturity of an athlete, youth represents the progression from childhood to adulthood. A youth is an adolescent whose body is continuing to grow into its adult state. A youth possesses all of the physical attributes of an adult, but not yet fully formed. A youth is also someone whose emotional development is not complete; it is not uncommon for athletes to reach their adult musculoskeletal development in advance of the completion of corresponding emotional growth.

Youth is usually associated with the biological process known as puberty, which begins at different times for both males and females. The general commencement of puberty for females in North America is age 10; for males, puberty often begins at age 12 or 13. In the three to four years that follow the onset of puberty, the human body undergoes its most rapid growth, second only to the growth rate experienced in a newborn child. It is the rapidity of physical growth that necessitates a specific consideration of the injuries commonly sustained in youth sports.

All youth athletes who participate in sport are exposed to the same physical forces and the same general types of injury as are adult athletes. The mechanics of the execution of the various maneuvers in any sport do not particularly change when the sport is played at a younger age; given the smaller athletes, there are often lesser amounts of mass making contact with one another, resulting in lesser forces in sports where contact is either desired or incidental. The risk of injury to a youth athlete in both contact sports and non-contact sports will usually stem from one of three causes—poor technique, often a function of substandard coaching, growth-related weaknesses in the youth musculoskeletal structure, and overuse or repetitive strain.

During adolescence, the bones, skeletal muscles, and connective tissues continue to grow. The most prominent aspect of this phase is the presence of growth plates near the epiphysis, the end of the long bones of the body, including the femur (thigh), the tibia and fibula (shin), and the humerus (upper arm). The growth plate is a softer, cartilage-like region of growing bone cells; at maturity, the growth plate will entirely ossify, or harden, into a permanent and seamless component of the entire bone. The growth plate is at elevated risk of injury during contact sport, as it is more prone to fracture if it receives significant trauma. A damaged growth plate that is not repaired may disturb future growth in the limb.

A related condition common to young athletes is Osgood-Schlatter disease (OSD), which is a condition where the patellar tendon, which attaches the kneecap to the tibia, is growing at a different rate than the bone structure. OSD becomes painful to athletes who are engaged in repetitive motions such as running. The condition is usually treated with rest; OSD will ultimately be outgrown by the athlete.

Concussion is an injury caused by the receipt and absorption of a blow to the head, often causing damage to both the skull and the surface of the brain. A concussion can cause pain, dizziness, and nausea, and an athlete who has sustained a concussion should have a through neurological examination prior to the resumption of a contact sport. Concussions are often the result of both poor coaching technique in contact sports such as American football and ice hockey, where the player is improperly instructed to position their body with the head leading the body on contact with an opponent.

A further coaching-related athletic injury among youths is the wide range of problems associated with overuse and repetitive strains placed on the not yet mature bodies of the athlete. In sports such as track running, distance running, and figure skating, where the legs of the athlete are subjected to continual stress, the athlete's training program must be carefully constructed to avoid the excess training volumes and intensities that lead to stress fractures; over 60% of stress fractures sustained by young athletes occur in the lower leg, commonly in the tibia (shin) between 1 in to 3 in (3–10 cm) above the ankle. Although not strictly a physical injury, these circumstances are also ripe to produce the debilitating mental state referred to as burn out, when the young athlete loses interest in training due to the combination of physical and mental overload.

The most common of the unavoidable athletic injuries in youths is the buckle or greenstick bone fracture. These fractures most often result when the young athlete puts out a hand to avoid a fall, with the impact radiating into the small carpal bones of the wrist; the bone, not yet fully formed or as dense as it will be in adulthood, does not fracture completely, but bends under the forces on impact. Most buckle fractures will heal through immobilization, by splint or cast. A common carpal bone to sustain fracture is the scaphoid (navicular) bone, located below the thumb joint in the wrist.

Throwing sports place significant forces on all of the muscle and skeletal structures involved in generating the forces necessary to throw the desired object. The most common and the most significant of these injuries with respect to the long-term health of the athlete are those caused to either the throwing shoulder or the elbow of young baseball pitchers. The development of a curve ball, a pitch that requires a vigorous overhand shoulder motion, accompanied by a forceful twisting of the elbow, places particular stress on the rotator cuff, the four muscles that are positioned on the top of the shoulder, providing strength and stability to the joint; the elbow motion creates powerful forces in very small tissues, the ulnar cruciate ligament, and the epicondyle tissues that encapsulate the elbow joint. The repetitive stress of throwing these pitches often leads to the development of strains or tears in one or more of the shoulder and elbow joints.

A common and dangerous injury to young athletes is environmental in nature. In outdoor sports played in warm weather, young athletes are exposed to heightened risk of the development of one of the progressive heath illnesses, heat cramps, heat exhaustion, or heat stroke. As young athletes may not possess the maturity to abide by a self-directed hydration plan, no warm weather youth sports should ever be undertaken without both ample and appropriate fluids, as well as heat-combative first aid materials.

**SEE ALSO** Genetics; Growth plate injuries; Knee: Genetic and non-athletic conditions affecting performance; Musculoskeletal injuries; RICE (Rest/Ice/Compression/Elevation) treatment for injuries.

# Youth sports performance

Youth sports performance is a multidimensional concept. At a participatory sports level, performance is focused on teaching the basic skills necessary to play a particular game, with the emphasis on the personal enjoyment of the youth, as an incentive to continue participation at either a higher level or as the athlete grows. At an elite-performance level, a range of issues are engaged, most of which center on the fact that a young athlete is not a miniature adult athlete, but rather an individual with needs that are unique to youth sports.

A youth is a person in the midst of physical and emotional transformations from child to adult. In virtually any sport, it is physically impossible for the youth to replicate adult performance, as the adolescent body is not fully developed in all aspects of the musculoskeletal system. For these reasons, the performance of a young athlete will be founded on a number of factors.

Young athletes are bombarded with media representations of professional athletes and how a particular sport should be played. Coaching a young athlete, in both individual and team sports, to train and to perform within their physical limitations is fundamental to ensuring sport enjoyment, a progressive skill improvement, and a reduction in the risk of injury.

Young athletes are less likely than adults to be able to self-motivate. Young athletes are more likely to become frustrated if they are unable to quickly master a particular sports technique. Motivation for the young person, particularly the correction of errors accompanied by positive reinforcement from coaches or supportive adults, is a useful method to keep the young athlete inspired to continue, particularly with training.

Stress is in many respects a far more debilitating factor with respect to the sports performance of the young athlete than with respect to an adult. Young people are subjected to stresses that emanate from a variety of sources—the stereotypical over-zealous parents and demanding, tyrannical coaches are not caricatures, but all too common examples of stress-generating forces. The peers of the athlete are also a part of the young athlete's environment that may exert an influence over how the athlete views his or her own performance as well as how he or she in fact performs.

These stress factors do not always present themselves directly, but in the manner in which the athlete responds to stress over time. Eating disorders, particularly among female athletes, are a common result of the negative self-image created in the athlete's mind concerning the ability to successfully compete. It is estimated that as many as 10% of all male high school athletes in the United States, and a lesser number of female athletes, experimented with anabolic steroids to improve their physical ability to perform.

When performance is overemphasized in a young athlete, the risk of burn out is heightened; burn out is a combination of physical and mental fatigue, usually induced in young athletes by a combination of competitive pressure and over-training.

Various scientific studies concerning how to ensure optimal youth sports performance suggest that making sure the athlete has an opportunity to play a number of different sports in adolescence is important. The thesis supporting a youth engaging in multiple sports applies to both the physical and mental aspects of sport. When youth have been encouraged to diversify their sports performance, there exists a much higher prospect of adult sports participation. When the young person plays a number of

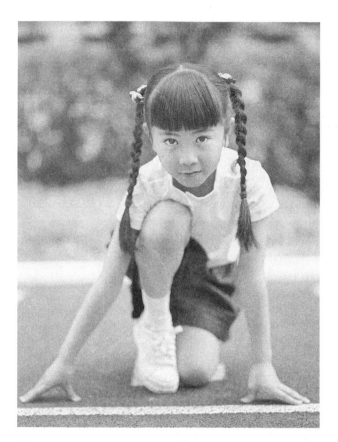

Coaching a young athlete to train and to perform within their physical limitations is fundamental to ensuring sport enjoyment. © MICHAEL PRINCE/CORBIS

# Youth sports training

The training and preparation of young athletes for sports competition involves a wide-ranging series of considerations. Training is a concept involving both the physical preparation of the athlete, as well as the teaching and the implementation of sport-specific techniques through coaching and practice. The physical elements of training must be delivered in a coordinated fashion, as a part of a comprehensive mental preparation of the athlete, including the use of a variety of sports psychology tools to focus and to motivate the athlete in training and competition.

Youth sports involve the consideration of physical and mental training issues that are absent in adult athletic training. As a youth, by definition, is an adolescent person, typically one who has entered puberty, a young athlete is generally in the midst of the most rapid physical growth cycle that he or she will ever experience, with the exception of infancy. All youth sports training must take into account the fact that as the athlete's body is growing, the bones and connective tissues are especially vulnerable to injury, particularly those related to overuse of a particular joint, or the forces generated by the repetitive stress of various sports accumulating to cause injury to an immature musculoskeletal structure.

The training of young athletes must also make provision for the fact that an athlete in the 12 to 16-year-old age range is unlikely to have the same level of emotional maturity as an adult athlete with respect to the reaction to coaching criticism, or the impact of the demands of high-level competition. Effective communication between the young athlete and coach is fundamental to successful training. The coach must engender an environment that encourages the athlete to raise any question or concern regarding training.

The unique features of the training programs developed for young athletes place a primary importance on the creation and implementation of a program that is based on the principle known as the periodization of training. The division of the training year (or any other significant period) is a recognition that athletes generally cannot train at a constant level; there are natural cycles to a training period that usually are tied to a specific goal or objective, and subsequent periods of rest or reduction in training intensity. All athletes, irrespective of their talent level, tend to benefit from training that provides a specific focus, with an opportunity to reflect on progress at the conclusion of the training segment to permit a readjustment on future training. The

sports through the course of the year, he or she is mentally refreshed and each sport is regarded as something of a new challenge. Athletes who play multiple sports also tend to develop a more balanced musculature, with less risk of injury due to repetitive stress or the overuse of a particular muscle structure.

Scientific research also reveals that in multidimensional sports such as the triathlon, while the elite-level athletes may come from one of the three particular disciplines of the sport, the athletes competing in the triathlon at a master's level (age 40 years and over) rarely specialized in swimming, cycling, or running as young athletes. In a similar fashion, studies conducted with respect to the typical participants in a marathon, over 40% of men and over 60% of female entrants did not run in any organized fashion prior to age 20. It is important that the young athlete not be directed into one sporting interest at the exclusion of all others to avoid a competitive plateau in the main activity, injury, or a change of interests.

SEE ALSO Motivational techniques; Sport performance; Sports coaching; Youth sports training.

unique physical and mental training circumstances of young athletes make periodization of the utmost importance.

The periodization of the training schedule for a young athlete with respect to a single sport will include designated preseason, competitive season, and off-season periods. Given that many young athletes may participate in more than one competitive sport, both the preseason and the off-season for one sport may represent the opposite segments respecting the athlete's other sports. The periods may also be further subdivided based on either known competitions or a desire to peak for them. In team sports, the usual competitive season is a progression from an opening game of the year to a season-ending playoff. In individual sports, such as track and field events, the competitive season may be a series of peaks, depending on the relative importance of the individual meets that form the season.

The determination of appropriate training periods provides the younger athletes with a measure of structure to their training that they might not be able to direct on their own. This issue is of paramount importance when the young athlete may be engaging in significant training intensity and training volume, such as that contemplated by two-a-day workouts in sports such as football or track and field.

The provision of effective direction to a young athlete with respect to diet and proper nutritional habits, including hydration, is an essential aspect of youth training. While all athletes are subject to dietary temptations, especially if they are training at a high level, young athletes have the dual concerns of proper nutrition to support their regular adolescent growth, coupled with the additional physical stresses of training. The successful motivation of young athletes to maintain proper diet will include the education of both the youth and their parents regarding nutritional practices, including the designation of a meal during the week when the athlete can go beyond the usual dietary boundary to a limited extent.

Of critical importance to the formulation of training periods is the insertion of periods of downtime, especially with respect to competition. The risk of mental fatigue, associated with high-level competition, travel to competition, and intense training to prepare for competition can be difficult for a young person to bear. This concern is especially pronounced in young athletes who either play more than one competitive sport, or who play a competitive sport on a year-round basis. Even for the competitive youth athlete, sport must remain fun.

In North America, the youth year-round sports trend is a relatively recent phenomenon. Until the 1980s, the American high school sports seasons had both a rhythm and a regularity that tended to encourage young athletes to play more than one sport. In the fall, the key boys' sports were football, volleyball, cross-country running, and soccer; for girls, it was soccer and volleyball. In the winter months, basketball was the primary sports for both genders, with other individual sports such as wrestling and swimming. In the spring months, a wide variety of sports were played, including lacrosse, track and field, and other outdoor activities. The summer months were typically devoted to organized sports such as baseball.

The rise of organizations such as AAU (Amateur Athletic Union) basketball in the summer months and year-round soccer training, or the increase in summer skills camps and schools in sports such as ice hockey have distorted the previous rhythm of the youth athletic year in North America. The drive to secure an athletic scholarship for a university education has placed a premium on year-round play. The risk of developing single-sport specialists at age 15 is that the athlete may not be competitive at age 20, and give up sports entirely.

Once the training periods and the related objectives are established, the training must be progressive, but at all times connected to the overarching notion that young athletes are not to be trained like adults, with simple reductions in training volume to account for their younger age. The development of the physical fitness of a young athlete, separate from the sport-specific skill development, must ensure that the characteristics of the musculoskeletal system of the young athlete are respected. All aspects of this physical training, in each of the components of strength, flexibility, endurance, and speed, must be addressed using less intensity and less volume that would be applied to a corresponding adult.

Keeping in mind the need to protect against injury to the young athlete, the training sessions must have a measure of fun. Young athletes are especially susceptible to burn out, the accumulation of physical demands and mental stress, when the sport takes on the aspects of classic 9-to-5 drudgery. A burned out athlete is a damaged athlete; the successful coach and corresponding training program will provide opportunities for the young athlete to have fun without the pressures of achieving a training goal. In individual sports, a day off to play an entirely different game is a common technique; in team sports, fun competitions are used.

Technique is essential to any sport success at any age; the teaching of the proper techniques to young people is critical for both safety and ultimate success. Technical instruction with young players must begin with a reinforcement of the particular rules of the sport. Rules instruction is of particular importance in contact sports, where the young players may have seen professional level competition and seek to emulate the actions of those players in their own training and play. American football has numerous opportunities to make contact with an opponent, within prescribed rules. Once the rules are entirely understood, the young player can be taught to execute the physical maneuvers in a safe manner.

With most athletes, physical techniques are not ideally taught through the simple demonstration of the entire sequence, with a direction to imitate it. Young players inevitably require progressive instruction, with the overall technique broken into its physical components, such as footwork, body position, hand position, and the sequence of movements to reach a result. An example is the basketball technique known as the box out, where a defensive player moves his or her body to prevent an offensive player from securing a rebound on a missed shot at the defender's goal. Instruction in the proper execution of the box out would begin with what the rules of the game permit by way of bodily contact; the coach would then identify any gray areas concerning what a referee might regard as incidental physical contact. Once an understanding of the appropriate rule is established, the players would be taken through a series of non-contact drills to assist them in developing the necessary spatial sense to the relationship between their position on the floor, the likely position of an opponent, and that of the goal and backboard. The next stage in the progression is the reinforcement of their desirable body position as the ball is being shot toward the goal. The teaching sequence culminates with a live practice of the technique involving an opponent if every other component has been executed correctly.

**SEE ALSO** Genetic prediction of performance; Growth; Youth sports injuries; Youth sports performance.

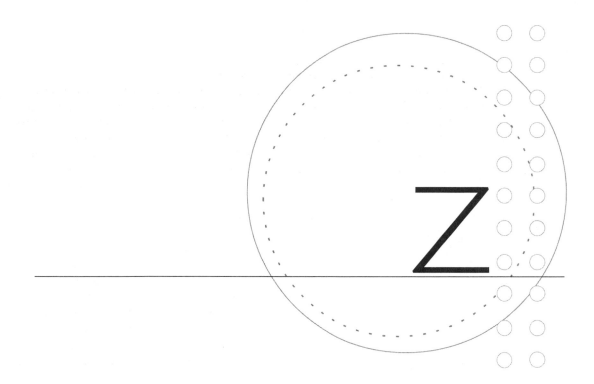

# Frank Joseph Zamboni Jr.

1901–7/27/1988
AMERICAN
MANUFACTURER, MOBILE ICE RESURFACING
EQUIPMENT

The Zamboni is one of the most identifiable pieces of equipment used in the sporting world. The mobile and mechanized ice resurfacing machine is a fixture at virtually every artificial ice surface in North America.

While the Zamboni is closely associated with ice hockey and the resurfacing of the rink between the periods of a professional game, the machine was created out of powerful commercial need to keep artificial ice functional in the southern California climate.

Frank Zamboni and ice making became associated with one another in 1921, when the 20 year old Frank entered the refrigeration business in Paramount, California, supplying ice for the then state of the art domestic ice box, soon to be supplanted by the more modern refrigerator.

Frank used his experience gained in the ice manufacturing business to open the Iceland Skating Rink in Paramount. At that time, artificial ice rinks were resurfaced by the manual labor of a team of men who scraped and then hosed down the surface by hand. Frank determined that there must be a more efficient way to resurface the ice.

Between 1942 and 1948, Frank built three primitive ice resurfacing machines using a variety of home-made and scrap automotive parts. In 1949, he succeeded in constructing a functional machine that was the forerunner to the modern Zamboni. People magazine described the device as a hideous, Rube Goldberg contraption with a wooden bin, a maze of pulleys, and crude four-wheel drive. Aesthetics aside, the Zamboni could clean ice well enough to resurface the Iceland rink in fifteen minutes.

The function of the Zamboni was simple. The purpose in ice resurfacing was to smooth out the ridges and divots created in the ice surface by skaters. The Zamboni machinery consists of a sharp blade, designed to shave the ice to a consistent and uniform surface; once shaved, the ice scrapings are scooped into a vat located within the Zamboni to be melted for reuse. The machine then sprays a fine layer of hot water over the ice. The surface then melts and is refrozen, creating a smooth skating surface through one pass of the Zamboni.

Other than securing a patent for his creation, Zamboni made no effort to market the device until 1950, when skating star Sonja Henie rented Iceland as a practice rink for her touring ice show. Henie was so impressed with the new machine that she paid Frank $5,000 to build her one. A short time later, the Ice Capades figure skating show put in an order for a machine, and Zamboni suddenly found himself in the business of manufacturing ice machines.

The machine manufacturing company business exploded into an international business concern when the U.S. Olympic Committee placed an order for four custom built machines for the 1960 Winter Olympics held at Squaw Valley, California. During the Olympic telecasts, the newly christened Zamboni was seen chugging its way across the world's television screens.

The Zamboni has proven to be a highly durable ice resurfacer—a 1955 Zamboni is still in use at a New Hampshire skating rink. Although there are commercial competitors, the Zamboni is regarded as the best ice resurfacing technology in the world. The Zamboni has achieved the status of a sport legend, all the more remarkable given that the Zamboni is a supporting actor in the world of ice sports, and not a prime actor. Ice hockey teams in particular have elevated the Zamboni; contests are often staged where the winner is given a Zamboni ride.

The Zamboni, a product of the determination of Frank Zamboni to bring efficiency to his ice skating business, is now a sports icon.

SEE ALSO Figure skating; Ice hockey rinks.

# Emil Zátopek

9/19/1922–11/22/2000
CZECH
LONG DISTANCE RUNNER

Emil Zátopek was an outstanding long distance runner during the 1940s and 1950s. He is most famous for his triple gold medal performance in the 1952 Summer Olympics held in Helsinki, Finland. There, he was first in the 5,000-m and 10,000-m events and, in his first attempt at distance running, the marathon.

Born in Czechoslovakia, now the Czech Republic, Zátopek began his running career in 1940, at the age of 16. Then, he was employed at a Bata shoe factory. The company sponsored a 1,500 m race, which Zátopek entered. Having never trained before, he finished second out of 100 competitors. His interest in running was sparked.

Only four years later, he broke his country's records for 2,000 m, 3,000 m, and 5,000 m events. In 1946, he was a member of the Czech national track and field team that competed at the European Championships. There, he finished fifth in the 5,000 m in a national record time.

Zátopek truly came into international prominence at the 1948 Olympics in London, England, where he won the gold medal in the 10,000 m (only the second time he had raced at that distance) and the silver medal in the 5,000 m.

This began a remarkable decade of running. In 1949, Zátopek twice set new world records at 10,000 m. He bettered his own record three more times during the next four years. In 1949, he won eleven 10,000 m races in succession, part of a streak of thirty-eight consecutive 10,000 m victories. During the 1950s, he established world records at 5,000 m (in 1954), 20 km (two times during 1951), 25 km (in 1952 and 1955), and 30 km (in 1952).

Zátopek was the first person to run 10,000 m in less than 29 minutes. As well, during 1951, he twice established world records for the distance run during 60 minutes, exceeding 20 km each time (a pace of 3 minutes per kilometer, or slightly over 4.5 minutes per mile).

His triple gold medal-winning effort in the 1952 Olympics was all the more remarkable as it came after he had been advised by a doctor not to compete due to possible lingering effects of a gland infection two months earlier. His 10,000 m victory was impressive; he passed all but two runners in the field during the race and won by 50 m. Three days later, in the 5,000 m, he came from 50 m behind in the final lap to win by several meters. Finally, he won the marathon by more than 2.5 minutes; his winning time of 2 hours, 23 minutes, 3 seconds was an Olympic record.

His three victories came within a span of eight days. And, on the afternoon when Zátopek captured the 5,000 m, his wife Dana won a gold medal for the Czech Republic in the javelin throw.

The 1956 Olympics held in Melbourne, Australia, was Zátopek's last. Running the marathon only weeks after a hernia operation, he finished sixth. The following year, he retired from competition.

In his last year of life his health declined, and he was hospitalized for a broken hip and pneumonia. Following a stroke on October 30, he was hospitalized yet again, where he died on November 22 at the age of 78.

He received full state honors at his funeral, which was attended by thousands of Czech citizens.

At only 5 ft 8 in (1.7 m) and 145 lb (65.7 kg), Zátopek had an unusual running style. In contrast to the smooth and steady cadence of most other elite runners, he ran in a style that even today is considered to be inefficient. His head would roll

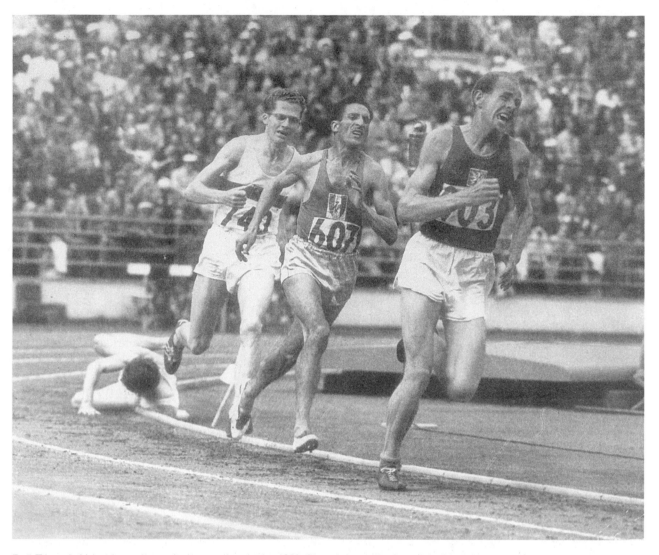

Emil Zátopek (right, shown here winning an event in the 1952 Olympics) was the first triple Olympic record holder, taking gold in the 5000 m, 10,000 m, and marathon events.

and his upper body would pivot horizontally about his waist as he ran. As well, he often grimaced and made loud wheezing and panting noises during a race. The latter noises earned him the nicknames "The Czech Locomotive" and "bouncing Czech."

However at odds with running dogma Zátopek's running style may have been, his results spoke volumes about his excellence as a runner. Moreover, his training regimen, which consisted of running laps at near-race speed, introduced the concept of speedwork into track training.

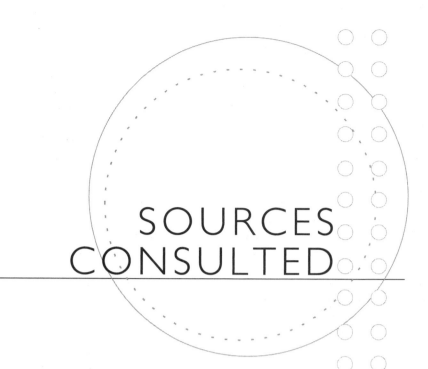

# SOURCES CONSULTED

## Books

Adair, Robert Kemp. *The Physics of Baseball*. New York: Perennial, 2002.

Allman, William F., and Eric W. Schrier, eds. *Newton at the Bat: The Science in Sports*. Ann Arbor: Books on Demand, 1994.

Armenti, Angelo, Jr., ed. *The Physics of Sports*. Woodbury: American Institute of Physics (AIP Press), 1992.

Axelrod-Contrada, Joan. *Mia Hamm: Soccer Player*. Ferguson Publishing, 2005.

Beckham, David. *My Side*. Collins Willow, 2004.

Beckham, David, and Tom Watt. *Beckham: Both Feet on the Ground: An Autobiography*. Harper Paperbacks, 2004.

Beckham, Ted. *David Beckham*. Boxtree, 2005.

Benoit Samuelson, Joan, and Gloria Averbuch. *Joan Samuelson's Running for Women*. Rodal Press, 1995.

Benoit, Joan. *Running Tide*. Knopf, 1987.

Bezruchka, Stephen. *Altitude Illness: Prevention & Treatment (Mountaineers Outdoor Expert)*. Mountaineers Books, 2005.

Bishop, Jan Galen. *Fitness through Aerobics*, 6th ed. Benjamin Cummings, 2004.

Bradley, Nick. *The 7 Laws of the Golf Swing*. DK Adult, 2005.

Burke, Edmund R. *Science of Cycling*. Champaign, IL: Human Kinetics, 1986.

———. *High-Tech Cycling*. Champaign, IL: Human Kinetics, 2003.

Carr, Gerald A. *Fundamentals of Track and Field*. Champaign, IL: Human Kinetics, 1999.

Coakley, Jay J. *Sports in Society: Issues and Controversies*, 8th ed. McGraw-Hill, 2004.

Cobb, Cathy, and Monty L. Fetterolf. *The Joy of Chemistry: The Amazing Science of Familiar Things*. Prometheus Books, 2005.

Cross, Rod, and Crawford Lindsey. *Technical Tennis: Racquets, Strings, Balls, Courts, Spin, and Bounce*. USRSA, 2005.

Eberhardt, Jared and Eric Kotch. *Blower: Snowboarding Inside Out*. Booth-Cliborn, 2002.

Griffith, H. Winter. *The Complete Guide to Sports Injuries*. Perigee Books, 2004.

Harris, Harry. *Pele: His Life and Times*. Welcome Rain, 2003.

Herman, Ellie. *Pilates for Dummies*. For Dummies, 2003.

Hines, James R. *Figure Skating: A History*. University of Illinois Press, 2006.

Jay, Timothy J. *Football Physics: The Science of the Game*. Emmaus, PA: Rodale, 2004.

Jorgensen, Theodore P. *The Physics of Golf*. Woodbury, NY: American Institute of Physics, 1994.

Kerrigan, Nancy, with Mary Spencer. *Artistry on Ice: Figure Skating Skills and Style*. Champaign, IL: Human Kinetics, 2003.

———. *Artistry on Ice: Figure Skating Skills and Style*. Human Kinetics Publishers, 2002.

King, Michael, and Yolanda Green. *Pilates for Pregnancy*. Ulysses Press, 2002.

Klaus, Susanne. *Adipose Tissue (Medical Intelligence Unit)*. Landes Bioscience, 2001.

Knudson, Duane. *Biomechanical Principles of Tennis: Using Science to Improve Your Strokes*. USRSA, 2006.

Lindsey, Crawford, Howard Brody, and Ron Waite. *The Physics and Technology of Tennis*. USRSA, 2004.

Lyon, Daniel. *The Complete Book of Pilates for Men: The Lifetime Plan for Strength, Power & Peak Performance*. Regan Books. 2005.

Martin, Danny, and Matt Diehl. *No-Fall Snowboarding: 7 Easy Steps to Safe and Fun Boarding*. Fireside, 2005.

Martin, John Stuart. *The Curious History of the Golf Ball, Mankind's Most Fascinating Sphere*. New York: Horizon Press, 1968.

Maxwell, Doug. *Canada Curls: The Illustrated History of Curling in Canada*. Whitecap Books, 2002.

Mazzeo, Karen S. *Fitness Through Aerobics, Step Training, Walking*. Brooks Cole, 2006.

McCord, Gary. *Golf for Dummies*. For Dummies, 2006.

Miller, Billy. *Ultimate Snowboarding*. Carlton Books, 2002.

Miller, Mark D., and Brian D. Cole. *Textbook of Arthroscopy*. WB Saunders Company, 2004.

Miller, Mark D., Daniel E. Cooper., and Jon J.P. Warner. *Review of Sports Medicine & Arthroscopy*. WB Saunders Company, 2002.

Nicklas, Barbara. *Endurance Exercise and Adipose Tissue*. CRC, 2001.

Nicklaus, Jack. *Golf My Way: The Instructional Classic, Revised and Updated*. Simon & Schuster, 2005.

Parent, Joseph. *Zen Golf: Mastering the Mental Game*. Doubleday, 2002.

Plante. Jacques. *Behind the Mask*. XYZ Publishing, 2003.

———. *Step by Step Hockey Goaltending: The Complete Illustrated Guide*. Studio 9 Books & Music, 2003.

Player, Gary. *The Golfer's Guide to the Meaning of Life: Lessons I've Learned from My Life on the Links*. Rodale Books, 2001.

Pound, Richard W. *Inside the Olympics: A Behind-the-Scenes Look at the Politics, the Scandals, and the Glory of the Games*. John Wiley & Sons, 2004.

Radcliffe, Paula. *Paula: My Story So Far*. Pocket Books, 2006.

Renner, Bill. *Kicking the Football*. Champaign, IL: Human Kinetics, 1997.

Sanderfoot, Alan. *What Color is Your Swimming Pool? A Homeowner's Guide to Troublefree Pool, Spa, & Hot Tub Maintenance*. Storey Publishing, 2003.

Schnakengerg, Robert. *Mia Hamm (Women Who Win)*. Chelsea House, 2000.

Scholz, Guy H., and Cheryl L. Bernard. *Between the Sheets: Creating Curling Champions*. Hillsboro Press, 2005.

Sherrow, Victoria. *Tennis (History of Sports)*. Lucent Books, 2002.

Shulman, Carole. *The Complete Book of Figure Skating*. Champaign, IL: Human Kinetics, 2002.

Shulman, Carole. *The Complete Book of Figure Skating*. Human Kinetics Publishers, 2001.

Starkey, Chad. *Athletic Training and Sports Medicine*. 4th ed. Jones and Bartlett Publishers, 2005.

Streeter, Michael. *Ice Skating (Sports Injuries: How to prevent, Diagnose & Treat)*. Mason Crest Publishers, 2004.

Tamminen, Terry. *The Ultimate Guide to Above-Ground Pools*. McGraw-Hill Professional, 2004.

U.S. Olympic Committee. *A Basic Guide to Speed Skating*. Griffin Publishing, 2001.

Valiante, Gio. *Fearless Golf: Conquering the Mental Game*. Doubleday, 2005.

Waitz, Grete and Gloria Averbuch. *On the Run*. Rodal Press, 2000.

Watts, Robert G. *Keep Your Eye on the Ball: Curve Balls, Knuckleballs, and Fallacies of Baseball*. New York: W.H. Freeman, 2000.

Weeks, Bob. *Curling for Dummies*. Toronto: CDG Books, Canada, Ltd., 2003.

Wegner, O., and Stephen Ferry. *Play Better Tennis in Two Hours*. International Marine/Rugged Mountain Press, 2004.

Woods, Tiger. *How I Play Golf*. Warner Books, 2001.

Zumerchik, John. *Newton on the Tee: A Good Walk Through the Science of Golf*. New York: Simon & Schuster, 2002.

## Periodicals

Adlington, Gregory S. "Proper Swing Technique and Biomechanics of Golf." *Clinics in Sports Medicine* 15:1, January 1, 1996, pp.9.

Ball, T.C., S.A. Headley, P.M. Vanderburgh, and J.C. Smith. "Periodic carbohydrate replacement during 50-min of high-intensity cycling improves subsequent sprint performance." *International Journal of Sports Nutrition*. 5:151-158, 1995.

Bartlett, Mark. "Tennis Racquet - Materials, Design, Evoultion and Testing." *Materials World* 8:15-16, June, 2000.

Below, P.R., R. Mora-Rodriguez, J. Gonzalez-Alonso, and E.F. Coyle. "Fluid and carbohydrate ingestion independently improve performance during 1-h of intense exercise." *Medicine and Science in Sports and Exercise*. 27:200-210, 1995.

Brancazio, Peter J. "The Science of Acrobatics." *Sportscience: Physical Laws and Optimum Performance*. New York: Simon & Schuster, 1984, 149-159.

Buskirk, E.R., and J. Mendez. "Sports Science and Body-Composition Analysis - Emphasis on Cell and Muscle Mass." *Medicine and Science in Sports and Exercise*. 16:6 584-593, 1984.

Chigbo, Okey. "The Go-To-Guy, Richard Pound." *CA Magazine* August, 2000.

Chilineck, Philip D. "Effect of Physical Activity on Bone Mineral Density Assessed by Limb Dominance Across the Lifespan." *American Journal of Human Biology* 12:633-637, July 25, 2000.

Committee on Sports Medicine and Fitness. "Medical Concerns in the Female Athlete." *Pediatrics* 106:610-613, September, 2000.

Duma, Bob. "Report: Etching Caused by Water Chemistry." *Aquatics International* 16:10-12, November 1, 2004.

Ellick, Adam B. "Emil Zatopek 1922-2000." *Running Times* March 2001.

Ganguli, Ishani. "Luge and the Lab." *The Scientist* February 28, 2006.

Groslambert, A. "Effects of Autogenic and Imagery Training on the Shooting Performance in Biathlon." *Research Quarterly for Exercise and Sport* 74:337-342, September 1, 2003.

Jackson, Harry. "Ice Skating Injuries: What to Expect." *St. Louis Post-Dispatch* January 20, 2006.

Mason, Francene. "High Altitude Illness: Avoiding the Perils of the Peaks." *AMAA Journal* 18:13-15, June 22, 2005.

## Websites

*Agency for Toxic Substances and Disease Registry (ATSDR).* "Agency for Toxic Substances and Disease Registry (ATSDR)." <http://www.atsdr.cdc.gov> (accessed on May 15, 2006.)

*AIDS Research Institute (ARI).* "AIDS Research Institute (ARI)." <http://ari.ucsf.edu> (accessed on May 15, 2006.)

*American Academy of Orthopaedic Surgeons.* "Arthroscopy." 2000. <http://orthoinfo.aaos.org/brochure/thr_report.cfm?Thread_ID=33&top> (accessed on January 22, 2006.)

*American Association for the Advancement of Science (AAAS).* "American Association for the Advancement of Science (AAAS)." <http://www.aaas.org> (accessed on May 15, 2006.)

*American College of Cardiology.* "American College of Cardiology." <http://www.acc.org> (accessed on May 15, 2006.)

*American Heart Association.* "American Heart Association." <http://www.amhrt.org> (accessed on May 15, 2006.)

*American Institute of Physics (AIP).* "American Institute of Physics (AIP)." <http://www.aip.org/aip/> (accessed on May 15, 2006.)

*American Journal of Preventive Medicine.* "American Journal of Preventive Medicine." <http://www.elsevier.com/locate/amepre> (accessed on May 15, 2006.)

*Annual Review of Public Health.* "Annual Review of Public Health." <http://arjournals.annualreviews.org/loi/publhealth> (accessed on May 15, 2006.)

*BBC Sport.* "Marathon Agony for Radcliffe." August 22, 2004. <http://news.bbc.co.uk/sport1/hi/olympics_2004/athletics/3589138.stm> (accessed on January 19, 2006.)

*BBC Sport.* "Rider's legends: Lasse Viren." September 19, 2000. <http://news.bbc.co.uk/sport1/hi/olympics2000/fans_guide/859597.stm> (accessed on February 4, 2006.)

*Brian Beckman, Miata.net, Eunos Communications LLC.* "Physics of Racing Series." <http://www.miata.net/sport/Physics/> (accessed on May 11, 2006.)

*British Medical Journal.* "British Medical Journal." <http://bmj.bmjjournals.com> (accessed on May 15, 2006.)

*Bryan Yager, NASA Advanced Supercomputing Division, National Space and Aeronautics Administration.* "Racing Physics." <http://www.nas.nasa.gov/About/Education/Racecar/physics.html> (accessed on May 11, 2006.)

*BUPA.* "Beta 2 Agonists." July, 2001. <http:www.bupa.co.uk/health_information/html/medicine/beta2_agonists> (accessed on January 18, 2006.)

*CBC.* "Luge History." 2006. <http://www.cbc.ca/olympics/sports/luge/history.shtml> (accessed on February 1, 2006.)

*CDC (Centers for Disease Control and Prevention).* "CDCSite Index A-Z." <http://www.cdc.gov/az.do> (accessed on May 15, 2006.)

*CEWEC Clinic Travel Medicine Center.* "Altitude Illness." May, 2005. <http://www.ciwec-clinic.com/altitude/> (accessed on January 21, 2006.)

*Cliff Richard Tennis.* "Planet Tennis: The History of Tennis." 2000. <http://www.cliffrichardtennis.org/planet_tennis/history.htm> (accessed on February 2, 2006.)

*Emedicine.* "Altitude Illness - Cerebral Syndromes." October 6, 2004. <http://www.emedicine.com/emerg/topic22.htm> (accessed on January 20, 2006.)

*Hazardous Substances & Public Health.* "Hazardous Substances & Public Health." <http://www.atsdr.cdc.gov/HEC/HSPH/hsphhome.html> (accessed on May 15, 2006.)

*HealthAtoZ.* "Aerobic Exercise." June 2005. <http://atoz.iqhealth.com/Atoz/fitness/cardiocraze/aroexcer.html> (accessed on January 21, 2006.)

*Hockey Fans.* "Jacques Plante." <http://www.hockey-fans.com/players/plante.php> (accessed on February 3, 2006.)

*How Stuff Works.* "How Swimming Pools Work." <http://home.howstuffworks.com/swimming-pool.htm> (accessed on February 7, 2006.)

*International Society for Infectious Diseases.* "International Society for Infectious Diseases." <http://www.isid.org> (accessed on May 15, 2006.)

*Internet Society for Sport Science.* "Adipose Tissue." July 10, 1998. <http://www.sportsci.org/encyc/adipose/adipose.html> (accessed on January 20, 2006.)

*Maine Women's Hall of Fame.* "Joan Benoit Samuelson." <http://www.uma.edu/libraries/MWHOF_Website/alibjsamuelson.html> (accessed on February 5, 2006.)

*Morbidity and Mortality Weekly Report.* "Morbidity and Mortality Weekly Report." <http://www.cdc.gov/mmwr> (accessed on May 15, 2006.)

*National Academies.* "Health & Medicine at the National Academies." <http://www.nationalacademies.org/health/> (accessed on May 15, 2006.)

*National Human Genome Research Institute (NHGRI).* "National Human Genome Research Institute (NHGRI)." <http://www.nhgri.nih.gov> (accessed on May 15, 2006.)

*National Institute of Environmental Health Sciences (NIEHS).* "National Institute of Environmental Health

Sciences (NIEHS)." <http://www.niehs.nih.gov> (accessed on May 15, 2006.)

*National Institutes of Allergy and Infectious Diseases, Division of AIDS.* "National Institutes of Allergy and Infectious Diseases, Division of AIDS." <http://www.niaid.nih.gov/daids/default.htm> (accessed on May 15, 2006.)

*National Institutes of Health.* "National Institutes of Health." <http://www.nih.gov> (accessed on May 15, 2006.)

*National Library of Medicine.* "Environmental Health and Toxicology." <http://sis.nlm.nih.gov/enviro.html> (accessed on May 15, 2006.)

*National Medical Society.* "Library of the National Medical Society." <http://www.medical-library.org/> (accessed on May 15, 2006.)

*National Public Health Institute.* "National Public Health Institute." <http://www.ktl.fi/portal/english> (accessed on May 15, 2006.)

*National Toxicology Program.* "National Toxicology Program." <http://ntp-server.niehs.nih.gov> (accessed on May 15, 2006.)

*Nation's Health.* "Nation's Health." <http://www.apha.org/tnh/> (accessed on May 15, 2006.)

*Nature.* "Nature." <http://www.nature.com> (accessed on May 15, 2006.)

*Net Doctor.* "Arthroscopy." September 15, 2005. <http://www.netdoctor.co.uk/health_advice/examinations/arthroscopy.htm> (accessed on January 22, 2006.)

*NIAAA - National Institute on Alcohol Abuse and Alcoholism.* "NIAAA - National Institute on Alcohol Abuse and Alcoholism." <http://www.niaaa.nih.gov> (accessed on May 15, 2006.)

*NIBIB - National Institute of Biomedical Imaging and Bioengineering.* "NIBIB - National Institute of Biomedical Imaging and Bioengineering." <http://www.nibib1.nih.gov> (accessed on May 15, 2006.)

*NIDA - National Institute on Drug Abuse.* "NIDA - National Institute on Drug Abuse." <http://www.nida.nih.gov> (accessed on May 15, 2006.)

*NIGMS - National Institute of General Medical Sciences.* "NIGMS - National Institute of General Medical Sciences." <http://www.nigms.nih.gov> (accessed on May 15, 2006.)

*NIMH - National Institute of Mental Health.* "NIMH - National Institute of Mental Health." <http://www.nimh.nih.gov> (accessed on May 15, 2006.)

*NINDS - National Institute of Neurological Disorders and Stroke.* "NINDS - National Institute of Neurological Disorders and Stroke." <http://www.ninds.nih.gov> (accessed on May 15, 2006.)

*Office of Public Health and Science.* "Office of Public Health and Science." <http://phs.os.dhhs.gov/ophs> (accessed on May 15, 2006.)

*Office of Research on Women's Health.* "Office of Research on Women's Health." <http://www4.od.nih.gov/orwh> (accessed on May 15, 2006.)

*Pharma-Lexicon International.* "MediLexicon." <http://www.medilexicon.com/> (accessed on May 15, 2006.)

*Princeton University.* "Outdoor Action Guide to High Altitude: Acclimatization and Illnesses." July 7, 1999. <http://www.princeton.edu/~oa/safety/altitude.html> (accessed on January 21, 2006.)

*Running Past.* "Profiles: Emil Zatopek." <http://www.runningpast.com/emil_zatopek.htm> (accessed on February 4, 2006.)

*Science Magazine.* "Science Magazine." <http://www.sciencemag.org> (accessed on May 15, 2006.)

*Sk8stuff.* "An Introduction to Figure Skating." February 24, 2004. <http://www.sk8stuff.com/f_basic_ref/intro_to_figure_skating.htm> (accessed on January 28, 2006.)

*Spine Universe.* "The Truth about Cortisone Shots." October 8, 2005. <http://www.spineuniverse.com/displayarticle.php/article1349.html> (accessed on January 22, 2006.)

*Springboard4Health.* "Adipose Tissue aka Body Fat." 2004. <http://www.springboard4health.com/notebook/health_adipose.html> (accessed on January 19, 2006.)

*Substance Abuse & Mental Health Services Administration (SAMHSA).* "Substance Abuse & Mental Health Services Administration (SAMHSA)." <http://www.samhsa.gov/index.aspx> (accessed on May 15, 2006.)

*Texas Heart Institute.* "Beta-Blockers." August, 2005. <http://www.tmc.edu/thi/betameds.html> (accessed on January 18, 2006.)

*United States Biathlon Association.* "About Biathlon." <http:www.usbiathlon.org/> (accessed on January 26, 2006.)

*Wellcome Library for the History and Understanding of Medicine.* "The guide to history of medicine resources on the Internet." <http://medhist.ac.uk/> (accessed on May 15, 2006.)

*Womens Soccer World.* "Hamm, Mia." May 23, 1999. <http://www.womensoccer.com/biogs/hamm.html> (accessed on January 30, 2006.)

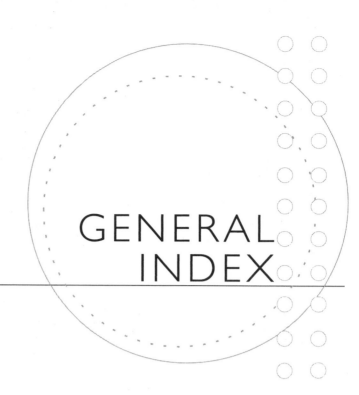

# GENERAL INDEX

Bolded page numbers refer to the main entry on the subject. Page numbers in italics refer to illustrations.

## A

AAA (American Arbitration Association), 1:23–24

AAFC (All-American Football Conference), 1:108, 277, 2:497

AAU (Amateur Athletic Union), 2:811

ABA (American Basketball Association), 2:466

Abbott, Senda Berenson, 1:**1–2**, 70, 2:488

ABC (American Broadcasting Company), 2:462

Abdominal muscles, 2:538, 762

Abdominal pain, exercise-related transient, 2:588–589

Abdul-Jabbar, Kareem, 1:**2–4**, *4*, 71
  Adidas shoes, 1:185
  Wooden, John Robert, 2:795

Abrasions, cuts, lacerations, 1:**4–6**, *5*
  aging, 1:19
  boxing, 1:104
  road rash, 2:573

Abscess, 1:402

Acceleration
  gymnastics landing force, 1:332–333
  motorcycle, 2:478
  tackling techniques, 1:282–283

Acclimatization, 1:**6–7**, *7*, 223
  altitude illness, 1:22
  cold weather, 1:224
  erythropoietin, 1:7, 2:655
  exercise physiology, 2:535
  heat, 1:6–7, 224, 241, 2:746, 769

high altitude, 1:6–7, 224, 2:523, 596
hydration, 1:235, 378
Ironman competitions, 1:409
Nordic skiing, 2:636
soccer, 2:654–655
tennis, 2:723
ventilatory, 1:366

Accredited testing facilities, 1:232

Acetaminophen, 2:517

Acetazolamide, 1:22, 203

Acetylsalicylic acid, 1:209, 2:503–504

Achilles (Greek warrior), 1:8

Achilles tendon injuries, 2:651–652, 717

Achilles tendon rupture, 1:**7–9**, 96, 451, 2:717
  American football, 1:280
  ankle injuries from, 1:31
  basketball injuries, 1:73
  foot injuries from, 1:152
  from running, 2:593–594

Achilles tendonitis, 1:*9*, **9–10**, 451, 2:593–594, 717

ACL injuries, 1:**10–12**, *12*, 96–97
  basketball, 1:74
  cycling, 1:178
  in female athletes, 1:10–12, 74, 96–97, 257, 297, 431
  figure skating, 1:268, 269
  football (American), 1:280, 281–282
  gymnastics, 1:332
  hamstring imbalance in, 1:341, 430, 2:557
  knee braces for, 2:514
  soccer, 2:652
  tendonitis, 1:269, 280

Acquired immunity, 1:400

Acromegaly, 1:325

Acromioclavicular joint, 2:619, 621, 653

ACTH (Adrenocorticotropin), 1:143, 372

Acting career, 1:107

Activation level, 2:674

Active hyperemia, 2:637

Active ingredients, 1:**12–13**

Active recovery, 2:575

Active stress, 1:7

Acupressure, 2:459

Acupuncture, 1:**13–14**, *14*
  achilles tendonitis, 1:10
  herniated disks, 1:363

Adams, Victoria, 1:79

Adaptogens, 1:143–144

Addiction, 2:556, 688

Adenosine, 1:112

Adenosine triphosphate (ATP)
  carbohydrate stores, 1:126, 127, 128–129
  cramps, 1:159
  creatine supplements, 1:160, 161
  fat oxidation, 1:253
  fluid replacement, 1:134
  free fatty acids, 1:290–291
  glycerol, 1:307
  glycogen, 1:308
  lactic acid, 1:437–438
  low-carbohydrate diet, 1:192
  oxygen, 2:523
  phosphocreatine, 2:532–533
  role of, 2:531–532
  in skeletal muscle, 2:627, 628
  slow twitch *vs.* fast twitch fibers, 2:480–481

ADH (Antidiuretic hormone), 1:202–203, 2:656, 726

American Tennis Association (ATA), 1:303

America's Cup, 1:405, 2:603

AMF-Voit, 1:414

Amino acid supplements, 1:**24–25**

Amino acids, 1:**25–26**
deconstruction of, 2:555
dehydration, 2:554
essential, 1:24–25
in fasting, 2:628
glutamine supplements, 1:306
in strength training, 2:691–692

Aminoglycosides, 1:212

Ampex Corporation, 1:304

Amphetamines
doping tests, 1:205
for sleep deprivation, 2:641
stimulant action of, 2:688
Tour de France use, 1:183

Amputee disability classification, 1:198, 2:526

Anabolic prohormones, 1:**26–27,** 146–147

Anabolic steroids, 1:**27–29,** *28*
American football use, 2:497
CASPER, 1:146–147
doping tests, 1:205, 2:519–520
East German athletes, 1:219
Ender, Cornelia, 1:219
Francis, Charlie, 1:287–288
Johnson, Ben, 1:*28,* 28–29, 287–288, 520, 2:737
protein synthesis, 2:484
roid rage, 1:29, 2:556
sexual disorders from, 2:612
weightlifting use, 1:27–28, 2:784

Anabolism, 1:26, 2:484

Anaerobic exercise
basketball, 1:78
ice hockey, 2:715
middle-distance races, 2:596
recovery from, 1:239–240
resistance training, 2:569
short, high intensity, 2:615
tennis, 2:723
triathlon, 2:742
volleyball, 2:760
*See also* Plyometrics

Anaerobic system
alactic, 1:128, 129
canoeing and kayaking, 1:123–124
endurance, 1:220, 221
fluid replacement, 1:134
football (American), 1:278
freestyle skiing, 2:634
intermittent exercise, 1:238
jump rope training, 1:420
lactic, 1:123–124, 220, 309
phosphocreatine, 2:532–533
wrestling, 2:801

Analgesics, 1:209, 401, 2:549, 696

Anaphylactic reaction, 1:401–402

Andrews, James R., 1:**29–30**

Androgen insensitivity syndrome (AIS), 2:612–613, *613*

Androstenedione, 1:27, 146, 2:744

Anemia, 1:228

Angiotensin, 1:380–381

Angular momentum, 1:279, 334, 2:660

Ankle
anatomy and physiology, 1:**30–31,** 274, 450
popping and cracking noises, 1:415

Ankle braces, 1:11, 31

Ankle fractures, 2:645

Ankle injuries, 1:30–31
cheerleading, 1:141
gymnastics, 1:331, 332
incidence, 2:485
snowboarding, 2:645

Ankle sprains, 1:30–31, **31–33,** *32*
basketball, 1:72–73
football (American), 1:280
RICE for, 2:572
soccer, 2:651

Anne (Princess), 2:612

Anorexia nervosa, 1:142, 212–213, 2:556, 781

Anterior cruciate ligament anatomy, 1:430

Anterior cruciate ligament injuries. *See* ACL injuries

Anti-depressants, 2:612

Anti-Doping Agreement. *See* International Anti-Doping Agreement

Anti-inflammatory medications, 1:401, 2:549

Antibiotics
ear, 1:211–212
eyedrop, 1:247
phytochemical, 2:537

Antidiuretic hormone (ADH), 1:202–203, 2:656, 726

Antifungal agents, 1:43–44

Antigens, 1:400

Antihistamines, 1:402, 2:490

Antioxidants, 1:**33–34,** 83
as cardioprotection, 1:132
phytochemical, 2:537
in sport nutrition, 2:669
*See also* Free radicals

APFA (American Professional Football Association), 2:496

Apnea
competitive, 1:289
sleep, 2:640

Appetite suppressants, 1:193

Aquapacer, 2:466–467

Arbitration
American Arbitration Association, 1:23–24
Court of Arbitration for Sports, 1:24, 157–158

Archery, 1:**35–36,** *36*

Archimedes principle, 1:95

Ariel, Gideon, 2:752

Arledge, Roone, 2:462

Arm exercises, 1:105

Arm injuries, 1:332

Armstrong, Lance, 1:**36–39,** *38, 39, 175*
blood-doping investigation, 1:91
femur size, 1:97
physiological tests of, 1:*182,* 182–183
popularity in France, 1:181
slow twitch fibers, 1:39, 182, 220
Tour de France victories, 1:173

Army football team, 2:576

Around Oahu Bike Race, 1:149–150, 408

Arrhythmia, 1:132–133, 188

Arrows, 1:35

Arteries, 1:136

Arthritis, 1:415

Arthroscopy, 1:**40–41,** *41,* 2:677–678
development of, 1:29–30
osteoarthritis, 2:517
osteochondritis dissecans, 2:518
Samuelson, Joan Benoit, 1:81

Articular cartilage. *See* Cartilage

Artificial legs, 2:553

Artificial limbs. *See* Prosthetics

Artificial turf, 1:250, 262, 2:647

Artistic gymnastics, 1:328

Ascorbic acid. *See* Vitamin C

ASDA (Australian Sports Drug Agency), 1:46–47

Asghar, Ibrahim, 2:*783*

Ashe, Arthur, 2:721

Aspirin, 1:209, 2:503–504, 537, 624

Association for Intercollegiate Athletics for Women (AIAW), 2:495–496

Astaphan, Jamie, 1:288

Asthma
exercise-induced, 1:**41–42,** *42*
exercise-induced bronchospasm in, 1:106
medications, 1:82, 2:549, 570, 696, 725
sports participation, 2:680–681

AstroTurf, 1:250

ATA (American Tennis Association), 1:303

Athens Paralympics, 2:527, 531

Athlete Location Form, 1:42–43

Athlete's foot, 1:43–44

Athletic injuries. *See* Sports injuries

Athletic performance
aging, 1:**20–21**
defined, 2:506, 549
genetic prediction of, 1:**300–301,** *301*
glycogen and, 1:308

gene, 1:208, 302–303, 2:486, 799
Griffith-Joyner, Delorez Florence, 1:321
in ice hockey, 2:547
injections of, 1:401
International Anti-Doping Agreement, 1:**403**
International Intergovernmental Consultative Group on Anti-Doping in Sport, 1:405–406
penalties, 2:521
prohibited substances, 2:550–552, *552*, 696, 724–725, 798, 799
restricted substances, 2:**569–570,** 695–696
USADA, 2:747–748
USADA research on, 2:747
*See also* Erythropoietin; Therapeutic use exemption; specific drugs

Doping control officer, 1:207

Doping control station, 2:521

Doping tests, 1:**205–208,** *207, 228*
anabolic steroids, 1:205, 2:519–520
arbitration in, 1:24
Athlete Location Form for, 1:42–43
Australian Sports Drug Agency, 1:46–47
Change of Plan Form, 1:139
competition, 1:206
Court of Arbitration for Sports, 1:157–158
cycling, 1:174–175
for erythropoietin, 1:90–91
event testing, 1:**231–233**
history, 2:797
in-competition, 2:519
Lund, Zach, litigation, 1:24
nandrolone, 2:489, 520–521
out-of-competition, 1:206–207, 2:**519–521,** 570, 747
Paralympics, 2:526–527
professional sports associations, 2:520, 521
random, 2:520
standards, 2:520–521
testosterone, 2:724
*See also* World Anti-Doping Agency

Dose and dosage, drug, 1:**208–209**

Doubleday, Abner, 1:61

Down force, 1:47, 49, 285, 2:491

Down syndrome, 2:665

Downhill skiing, 1:349, 442, 2:632–633
*See also* Alpine skiing

Downswing, 1:317

Dr. Dunkenstein. *See* Griffith, Darrell

Drafting
cycling, 1:37–38, 173–174
NASCAR auto racing, 2:492

Drag
aerodynamics of, 1:47
bobsled, 1:93
canoe and kayak, 1:122
cycling, 1:183
discus, 1:201

Formula 1 auto racing, 1:285
parachute, 2:638
resistance training, 2:569, 602
rowing hydrodynamics, 2:581
sailboat, 2:607
swim suit, 1:88, 249
swimming, 2:705–706

Drag racing, 1:50, 154, 2:478

Dragneva, Izabela, 2:*552*

Dragon boat racing, 1:123, 125

Drake, Francis, 1:98

Drake, Jim, 2:788

Draw stroke, 1:124

"Dream team," 1:72, 417

Dressage, 1:229

Drive shots, cricket, 1:166

Driver's championship, 1:49

Dropkick, rugby, 2:**585–587,** *586*

Drug testing. *See* Doping tests

Drugs
active ingredients of, 1:**12–13**
asthma, 2:549, 570, 696, 725
*vs.* dietary supplements, 1:196
dose and dosage, 1:**208–209**
effectiveness of, 1:209
over-the-counter, 1:208–209
prescription, 2:527, **548–549**
restricted use of, 2:569–570
sexual disorders from, 2:612
sleep disturbances from, 2:640
therapeutic use exemption, 2:527, 549, 570
therapeutic use exemption for, 2:696, 724–725
tolerance to, 1:209
*See also* Doping; specific drugs

Dry land training
canoe and kayak, 1:124
ice hockey, 1:396, 2:715
swimming, 2:703

Drysuits, 2:784

DSHEA. *See* Dietary Supplement Health and Education Act

Dual moguls, 2:633

Dubin Inquiry, 1:287–288

Dueling swords, 1:257

Dundee, Angelo, 1:104

Dunk shot. *See* Slam dunk

Dunkenstein, Dr. *See* Griffith, Darrell

Dynamic stretching, 2:805

# E

Ear drops, 1:**211–212**

Ear infections, 1:211–212

Ear wax, 1:212

Earnhardt, Dale, 2:491

East German athletes, 1:219

Eastern healing therapies, 1:**13–14,** *14*

Eating disorders, 1:**212–213,** *213*
cheerleaders, 1:142

compulsive exercise with, 1:152
in female athletic triad, 1:152, 298, 2:613
gymnastics, 1:212, *213*, 329–330, 428, 2:556
sports participation with, 2:680
weight loss, 2:781
in young athletes, 2:809

ECA stack, 2:624

Eccentric muscle contractions, 1:189, 2:544

Eccrine gland sweat secretion, 1:**213–214**

Echinacea, 1:361

ECO Challenge, 1:246

Ectomorphs, 1:94, 2:464

Eczema, 2:733

Eddy resistance, 2:705–706

Edema
cerebral, 1:22
pulmonary, 1:22, **365–366,** *366*

Education, sports medicine, 2:**681–682,** *682*

Eformoterol, 1:82

Eggs, 1:25

Einhoven, William, 1:353

Elastic muscle strength, 2:689, 690

Elbow
anatomy and physiology, 1:**214–216,** *216*
golfer's, 1:218, 314
Little Leaguer, 1:217
range of motion, 2:563
tennis, 1:218, 314

Elbow fractures, 1:217

Elbow injuries, 1:**216–218,** *217*
baseball, 1:66–68
contact sports, 1:216
football (American), 1:281
golf, 1:314
gymnastics, 1:331
osteochondritis dissecans, 2:517
from strength sports, 1:216
from striking motions, 1:216
tendinitis, 2:717
from throwing technique, 1:215
in young athletes, 2:809
*See also* Ulnar collateral ligament (UCL) injuries

Electrocardiograms, 1:*353*, 353–354, 2:738

Electroencephalography, 1:86

Electrolyte balance/imbalance
heat cramps, 1:356
sports drinks for, 1:111
water, 2:770

Electrolyte replacement, 1:271, 356
*See also* Fluid replacement

Electromyelography, 1:86

Electronic timing, 2:707, 735

*Eleutherococcus senticosus*, 2:522

Elevation. *See* RICE

Keel, 2:605, 607

*Keratoconjunctivitis sicca*, 1:246

Kersee, Bob, 1:320–321, 418

Kersee, Jackie Joyner. *See* Joyner-Kersee, Jackie

Ketoacidosis, 2:532

Kick
field goal, 1:279–280
scissor, 1:367–368

Kick wax, 2:630, 631, 635

Kickboxing, cardio-, 1:129, 131

Kidney function. *See* Renal function

Kidney stones, 1:113–114

Killy, Jean-Claude, 1:349

Kilocalories, 1:116, 117–118

Kinesiology, 2:681

Kinesthetic senses, 1:58

Kinetic energy
golf swing, 1:316
linear, 1:279–280

Kittinger, Joseph, 2:638

Klein, Gary Gordon, 1:**428**

Klein Bike Company, 1:428

Klister wax, 2:631, 635

Klochvova, Yona, 2:700

Knee
anatomy and physiology, 1:10,
**428–430**, *429*, 433, 449–450
genetic and non-genetic conditions
of, 1:**430–432**
popping and cracking noises, 1:415
structural imbalances, 1:431, 433

Knee braces, 2:514

Knee injuries, 1:*432*, **432–434**, *433*
arthroscopy, 1:29–30
basketball, 1:73–74
cartilage, 1:415
cheerleading, 1:141
cycling, 1:178
in female athletes, 1:297
figure skating, 1:268
football (American), 1:278, 281–282
gymnastics, 1:331
hyperextension, 1:331, 434, 2:563
ice hockey, 1:392
incidence, 2:485
jumper's knee, 1:73–74, 433, 2:558,
717
osteoarthritis, 2:516
osteochondritis dissecans, 2:517,
518
overuse, 1:433
soccer, 2:652
sprains, 2:684
water skiing, 2:775
*See also* ACL injuries

Knee lifts, hurdles, 2:592

Knee prosthetics, 2:553

Knee replacement, 2:516

Kneeboarding, 1:245–246, 2:766, 774

Knight, Phil, 1:98

Knockouts, 1:101

Knuckles, 1:415

Kodokan judo. *See* Judo

Korbut, Olga, 1:328

Korda, Petr, 2:489

Kostadinova, Stefka, 1:368

Kumite, 1:426

Kuzenkiova, Olga, 1:*339*

Kwan, Michelle, 1:269

## L

Lacerations. *See* Abrasions, cuts,
lacerations

Lacrosse, 1:**435–437**, *436*, *437*
box, 1:396, 436–437
Brown, James Nathaniel, 1:106–107
elbow injuries from, 1:216
field, 1:435–436

Lactate. *See* Lactic acid

Lactic acid
athletic performance, 1:**437–438**
buildup, 1:39, 114, 183
cramps from, 1:160
energy production, 1:128, 129,
437–438
glycogen, 1:438
intermittent exercise for, 1:238
liver function, 1:443

Lactic anaerobic system, 1:123–124,
220, 309

Ladder drills, 2:723

Ladies Professional Golf Association
(LPGA), 1:304, 2:662–663

Landers, Pete, 2:659

Landing forces
gymnastics, 1:331, **332–334**, *333*,
335
sky diving, 2:639

Landy, John, 1:60, 2:596

Laryngitis, 2:750

Lateral epicondyle tendon, 1:215

Lateral epicondylitis, 1:218, 314, 2:717

Lateral movements, 2:694, 712

Lauterbur, Paul Christian, 1:**438–439**

Law of inertia, 1:282, 2:533

Laws of motion, 1:282–283, 2:533

Laxatives, 1:213

Layden, Elmer, 2:576

Lazutina, Larissa, 1:157

LDL. *See* Low density lipoproteins

Lean muscle mass, 1:94, 2:734, 779, 780

Leaps
figure skating, 1:*266*, **266–267**
*See also* Jumping

Learning disabilities, 2:665

Leavitt, J. Noxon, 1:**439**

Ledley, Robert Steven, 1:**439–440**

"Leg before wicket," 1:164, 166

Leg exercises
ice hockey, 1:396
shot put, 2:618
swimming, 2:707
synchronized swimming, 2:709
treadmill, 2:738–740
vertical jump, 2:753
water skiing, 2:775–776

Leg injuries
cycling, 1:178
incidence, 2:485
lower leg, 1:**450–452**, *451*, 2:485,
566, 645, 651, 775
upper leg, 2:**728–729**
*See also* Foot injuries;
Knee injuries

Legs
artificial, 2:553
bow, 2:516
lower leg anatomy, 1:449–450, *450*
strength training, 1:105, 179
unequal length of, 2:552, 566, 592
upper leg anatomy, 2:728

Lemond, Greg, 1:38, 173, 440

Lennon, Boone, 1:**440**

Lens, contact, 1:**154–155**

Leslie, Lisa Deshaun, 1:77, **440–442**

Lettner, Rudolph, 1:**442**

Leucine, 2:484

Leukemia, 1:400

Leukocytes. *See* White blood cells

Leukotriene, 1:157

Level I injuries, 2:678

Level II injuries, 2:678

Level III injuries, 2:678

Lewis, Carl, 2:749

LH (Luteinizing hormone), 2:743

"The Libero," 2:759

Licorice, 1:362

Lidocaine, 1:13

Life expectancy, 1:444

Life, quality of, 1:444

Lifestyle
juvenile obesity, 1:422–423
recreational sports, 2:563

Lift
automobile racing, 1:47
discus, 1:201
golf ball, 1:313
sailboat, 2:606

Lifting
figure skating, 1:268
injuries from, 1:446
power, 2:665, 783

Ligament injuries
from artificial turf, 1:250
gymnastics, 1:331
popping and cracking noises from,
1:415
wrist, 2:802
*See also* ACL injuries; Sprains

Triglycerides
in adipose tissue, 1:15–16, 95
fat oxidation, 1:253
liver function, 1:442–443

Triiodothyronine (T3), 1:372

Trillant, Andrew, 1:29

Triple axel, 1:266–267, 410

Triple jump, 2:737, *744*, **744–745**

Triple lutz, 1:454

Triplett, Norman, 2:472

Trochanteris bursitis, 1:368

Tubing, exercise, 1:69

Turf, artificial, 1:250, 262, 2:647

Turf toe, 1:250

The Turners, 1:412

Turns, swimming, 2:706

Turnverein, 1:412

Twain, Mark, 2:698

12 Rules of the Marquees, 1:101

24-second clock rule, 1:83–84, 2:466

Twitches, muscle, 2:479

Two-a-day practice sessions,
2:**745–746**

Tympanic thermometers, 1:155

Type 1 diabetes, 2:510

Type 2 diabetes, 1:422, 2:511

Type A personality, 2:674–675, 693

Type B personality, 2:674–675

Type I fibers. *See* Slow twitch fibers

Type II fibers. *See* Fast twitch fibers

# U

U. S. Anti-Doping Agency (USADA),
2:727, **747–748**

UCL injuries. *See* Ulnar collateral ligament (UCL) injuries

UCLA Bruins, 2:795–796

UEFA (Union of European Football
Associations), 1:233, 405, 2:647

Ulanov, Alexei, 1:*265*

Ulnar bone, 1:214

Ulnar collateral ligament anatomy,
1:96, 215

Ulnar collateral ligament (UCL) injuries, 1:217
arthroscopy, 2:677
baseball, 1:67, 68
football (American), 1:280

Ulnar nerve, 1:215

Ulnohumeral joint, 1:214, 215

Ultimate Frisbee, 1:293

Ultra marathon running, 1:246

Ultrasound, 1:10, 363, 2:539

Ultraviolet (UV) rays, 1:149

UNESCO (United Nations Education,
Science and Cultural Organization),
1:406

Unexplained performance syndrome,
2:556

Union Internationale de Pentathlon
Modern et Biathlon, 1:84

Union of European Football Associations (UEFA), 1:233, 405, 2:647

United Nations Education, Science
and Cultural Organization
(UNESCO), 1:406

United States Anti-Doping Agency
(USADA), 2:729, **747–748,** 799

United States Department of Agriculture (USDA), 2:504–505, 506–507

United States Golf Association, 1:310,
312

United States Lawn Tennis Association (USLTA), 1:303

United States Olympic Committee
(USOC), 1:24, 2:**748–749**

United States Postal Service Pro
Cycling Team (USPSPCT), 1:37–38

United States Track and Field Association (USTAF)
hydration guidelines, 1:379
marathons, 2:791
therapeutic use exemptions, 2:696

United States Volley Ball Association
(USVBA), 2:758

Universal line machines, 2:752

University sports. *See* Intercollegiate
sports

University of Texas, Human Performance Laboratory, 1:182

Unsaturated fats, 1:252, 254

Upper leg injuries, 2:**728–729**

Upper respiratory tract infections,
2:**749–750**

Uppercut, 1:102, 130–131

Urine color, 2:726, 746

Urine production, 1:202–203

USA Table Tennis Association
(USATTA), 2:711

USA Volleyball, 2:758

USADA (U. S. Anti-Doping Agency),
2:727, **747–748,** 799

USDA (United States Department of
Agriculture), 1:118, 2:504–505,
506–507

USLTA (United States Lawn Tennis
Association), 1:303

USOC (United States Olympic Committee), 1:24, 2:**748–749**

USTAF (United States Track and Field
Association), 1:379, 2:696, 791

# V

Vaccination, 1:400

Variable resistance exercise,
2:**751–752**

Variable weight diving, 1:290

Vasicinone, 2:624

Vasoconstriction, 2:727

Vasodilation, 2:727, 807

Vasodilators, 1:381

Vault, pole. *See* Pole vault

Vaulting, gymnastics, 1:**334–335**, *335*,
412

Vegas line, 2:497

Velcro, 1:186

Velocio, 1:172

Velocity
banks and curves, 2:533–534
tackling techniques, 1:282–283

Velodrome, 1:173, 177

Ventilatory acclimatization, 1:366

Ventricular fibrillation, 1:132

Venture (Aerodynamics), 1:48

Vertebrae alignment, 1:144–146

Vertical jump, 2:**752–753**

Vesicles, 1:88

Vestibular system, 1:58

Viagra, 2:612

Viatu, Casey, 1:416

Videotape recorders, 1:304

Villeneuve, Giles, 1:50

Viren, Lasse, 1:89, 2:**753–754**, *754*

Vision-impaired disability classification, 1:198, 2:526

Vision loss, 2:680

VISTA conferences, 2:526

Visualization, 2:**754–755**
biofeedback, 1:87
bowling, 1:100
shooting, 2:615
sport psychology, 2:673–674

Vitamin A, 1:33, 83

Vitamin A deficiency, 2:458

Vitamin B-complex, 1:**53–54,** 2:669

Vitamin B-complex deficiency, 1:54,
2:458

Vitamin B1, 1:53

Vitamin B2, 1:53

Vitamin B3, 1:53

Vitamin B6, 1:53, 197, 2:744

Vitamin B9, 1:54

Vitamin B12, 1:53

Vitamin C, 1:33, 132, 2:**755–756**

Vitamin C deficiency, 1:196, 2:458, 756,
777

Vitamin D
bone development, 1:98, 323, 2:518
calcium with, 1:113, 2:468
cortisone injections, 1:157
glucocorticoids, 1:305
phosphates, 2:532
in sport nutrition, 2:669
stress fractures, 2:566

# X

X Games, 2:625, 766
X rays, 2:677
Xiang, Liu, 2:*591*

# Y

Yacht racing, 1:405, 2:603
Yams, wild, 2:**787–788,** *788*
Yana, Tie, 2:*712*
Yellow dock, 1:362
YMCA (Young Men's Christian Association), 2:487
Yo-yo dieting, 1:193
Yoga, 2:**805–806,** *806*
    cycling, 1:174
    flexibility from, 2:695
    low-impact cardiovascular exercise, 1:448
    for piriformis syndrome, 2:539
    resistance training, 2:568
Yogurt, 1:197
Yohimbine, 2:**806–807**
Young, Steve, 2:767

Young athletes
    contact sports for, 2:812
    defined, 2:808, 809
    diet for, 2:811
    eating disorders in, 2:809
    foot stress fractures in, 2:694
    football-related concussion, 1:20
    medical conditions of, 2:679
    motivational techniques, 2:809
    nutrition for, 2:507
    Osgood-Schlatter disease, 2:515
    participation by, 2:731
    periodization of training for, 2:810–811
    plyometrics for, 2:544
    resistance training, 2:568
    scholarships, 2:811
    sleep for, 2:640
    sport coaching for, 2:808, 810
    sport performance of, 2:808, *810*
    sports training, 2:810–812
    strength training for, 2:**690–691**
    stress in, 2:809
    throwing technique for, 2:808–809
    volleyball training, 2:762
    warm weather exercise, 2:809
    *See also* Adolescents; Children

Young Men's Christian Association (YMCA), 2:487
Youth sport performance, 2:**809–810,** *810*
Youth sports injuries, 2:803, **808–809**
Youth sports training, 2:**810–812**
*Yurchenko,* 1:335

# Z

Zamboni, Frank Joseph, 1:393, 2:**813–814**
Zamboni machines, 1:393, 2:813–814
Zátopek, Dana, 2:814
Zátopek, Emil, 1:237, 2:594, **814–815,** *815*
Zinc, 1:197, 2:468, 744
Zinc oxide, 1:13
ZMA, 2:744
Zmelik, Robert, 1:187
Zoloft, 2:612
Zsivoczky, Attila, 1:*367*